59-
4

Pediatrics, Neurology, and Psychiatry— Common Ground

Behavioral, Cognitive, Affective, and Physical Disorders in Childhood and Adolescence

Joel Herskowitz, M.D.

Assistant Professor of Pediatrics and Neurology,
Boston University School of Medicine; Pediatric
Neurologist, Departments of Pediatrics and
Neurology, Boston City Hospital

N. Paul Rosman, M.D.

Professor of Pediatrics and Neurology, Director of
Pediatric Neurology, Associate Director of Pediatrics,
Boston University School of Medicine; Director of
Pediatric Neurology, Associate Director of Pediatrics,
Boston City Hospital

WITH THE CONSULTATION OF

Alan N. Marks, M.D.

Associate Clinical Professor of Psychiatry, Assistant
Professor of Pediatrics, Tufts University School of
Medicine; Director of Inpatient Child Psychiatry,
Division of Child Psychiatry, Tufts-New England Medical
Center Hospital

WITH A FOREWORD BY

T. Berry Brazelton, M.D.

Associate Professor of Pediatrics, Harvard Medical School;
Chief, Child Development Unit, Children's Hospital Medical
Center

Pediatrics, Neurology, and Psychiatry— Common Ground

Behavioral, Cognitive, Affective, and Physical Disorders in Childhood and Adolescence

MACMILLAN PUBLISHING CO., INC.
New York

Collier Macmillan Canada, Inc.
TORONTO

Baillière Tindall
LONDON

Macmillan Publishing Co., Inc.
866 Third Avenue, New York, New York 10022

Collier Macmillan Canada, Inc.
Baillière Tindall · London

Library of Congress Catalog Card Number 82-15280
ISBN 0-02-354620-4

Printing: 1 2 3 4 5 6 7 8   Year: 2 3 4 5 6 7 8 9 0

To

    our parents—**Reida and Irwin,**
                  Cecelia and Murray

      our wives—**Raymonde, and**
                  Syrille

  our children—**Laurel and Sylvan,**
                  Michael, Adam, and Elizabeth

Foreword

As we have become better able to conquer more and more infectious, inflammatory, and neoplastic disease entities, the challenges to handle some of the subtler, more complex disorders of the central nervous system increasingly become a focus. At a time when the great majority of high-risk premature infants will survive and a large proportion will appear to have normal brain function, we can afford to develop an expectancy for optimality in all areas of child development. With a new look at the plasticity of the central nervous system, indicated by these infants' recovery from known CNS insults, we are developing an expectation for recovery of other cognitive, affective, and neuromotor processes that previously have been labeled as "fixed." The appropriate treatment for disorders of neuromotor, cognitive, and affective systems most often involves a multidisciplinary team approach. In this volume the authors bring together the talents of three disciplines toward nervous system structure and function. The main value of this book is its translation of a neurologic point of view into clear language available to pediatricians, psychiatrists, psychologists, nurses, and therapists from other disciplines. Each chapter lays out an approach to diagnosis and treatment of clinical problems—some of them more obviously neurologic than others: autism, sleep disorders, hyperactivity and attentional disorders, learning disabilities, child abuse and neglect, and drug abuse. Particularly with movement disorders, coupling this approach with the new therapeutic techniques that are evolving in the area of physiotherapy (for example, those of Bobath and Ayres) might result in more incisive therapy for central nervous system disease entities once considered fixed. As new investigative tools such as brain-mapping procedures (of Duffy and colleagues) evolve, they can lead us to a clearer etiologic and functional understanding of many such disorders of CNS function.

Meanwhile, our search must be for a preventive approach to such disorders, particularly their affective components, since an expectation for failure and a poor self-image all too frequently accompany these entities. Children

in these chapters must all suffer from the accompanying image of themselves as failures. If we can make clear diagnoses at early ages, as described by the authors, we should also be able to identify affected children earlier as at risk for failure in these developmental processes. Attention to the child's affective development with an approach that is designed to support his strengths and his opportunities for organization in the face of a deficit should optimize his chance for success in spite of an identified handicap. Then, the successful functional outcome may well outweigh the underlying CNS deficit. By clarifying the diagnosis, as well as the present all-too-inadequate state of the art in treatment of neurologic, neuropediatric, and neuropsychiatric disorders, the authors have brought out the need for early identification and prevention in the areas they have approached.

This book presents an excellent reference outline of the present state of the art of treatment. It leaves me, as a pediatrician, ready to reevaluate each entity from the point of view of preventive primary care. Couldn't we do better than to allow a child with a rather minor learning deficit to grow up with a permanently damaged image of himself, with an expectation for failure that far outweighs the burden of the deficit? His failure in learning becomes magnified by the functional patterns of an expectation to fail. This volume, in combining the points of view of neurology, pediatrics, and child psychiatry, becomes a base for reevaluating the state of the art of diagnosis and therapy of each of the entities approached in this book. Each case that the authors describe as examples should kindle a longing in the reader to develop a more preventive, holistic approach to the treatment of these disorders. This book should be a milestone toward the combined approach of three closely related fields—pediatrics, neurology, and child psychiatry.

T. Berry Brazelton, M.D.

Associate Professor of Pediatrics,
Harvard Medical School; Chief,
Child Development Unit, Children's
Hospital Medical Center

Preface

As pediatricians and neurologists have become increasingly concerned with problems of behavior, learning, and other aspects of development, psychiatrists have increasingly sought biologic contributions to many such problems. Despite these trends, a book bringing together knowledge from all three specialties in approaching problems of behavior, cognition, affect, and physical function in childhood and adolescence has been lacking. This book is our response to this need. It is devoted to the common ground shared by Pediatrics, Neurology, and Psychiatry and is intended to provide an approach to problems that cut across the lines of professional disciplines.

Part One of the book, "General Considerations," is its foundation. It provides an overview of nervous system structure and function, definitions of behavior, and an outline of the clinical diagnostic process: history, examination, and investigation.

Part Two, "Major Clinical Problems," is the core of the book. It consists of 17 clinically oriented chapters, each dealing with one problem or a related group of problems. Included are Hyperactivity and Attentional Disorders, Psychosis, Memory Disturbances, Aggressive and Violent Behavior, Learning Disabilities and Disorders of Speech and Language, Mental Retardation, Depression, Sleep Disorders, Child Abuse, Seizures and Other Paroxysmal Disorders, Hysteria, Disorders of Movement, Headaches, Disorders of Eating and Elimination, Behavioral Regression, Drug Abuse, and Chronic Illness and the Dying Child. The format of each clinical chapter is as follows: Definition, Diagnosis, Differential Diagnosis, Etiology, Treatment, and Outcome. A structured, comprehensive approach to diagnosis and treatment is emphasized. Rather than an exhaustive discussion of each topic, selected aspects considered of greatest importance have been presented.

Each chapter within Part Two has a section on Correlation, which presents selected relevant Anatomic, Biochemical, and Physiologic aspects of the problems considered. More than 100 tables highlight key information so that it may be most readily available to the practitioner. The Index, extensively cross-referenced, also has been prepared to be maximally useful. More than 100 illustrations have been included to amplify and clarify the text. An extensive and current bibliography, containing more than 800 Cited References, also includes Additional Readings that refer to papers of historic interest, review articles, and related topics for further exploration. In addition—constituting a "book within a book"—are over 100 wide-ranging cases, drawn from the authors' personal experience, which provide a direct view of the clinical diagnostic and therapeutic processes in practice.

Part Three, "Conclusion," considers issues of prevention, early intervention, and new directions in current and future research.

This book has been designed for use by medical and mental health professionals working with children—pediatricians, psychiatrists, neurologists, generalists, developmentalists, and psychologists—as well as pediatric nurse practitioners, social workers, teachers (particularly those in areas of counseling and special education), and physical, occupational, and speech and language therapists. By providing these professionals with an organic foundation within a developmental context and a structured approach to diagnosis and treatment, it is hoped that this book will assist them in dealing with complex and multifaceted problems of children and their families.

We would like to thank the following people for their contributions to the book: Dr. Joel J. Alpert for his support, encouragement, and helpful suggestions; Dr. Edward M. Kaye for help in preparing the cases; Dr. Raymonde Dumont-Herskowitz for her consultation regarding endocrinologic matters; Ms. Bonita Bröckl for assistance with the manuscript; and Mrs. Syrille Rosman for her help in a multiplicity of ways. Special thanks are due to Ms. Elizabeth Baker Volk and Mrs. Reida Postrel Herskowitz for their sustained and timely efforts in preparation of the manuscript. We have benefited greatly from the wisdom and perspective of our editor, Miss Joan C. Zulch, throughout this four-year project. Finally, we acknowledge with deepest gratitude the encouragement and understanding of our families.

Joel Herskowitz, M.D.
N. Paul Rosman, M.D.

Boston, Massachusetts

Contents

Part One

General Considerations

1 The Common Ground of Pediatrics, Neurology, and Psychiatry

Relationships among the specialties of pediatrics, neurology, and psychiatry continue to evolve. As medicine became increasingly specialized during the twentieth century, a state of separation, even isolation, of these disciplines from one another appeared to develop. Gradually, such separation lessened then ceased, after which these bodies of knowledge began to grow toward each other. Contact, initially quite limited, has grown. Interfaces have formed, and further interaction and communication have led to a recognition of common ground (see Fig. 1–1). This common ground, considerable in extent, underlies the concerns of many professionals devoted to the health of children, particularly pediatricians, neurologists, and psychiatrists.

Most recently, several trends occurring within pediatrics, neurology, and psychiatry have reflected their areas of mutual concern. As immunizations and antibiotics have brought major infectious diseases under increasingly effective control, pediatrics has become increasingly involved with problems of behavior, emotion, and learning. Neurology has expanded its emphasis beyond structural components of disease to focus on physiologic and biochemical disorders of the central nervous system, while becoming more attentive to the behavioral and psychologic aspects of such disorders. At the same time psychiatry has become more biologically oriented, incorporating structural, physiologic, and biochemical knowledge of nervous system functioning from neurology with developmental perspectives provided by pediatrics. This book is based upon and devoted to this common ground.

HEALTH AND DISEASE IN CHILDHOOD

Health, as has become widely recognized, is not merely the absence of disease. Rather, it is a state of physical, emotional, and social well-being in which the person—in this instance, the child—is able to participate actively in age-appropriate activities and to grow. Growth is indeed the ''job'' of childhood. It applies not only to physical development (in such terms as height, weight, and head circumference) but to cognitive, emotional, and social development as well. Disease can be considered to involve a breakdown

3

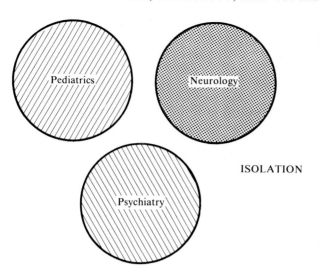

FIGURE 1–1. Evolving relationships between pediatrics, neurology, and psychiatry.

ISOLATION

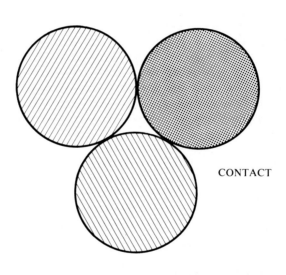

CONTACT

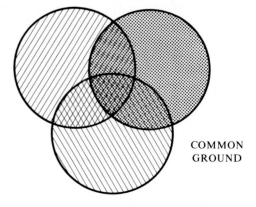

COMMON
GROUND

in one or more of these areas. The state of well-being is lost. Physical growth may suffer, emotional upset occur, or social adjustment be impaired.

Human beings exist in a state of delicate balance at multiple levels. A problem at one level of organization may have important repercussions at other levels. For example, substitution of a single amino acid in a polypeptide chain of hemoglobin can lead to sickling of red blood cells, which results in impaired blood flow to many organs, causing severe pain, tissue damage, and chronic disability or death. This disorder, sickle cell disease, like many others, can be viewed at several levels in a multiaxial framework from the molecular to the social.

The emotional and social consequences of disease will depend upon the age and developmental level of the child. Beginning with infancy, the child's affective development becomes increasingly complex, while social interactions progressively widen from the mother–child pair to nuclear family, school, and community. Therapy should be directed toward restoring normal function at those levels through a program that may involve directly treating the illness, altering the child's milieu, and helping the child and family adjust to the problem.

Ideally, recognition of a molecular defect would lead to correction of the problem at that level and at all higher levels as well. In fact, with early identification of such disorders as congenital hypothyroidism and phenylketonuria, treatment at the molecular level can prevent abnormal development. With sickle cell anemia, however, among other disorders, knowledge of the basic defect has not yet led to definitive treatment. Thus, therapy remains symptomatic and only partially helpful.

The clinical diagnostic process—history, examination, and investigation —is structured to deal with problems at multiple levels. Its goals are to establish as specific a diagnosis as possible, provide information as to prognosis, and formulate a comprehensive treatment plan. As an integral part of this process, it is important for the professional to gain an understanding of the psychosocial framework within which problems have been recognized and help sought. For example, headaches may have appeared or worsened with the onset of adolescence, upon changing schools, or with the death of a family member.

Indeed, it is always appropriate to ask, explicitly or implicitly, "Why has the child been brought for evaluation *now*?" Sometimes the child's problem is relatively minor, and parental anxiety has played the largest part in their seeking professional help. At other times a chronic problem (such as recurrent headaches) has become intensified, a long-standing difficulty (such as clumsiness) has caused the child increasing embarrassment, or new difficulties (such as fecal soiling, loss of consciousness, or involuntary movements) have appeared.

RECOGNITION AND EVALUATION

Entry into the clinical diagnostic process can itself be a complicated matter. The essential element is a symptom—a disturbance in function recognized by the child, parent, or other lay person—or a sign, an objective abnormality recognized by a professional. If the disturbance is not severe (for example, a mild headache), the child may consider it part of normal experience. Hence, such a symptom may be present for weeks or months without being recognized as a problem. If the child mentions it to a parent, one of several courses may be pursued. The parent may reassure the child that "it's nothing." The parent may recognize a possible problem but not feel it is serious enough to merit professional attention. Or the parent may seek evaluation of the child.

Simple reassurance by telephone, brief examination to exclude "something serious," or definitive assessment consisting of careful history and examination supplemented by well-chosen investigations may result from professional involvement. The professional person must always listen carefully to what the child and the parents are saying and give them confidence to speak about things that may be difficult to describe or that seem strange or "weird."

The case of a seven-year-old girl with migraine headaches illustrates several aspects of the processes of recognition and referral and the multifaceted nature of a seemingly straightforward problem. When this first-grade girl returned from school each day, she lay down for a two-hour nap. She did not complain to her mother that anything was bothering her, and she seemed otherwise well, although she appeared to lack energy for her usual activities.

She was seen by her pediatrician, who learned that the child's after-school fatigue was accompanied by headache. It was pounding in quality, involved the forehead on both sides, began gradually without warning, and was associated with an upset stomach. School performance had been considered satisfactory, but finishing assignments in class was chronically difficult for her, especially when it involved the use of pencil and paper.

On examination, the child was subdued and looked sad. Although her high intelligence was apparent in conversation, she could read barely at grade level. Handwriting was sloppy. Geometric figures were drawn slowly and crudely for her age. Examination was otherwise unremarkable.

She was considered to have a form of childhood migraine because of the characteristic pounding quality of her headaches, accompanying abdominal pain, and positive family history. Academic stress (associated with perceptual-motor dysfunction) was felt to be an important precipitant, with fatigue and depression secondary to the chronic school problems also contributing to the child's symptoms. Because she had been performing at grade level, her classroom teacher had not perceived a problem. Once the school-related stresses were recognized, additional testing was carried out to clarify further her areas of difficulty. She received individualized help within the classroom, her headaches disappeared, and she was able to resume her regular after-school activities.

This case illustrates the interplay that commonly occurs among different etiologic factors and also shows characteristic impairment at various levels of function: physical, academic, and social. The child's migraine syndrome clearly falls within the common ground of pediatrics, neurology, and psychiatry, as do such frequently encountered problems as hyperactivity, sleep disorders, and memory disturbances.

Because the "whole child"—not just the headache—was considered in this case, a broader, more definitive plan could be established rather than a narrow pharmacologic approach. Pain is, after all, a signal that something is wrong; but it does not necessarily specify where. Thus, diagnostic and therapeutic considerations best include multiple levels of possible dysfunction.

Whether or not the evaluation and management of the child with a behavioral or emotional problem will involve persons from different disciplines will depend upon the nature of the problem and its severity. When several specialists are involved, one person (usually the pediatrician) should be identified as the team leader, acting with—and on behalf of—the parents, who generally make the final decisions for the child.

The parents should be informed not only of the problems that are being evaluated but also of the principal diagnostic possibilities that exist, the consultants to be involved, and the evaluation planned. The parents may find it reassuring to learn, for example, that neurologic consultation does not imply that their child is brain-damaged and that investigations such as electroencephalogram or computerized tomographic scan are not painful and pose no significant risk to the child. Nor does psychiatric diagnostic referral mean that the child is "crazy," that the parents are failures, or that decades of treatment are required. Through such open communication, parents will be in an optimal position to participate in an informed and active fashion in the diagnostic process, understand the information gained, and act upon the recommendations (treatment options) that result.

SUMMARY

The disciplines of pediatrics, neurology, and psychiatry—relatively isolated from one another earlier in this century—have come together increasingly. Such progress appears to be based upon recognition of the common ground they share in dealing with many of the behavioral and emotional problems of infancy, childhood, and adolescence. It further reflects the increasing developmental and behavioral concerns of pediatrics and neurology and the growing biologic orientation of psychiatry.

Health, more than merely the absence of disease, implies active functioning and growth at many levels. Since disease usually interferes with the child's function at several levels, a comprehensive approach to diagnosis and treatment involving several disciplines is often appropriate. With effective communication between the primary medical provider, other professionals, and the parents as active participants in decision-making, the health of the child can be maximized.

2 Structure and Function of the Nervous System: An Overview

This chapter sets forth fundamental anatomic, biochemical, and physiologic aspects of the nervous system. This overview is intended not to be exhaustive but to provide a framework with which to approach the clinical chapters that follow.

Anatomy will be discussed from the standpoints of basic structure of the nervous system, functional anatomy, and developmental anatomy. Basic structures will include the central nervous system, peripheral nervous system, cerebrospinal fluid system, and vascular system. Functional anatomy will focus upon the reticular activating system, autonomic nervous system, limbic system, motor systems, sensory systems, and associational systems. Developmental anatomy will include discussion of neural tube development and brain growth: macroscopic (gyral) development and microscopic development, including myelinogenesis.

Biochemical aspects covered will be neurotransmitters, neuroendocrine hormones, other peptides, and energy metabolism of brain. Physiologic topics will include membrane physiology, synaptic function, and the neuromuscular unit.

ANATOMY

BASIC STRUCTURE

Central Nervous System. The central nervous system consists of the brain and the spinal cord. Both are encased within a bony, protective structure (the skull and the spine, respectively) and are covered by the three-layered meninges (pia, arachnoid, and dura). The brain consists of two hemispheres connected deeply by a broad white band, the corpus callosum. Below the corpus callosum are several paired and unpaired structures: the diencephalon (which includes the thalamus and hypothalamus), the basal ganglia (caudate nucleus, putamen, and globus pallidus), and the pituitary gland. From here the brain narrows further, funneling down to form the

8

brainstem (midbrain, pons, and medulla), and then passes through the foramen magnum to leave the cranium. The continuation of the central nervous system is the spinal cord.

The hemispheres are labeled right and left from an anatomic perspective. The interhemispheric fissure separates the two hemispheres. Each hemisphere is subdivided into lobes: frontal, parietal, temporal, and occipital (see Fig. 2–1). The sylvian fissure, angling back toward the occipital lobe, separates the temporal lobe from the frontal and parietal lobes above. The central sulcus, or fissure of Rolando, separates the frontal lobe from the parietal lobe. The parietal–occipital and temporal–occipital boundaries are less obvious. The lobes of the brain are further divided by sulci into convolutions, or gyri.

On cut section of the brain, its division into gray and white matter is readily evident. The outermost portion of the brain is gray matter, several millimeters thick, which constitutes the cortex (derived from the Latin word for

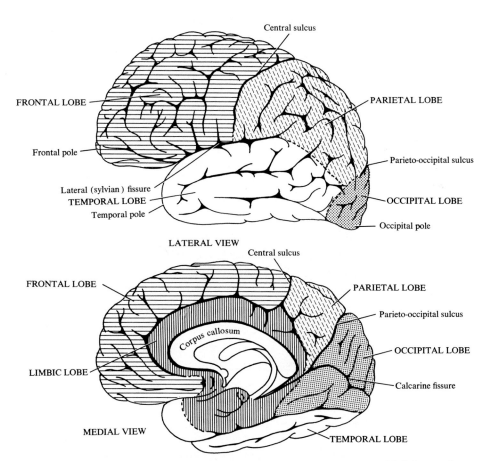

FIGURE 2–1. Left cerebral hemisphere (lateral and medial views) with lobes and major fissures and sulci identified. (From Pansky, B., and Allen, D. J. *Review of Neuroscience.* Macmillan Publishing Co., Inc., New York, 1980.)

bark). The underlying tissue is white matter, which derives its color from myelinated nerve fibers originating in the cortex.

The basal ganglia (caudate nucleus, putamen, and globus pallidus) and the thalamus are paired structures situated at the base of the brain (see Fig. 2–2). The putamen and the globus pallidus make up the lenticular nucleus. The caudate nucleus, divisible into head, body, and tail portions, and the putamen constitute the striatum.

The brainstem is subdivided into mesencephalon (or midbrain), pons, and medulla (or medulla oblongata). Each portion of the brainstem has easily recognizable gross anatomic features and a distinctive appearance on cut section (see Fig. 2–3). The midbrain is notable for pealike colliculi (Latin for *little hills*) dorsally, two footlike cerebral peduncles ventrally, and a black band (the substantia nigra) proximally within each peduncle. The pons (Latin for *bridge*) is evident as the midportion of the brainstem connecting it with parts of the enwrapping cerebellum. The medulla, the lowermost portion of the brainstem, is characterized on inspection by two sets of bulges, the inferior olives and the pyramids. They lie laterally and medially, respectively, on each side of the midline. Viewed ventrally, the crossing, or decussation, of the pyramids is visible to the unaided eye.

The spinal cord begins at the level of the foramen magnum and extends down to about the level of the second lumbar vertebra. It is divided into cervical, thoracic, lumbar, sacral, and coccygeal segments. Though less so than the brainstem, each segment of the spinal cord has a relatively distinctive appearance. Identifying features include prominent enlargments in the cervi-

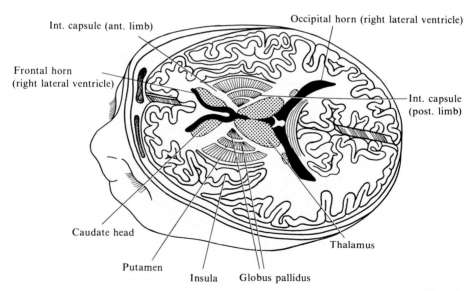

FIGURE 2–2. Horizontal section through brain demonstrating relationships of basal ganglia, thalami, internal capsules, and lateral ventricles. (From Pansky, B., and Allen, D. J. *Review of Neuroscience.* Macmillan Publishing Co., Inc., New York, 1980.)

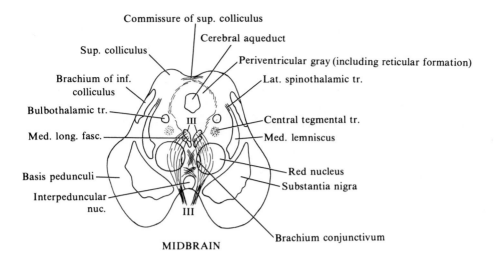

MIDBRAIN

Commissure of sup. colliculus
Cerebral aqueduct
Sup. colliculus
Periventricular gray (including reticular formation)
Brachium of inf. colliculus
Lat. spinothalamic tr.
Bulbothalamic tr.
III
Med. long. fasc.
Central tegmental tr.
Med. lemniscus
Red nucleus
Basis pedunculi
Substantia nigra
Interpeduncular nuc.
III
Brachium conjunctivum

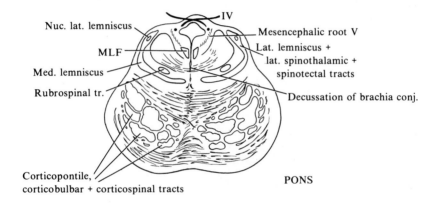

PONS

Nuc. lat. lemniscus
IV
Mesencephalic root V
MLF
Lat. lemniscus + lat. spinothalamic + spinotectal tracts
Med. lemniscus
Rubrospinal tr.
Decussation of brachia conj.
Corticopontile, corticobulbar + corticospinal tracts

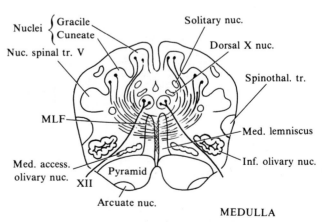

MEDULLA

Nuclei { Gracile Cuneate
Solitary nuc.
Nuc. spinal tr. V
Dorsal X nuc.
Spinothal. tr.
MLF
Med. lemniscus
Med. access. olivary nuc.
XII
Pyramid
Inf. olivary nuc.
Arcuate nuc.

FIGURE 2–3. Cross-sections at three levels of brainstem showing characteristic configuration and major structures. (From Pansky, B., and Allen, D. J. *Review of Neuroscience.* Macmillan Publishing Co., Inc., New York, 1980.)

11

cal and lumbar areas, which give rise to nerves to the upper and lower limbs, respectively.

Peripheral Nervous System.   The peripheral nervous system consists of nerves of cranial and of spinal origin. The twelve pairs of *cranial nerves* are conventionally listed and numbered in rostral-to-caudal order as follows: olfactory, optic, oculomotor, trochlear, trigeminal, abducens, facial, vestibulocochlear (or auditory), glossopharyngeal, vagus, accessory (or spinal accessory), and hypoglossal. Departure of the cranial nerves from the brainstem as seen from its ventral surface is illustrated in Figure 2–4.

Several relationships are of special significance. The oculomotor nerve (III) lies close to the temporal lobe in its medial and inferior frontal portions. The abducens nerve (VI), leaving the brainstem at the pontomedullary junction, pursues a long intracranial course before leaving the cranium to reach the orbit.

The peripheral nerves of spinal origin are made up of ventral and dorsal roots that come together alongside the spine. The thirty-one pairs of *spinal nerves* consist of eight cervical, twelve thoracic, five lumbar, five sacral, and one coccygeal pair. Spinal nerves are named and numbered according to

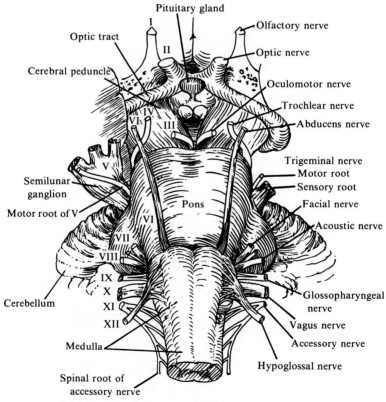

FIGURE 2–4. Ventral surface of brainstem showing exit of cranial nerves. (From Chusid, J. G. *Correlative Neuroanatomy and Functional Neurology,* 17th ed. Lange Medical Publications, Los Altos, Calif., 1979.)

their level of departure from between adjacent vertebrae (see Fig. 2–5). The different rates of growth of the bony spine and the spinal cord itself result in a difference between bony spinal level and spinal cord level. This discrepancy can be a source of considerable clinical confusion.

Cerebrospinal Fluid System. The cerebrospinal fluid system consists of four ventricles, connecting channels, cerebral cisterns, and subarachnoid spaces. Each of the two lateral ventricles lies within a cerebral hemisphere and is connected to the third ventricle through a foramen of Monro. The third ventricle lies in the midline between the halves of the thalamus and hypothalamus. The aqueduct of Sylvius, normally only a few millimeters wide, conducts cerebrospinal fluid from the third ventricle to the fourth (see Fig. 2–6).

Cerebrospinal fluid (CSF) within the fourth ventricle communicates with the cranial and spinal subarachnoid spaces via the two foramina of Luschka (each lying laterally within the fourth ventricle) and the foramen of Magendie, situated in the midline (see Fig. 2–7). CSF leaving the fourth ventricle travels around the base of the brain within the cerebral cisterns and up over the cerebral convexities to the superior sagittal sinus, where it is resorbed through the arachnoid granulations to join with venous blood. CSF exiting from the fourth ventricle also descends in the subarachnoid space. Spinal CSF returns to the base of the brain and then circulates up over the hemispheres to the superior sagittal sinus. Because the spinal subarachnoid space extends considerably beyond the spinal cord, lumbar puncture is carried out below the second or third lumbar vertebra to avoid injury to the spinal cord.

Cerebrospinal fluid is formed at a rate of approximately one-third ml per minute (or one ounce in one and one-half hours). The total volume of CSF within the entire system is 30–150 ml depending upon the age of the child.

Vascular System. Blood supply to the brain is provided primarily by the anterior, middle, and posterior cerebral arteries. The areas of brain subserved by these arteries are shown in Figure 2–8. The anterior and middle cerebral arteries are the end branches of the internal carotid artery. The posterior cerebral arteries are derived from the unpaired basilar artery, itself formed by the two vertebral arteries. The vertebral-basilar system lies upon the ventral surface of the brainstem. At the base of the brain, these three major vessels (anterior, middle, and posterior cerebral arteries) and communicating branches come together, forming the circle of Willis (see Fig. 2–9).

The meninges are supplied largely by the middle meningeal arteries. They stem from the external carotid arteries and branch into anterior and posterior divisions, which often cause grooves evident in lateral views of skull x-rays.

Blood leaves the brain through a specialized venous system. In addition to superficial and deep cerebral veins, blood is drained into sinuses formed from the dura. The dural sinuses ultimately communicate with the right heart by way of the internal jugular vein.

Blood supply to the spinal cord is provided through an unpaired anterior spinal artery and the paired posterior spinal arteries.

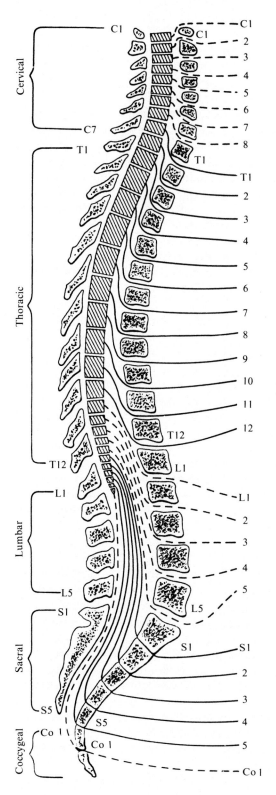

FIGURE 2–5. Relationships of spinal cord segments, spinal nerves, and vertebral bodies. (From De-Jong, R. N. *The Neurologic Examination,* 4th ed. Harper and Row Publishers, Hagerstown, Md., 1979.)

14

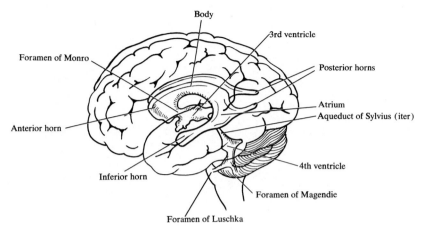

FIGURE 2–6. Lateral view of brain showing ventricular system and connecting channels. (From Pansky, B., and Allen, D. J. *Review of Neuroscience*. Macmillan Publishing Co., Inc., New York, 1980.)

FUNCTIONAL ANATOMY

Reticular Activating System. The reticular activating system mediates levels of consciousness (state of arousal) from sleep to wakefulness. Its anatomic basis is the reticular formation, a patchy collection of neurons within the core of the brainstem (see Fig. 2–3). The reticular formation extends from the medulla to the thalamus, where so-called nonspecific thalamic nuclei serve as relays for widespread cortical excitation. The role of the hypothalamus in sleeping and waking is discussed in Chapter 9.

The reticular formation is richly connected by afferent and efferent pathways to neural structures both rostrally (cerebral cortex) and caudally (peripheral nerves of spinal origin). It thus functions as the anatomic structure that if stimulated maintains wakefulness (or, conversely, if not stimulated, leads to sleep). That pain fibers reaching the midbrain reticular formation are especially numerous has suggested a structural basis for arousal through noxious stimulation (Plum and Posner, 1980).

Autonomic Nervous System. The autonomic nervous system is involved primarily in maintenance and survival activities of the organism. Processes of maintenance such as digestion, respiration, and circulation are largely the domain of the *parasympathetic nervous system*. Survival activities, "fight or flight" measures, are mediated through the *sympathetic nervous system*.

Parasympathetic outflow from the central nervous system is both cranial and spinal (see Fig. 2–10). Cranial nerves III, VII, IX, and X include parasympathetic fibers that mediate pupillary constriction, taste, and cardiodeceleration, among other functions. Spinal outflow is through sacral segments 2 through 4, which are involved in bowel and bladder function (see Chapter 10).

Cells of the intermediolateral cell column of the spinal cord give rise to the sympathetic outflow. This column extends from the first thoracic spinal segment (T_1) to the second or third lumbar level (L_2 or L_3). The first four or five segments of the thoracic spinal cord contribute preganglionic fibers to

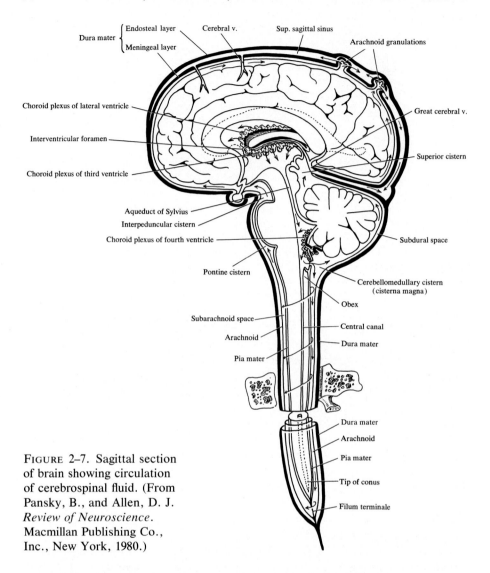

FIGURE 2–7. Sagittal section of brain showing circulation of cerebrospinal fluid. (From Pansky, B., and Allen, D. J. *Review of Neuroscience*. Macmillan Publishing Co., Inc., New York, 1980.)

three cervical ganglia (superior, middle, and stellate), which lie adjacent to the spine. Postganglionic fibers travel from these ganglia to the heart and involuntary muscles of the eye. Here they are involved in cardioacceleration and in pupillary dilatation, respectively. Sympathetic fibers also allow for tonic contraction of the upper lid (thereby helping to keep the eyes fully open) and are involved in thermal regulation of the face through influences on sweating and vasodilation.

Limbic System.   The limbic system consists of a phylogenetically old group of brain structures involved in memory, affect, and olfaction in addition to survival-related behaviors such as mating, fighting, and fleeing. The limbic system lies deep within the brain along its medial aspect and is made up of several C-shaped structures (see Chapters 5 and 15). The hippocampus, fornix, and mammillary body of the hypothalamus form one C (see

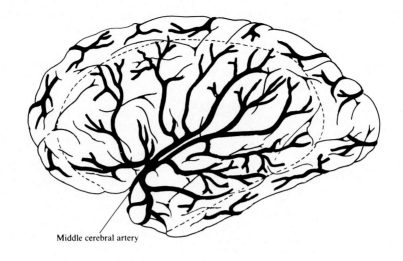

Middle cerebral artery

ARTERIAL SUPPLY— LATERAL VIEW

CEREBRAL CORTEX

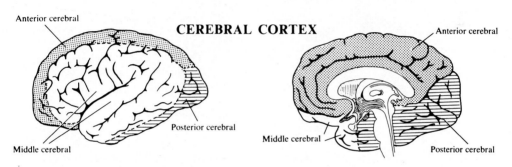

Anterior cerebral

Middle cerebral

Posterior cerebral

Anterior cerebral

Middle cerebral

Posterior cerebral

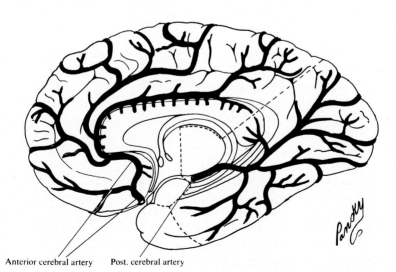

Anterior cerebral artery   Post. cerebral artery

ARTERIAL SUPPLY—MEDIAL VIEW

FIGURE 2–8. Arterial supply to the cerebral hemispheres. (From Pansky, B., and Allen, D. J. *Review of Neuroscience*. Macmillan Publishing Co., Inc., New York, 1980.)

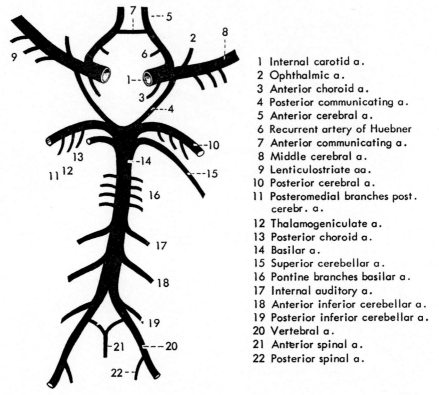

1 Internal carotid a.
2 Ophthalmic a.
3 Anterior choroid a.
4 Posterior communicating a.
5 Anterior cerebral a.
6 Recurrent artery of Huebner
7 Anterior communicating a.
8 Middle cerebral a.
9 Lenticulostriate aa.
10 Posterior cerebral a.
11 Posteromedial branches post.
   cerebr. a.
12 Thalamogeniculate a.
13 Posterior choroid a.
14 Basilar a.
15 Superior cerebellar a.
16 Pontine branches basilar a.
17 Internal auditory a.
18 Anterior inferior cerebellar a.
19 Posterior inferior cerebellar a.
20 Vertebral a.
21 Anterior spinal a.
22 Posterior spinal a.

FIGURE 2–9. Major arteries at the base of the brain, including the circle of Willis. (From Gilroy, J., and Meyer, J. S. *Medical Neurology,* 3rd ed. Macmillan Publishing Co., Inc., New York, 1979.)

Fig. 2–11). The cingulate gyrus, isthmus, parahippocampal gyrus, and amygdaloid nucleus form another. A third limbic C is made up of the amygdala, stria terminalis, and septal nuclei.

Motor Systems.   The neurologic basis for movement can be broken down into three systems—pyramidal, extrapyramidal, and cerebellar—which work closely together and are themselves dependent upon sensory input. A more detailed description of these motor systems is presented in Chapter 13 (CORRELATION: ANATOMIC ASPECTS).

The *pyramidal system,* also known as the voluntary motor system, originates in pyramidal neurons within the motor cortex of the frontal lobe (see Fig. 2–12). This precentral cortex is structured somatotopically such that stimulation of a specific portion of the motor strip will result in movement of a contralateral body part (see Fig. 2–13). Pyramidal fibers travel through the diencephalon to the brainstem, where most of these fibers decussate in the medulla. The pyramidal system continues in the spinal cord as the lateral corticospinal tracts. These tracts end upon anterior horn cells that give rise to ventral roots, which constitute the voluntary motor components of spinal nerves.

The *extrapyramidal motor system* consists of the basal ganglia (caudate

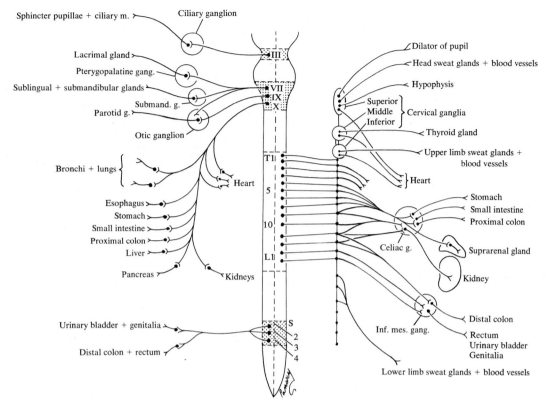

FIGURE 2–10. Autonomic (parasympathetic and sympathetic) nervous system connections to peripheral organs. (From Pansky, B., and Allen, D. J. *Review of Neuroscience*. Macmillan Publishing Co., Inc., New York, 1980.)

nucleus, putamen, globus pallidus) and their interconnections (see Fig. 2–2). These structures function unconsciously to determine the interplay between muscle groups or different muscles, thereby influencing posture and movement. The function of this system and its constituent parts has been suggested by disorders that preferentially affect certain of the basal ganglia. These include Huntington disease (caudate nucleus and putamen) and kernicterus (globus pallidus) (see Chapter 13).

The cerebellum is the focal point of the *cerebellar system,* intimately involved with voluntary movements although its function, too, is unconscious. Situated upon the brainstem, the cerebellum is involved in matching the present position of the body with the anticipated or desired position. It is basically a somatic afferent organ, the "head ganglion of proprioception." Of its afferent inputs, the spinocerebellar tracts are of particular importance.

Sensory Systems.   The millions of nerve fibers bringing visual information to the brain and the amount of cerebral cortex devoted to visual function reflect the importance of the *visual system* in man.

Several steps are involved in the propagation of visual impulses from eye to brain (see Fig. 2–14). Light first passes through the cornea and the lens to

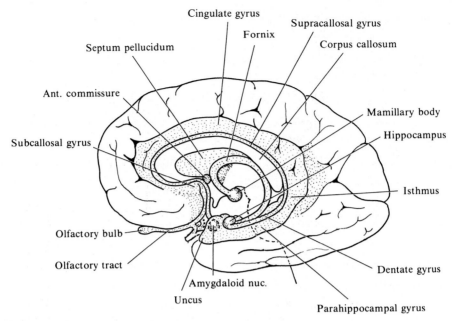

FIGURE 2–11. Sagittal section of brain showing major structures of limbic system. (From Pansky, B., and Allen, D. J. *Review of Neuroscience.* Macmillan Publishing Co., Inc., New York, 1980.)

the retina where photosensitive neurons (rods and cones) are stimulated. Visual information collected from throughout the retina leaves the eye via the optic nerve. Its point of exit, the optic papilla, is seen upon ophthalmoscopic examination just medial (or nasal) to the posterior pole of the eye (see Fig. 2–15).

The optic nerves form the optic chiasm (from the Greek for the letter X) at the base of the brain. Here, optic nerve fibers cross such that fibers from the left half of each retina, namely, nasal fibers from the right eye, temporal fibers from the left, travel together as the left optic tract and corresponding portions of the retina make up the right optic tract. (The left half of the retina receives visual input from the right half of the visual field, and vice versa.) Each optic tract is connected with the lateral geniculate body of the thalamus and the superior colliculus and pretectal nuclei of the midbrain. The latter structures are involved in pupillary reactions to accommodation and light. From the lateral geniculate bodies, fibers sweep around the walls of the lateral ventricles as the geniculocalcarine tracts to terminate in the occipital lobes. Within the occipital cortex, visual fields are represented topographically in upside-down and reversed fashion.

The *auditory system* consists of three major elements: peripheral end organ (the inner ear), cranial nerve (the vestibulocochlear, or auditory, nerve), and central structures (nuclei of the brainstem and temporal lobe).

The external ear directs sound to the tympanic membrane. Movement of the tympanic membrane is transmitted to the ossicular chain (malleus, incus, and stapes) within the middle ear. Movements of the ossicles are transmitted

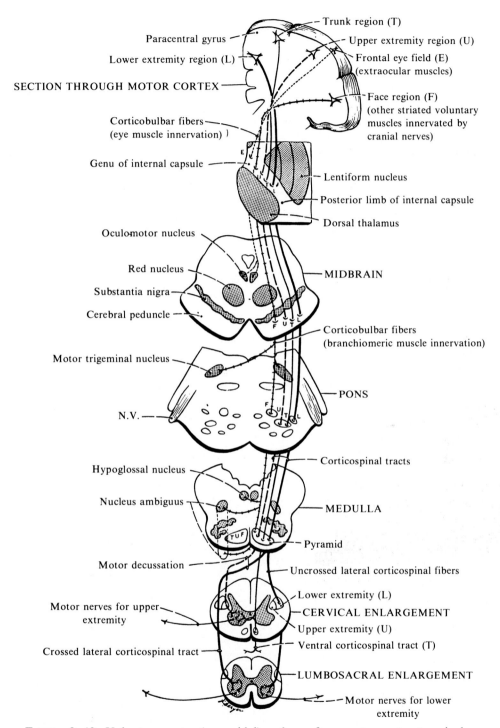

FIGURE 2–12. Voluntary motor (pyramidal) pathway from motor cortex to spinal cord. (From Crosby, E. C.; Humphrey, T.; and Lauer, E. W. *Correlative Anatomy of the Nervous System.* Macmillan Publishing Co., Inc., New York, 1962.)

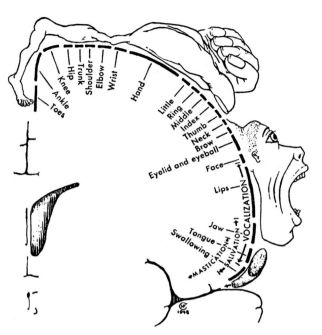

FIGURE 2–13. Motor homunculus depicting somatoto-
pic organization. (From Penfield, W., and Rasmussen,
T. *The Cerebral Cortex of Man.* Macmillan Publishing
Co., Inc., New York, 1950.)

to perilymphatic fluid within the snail-like cochlea of the inner ear. The cochlea contains the organ of Corti, whose hair cells respond to movements of
endolymphatic fluid. The hair cells are innervated by distal processes of bipolar neurons located in the spiral ganglion. Their central processes make
up the vestibulocochlear nerve.

The vestibulocochlear nerve enters the brainstem and synapses with the
cochlear nuclei in the medulla (see Fig. 2–16). Fibers from the cochlear nuclei travel upward in the lateral lemniscus (from the Latin *lemniscus,* meaning "ribbon") to synapse with the inferior colliculus of the midbrain. From
the inferior colliculus, axons go to the medial geniculate body, a specific sensory nucleus of the thalamus. Fibers radiate from there to the auditory receptive area of the cerebral cortex, the anterior transverse gyrus of the temporal lobe (Heschl's gyrus) (see Chapter 17).

Somatic sensation is mediated through several major pathways. Perception of pain and temperature for the body is subserved by sensory fibers
whose cell bodies are located in dorsal root ganglia alongside the spinal cord.
These fibers enter the dorsal horns of the spinal cord, where they synapse
with other neurons whose fibers cross the midline to form the lateral spinothalamic tracts (see Fig. 2–17). These tracts proceed rostrally to end in the
ventral posterolateral nuclei of thalamus. From there fibers travel upward to
terminate in the somesthetic area of parietal lobe, the postcentral cortex.
Pain and temperature sensation for the face is subserved by the fifth cranial
nerve, the trigeminal.

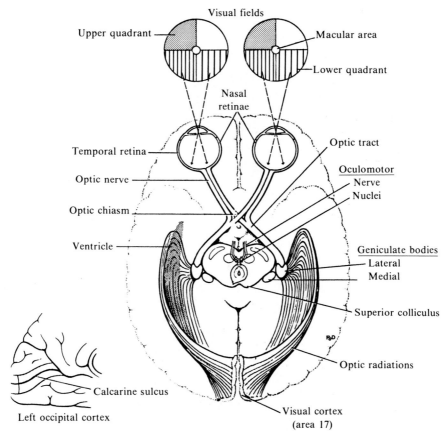

FIGURE 2–14. Visual pathways as seen from the ventral surface of the brain. (From Carpenter, M. B. *Core Text of Neuroanatomy*, 2nd ed. © 1978, The Williams & Wilkins Company, Baltimore.)

Proprioception, or position sense, is mediated through a different pathway (see Fig. 2–18). Sensory fibers (also derived from neurons within dorsal root ganglia) enter the posterior funiculi (posterior columns) of the spinal cord and, without synapsing or crossing the midline, pass upward as the gracile and cuneate fasciculi to end in the gracile and cuneate nuclei of the medulla. Fibers derived from these nuclei form the medial lemnisci, which decussate within the medulla and end in the ventral posterolateral nuclei of the thalamus, as do pain and temperature fibers. From there, as with pain and temperature fibers, those carrying proprioceptive impulses terminate in the postcentral gyrus of the parietal lobe. This pathway subserves not only proprioception but two-point discrimination and stereognosis as well.

Associational Systems. The primary receptive areas of the brain are the calcarine cortex of the occipital lobe (visual), the anterior transverse gyrus of the temporal lobe (auditory), and the postcentral gyrus of the parietal lobe (somesthetic). Each primary receptive area receives impulses from specific thalamic nuclei (lateral geniculate body, medial geniculate body, and ventral posterolateral nucleus, respectively).

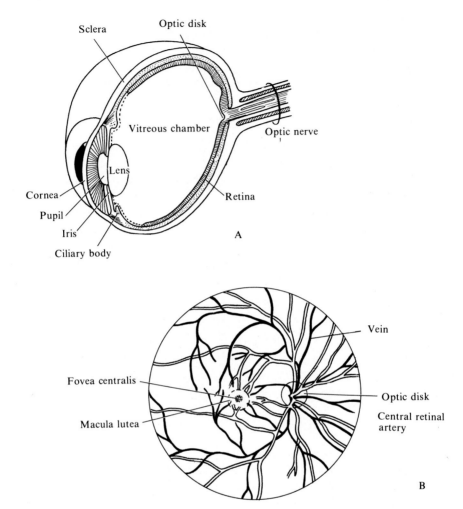

FIGURE 2–15. *A*. Cross-section of eye showing major structures. *B*. Diagram of retina as seen by ophthalmoscopic examination. (From Pansky, B., and Allen, D. J. *Review of Neuroscience*. Macmillan Publishing Co., Inc., New York, 1980.)

Adjacent to these primary receptive areas are *sensory association areas*. The somesthetic association area lies just posterior to the postcentral gyrus of the parietal lobe (see Figs. 2–1 and 2–19). The visual association area surrounds the primary visual cortex of the occipital lobe. The auditory association area lies behind the primary auditory cortex within the temporal lobe. Another association area, the angular gyrus, is located just behind the posteriormost portion of the sylvian fissure, lying virtually at the intersection of the three primary sensory receptive areas noted above.

DEVELOPMENTAL ANATOMY

Neural Tube Development.   The brain and spinal cord develop from the neural tube. During the third week of intrauterine development, the nervous system is evident as a neural plate, a thickened portion of ectoderm (see Fig.

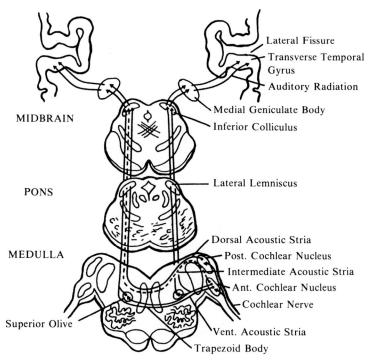

FIGURE 2–16. Auditory pathways from eighth cranial (cochlear) nerve to temporal auditory cortex. (From Clark, R. G. *Essentials of Clinical Neuroanatomy and Neurophysiology,* 5th ed. F. A. Davis Company, Philadelphia, 1975.)

2–20). Folds subsequently develop along the lateral margins of the neural plate, while an indentation forms along its midportion to create the neural groove (see Fig. 2–21). Deepening of the groove and fusion of the folds that border the neural plate result in formation of the neural tube. The midportion of the neural tube is formed first, then its ends. Closure of the anterior end occurs about the twenty-third day of gestation, closure of the posterior portion some two days later. Failure of closure will result in a form of spina bifida.

The anterior portion of the neural tube is destined to become the brain, the caudal portion the spinal cord (see Fig. 2–22). Initially, the anterior neural tube gives rise to three primary brain vesicles: forebrain, midbrain, and hindbrain. The forebrain develops two lateral bulges from which the two cerebral hemispheres are derived. The cavities within the anterior neural tube become the ventricular system of the brain. From the hindbrain originate the pons, medulla, and cerebellum. Between forebrain and hindbrain is the midbrain, which undergoes the least change among the primary brain vesicles.

Macroscopic Brain Development. Continued growth of the fetal cerebral hemispheres leads to changes in the configuration of the brain. In contrast to the relatively smooth cortical surface of early fetal life, convolutions de-

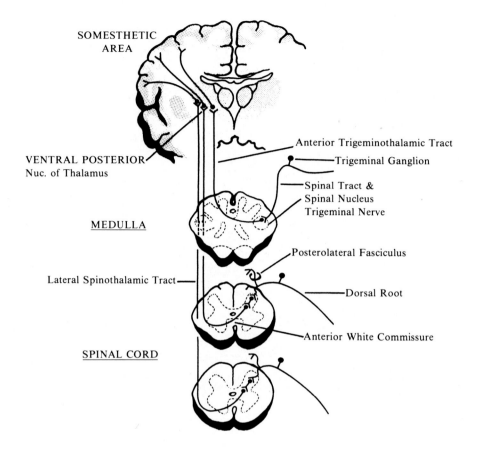

PAIN-TEMPERATURE

FIGURE 2–17. Pain and temperature pathways from spinal cord to parietal cortex. (From Clark, R. G. *Essentials of Clinical Neuroanatomy and Neurophysiology,* 5th ed. F. A. Davis Company, Philadelphia, 1975.)

velop as a consequence of cortical growth that causes folding of brain tissue and formation of gyri (see Figs. 2–23 through 2–25) (Chi *et al.,* 1977). This tremendous amount of growth and infolding—especially striking during the last third of gestation—causes part of the cortex to become buried within the brain, inapparent upon gross inspection (unless the lips of the sylvian fissure are pulled apart) (see Fig. 2–24). This buried island of cortex is the insula, which belongs to the parietal lobe superiorly and to the temporal lobe inferiorly.

Microscopic Brain Development. By the first month of gestation, the neural tube is organized into three concentric layers: ependymal, mantle, and marginal. Ependymal cells line the neural tube. Also within the ependymal layer are stem cells, which proliferate to form rudimentary dorsal and ventral horns of the spinal cord (see Fig. 2–26). Similar events take place within the brainstem as well, although stretching out of the ependymal roof plate of the fourth ventricle causes the would-be dorsal (sensory) horns to lie

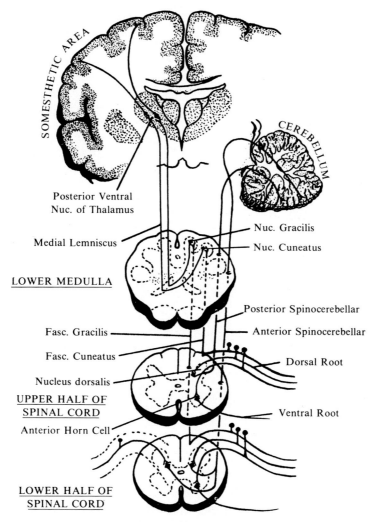

PROPRIOCEPTION-STEREOGNOSIS

FIGURE 2–18. Pathways for proprioception and stereognosis from spinal cord to somesthetic area of parietal lobe. (From Clark, R. G. *Essentials of Clinical Neuroanatomy and Neurophysiology,* 5th ed. F. A. Davis Company, Philadelphia, 1975.)

laterally. The mantle layer gives rise to gray matter as neurons migrate outward during gestation to form the multilayered cortex (Volpe, 1977). The marginal layer is destined to be white matter, containing myelinated nerve fibers that emanate from cells within that layer.

Myelinogenesis. The covering of nerve fibers with myelin makes possible orderly and efficient transmission of nerve impulses. Within the central nervous system, myelination is carried out by oligodendroglia, within the peripheral nervous system by Schwann cells. It is myelin that gives white matter its color.

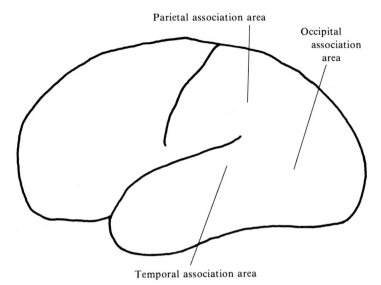

Parietal association area

Occipital
association
area

Temporal association area

FIGURE 2–19. Sensory association areas of cerebral cortex.

The process of myelination proceeds both centrally and peripherally, in an ordered fashion that begins in utero and continues for many years postnatally (Yakovlev and LeCours, 1967). For example, acoustic fibers are myelinated by the third trimester of gestation, whereas associational tracts continue to become myelinated beyond the first decade of life (see Fig. 2–27).

BIOCHEMISTRY

Neurotransmitters.   Neurotransmitters are chemical substances produced by neurons. They are released at nerve endings upon stimulation and act upon other cells (nerve, muscle, or other) to cause membrane changes. Acetylcholine, for example, is a neurotransmitter that acts in an excitatory fashion upon a receptor membrane, destabilizing it and—under some circumstances—initiating a propagated electrical impulse. This process is described in further detail below in the section on PHYSIOLOGY.

Among an ever increasing list of neurotransmitters are also included dopamine, norepinephrine, serotonin, and gamma aminobutyric acid (GABA). Whereas acetylcholine is an excitatory neurotransmitter, GABA appears to be inhibitory, stabilizing the postsynaptic cell membrane by increasing the negative charge within the cell.

Neuroendocrine Hormones.   Hormones, like neurotransmitter substances, are chemical messengers. Hormones, however, usually act at relatively distant sites after having been delivered directly to the bloodstream. An example is insulin, which is produced by islet cells of the pancreas and travels widely throughout the body via the bloodstream to facilitate entry of glucose into cells.

The pituitary gland and hypothalamus are the major neuroendocrine

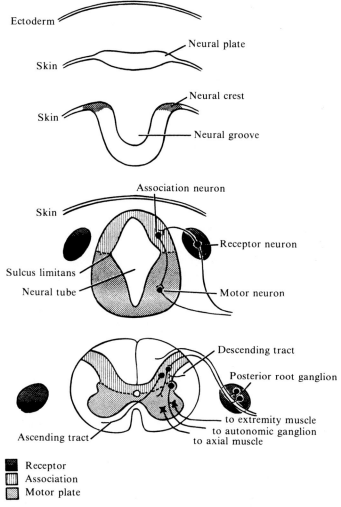

Receptor
Association
Motor plate

FIGURE 2–20. Development of the spinal cord from neural ectoderm. (From Lemire, R. J.; Loeser, J. D.; Leech, R. W.; and Alvord, E. C., Jr. *Normal and Abnormal Development of the Human Nervous System*. Harper and Row, Publishers, Hagerstown, Md., 1975.)

organs within the brain (see Chapter 6: CORRELATION). Specialized cells of the anterior pituitary produce thyroid-stimulating hormone (TSH), adreno-corticotropic hormone (ACTH), luteinizing hormone (LH), growth hormone (GH), prolactin, melanocyte-stimulating hormone (MSH), follicle-stimulating hormone (FSH), and beta-lipotropin. These pituitary hormones are released in response to neurohormones made by the hypothalamus: thyrotropin-releasing factor (TRF), corticotropin-releasing factor (CRF), luteinizing hormone-releasing factor (LHRF), growth hormone release-inhibiting factor (somatostatin), and prolactin release-inhibiting factor (PIF).

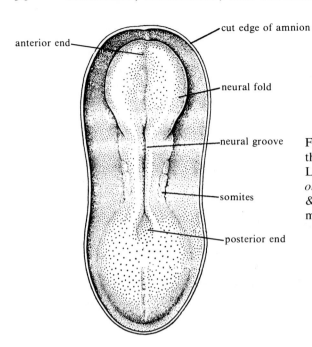

FIGURE 2–21. Formation of the neural groove. (From Langman, J. *Medical Embryology.* © 1963, The Williams & Wilkins Company, Baltimore.)

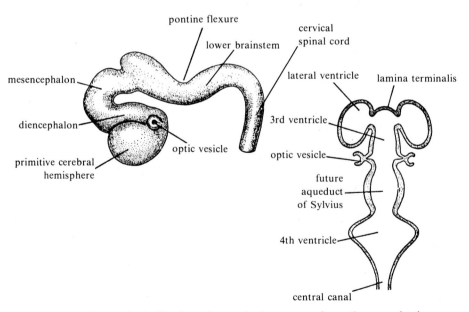

FIGURE 2–22. Formation of brain and ventricular system from the neural tube. (From Langman, J. *Medical Embryology.* © 1963, The Williams & Wilkins Company, Baltimore.)

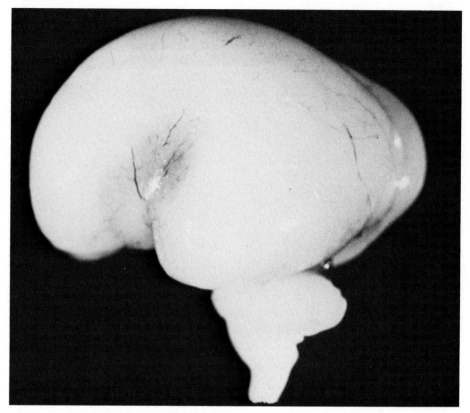

FIGURE 2–23. Fetal brain early in gestation showing early formation of sylvian fissure without other evidence of gyrus formation.

The posterior pituitary does not itself manufacture hormones. It receives vasopressin (also known as antidiuretic hormone, or ADH) and oxytocin from the hypothalamus, where they are made. These hormones reach the posterior pituitary from the hypothalamus along nerve fiber tracts that traverse the infundibulum.

Other Peptides. Included in this category are endogenous opioids (such as enkephalins and endorphins) and gastrointestinal peptides (such as cholecystokinin) produced within and acting upon the central nervous system (Krieger and Martin, 1981) (see Chapter 19).

Energy Metabolism. The brain depends upon the metabolism of carbohydrates for energy under most circumstances, although at times fat may be utilized by the brain as an energy source. Under aerobic conditions (that is, in the presence of oxygen), carbohydrates are broken down into glucose subunits, then further metabolized to acetyl coenzyme A, which enters the Krebs tricarboxylic acid cycle. Through the so-called respiratory chain of reactions, energy from the oxidation of glucose is stored by the formation of adenosine triphosphate (ATP). Under anaerobic conditions, glucose is me-

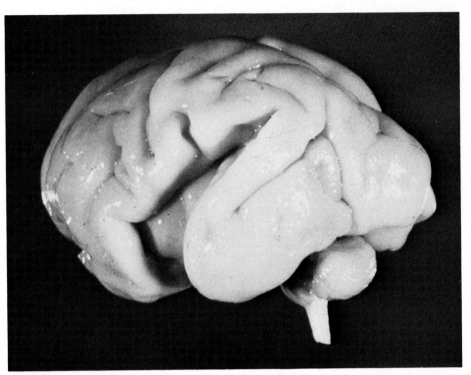

FIGURE 2–24. Fetal brain in mid-gestation showing formation of major gyri with insular cortex incompletely buried.

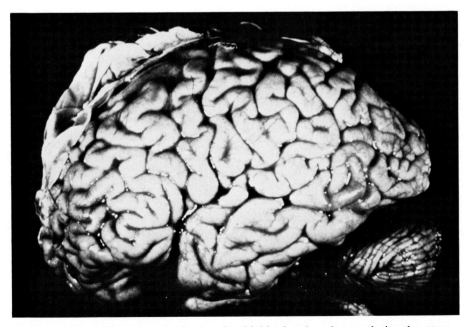

FIGURE 2–25. Fully mature brain showing highly developed convolutional pattern. Insular cortex is no longer visible.

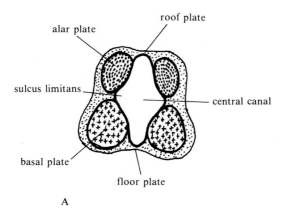

A

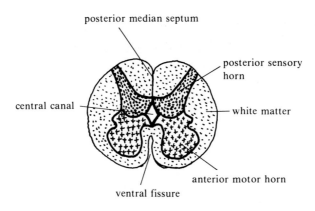

B

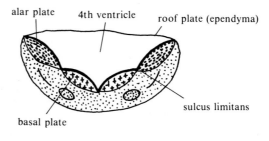

C

FIGURE 2–26. Development of spinal cord (*B*) and brainstem (*C*) from earlier embryonic structure (*A*). (From Langman, J. *Medical Embryology.* © 1963, The Williams & Wilkins Company, Baltimore.)

MYELOGENETIC CYCLES

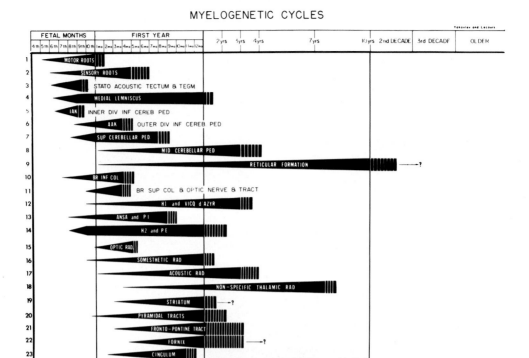

FIGURE 2–27. Development of myelinated pathways within the central nervous system. (From Yakovlev, P. I., and Lecours, A.-R. The myelogenetic cycles of regional maturation of the brain. In *Regional Development of the Brain in Early Life*. Minkowski, A., ed. Blackwell Scientific Publications. Oxford, 1967.)

tabolized less efficiently so that fewer ATP molecules are produced per unit of glucose.

PHYSIOLOGY

Membrane Physiology. Under normal resting conditions, the inside of the cell is negatively charged compared with the outside. This charge differential (−70 to −90 millivolts) is maintained primarily by sodium (Na^+) being actively pumped out of cells. This process, which requires energy, keeps sodium concentration much higher outside the cell than inside. Entry into the cell of chloride ion (Cl^-) and exit of potassium ion (K^+) along an osmotic gradient also help to maintain the electronegativity of the cell interior.

When sodium in sufficient amount enters a nerve cell, the charge of the cell membrane becomes reversed. It is now positive on the inside, negative on the outside. This depolarization reduces the stability of adjacent nerve cell membranes; and as they, too, undergo depolarization, an electrical impulse is generated.

Once the cell interior reaches a certain level of positive electrical charge, no further sodium rushes in; hence, impulse propagation is no longer fostered. The resting membrane potential can then be reestablished through sodium being pumped out of the cell.

The excitability of nerve cells depends upon several factors. A high concentration of potassium ion outside the cell will retard its exit from inside. Consequently, the resting membrane potential will be lessened, the cell membrane destabilized, and propagation of a nerve impulse more likely to occur. Conversely, a low concentration of extracellular potassium leads to increased negativity inside the cell and stabilization of the cell membrane.

Calcium (Ca^{++}) appears to influence sodium ion flow by blocking "pores" or channels that normally permit sodium influx. Low serum calcium thus will foster sodium influx and result in overexcitability of cell membranes, which may be manifested clinically by hyperreflexia, tetany, or seizures. Elevated serum calcium, by contrast, typically is associated with depression of many functions of the nervous system.

Because energy is required to pump sodium out of cells in order that negativity be maintained within, interruption of energy sources—resulting in inadequate supply of glucose, oxygen, or both—may lead to membrane instability and altered function manifested, for example, as convulsions.

Synaptic Function.   The synapse is the junction between two neurons. It consists of the presynaptic neuron, synaptic cleft, and postsynaptic neuron. Depolarization of the presynaptic neuron is associated with discharge of neurotransmitter into the synaptic cleft. The neurotransmitter then acts upon the postsynaptic membrane to increase or decrease the charge differential across the membrane. An excitatory neurotransmitter will cause depolarization of the postsynaptic membrane. When depolarization caused by the effect of one or more excitatory neurons exceeds a certain threshold, propagation of an electrical impulse will result. An inhibitory neurotransmitter will render the postsynaptic membrane less excitable, thereby inhibiting impulse transmission. Thus electrical and biochemical information are exchanged at the synapse.

Termination of neurotransmitter activity at the synapse differs among neurotransmitters. For example, acetylcholine is broken down by the enzyme acetylcholinesterase within the synaptic cleft. Monoamine neurotransmitters such as norepinephrine and dopamine, by contrast, are inactivated primarily by re-uptake of neurotransmitter by the presynaptic neuron. Additionally, some breakdown of monoamine neurotransmitter also occurs within the synaptic cleft (through the action of catechol-O-methyltransferase) and within the presynaptic neuron (by monoamine oxidase).

Neuromuscular Unit.   The neuromuscular unit consists of an anterior horn cell, the motor nerve roots originating from that cell, and all muscle fibers upon which these motor nerve roots end. Between nerve and muscle fiber is the motor end plate, a specialized portion of the muscle fiber designed to convert the electrical energy of a neural impulse into the mechanical energy of muscle contraction. The molecular basis of muscle contraction is discussed in Chapter 13 (CORRELATION: PHYSIOLOGIC ASPECTS).

SUMMARY

This chapter has presented an overview of the structure and function of the nervous system, focusing upon major anatomic, biochemical, and physiologic aspects and providing a foundation for approaching the clinical problems to be presented in Part Two.

CITED REFERENCES

Chi, J. G.; Dooling, E. C.; and Gilles, F. H. Gyral development of the human brain. *Ann. Neurol.*, **1:**86–93, 1977.
Krieger, D. T., and Martin, J. B. Brain peptides. *N. Engl. J. Med.*, **304:** 876–85, 944–51, 1981.
Plum, F., and Posner, J. B. *The Diagnosis of Stupor and Coma,* 3d ed. F. A. Davis Co., Philadelphia, 1980.
Volpe, J. J. Normal and abnormal human brain development. *Clin. Perinatol.*, **4:** 3–30, 1977.
Yakovlev, P. I., and Lecours, A.-R. The myelogenetic cycles of regional maturation of the brain. Pp. 3–65 in *Regional Development of the Brain in Early Life*. Minkowski, A., ed. Blackwell, Oxford, 1967.

ADDITIONAL READINGS

Carpenter, M. B. *Core Text of Neuroanatomy,* 2nd ed. Williams & Wilkins, Baltimore, 1978.
Cooper, J. R.; Bloom, F. E.; and Roth, R. H. *The Biochemical Basis of Neuropharmacology,* 3rd ed. Oxford University Press, New York, 1978.
Crosby, E. C.; Humphrey, T.; and Lauer, E. W. *Correlative Anatomy of the Nervous System.* Macmillan Publishing Co., Inc. New York, 1962.
Fishman, R. A. *Cerebrospinal Fluid in Diseases of the Nervous System.* W. B. Saunders Co., Philadelphia, 1980.
Krieger, D. T., and Hughes, J. C., eds. *Neuroendocrinology.* Sinauer Associates, Inc., Sunderland, Mass., 1980.
Langman, J. *Medical Embryology,* 3rd ed. Williams & Wilkins, Baltimore, 1975.
Lehninger, A. L. *Biochemistry: The Molecular Basis of Cell Structure and Function,* 2nd ed. Worth, New York, 1975.
Luria, A. R. *The Working Brain: An Introduction to Neuropsychology.* Haigh, B., trans. Basic Books, Inc., New York, 1973.
Magoun, H. W. *The Waking Brain,* 2nd ed. Charles C Thomas, Springfield, Ill., 1963.
Netter, F. H. *Nervous System.* Vol. I of *The Ciba Collection of Medical Illustrations.* Ciba Pharmaceutical Company, Summit, N.J., 1953.
Pansky, B., and Allen, D. J. *Review of Neuroscience.* Macmillan Publishing Co., Inc., New York, 1980.
Papez, J. W. A proposed mechanism of emotion. *Arch. Neurol. Psychiat.*, **38:** 725–43, 1937.
Penfield, W., and Rasmussen, T. *The Cerebral Cortex of Man: A Clinical Study of Localization of Function.* Macmillan Publishing Co., Inc., New York, 1950.
Scientific American. The brain. *Sci. Am.*, **241:** 45–232, 248, 249, September 1979.
Young, J. Z. *Programs of the Brain.* Oxford University Press, Oxford, 1978.

3 Behavior: Its Definition and Development

Behavior is first and foremost movement. Whether one speaks of the infant kicking his limbs in excitement, the toddler imitating mother doing housework, the school-age child learning to write, or the teenager holding down a part-time job, the common thread is movement. Movement is even part of life before birth, when behavior ranges from random to semipurposeful activity.

Behavior as movement cannot be considered apart from development, the appearance and transformation over time of physical, emotional, and social activities. The environmental context must also be taken into account. In the newborn child, behaviors of sucking, clinging, and crying are inbuilt, though they depend upon internal and external factors. In the toddler, walking is essentially preprogrammed, but using a spoon involves newly gained fine motor skills and perception of ''grown-up'' eating patterns. The school-age child, already competent in basic activities such as walking and talking, is concerned with acquiring and refining communication skills: reading, spelling, and writing. The adolescent's behavior reflects age-appropriate strivings toward physical, emotional, and financial independence as adulthood is approached.

The unifying feature of behavior from infancy to adolescence thus is movement, whether reflexive or purposeful. This chapter will pursue further the definition of behavior, consider its biologic basis, and present an overview of the development of behavior in infancy and early childhood.

DEFINITIONS OF BEHAVIOR

Behavior, a characteristic of all living things, encompasses the entirety of responses to internal and external environments. Human behavior can be considered the activities of an individual within personal and social contexts at levels ranging from the molecular to the societal.

Several authors in the field of development have addressed themselves to the definition of behavior. Gesell (1945) termed the earliest behavior "an endogenous kind of animation which undergoes progressive changes in embryo and infant." He noted that movements in response to touch had been seen in an 8½-week-old fetus that had been removed with the uterus at hysterectomy. He considered behavior to be an intrinsic part of growth, which he described as "an organizing process which creates patterns of structure and function."

Skinner (1953) defined behavior as "the coherent, continuous activity of an integral organism." He further characterized human behavior as being flexible and relatively changeable, contrasting these attributes with a steam engine, described by Coleridge as "a giant with one idea." Yet, noted Skinner, as "machines have become more lifelike, . . . living organisms have been found to be more like machines."

Part of this machinery is the reflex, simple or conditioned. With classical pavlovian conditioning, a conditioned stimulus (such as ringing a bell) replaces an unconditioned stimulus (such as placing food before a laboratory animal) in producing a reflex response (in this instance, salivation). Such conditioned reflexes are unconscious, stereotyped, and relatively unmodifiable behaviors (Skinner, 1953).

Operant conditioning, by contrast, does not depend upon intrinsic reflex behaviors in response to a stimulus, but allows for the shaping of behavior. With operant conditioning, a stimulus is followed by a period during which behavior is shaped as the desired behavior is rewarded. For example, after a light of a particular color is presented to an experimental animal (e.g., a bird), if one object is chosen rather than another, food is given as a reward.

An everyday example of operant conditioning provided by Skinner is picking apples (*behavior*) depending upon their color (*stimulus*) to achieve the desired sour or sweet taste (*reinforcement*). Toilet-training is another example of operant conditioning. The urge to defecate is the stimulus for appropriate use of the toilet, and reinforcement at first takes the form of parental praise. In this instance, operant behavior competes with and eventually supervenes over reflex bowel action.

Bowlby (1969) has emphasized the goal-oriented nature of behavior. In his studies on attachment, he described actions varying with the age of the child by which the child can maintain contact with the mother. These actions are initially instinctual (e.g., sucking, grasping, clinging) and progress to more complex behaviors such as visual tracking (with head and eyes), locomotion (crawling and walking), and language (e.g., speaking with or calling the mother who is out of sight). Memory, too, can be considered in this category of attachment behavior, since it provides for continued psychologic, if not physical, contact.

Cognitive development has been the focus of Piaget's investigations. He has described a developmental progression from sensorimotor to preconceptual to conceptual phases of cognition (Piaget, 1952; Maier, 1969; Ginsberg and Opper, 1969). The sensorimotor phase, taking place during the first two years of life, includes countless "experiments" conducted by the baby that provide a rudimentary grasp of the world. The preconceptual phase usually occurs between 2 and 11 years of age and involves intuitive thought and concrete operations. The conceptual phase, beginning at 11 to 15 years, is a stage of formal operations in which symbolic rather than concrete thinking comes to be used.

Yakovlev (1948) stressed the fundamental role of movement in behavior and described three major areas, or spheres, of motility: visceration, expression, and effectuation.

Visceration is concerned with activities ranging from the conscious to the unconscious that play a role in maintenance of the organism. These include the processes of respiration, circulation, ingestion, digestion, and excretion of food, all of which are involved in providing energy for maintaining the organism in its many spheres of activity.

Expression involves the manifestation of internal (visceral) states, including emotional expression. In the infant, alert attentiveness is evidence of satisfaction of bodily needs (contact, food, warmth, sleep). Crying can be a manifestation of hunger. Facial movements reflect an unhappy state, as respiratory and laryngeal movements become coordinated to generate a hungry cry. This vocalization is a crude form of speech, later to undergo extraordinary refinement as the child grows. Use of the arms in gesture is another manner of expression. Semipurposeful flailing of the arms in a happy, excited baby is quite a different statement from the pushing away of the breast by an irritable infant.

Effectuation involves changing the world of matter through the use of the body, tools, or machines. The bipedal status of man has freed the forelimbs for use in shaping the environment, and instruments and machines have extended the capabilities of the hand.

Yakovlev described a unity of form and function of the nervous system as it pertains to behavior, that is, to the three spheres of motility. The *innermost* portion of the nervous system is gray matter comprising the sympathetic and parasympathetic divisions of the autonomic nervous system, involved in maintenance activities of the organism, *visceration*. An *intermediate* system, lying superficial to the innermost, includes the basal ganglia and portions of limbic cortex. It subserves functions of vocalization, gesture, muscle tone, posture, and outward *expression* of visceral states: emotion. The *outermost* system originates in the well-myelinated, relatively large neurons of the cerebral cortex, especially portions that have developed late from an evolutionary standpoint. Pyramidal fibers are considered part of this system, whereas fibers originating within the basal ganglia are part of the intermediate system. The cerebral cortex, as the locus for fine movements of the hands and for higher cognitive processes, is the embodiment of the sphere of *effectuation*.

Bronson (1965) has presented a conceptual model of central nervous system structure and function that is likewise hierarchical, with three levels that are structurally and functionally interconnected. Level one consists of the brainstem; level two, subcortical structures including the thalamus and basal ganglia; and level three, the neocortex.

TABLE 3–1. **Development in the Infant and Young Child***

Gross Motor

Newborn	Complete head lag when pulled to sit; reflex walking
5–6 months	Bears weight on lower limbs nearly fully; rolls prone to supine (belly to back); lifts head off horizontal when about to be pulled up; no head lag with pull to sit
6–7 months	Sits in tripod position (hands placed forward for support)
8–9 months	Crawls backward; sits steadily for several minutes and can use hands while sitting; pulls self to stand
9–10 months	Crawls forward on abdomen; attains sitting position by self
12 months	Walks with one hand held
15 months	Walks without assistance
15–18 months	Seats self in chair; pulls wheeled toy
2 years	Walks backward; runs; goes up and down stairs alone
2½ years	Jumps with both feet
3 years	Rides tricycle; stands on one foot for 2 or 3 seconds
4 years	Hops on one foot
5 years	Skips on both feet; rides bicycle

Fine Motor

Newborn	Grasp reflex (for first two to four months)
3–5 months	Looks at hands; reaches for dangling object; grasps an object voluntarily
6 months	Drops one cube when another is given; holds bottle
7 months	Transfers objects from hand to hand; takes second cube without dropping first; rakes raisin to pick it up
9 months	Uses crude pincer grasp to pick up raisin
10 months	Uses neat pincer grasp
11–12 months	Gives toy to examiner
12–15 months	Throws objects to floor; builds tower of two or three 1-inch cubes; holds two cubes in one hand; scribbles spontaneously
18 months	Builds tower of three or four cubes
2 years	Builds tower of six or seven cubes; turns doorknob; scribbles vertically and in circle after demonstration
2½ years	Neater pencil grasp; builds eight-cubed tower
3 years	Builds tower of nine or ten cubes; unbuttons; copies a circle

Speech and Language

0–2 months	Moves limbs, head, eyes in response to voice or noise; vocalizes
2 months	Makes squeals of pleasure; exhibits differentiated crying
2–3 months	Coos
4 months	Laughs aloud
5–7 months	Babbles (produces two-syllable utterances: "mama," "baba")
9–11 months	Says "mama," "dada" nonspecifically; inhibits activity in response to "No!"
12–15 months	Uses two or three words meaningfully; knows animal sounds
15–18 months	Shows body parts; follows two simple directions; uses jargon with many intelligible words
20–24 months	Uses two- or three-word phrases

40

TABLE 3–1. (*Continued*)

*Speech and
Language
(Continued)*

2 years	Uses "I," "me," "you," "mine"; uses first name when referring to self
$2\frac{1}{2}$ years	Understands two prepositions
3 years	Gives first and last name; understands three prepositions; follows two-step commands; uses plurals

*Social and
Emotional*

0–2 months	Becomes quiet when picked up; maintains brief eye contact when feeding; smiles to stimulation (talk or touch)
3–5 months	Laughs; cries when left alone or put down; indicates awareness of strange surroundings; reaches out to familiar persons; smiles spontaneously; smiles at image in mirror; watches adults walk across a room
6–8 months	Laughs at pat-a-cake and peek-a-boo games; withdraws or cries when stranger approaches; pats and touches image in mirror
9–11 months	Plays pat-a-cake and peek-a-boo; offers toy but does not release it; displays discomfort when separated from mother in a strange environment
11–15 months	Offers and gives toy to adult
16–19 months	Uses mother as secure base; checks back with her frequently
20–23 months	Plays near other children (parallel play); puts toys away on request
24–27 months	Imitates housework
28–31 months	Notes sexual differences
32–35 months	Separates easily from mother in strange environment; identifies own sex; begins to understand taking turns

Cognitive

3–5 months	Watches place where a moving object has disappeared
6–8 months	Attains partially hidden object; looks to floor when something falls; removes cover placed over face
9–12 months	Pulls string to secure ring; attains completely hidden object
13–15 months	Repeatedly finds toy hidden under one or several covers; inverts a small bottle to retrieve raisin inside; uses stick to try to attain object out of reach
19–23 months	Deduces location of hidden object from indirect visual cues
24–29 months	Matches colored blocks; understands concept of one
30–36 months	Repeats two digits; matches four shapes (circle, square, cross, star); identifies objects by their use (car, penny, bottle)

* Adapted from Illingworth, R. S. *The Development of the Infant and Young Child: Normal and Abnormal,* 7th ed. Churchill Livingstone, Edinburgh and New York, 1980.

Level one, the brainstem, projects upward to affect the general level of alertness and responsiveness of the organism. Level two provides for further focusing of attention and for motivational and emotional orientations that support goal-oriented behavior. Level three structures mediate development of cognitive, perceptual, and motor capacities. Bronson linked three types of learning with this hierarchical model: classical (pavlovian) conditioning with level one, instrumental learning (operant conditioning) with level two, and latent (higher cognitive) learning with level three.

Thus does the structure of the central nervous system reflect, and provide for, different levels of movement and behavior.

DEVELOPMENT OF BEHAVIOR

Behavior grows with the child. Like physical growth (manifested by changes in height, weight, and head circumference), development of behavior can be approached most usefully by consideration of separable (though certainly not unrelated) developmental areas. These include gross motor, fine motor, speech and language, social and emotional, and cognitive aspects of behavior.

In considering a child's development, one should keep in mind that under normal circumstances, development does not proceed at the same rate in each area. The more rapid acquisition of gross motor skills as contrasted with language skills illustrates this principle (see Table 3–1).

The importance of clarifying areas of strength and weakness, and particularly of determining whether a child is globally delayed or behind in only one area (or relatively few), is emphasized in Chapters 5, 8, and 18. It should be emphasized further that the child's accomplishment of a given developmental task "on schedule" may not itself provide the fullest picture of behavior. The quality of performance of the task must also be considered. Does the child carry out the task with vigor, or must coaxing be employed? Is the task done with a minimum of demonstration, or is detailed instruction required? How attentive is the child to detail? How persistent or easily frustrated?

SUMMARY

Behavior is, in essence, movement. It begins prenatally and continues throughout life, varying with the age and developmental stage of the child. Definitions of behavior have been considered, and the hierarchical models of Yakovlev and Bronson for relating structure and function of the nervous system are reviewed.

Developmental assessment should take into account different areas of development (gross motor, fine motor, speech and language, social and emotional, and cognitive). The child's profile of strengths and weaknesses should be determined and the quality of performance noted. Development of behavior in infancy and early childhood within these several areas is outlined.

CITED REFERENCES

Bowlby, J. *Attachment and Loss*. Vol. I: *Attachment*. Basic Books, Inc., New York, 1969.

Bronson, G. The hierarchical organization of the central nervous system: implications for learning processes and critical periods in early development. *Behav. Sci.*, **10:** 7–25, 1965.

Gesell, A. *The Embryology of Behavior*. Harper and Row, Publishers, New York, 1945.

Ginsburg, H., and Opper, S. *Piaget's Theory of Intellectual Development: An Introduction*. Prentice-Hall, Inc., Englewood Cliffs, N.J., 1969.

Illingworth, R. S. *The Development of the Infant and Young Child: Normal and Abnormal*, 7th ed. Churchill Livingstone, Edinburgh and New York, 1980.

Maier, H. W. *Three Theories of Child Development*, rev. ed. Harper and Row, Publishers, New York, 1969, pp. 80–157.

Piaget, J. *The Origins of Intelligence in Children*. International Universities Press, Inc., New York, 1952.

Skinner, B. F. *Science and Human Behavior*. Free Press, New York, 1953.

Yakovlev. P. I. Motility, behavior and the brain. *J. Nerv. Ment. Dis.*, **107:** 313–35, 1948.

4 Clinical Diagnostic Process: History, Examination, and Investigation

Through the clinical diagnostic process, problems are identified and characterized as to severity and cause (insofar as is possible) so that an optimal therapeutic plan can be established and prognosis determined. This chapter presents a general approach to assessment of the child brought for evaluation because of cognitive, behavioral, or affective problems. In Part Two, specific aspects of history, examination, and investigation will be presented as they pertain to various clinical problems. This chapter serves as a framework for diagnostic assessment.

HISTORY

The clinical diagnostic process is divided into three parts: history, examination, and investigation. In practice, it is often artificial to consider these elements completely separable. While the history is being obtained, information is being gathered as to the child's mental status: alertness, attentiveness, intelligence, affect, and interpersonal interactions, among other attributes. An ordered approach is nonetheless justified, because information pertaining to several areas cannot be elicited and recorded at once and because the standard structure of the clinical diagnostic process facilitates communication among professionals.

It is important to recognize that history-taking is not merely information-gathering. The professional's participation in the diagnostic process implies concern and an attempt at understanding (in a sense, sharing) the pain, disability, and confusion that may be experienced by the child and family. The importance of determining why help is being sought at a particular time was addressed in Chapter 1.

As the history is obtained, a bond is being formed between the professional and the child and family that can have major diagnostic and therapeutic implications. The trust that is established will allow the child and fam-

44

ily to discuss delicate matters of importance. It also will permit the most complete examination possible and may allow for appropriate investigations to be undertaken, even though certain of these may be unpleasant. Such trust will also allow the child and family to pursue additional consultation, if it is felt to be necessary, with assurance.

Perhaps most important, a relationship of trust will allow for the effective implementation of a treatment plan later to be drawn up with the child's confidence that it will significantly improve his or her life and probably that of the family as well.

The history is almost always the most important part of the clinical diagnostic process. Indeed, the diagnosis is established by careful history-taking in the large majority of cases, with examination and investigation accounting for the remainder.

The history provides a longitudinal perspective, which is of particular importance with problems such as headaches, seizures, mental retardation, and behavioral regression. With a seizure disorder, for example, a seizure will be apparent during the office assessment itself relatively infrequently. One must rely on information provided by the child, parent, or other observer as to frequency, response to medication, and other clinical features. Headache is almost exclusively a subjective category of complaint. Once the history has narrowed down the diagnostic possibilities, then examination and investigation are much more likely to confirm or establish a specific diagnosis.

The overall structure of the history is indicated in Table 4–1.

The *chief complaint* should be recorded whenever possible in the words of the child and the parents. In that way, one can better understand the child's and family's perception of the problem and ultimately formulate a treatment plan that is most relevant to their concerns.

The *history of the presenting problem* should focus upon the symptom or symptoms that have led to evaluation. For example, with the problem of

TABLE 4–1. **Outline of History**

Chief complaint
History of presenting problem
Past history
    Pregnancy, delivery, and development
    Significant illnesses
    Accidents, including head trauma
    Hospitalizations
    Operations
    Medications
    Allergies
    Immunizations
    Diet
Family history
Social history and personal profile
School history
Review of systems

headache, symptoms should be characterized as to onset, frequency, intensity, location, character of pain, associated symptoms, precipitating circumstances, and response to prior treatment (see Chapter 11). Each symptom should be traced from its time of onset to the present.

The psychosocial framework of the problem and the degree of associated disability should be determined. For example, headaches may have worsened upon entering junior high school or with impending divorce of the child's parents. Frequent headaches that do not interfere with academic performance or social activities may suggest the influence of stress.

Not every item listed as part of *past history* need be pursued in every instance, but each item will have relevance under certain circumstances. Immunization status, for example, will often be noncontributory. In the school-age child with behavioral deterioration suggesting subacute sclerosing panencephalitis (SSPE), however, history of immunization against measles will be quite pertinent (see Chapter 8).

It is generally useful to inquire about hospitalizations and operations. For example, a child being evaluated for headaches may have been admitted to hospital as an infant because of unexplained episodes of vomiting, which could be considered a migraine equivalent (see Chapter 11).

Early history—pregnancy, labor, birth, and development—is a cornerstone in the assessment of the pediatric patient. It should be noted, however, that reviewing details of early history sometimes lends considerable weight to events (such as a fall during the third trimester) that have no bearing upon current problems. On the other hand, reviewing early history, in addition to providing essential information, can provide the opportunity to extinguish smoldering embers of guilt, confusion, and responsibility. For example, a woman who feared that she had caused her child's neurofibromatosis (manifested by skin lesions and other stigmata) by spilling coffee on herself during pregnancy could be reassured of her blamelessness.

The importance of obtaining past records and reviewing them cannot be overemphasized. Evaluation may already have been carried out and the problem definitively diagnosed. Hence, complete reassessment may not be required. In some circumstances a written report or summary of prior evaluation may not be sufficient for the current problem, and the investigations themselves (such as x-rays, electroencephalograms, and computerized tomographic scans) should be obtained for review.

Family history will be relevant in the assessment of many behavioral and emotional disorders in childhood. Many conditions (such as Duchenne muscular dystrophy) behave in a clearly hereditary fashion (in this instance, X-linked recessive). Other problems—such as dyslexia and hyperactivity—follow a less well-defined pattern of inheritance. Clarifying a positive family history can enhance the parents' understanding of their child's behavior, which may be "cut from the same cloth" as that of a similarly affected parent whose problems may have escaped notice or proper attention.

When the problem appears to be familial, time should be set aside to detail the family tree. If the disorder might be of autosomal recessive inheritance (as it often is with genetic-metabolic disease), one should ascertain if the parents are consanguineous or of the same ethnic group, which would increase the likelihood of the disorder being expressed. Constructing a pedigree may be facilitated by having the parents ask other family members to provide missing information.

If the child is dysmorphic and chromosomal anomaly is being considered, a family history of mental retardation, infertility, spontaneous abortions, or stillbirths should be sought.

The *social history and personal profile* should flesh out the history, providing a picture of the person who has the problems. Hobbies, career aspirations, academic achievements, part-time employment, and athletic pursuits merit exploration, as they provide a view of life outside the office. A child's hobbies (such as coin collecting) or athletic interests may be nonacademic areas of excellence that can be built upon in a learning-disabled child who has experienced repeated frustrations and failures in school.

It can be valuable to learn of parents' projections or career aspirations for their child by asking, "What do you see for your child in 10 to 15 years?" Their expectations may be appropriate, unrealistically high (as with a mentally retarded child), or unknowingly low (as with a learning-disabled child who is, in fact, "college material"). Early events (seizures, borderline developmental status in infancy, illness, or prematurity) may have frightened the parents and led them to set their sights too low.

The *school history* should include at the very least academic performance, recent improvement or decline, and the child's attitude toward school (see Chapter 17).

The *review of systems* is a screen for problems that may not seem directly relevant to the chief complaint and the history of the presenting problem. Typical symptoms sought might include headache, personality change, sleep disturbance, weight loss or gain, enuresis, seizures, hearing difficulties, visual impairment, depression, heat intolerance, hyperactivity, and school problems.

EXAMINATION

Although the importance of the history has been emphasized earlier, the value of careful examination should not be underestimated. The examination often confirms the diagnosis suggested by the history. Less frequently it indicates the diagnosis where one had not been determined previously. The examination also provides objective data with which to compare (and validate) the observations of parents. And it represents another point in time for assessment of growth and development.

The examination should begin with a *general description* based primarily upon observation. One should resist the tendency to apply the hands immediately even for such conventional measures as checking the pulse or blood pressure, in order that the most striking aspects of the child's appearance and behavior be registered and recorded. Activity level, alertness, affect, curiosity, or extraordinary neatness might merit specific mention.

Engaging the child in introductory conversation will facilitate his or her adjustment to the examination and permit the examiner to learn the child's perception of why he or she has been brought for evaluation. Indeed, much of the information pertaining to the general description applies as well to the mental status examination, discussed below. By beginning the examination with general observations, however, one will be better able to gain a sense of the uniqueness of the child being examined.

The *general physical examination* should include vital signs (pulse rate, blood pressure, respirations, and temperature) and growth parameters (height, weight, and head circumference). Growth data should be plotted on standard charts, which permit visualization of significant deviations from the mean at a given time and of fall-off or increase in growth rate when previous measurements are compared with those of the present.

The examination then generally proceeds in an ordered fashion, usually rostrocaudally (from head to feet). The orderliness with which data are recorded may not reflect the order of the examination, for another guiding principle in pediatrics is that the least disturbing aspects of the examination are carried out first and the more difficult or upsetting parts (such as funduscopic examination or rectal examination) are saved until later.

Examination of the skin is important in a wide variety of clinical problems ranging from seizure disorder to child abuse. Inspection of readily accessible portions of the limbs or trunk alone should not be considered adequate. The entire skin should be inspected, for injuries to buttocks or perineum only then will become evident. Birthmarks (such as café-au-lait spots or hypopigmented macules) in nonexposed areas may provide important diagnostic clues in children with developmental delay or seizures (see Figs. 4–1 and 4–2).

The *neurologic examination* involves assessment of cranial nerves, motor function, sensation, coordination, reflexes, and mental status. The last-mentioned is discussed later as a separate entity.

All twelve *cranial nerves* should be tested whenever possible. The manner in which each cranial nerve is tested should be recorded. For example, the first cranial nerve (olfactory) may be tested by asking the child (whose eyes are closed) if he smells anything as cloves are brought toward his nose. A correct response might be recorded as follows: "Cr. n. I—smells cloves." Substances irritating to the nasal mucosa such as pepper or smelling salts should not be used to test olfaction, because pain receptors associated with the trigeminal nerve would then be involved.

The second cranial nerve (optic) is tested in several ways. Visual acuity can be assessed with either the hand-held Rosenbaum card or with the Snellen wall chart. Testing of visual fields will depend upon the age and cooperativeness of the child. Response to movement of the examiner's fingers is a relatively crude manner of testing, but it may nonetheless demonstrate a hemianopic field deficit in a young child. In the older child, much smaller objects such as a 4-mm white-headed pin can be used to map out visual fields by confrontation. Tangent screen testing can be carried out if further refinement is desired. Optokinetic nystagmus can be evaluated by rotation of a striped drum or use of an analogous device.

Ophthalmoscopic examination of the optic fundus is an essential part of the visual examination. The optic disks, maculae, vessels, and retinal background should be noted. Disks may be elevated and show blurred margins in

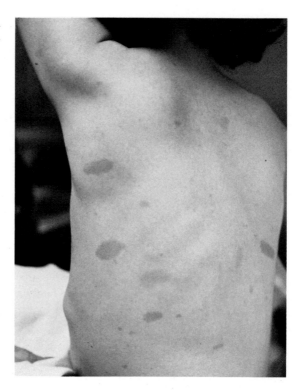

FIGURE 4–1. Multiple café au-lait spots of the trunk.

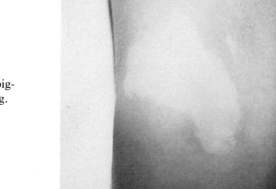

FIGURE 4–2. Hypopig-mented macule of leg.

association with increased intracranial pressure or optic neuritis, or they may be atrophic. Vessels may be diminished in number and attenuated in diameter. The maculae may be cherry red in color or scarred. The retina may show pigmentary degeneration or other retinopathy (see Fig. 4–3).

Pupillary reactions to light and accommodation are subserved by the second and third cranial nerves. The optic nerves mediate the afferent portion of the reflex; the oculomotor, the efferent (pupilloconstrictor) limb. The third cranial nerve (oculomotor) is also involved in extraocular movements in conjunction with the fourth (trochlear) and sixth (abducens) cranial nerves. Strabismus, or "squint," may be evidence of cranial nerve dysfunction or, more often, imbalance of eye muscles. With a third nerve palsy, the eye on the affected side is down and out (abducted) with accompanying ptosis (and usually pupillary dilation). With sixth nerve paralysis, the affected eye is deviated nasally and cannot be abducted fully, if at all.

The fifth cranial nerve (trigeminal) deals primarily with sensory function of the face and with muscles of mastication. Three branches of the trigeminal (ophthalmic, maxillary, and mandibular) subserve facial sensation. The corneal reflex is mediated by the fifth and seventh cranial nerves. Motor functions of the trigeminal nerve are tested by having the child bite down (while

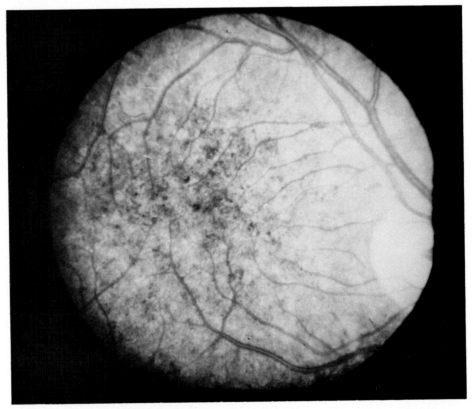

FIGURE 4–3. Photograph of optic fundus showing pigmentary changes characteristic of congenital rubella infection.

the examiner feels the masseter and pterygoid muscles), open the mouth against resistance, and move the jaw from side to side.

The seventh cranial nerve (facial) is involved primarily with facial movement and with taste over the anterior two-thirds of the tongue. Its motor functions are tested by having the child close the eyes forcibly (burying the lids), retracting the corners of the mouth (by saying the letter ''E''), and making the ''cords'' in the neck (the platysma muscle) stand out.

The eighth cranial nerve (auditory, or vestibulocochlear) is involved in hearing, balance, and eye movements. The child's responsiveness to conversational speech should be noted. Must the examiner raise his voice for the child to hear it? Does the child gaze intently at the speaker's lips? Whispering in each ear at increasing distances provides a semiquantitative means of assessing hearing, but by no means does this test (or cruder means of assessment such as banging a trash can) replace formal audiologic evaluation.

If hearing is impaired, then the tuning fork tests of Weber and Rinné can be carried out in the cooperative child. With the Weber test, the vibrating tuning fork is placed in the middle of the forehead. Lateralization will occur to the side of conductive hearing loss. With the Rinné test, the ringing tuning fork is placed upon the mastoid bone to determine if conduction of sound through bone is less than conduction through air (which would be normal). With conductive hearing loss (such as can occur in middle ear disease), bone conduction will typically be greater than air conduction. With sensorineural hearing loss, both air conduction and bone conduction are reduced, though air conduction continues to be greater than bone conduction.

The vestibular system is assessed along with cranial nerves III, IV, and VI when extraocular movements are evaluated. Nystagmus, spontaneous or gaze-evoked, can result from vestibular dysfunction. The oculocephalic maneuver and caloric testing are other ways to assess the vestibular portion of the eighth cranial nerve (see Chapter 19).

The ninth (glossopharyngeal) and tenth (vagus) cranial nerves function together to elevate the palate and mediate the gag response. The glossopharyngeal also subserves taste sensation over the posterior one-third of the tongue. The vagus is additionally involved in laryngeal function; hence a hoarse voice may reflect tenth nerve dysfunction.

The eleventh cranial nerve (spinal accessory) is tested by having the child shrug the shoulders and turn the head to each side against resistance.

The twelfth cranial nerve (hypoglossal) supplies the muscles of the tongue. It is examined by having the child stick his tongue straight out. Deviation to either side should be noted. Strength of the tongue can be assessed by having the child push it against the inside of his cheek against resistance provided by the examiner's fingers. The tongue should also be examined for fasciculations and for evidence of its having been bitten.

The *motor examination* is presented in detail in Chapter 13. A few points will be highlighted here. The extent of examination will depend upon the particular problem the child is experiencing. Assessment includes several parts: posture, spontaneous movement, tone, muscle bulk, strength, and functional testing.

Posture refers to position of body parts at rest. For example, following right hemisphere brain injury, the left arm often will be flexed at the elbow, wrist, and fingers.

Spontaneous movement may be increased and random as in Sydenham chorea or diminished as in Hallervorden-Spatz disease.

Tone, the resistance of muscles to passive stretch, may be categorized as normal, hypertonic (increased), or hypotonic (decreased). Tone of the extremities is assessed by testing passive movements at the elbow, wrist, hip, knee, and ankle. Increased tone at the ankle may be signified by tightness of the heel cord or by clonus (repetitive jerking upon brisk dorsiflexion). Increased tone in children is usually spastic in nature, often with a clasp-knife quality. Other forms of hypertonia are paratonia, cogwheel rigidity, and gegenhalten (see Chapter 13).

Muscles should be inspected for evidence of wasting or enlargement (see Fig. 4–4). The pattern of involvement should be noted: proximal, affecting neck, shoulders, and thighs; distal, affecting hands and feet. Palpation of muscles should determine their consistency, e.g., "doughy" or hard. Myotonia, or sustained muscle contraction upon active effort or passive percussion, should be sought.

Testing of individual muscle groups is a relatively simple and brief procedure and should not be restricted to children with apparent or suspected

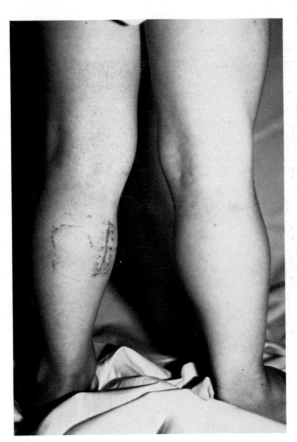

FIGURE 4–4. Enlarged calves due to pseudohypertrophied muscle.

motor difficulty. Testing should include the following: abduction of the arm at the shoulder, flexion and extension at the elbow, flexion and extension of the wrist, abduction of the fingers, hand grip, flexion of the hip upon the thigh, flexion and extension at the knee, and dorsiflexion at the ankle. Patterns of muscle weakness (proximal versus distal; left versus right) should be noted.

Muscle strength may be graded on a numerical basis (0–4). Normal strength is given a value of 4, whereas no movement at all—not even a flicker—is graded as 0. A score of 3 indicates that voluntary movement can be performed against resistance. A score of 1 indicates that some active movement can be carried out if the effects of gravity are eliminated. A score of 2 denotes that movement can be carried out against gravity but not resistance.

Functional muscle testing involves assessment of muscle groups in action. Activities to test proximal muscle function include deep knee bends, walking stairs two at a time, and arising to a stand from a sitting position on the floor. A Gowers sign, in which a seated child "climbs upon himself" to achieve a standing position, is evidence of proximal muscle weakness (see Fig. 4–5).

Examination of gait is an essential part of evaluating the motor system. Rhythmicity and fluidity of ambulation should be noted along with associated arm movements. Toe-walking, heel-walking, walking on the sides of

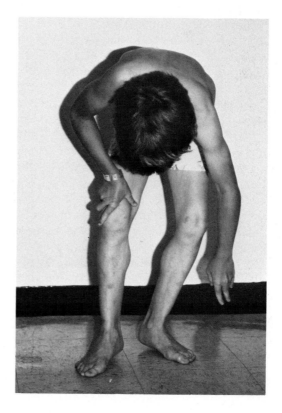

FIGURE 4–5. Boy with muscular dystrophy climbing upon himself to achieve standing position (Gowers sign).

the feet, and walking in tandem may bring out disturbances in gait or abnormalities of arm movement (such as posturing of one arm).

The *sensory examination* need not be exhaustive unless a specific sensory deficit is suspected. Under most circumstances, a screening examination that includes testing of perception of light touch, positional change, vibration, cold stimulation, and pinprick in all extremities will suffice.

Special sensory (higher cortical) functions include stereognosis, graphesthesia, right-left orientation, finger-naming, and visual-spatial ability (see Chapter 17). Stereognosis is the recognition of an object placed in one hand by manipulating it while the eyes are closed. Graphesthesia is the ability to identify a letter or number traced by the examiner's finger upon the child's palm. Finger-naming refers to the child's ability to identify and name fingers on his own hand and that of the examiner. Right-left orientation can be tested by requesting of the child, "Show me your right hand," "Place your right hand on your left knee," or "Touch my right hand." Visual-spatial ability can be assessed by asking the child to copy geometric figures, label maps, place pieces in formboards, and build standard constructions with one-inch cubes.

Testing of *coordination* routinely consists of several parts: finger-to-nose movements, rapid alternating movements, rhythmic tapping, and tandem gait. On finger-to-nose testing, the child is to touch alternately with the tip of his index finger the examiner's fingertip and the tip of his own nose. The task can be made more difficult if the examiner's finger is moved from one point to another.

Rapid alternating movements can be tested by having the seated child alternately slap the front and back of his hand against his thigh rapidly and repeatedly. Another means of assessing coordination involves the child's ability to reproduce rhythms tapped out by the examiner. Arms or legs may be tested in this manner.

Deep tendon *reflexes* should be elicited at the elbow (biceps, triceps), wrist (brachioradialis), knee (patella), and ankle. Reflexes are graded on a 0 to 4 basis with grades 2 and 3 generally considered normal. Reflexes that are graded as 0 (unelicitable) or 4 (clonic, or reduplicated) are nearly always abnormal. Deep tendon reflexes that are exaggerated on one side of the body or markedly increased in the legs as contrasted with the arms are also pathologic. In some normal persons, deep tendon reflexes are uniformly diminished (graded as 1) or, occasionally, unelicitable.

The Babinski sign, or extensor toe sign, is a pathologic reflex manifested by extension of the great toe (at times associated with fanning of the other toes) when the lateral surface of the sole is stroked firmly. A Babinski sign is abnormal except during the first year or so of life (until about the time the child begins to walk). The stimulus used to elicit the response should be mildly noxious: more than a tickle but less than a painful scrape that would necessitate withdrawal of the leg. A flexor response is normal.

Several other reflexes—suck, root, and grasp (palmar, plantar)—are normally present during the first three to four months of life. Their persistence suggests cerebral maldevelopment, their reappearance cerebral damage.

The *mental status examination* is an integral part of every pediatric examination. It consists of careful observation combined with more formal testing to assess the child's appearance, behavior, affect, content of speech, orientation, memory, attention, insight, judgment, abstraction, and intelligence. One or more of these elements may be sufficiently striking as to have been included in the general description as discussed earlier.

Speech and language are unique parameters of human functioning that are properly included as part of the mental status examination as well. The office assessment of speech and language function is presented in detail in Chapter 17. Its essential components are spontaneous speech, naming, repetition, comprehension, and written language. It is often worth recording a sample of the child's speech to document its structural complexity and vocabulary. More detailed assessment can be pursued as indicated.

Appearance refers to style and neatness of dress, grooming, and hygiene.

Behavior includes the degree of motor activity and cooperativeness. Is the child continually in motion, running around the room, or seated calmly in a chair? Is he easily engaged in conversation and testing, or is he negativistic and provocative?

Affect is the child's observed emotional state (e.g., anxious, relaxed, depressed, or happy). Affect should be distinguished from the feeling state of *emotion* and from *mood,* the pervasive and sustained emotional climate (see Chapter 6).

Content of speech can include delusions, hallucinations, illogicality, incoherence, or other evidence of a thought disorder. Delusions are false beliefs fixedly held. Hallucinations are perceptual experiences (e.g., visual, auditory, or tactile) without basis in external reality (see Chapter 5). More normally, speech will often contain information as to the child's interests, hopes, and fears.

Orientation refers to the child's knowledge of self, time, place, and circumstances of evaluation—why he or she has been brought for assessment.

Memory can be tested in several ways: immediate memory by the child's repetition of digits presented one second apart, short-term memory by having the child recall three or four objects or a short (one-paragraph) story after five to ten minutes, and long-term memory by the child's ability to remember details of a recent birthday or summer vacation (see Chapter 16).

Digit span is a measure of *attention* as well as of immediate memory. Attention can also be evaluated by having the child count backward from 100 by sevens or threes, recite the alphabet in reverse order, or write the numbers 1 through 100.

Insight refers to the child's perception of why he or she is being evaluated (also included earlier as part of orientation) and possible reasons for such difficulties.

Judgment is tested conventionally by the child's response to questions such as, "What would you do if you found a stamped, addressed letter on the sidewalk?" or "What would you do if you were in a movie theater and smelled smoke?" The answers to such questions depend in large part upon language skills and the child's perception of what the examiner would like to hear. As such, they reflect relatively little upon judgment as it pertains to everyday life, which involves the weighing of choices and the making of decisions.

Abstraction can be tested by interpretation of proverbs such as "A rolling stone gathers no moss," "Don't cry over spilled milk," or "A stitch in time saves nine." In younger children, conceptualization can be assessed by asking, "How are an orange and a baseball similar?" "What do a bird and an airplane have in common?" "How are a bicycle and a boat alike?"

Intelligence should be estimated as part of the mental status examination. Though formal psychometric testing is often required for the most accurate assessment, much can be learned about the child's intelligence through informal, semistructured conversation that explores the child's language, vocabulary, depth of knowledge, and logicality of thought. The draw-a-person test, scored by Goodenough-Harris standards, is a useful tool in assessing overall intelligence. Motorically impaired children or those with perceptual-motor dysfunction, however, will tend to do poorly on this test since it will give them falsely low scores. General principles in developmental assessment and an outline of development in infancy and early childhood were presented in Chapter 3.

INVESTIGATION

Investigation of the child with a behavioral or emotional problem may range from none at all to the most extensive studies. The number of tests available is almost limitless, and one should be guided as to the choice of tests by the following question: "Will the result of this investigation influence the management of this child?"

If the answer is "no," then the need for the test should be reevaluated. If the answer is "yes," other matters such as availability, time, discomfort, risk, and expense remain to be considered. For example, examination of cerebrospinal fluid is mandatory when meningitis is a clear possibility. But lumbar puncture is not justifiable as part of a child's investigation merely for the sake of "completeness." Since hypocalcemia is a readily treatable and specific cause for seizures, a blood test to check the calcium level is justified in the assessment of most children with a history of unexplained seizure. On the other hand, a computerized tomographic (CT) scan of the head is not justified in every child who has had a seizure since the likelihood of a result that would alter the child's management is small.

Though a test may not immediately or directly benefit the child, by helping to establish a specific diagnosis it may provide essential clarification for the parents and assist them in future family planning. For example, chromosome analysis of a mentally retarded child will not, itself, help that child; but the parents' willingness to have further children may depend upon the results of that test (if the disorder is associated with a recognizable chromosomal defect).

The hospitalized child usually will have a number of routine investigations. These generally will include a complete blood count (CBC), urinalysis, and tuberculin skin tests. Additional investigations will depend upon the nature of the problem or problems.

To maximize the amount of information gained through an investigation, careful planning is necessary. For example, when a lumbar puncture is to be performed and the presence of abnormal cells in the cerebrospinal fluid sought, the cytology laboratory should be notified in advance so that the specimen can be processed promptly. An extra tube of cerebrospinal fluid generally should be obtained and saved, for studies may need to be repeated or additional tests performed. Similarly, whatever blood is necessary for testing should be drawn at one time, if possible, in order to spare the child repeated venipunctures. Furthermore, if sedation for a CT scan, for example, is necessary, it may be best to schedule the child for an elective lumbar puncture immediately afterward. Table 4-2 lists some of the investigations that can be carried out involving blood, urine, and cerebrospinal fluid.

Radiologic investigation can be of great value in confirming or establishing a diagnosis. For example, plain skull x-rays may reveal splitting of cranial sutures with increased intracranial pressure, intracranial calcifications with toxoplasmosis or tuberous sclerosis, or a variety of fractures with trauma (see Chapters 11, 12, and 20) (see Fig. 4-6). Skeletal x-rays may disclose multiple fractures in the battered child or radiopaque epiphyseal lines with lead poisoning.

The CT scan has revolutionized neuroradiologic investigation (see Fig. 4-7). Intracranial mass lesions (such as tumors and hematomas), hydrocephalus, and dysplastic processes of brain are usually readily evident (Bachman *et al.*, 1977; Ferry, 1980). Pneumoencephalography, in which cerebrospinal fluid is withdrawn and replaced with air to permit visualization of intracranial structures, may still provide unique information, although the usefulness and availability of CT scanning have diminished greatly indications for its use. Cerebral arteriography remains a valuable measure pre-

TABLE 4-2. **Analysis of Body Fluids**

Blood	Sodium, potassium, chloride, bicarbonate, liver enzymes, ammonia, urea nitrogen, creatinine, glucose, calcium, magnesium, ceruloplasmin, copper, lead, anticonvulsant medication, erythrocyte sedimentation rate, connective tissue studies, alpha fetoprotein, pyruvic acid, lactic acid, amino acids, thyroxine, cortisol, toxic substances, lysosomal enzymes, chromosomes, antibody titers related to congenital infection (such as rubella, cytomegalic inclusion disease, toxoplasmosis)
Urine	Sugar, amino acids, organic acids, mucopolysaccharides, toxic substances, porphyrins, culture for cytomegalovirus and other viruses
Cerebrospinal fluid	White blood cells, red blood cells, protein, sugar, cultures, cytology for neoplastic cells, immunoglobulins, measles and rubella antibodies, treponemal antibodies

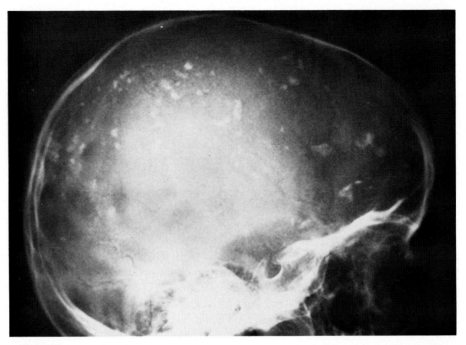

FIGURE 4–6. Plain radiograph of the skull showing scattered intracranial calcifications from congenital toxoplasmosis infection.

operatively, for example, with tumor, and in the evaluation of suspected vascular malformation or vasculitis.

Positron emission tomography (PET) of the brain, involving injection of radioisotopically labeled glucose for the study of regional metabolic activity, appears to be a diagnostic instrument of great promise (Ter-Pogossian *et al.*, 1980; Mazziotta *et al.*, 1981). Measurement of regional cerebral blood flow through inhalation of radioisotopically labeled gas is another neuroradiologic

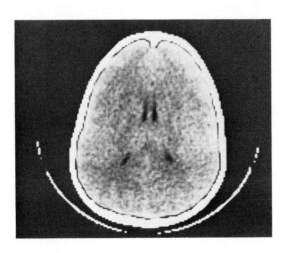

FIGURE 4–7. Normal plain computerized tomographic (CT) scan of the head.

investigation of incompletely explored clinical applicability (Lassen *et al.*, 1978).

Electroencephalography (EEG) is a valuable neurologic tool. Though it does not "tell all" about brain function, it can be definitively diagnostic (as in petit mal epilepsy), confirm a clinical diagnosis (e.g., of seizure disorder), help in localizing a pathologic process to a particular portion of brain, and suggest a category of brain dysfunction (for example, toxic-metabolic) (Lewis and Freeman, 1977).

Other electrophysiologic investigations include electromyography, nerve conduction studies, and evoked potential studies. Electromyography (EMG) involves insertion of a small, sharp recording needle directly into muscle. The pattern of electrical discharge upon insertion of the electrode, at rest, and with exertion is noted and compared with patterns seen in normal and pathologic states. Nerve conduction studies measure the velocity of an electrical impulse over a measured segment of nerve (see Chapter 8). Evoked potential studies involve noninvasive techniques to assess visual, auditory, and somesthetic pathways (Mizrahi and Dorfman, 1980). In studies of auditory-evoked potentials, for example, a click is produced and electrical wave forms from different parts of the auditory pathway (from end organ to cerebral cortex) recorded from scalp electrodes. Auditory-evoked potentials are especially useful in evaluating the young child with suspected hearing impairment. Visual-evoked responses are valuable in detecting interference in transmission of visual impulses characteristic of multiple sclerosis (see Chapter 8).

Biopsy may prove to be important in diagnosis. Valuable information may be derived from the examination of tissue (e.g., bone marrow, liver, skin fibroblasts, skeletal muscle, peripheral nerve, or brain) by histologic and histochemical methods, electron microscopy, and biochemical analyses (see Fig. 4–8). Lysosomal enzyme studies and electron microscopy of cultured skin fibroblasts have made brain biopsy only rarely necessary in the investigation of suspected metabolic disease of the nervous system.

Consultation itself may be considered a kind of investigation. Formal psychologic assessment will often be valuable (if not essential) in evaluating the child who is mentally retarded, emotionally disturbed, or otherwise behaviorally disordered. Psychiatric consultation can help to elucidate significant interpersonal dynamic issues that may contribute to or cause the problems in question and can provide recommendations as to treatment (particularly regarding psychotherapy and the use of psychoactive drugs). The genetic counselor can be of help both diagnostically and preventively by exploring family history in depth and by providing information as to the risk of having another affected child. The ophthalmologist can be of assistance in diagnosing many disorders, particularly when papilledema is suspected or when a neurodegenerative disease (such as Tay-Sachs disease, ceroid lipofuscinosis, and subacute sclerosing panencephalitis) is being considered.

The developmentally delayed child may benefit also from formal evaluation by a speech and language therapist, audiologist, physical therapist, or occupational therapist (who assesses fine motor and perceptual motor functions as well as skills of daily living). Such evaluation can be helpful not only

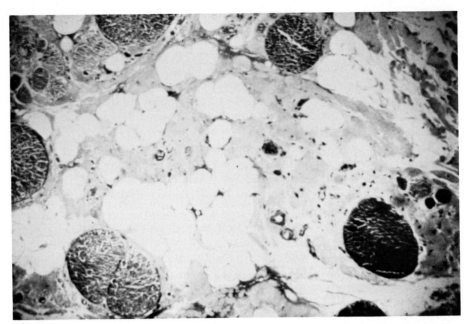

FIGURE 4–8. Muscle biopsy specimen in Duchenne muscular dystrophy showing marked variation in fiber size and infiltration with fat and fibrous tissue.

by characterizing the child's current level of function but also by establishing an individualized plan of remediation and follow-up assessment.

SUMMARY

The clinical diagnostic process consists of history, examination, and investigation. The history, by which the diagnosis is often established, begins with the chief complaint and traces it and associated symptoms from their onset to the present. The history also includes development, significant illnesses, hospitalizations, family history, personal profile, school history, and review of systems. History-taking is not merely information-gathering. It is the first step in the therapeutic process as well. Examination consists of four parts: general description, general physical examination, neurologic examination, and mental status examination. Investigation, if any, will depend upon the history and examination and the degree to which anticipated results might influence management. Consultation (psychologic, psychiatric, genetic, ophthalmologic) may extend the initial assessment. Through this process, the diagnosis is established as definitively as possible so that a comprehensive treatment plan can be made.

CITED REFERENCES

Bachman, D. S.; Hodges, F. J., III; and Freeman, J. M. Computerized axial tomography in neurologic disorders of children. *Pediatrics,* **59:** 352–63, 1977.
Ferry, P. C. Computed cranial tomography in children. *J. Pediatr.,* **96:** 961–67, 1980.

Lassen, N. A.; Ingvar, D. H.; and Skinhøj, E. Brain function and blood flow. *Sci. Am.,* **239:** 62–71, 188, October 1978.

Lewis, D. V., and Freeman, J. M. The electroencephalogram in pediatric practice: its use and abuse. *Pediatrics,* **60:** 324–30, 1977.

Mazziotta, J. C.; Phelps, M. E.; Miller, J.; and Kuhl, D. E. Tomographic mapping of human cerebral metabolism: normal unstimulated state. *Neurology* (New York), **31:** 503–16, 1981.

Mizrahi, E. M., and Dorfman, L. J. Sensory evoked potentials: clinical applications in pediatrics. *J. Pediatr.,* **97:** 1–10, 1980.

Ter-Pogossian, M. M.; Raichle, M. E.; and Sobel, B. E. Positron-emission tomography. *Sci. Am.,* **243:** 170–81, 210, October 1980.

ADDITIONAL READINGS

DeJong, R. N. *The Neurologic Examination,* 4th ed. Harper and Row, Publishers, New York, 1979.

DeMyer, W. *Technique of the Neurologic Examination,* 3rd ed. McGraw-Hill Book Company, New York, 1980.

Dodge, P. R. Neurologic history and examination. In *Pediatric Neurology,* 2nd ed. Farmer, T. W., ed. Harper and Row, Publishers, Hagerstown, Md., 1975, pp. 1–43.

Freeman, N. Children's drawings: cognitive aspects. *J. Child Psychol. Psychiatry,* **17:** 345–50, 1976.

Gordon, R.; Herman, G. T.; and Johnson, S. A. Image reconstruction from projections. *Sci. Am.,* **233:** 56–68, 138, October 1975.

Lewis, M. Child psychiatric consultation in pediatrics. *Pediatrics,* **62:** 359–64, 1978.

Paine, R. S., and Oppé, T. E. *Neurologic Examination of Children.* Wm. Heinemann, London, 1966.

Phelps, M. E.; Mazziotta, J. C.; Kuhl, D. E.; Nuwer, M.; Packwood, J.; Metter, J.; and Engel, J., Jr. Tomographic mapping of human cerebral metabolism: visual stimulation and deprivation. *Neurology* (New York), **31:** 517–29, 1981.

Simmons, J. E. *Psychiatric Examination of Children,* 2nd ed. Lea & Febiger, Philadelphia, 1974.

Strub, R. L., and Black, F. W. *The Mental Status Examination in Neurology.* F. A. Davis Co., Philadelphia, 1977.

Part Two

Major Clinical Problems

5 Autism, Schizophrenia, and Other Psychoses

Childhood psychosis is surely among the most difficult problems to confront a parent or a professional. Whether the problem is autism or schizophrenia, affected children usually appear physically normal, have developed normally for at least a time, and may even function normally (or better) in specific areas. These factors have stimulated, indeed goaded, persons coming in contact with such children into striving yet harder to find a key that might unlock the restricted, disordered personality and free the more normal child who seems to lie within.

The most recent decades have brought forth evidence for organic bases of, and contributions to, childhood psychoses. These data have added greatly to earlier developmental, psychosocial, and psychodynamic perspectives.

This chapter will look broadly at psychoses of childhood and adolescence with the primary focus upon infantile autism and childhood schizophrenia. Autism will be defined and differentiated from schizophrenia. Pertinent features of the clinical history and examination will be presented and the role of investigation explored. Causes of childhood psychosis and conditions that must be distinguished from it are discussed. Relevant anatomic, biochemical, and physiologic aspects will be presented. The following questions will be addressed specifically:

What is the definition of psychosis in childhood?

What is infantile autism?

Are autistic children schizophrenic?

How does infantile autism differ from autistic syndromes occurring in blind, deaf, or otherwise severely handicapped children?

In what ways do the brains of autistic children differ from those of normal children? What is the role of temporal lobe dysfunction?

What biochemical considerations are relevant to autism and schizophrenia?

Are all psychoses organically derived, or do some arise solely on a functional basis?

How may a behaviorally disturbed child with ''aphasia'' be distinguished from an autistic child?

What investigations are indicated in the diagnostic assessment of the child with autism? Schizophrenia?

What therapies will help the child with autism or schizophrenia?

Is institutionalization necessary or desirable?

What is the outcome in children with autism or schizophrenia?

AUTISM, SCHIZOPHRENIA, AND OTHER PSYCHOSES

DEFINITION

Childhood psychosis is a state in which impairment in behavior, relatedness, and communication leaves the child so disturbed and disordered that normal family, academic, and other social functions are impossible. The term *psychosis* is used to indicate both quantitatively and qualitatively the seriousness of the disturbance of behavior. It is strikingly abnormal at any age or stage of development.

The term *psychosis* must be used especially carefully with children, since it encompasses such different syndromes as *infantile autism* and *schizophrenia*. The diagnosis of infantile autism is based upon three major criteria: failure of normal speech and language development; gross and sustained impairment of interpersonal relationships; and onset of symptoms before 30 months of age. (Kanner, 1943; Creak *et al.*, 1964; Hauser *et al.*, 1975; *DSM-III*, 1980) (see Table 5–1).

Disturbance of speech and language development may be evident as failure to acquire speech. Several single words are expected to be used normally by 1 year of age and words in combination (phrases or short sentences) by 2 years. Other distortions of normal language development may take the form of echolalia, confusion of personal pronouns (as in the substitution of ''you'' for ''me''), and idiosyncratic use of words.

Interpersonal relationships are characterized by aloofness: lack of interest in and responsiveness to people. Kanner (1943) emphasized the disordered attachment by entitling his germinal paper ''Autistic Disturbances of Affective Contact.''

Onset before 30 months may be difficult to establish. Inexperienced or unobservant parents may have overlooked behavioral abnormalities for months. As a result, grandparents or neighbors may be primarily responsible for evaluation being sought.

Additional features that are frequently associated with infantile autism include pathologic preoccupation with particular objects without regard for

TABLE 5–1. **Essential Criteria for Diagnosis of Infantile Autism**

Failure of normal speech and language development
Gross and sustained impairment of interpersonal relationships
Onset of symptoms before 30 months of age

TABLE 5–2. **Behavioral Symptoms Frequently Accompanying Autism**

Pathologic preoccupation with objects (spinning or twirling objects)
Sustained resistance to change in environment (insistence upon sameness)
Distorted motility patterns (bizarre posturing, rocking, spinning)
Abnormal responses to perceptual stimuli (relative insensitivity to pain)
Excessive anxiety (provoked by commonplace phenomena) or lack of fear
Islands of normal or exceptional function

their usual functions (such as spinning or twirling objects); sustained resistance to change in the environment (associated with striving to maintain or restore sameness); distorted motility patterns (such as bizarre posturing, rocking, or spinning); abnormal responses to perceptual stimuli (such as relative insensitivity to pain); excessive anxiety (provoked by commonplace phenomena) or, conversely, inappropriate lack of fear; and "islands" of normal or exceptional function (intellectual or otherwise) against a background of serious retardation (see Table 5–2).

Because of its dissimilarity to psychotic disorders of later life, the *DSM-III* (1980) has classified infantile autism as a *pervasive developmental disorder* rather than a psychosis. The term *psychosis* is retained here as an indication of the severity of deviation from normal behavior as compared with other behavior disorders. Syndromes sharing some but not all features of infantile autism (e.g., beginning after 30 months of age) have been classified as *childhood onset pervasive developmental disorder* and *atypical pervasive developmental disorder*.

Schizophrenia typically has its onset in adolescence or early adulthood, but it may be encountered in the younger school-age child. The essential features of schizophrenia in childhood are (1) duration of at least six months; (2) deterioration from a previous level of functioning; and (3) characteristic disturbances of thought, perception, affect, volition, sense of self, relatedness, and motor activity (*DSM*-III, 1980). For the diagnosis of schizophrenia to be made, an associated or antecedent affective disorder must be absent (see Table 5–3). When symptoms have lasted continuously for less than six months, *schizophreniform psychosis* or *brief reactive psychosis* (with symptoms of less than two weeks) may be more appropriate diagnoses than schizophrenia.

Deterioration from a previous level of functioning in childhood will often take the form of worsened school performance. An adolescent employed on a part-time basis might, in addition, show impaired work performance.

TABLE 5–3. **Essential Criteria for Diagnosis of Schizophrenia**

Characteristic disturbances of thought, perception, affect, volition, sense of self, relatedness, and motor activity
Deterioration from a previous level of functioning
Duration of six months or longer
No associated or antecedent affective disorder

Characteristic disturbances in thinking may affect both the form and the content of thought. The commonest example of formal thought disorder is loosening of associations (or "derailment"). With loosening of associations, ideas slip off one track onto another that may be clearly but obliquely related or onto one that is completely unrelated. Other examples of formal thought disorder are incoherence (which can result from extreme loosening of associations) and neologisms ("new words").

Disturbances in content of thought are often prominent in schizophrenia. They usually take the form of *delusions,* which are false beliefs that are fixedly held. Characteristic delusions are ideas of reference (in which environmental events take on personal significance) and persecutory delusions (in which it is believed that persons are spying on, spreading false rumors about, or planning harm toward the individual). Thought broadcasting, thought insertion, and thought control are other characteristic delusions. Somatic, grandiose, or religious delusions as well as extreme illogicality are other manifestations of disturbance in content of thought.

Hallucinations are distortions in perception in which subjective sensory perceptions in one or more modalities (sound, sight, touch, smell, or taste) are experienced without basis in objective reality. Typical hallucinations are hearing voices, seeing persons, or feeling bugs crawling upon or within the skin. *Illusions,* by contrast, are false perceptions of objects or events that do exist or have occurred.

Disturbance of sense of self (loss of ego boundaries) often occurs as part of a schizophrenic syndrome. Disturbance in relationship to the external world may take the form of withdrawal. Such withdrawal in severe form has been termed *autism.* Hence the link (more apparent than real) between schizophrenia and infantile autism has been implied, often the source of confusion and misunderstanding.

Motor behavior may be disturbed in several ways in schizophrenic disorders. These include marked diminution in reactivity (when extreme, taking the form of catatonic stupor), maintenance of rigid posture (as with catatonic waxy inflexibility), or purposeless and stereotyped behavior (as with catatonic excitement). The effects of prescribed or illicitly taken drugs must always be considered in assessing motor disturbance in a person with schizophrenic psychosis. With phenothiazines, for example, effects include dystonia, akathisia, and tardive dyskinesia (see Chapter 13).

The differences between childhood schizophrenia and infantile autism are summarized Table 5–4 (Kolvin *et al.,* 1971; Rutter, 1977; Schopler and Dalldorf, 1980). Schizophrenia characteristically pursues an episodic course with remissions and relapses. Infantile autism, on the other hand, usually takes a stable or very slowly improving course. Another important difference is that delusions or hallucinations are typical in schizophrenia but occur only rarely among autistic persons even in childhood.

DIAGNOSIS

In this section on diagnosis, the clinical process will be described first as it pertains to autism, then to schizophrenia.

Clinical Process. *History.* The *autistic child* may be brought to profes-

TABLE 5–4. **Distinctions Between Infantile Autism and Schizophrenia**

Clinical Aspect	Autism	Schizophrenia
Onset	Before $2\frac{1}{2}$ years	Later than 7 years
Sex preponderance	Male	None
Family history	Usually not	Sometimes
Course	Usually stable	Often relapsing, remitting
Delusions and hallucinations	Rare	Frequent
Intellectual subnormalcy	Usual	Uncommon
Seizures	Not uncommon	Rare
Pre- or perinatal difficulties	Frequent	Infrequent
Nonrighthandedness	Frequent	Infrequent

sional attention for a number of reasons. "He's three years old and still not talking." "She shrieks whenever anything in her daily routine is changed." "He can spend literally hours twirling a hair between his fingers in front of his eyes."

In assessing the child with autistic features of behavior, the presence or absence of the major criteria for diagnosis of autism as well as characteristic associated features should be noted. Specific mention should be made of language development, interpersonal relationships, and age of onset.

Language development of the autistic child can be abnormal in several ways. Speech delay is common, with lack of single words by two years or of word combinations by three years. Idiosyncratic, overly concrete usage of words may occur. For example, the word "yes" may mean quite specifically and exclusively, "Pick me up and carry me on your shoulders." Reversal of pronouns ("you" instead of "me") and echolalia are also characteristic. The abnormality of these speech and language behaviors lies not so much in their occurrence as in the persistence of these immature patterns.

Impaired interpersonal relationships may have become evident in several ways (Kanner, 1943; Rutter, 1977). Anticipatory posturing may have been absent in the two- to four-month-old infant when the parents reached over to pick up the child. Reaction to strangers may have been diminished or may never have developed. Autistic children are unlikely to wave "bye-bye," play "peek-a-boo," or imitate housework. Imaginative play, such as manipulating dolls and cars, is generally lacking. Play is characteristically stereotyped and repetitive. Autistic children do not greet their parents' return from work or from shopping in a typical fashion, nor do they seek solace from parents if injured or upset. In guiding an adult to a desired object, the child may take the person by the wrist as if the arm were not attached to a body. An autistic child may point with the whole hand rather than with the extended index finger.

As noted above, recognition of onset of abnormal behavior before $2\frac{1}{2}$ years of age will depend upon the parents' knowledge of normal development in early childhood and their perception of their own child's behavior as compared with these norms. Preschool screening programs often provide the stimulus for further evaluation based upon recognition of speech delay or bizarre behavior.

Associated features might include pathologic preoccupation with objects, sustained resistance to environmental change, distorted motility patterns (such as spinning, rocking, or head banging), abnormal responses to perceptual stimuli, excessive anxiety, and overall developmental retardation with preserved islands of normalcy or superior functioning.

Developmental history should include past milestones as well as current level of function in various areas (speech and language, gross and fine motor, social and adaptive skills). The tempo of development should be noted (see Chapter 8). This developmental focus is important in differentiating infantile autism from syndromes of mental retardation, specific language disability, deafness, and disintegrative psychosis (see DIFFERENTIAL DIAGNOSIS).

Questions might include the following: When did you first suspect that your child might not be developing normally? Has your child acquired any skills that later have been lost? Are there any things that your child does especially well—better than others his age? What does he do at age level? How does he react to sounds? Does he make his wants known clearly even without words?

The past history should include standard inquiry as to pregnancy and birth. Specific information should be sought as to maternal exposure to rubella, indications of fetal distress (such as meconium-stained amniotic fluid, severe vaginal bleeding, or emergency cesarean section), neonatal resuscitation, or prolonged nursery stay. Head trauma, seizures, and hospitalizations should also be noted. Exclusive use of one hand prior to three or four years of age suggests damage or dysfunction of the ipsilateral cerebral hemisphere.

Social history should note important separations or other major events in the child's life. These may include prolonged or repeated hospitalizations (of mother or child), multiple changes of primary caretaker, or terrifying events.

Schizophrenia with onset in childhood (especially adolescence) characteristically presents with deterioration in a previous level of functioning. This change may take the form of decline in school achievement, withdrawal from usual friends, dropping out of athletics, or worsening of job performance.

Delusions may take several forms in the schizophrenic child. With delusions of thought control, an outside party or force is felt to influence completely the person's mind. With thought broadcasting, the person's thoughts are considered to be propagated directly to the external environment. Delusions may be somatic, as with the fixed belief that "my head is dented in like a ping-pong ball."

Hallucinations are not likely to be mentioned spontaneously by the child. Careful and delicate questioning is usually required to establish their occurrence, although sometimes the examiner may observe the child to be hallucinating. Rather than an abrupt and possibly frightening inquiry ("Have you been hearing voices?"), a gentler approach is preferable. Acknowledging the common experience of hearing music and conversations in one's imagination, the interviewer can ask about auditory, visual, or other hallucinations. An unhurried approach to this portion of the interview is important, for the child's impulse in responding to such questions will usually be denial. A pause or look into the distance may suggest that the child is recalling a hallucinatory experience.

Further characterization of the hallucinations should be undertaken. Auditory hallucinations may be threatening or controlling. They may involve a running commentary on the person's activities. Such hallucinations may direct the child to hurt himself or others. Visual hallucinations can be highly structured (involving people, for example) or relatively amorphous (e.g., consisting of sparkling lights or patterned displays). Olfactory hallucinations may be readily identifiable (for example, the smell of burning rubber) or just indescribably bad.

The personality and social adjustment of the child (or adolescent) prior to onset of psychotic symptoms should be explored. The tendency for withdrawal should be noted. Important life events such as a family move, death of a relative, or change in school should be sought. The child's reactions to such events should be clarified. The child's maturational stage with regard to puberty should also be noted.

Review of systems in the schizophrenic child should include questioning as to headaches, visual disturbance, personality change, coordinational problems, depression, or drug use.

Family history of the psychotic child, whether autistic or schizophrenic, may provide a clue as to a genetically determined metabolic basis for the disorder. This group of disorders includes Wilson disease (hepatolenticular degeneration), homocystinuria, and metachromatic leukodystrophy. These disorders are all autosomal recessive in inheritance; hence, the chance of occurrence is especially high when parents are consanguineous.

When genetic or metabolic disorder is being considered, construction of a formal family pedigree may be of great value in identifying affected persons who might otherwise have been overlooked. Inquiry should include the occurrence of language disorder or mental retardation in the family of the autistic child. In assessing the schizophrenic child, questioning should include asking whether mental illness has occurred in family members and whether any persons have had psychiatric hospitalization, received electroconvulsive therapy, been under the care of a psychiatrist, or taken psychoactive medication.

Examination. The *general description* should tell how the psychotic child strikes the observer. Aloof? Bizarre? Actively hallucinating? Frightened? Frightening? Depressed? Catatonic? The child's anxiety at being in unusual surroundings with strange people may make his behavior upon first impression seem particularly disturbed or unusual. Hence the examiner should not rely too heavily upon this first impression but should observe and record the process of behavior and interaction as it evolves during the interview and examination.

The *general physical examination* of the child with *infantile autism* is likely to be essentially normal, although an increase in the number of minor physical anomalies has been reported among autistic children as compared with siblings and unrelated control groups (Campbell *et al.*, 1978). These anomalies include two or more hair whorls, epicanthal folds, low-set ears, adherent ear lobes, single transverse palmar creases, and partial syndactyly of the toes. Macrocephaly has occasionally been noted; its significance is also obscure (Hauser *et al.*, 1975).

The *general physical examination* of the child with a *schizophrenic syndrome* should seek evidence of organic psychosis. Such a clinical picture might be produced by metabolic disorder (hypo- or hyperthyroidism), drug ingestion (amphetamines, hallucinogens), or multisystem disease (adrenoleukodystrophy, Wilson disease, systemic lupus erythematosus).

The pulse rate may be increased with hyperthyroidism, amphetamine use, or marijuana use. The skin may show evidence of drug ingestion (needle tracks, abscesses), adrenoleukodystrophy (pigmentation of gums and areolae), or systemic lupus erythematosus (a reddened "butterfly" eruption). The skin may be warm and moist with hyperthyroidism, dry and roughened with hypothyroidism. Eye examination may disclose a greenish-brown discoloration around the cornea (Kayser-Fleischer ring) or scleral icterus with Wilson disease (hepatolenticular degeneration).

The *neurologic examination* of the child with *autism* should include particular attention to speech and language functions, hearing ability, motor activities, and the possible occurrence of seizures.

Whereas the general examination of the autistic child is often (if not usually) normal, the neurologic examination will often be abnormal. For example, five of the eighteen patients reported by Hauser and colleagues (1975) had focal neurologic findings. These included extensor plantar responses, hyperreflexia, and visual neglect. Eight children were left-handed and three had not established hand preference.

Damasio and Maurer (1978) described frequent extrapyramidal findings (dystonia, dyskinesia, and choreoathetosis) among autistic children. They also have called attention to facial asymmetry occurring with affective display (such as smiling or crying) or with speaking.

In evaluating the autistic child, the examiner should pay particular attention to speech and language function (see Chapter 17). Is speech produced spontaneously or only by echoing? What is the character of spontaneous speech: words, phrases, sentences, repetitive jingles, gibberish, or noises such as clicking? Is articulation clear? Is musicality (rhythm and melody) of speech normal? Do words have overly concrete or idiosyncratic meanings? Are the pronouns "I" and "you" used correctly, or are they reversed? Does the child communicate by gesture? Is comprehension impaired as well as expression? Samples of the child's speech should be written down verbatim or portions tape-recorded.

The language of a *schizophrenic child* may provide evidence for disordered thinking. Words may be made up, that is, neologisms. Sentences may have no apparent relationship to one another except their sounds. For example, one sentence may end with "Mars and Venus (venous)" and the next one begin with "Blood . . ." Such "clang" associations are a form of derailment, in which ideas slip off one track onto another that is loosely associated.

The ophthalmologic part of the neurologic examination of the psychotic child should include particular attention to the optic fundi. Papilledema may occur secondary to brain tumor or other mass lesion giving rise to increased intracranial pressure. Headache, typically associated with increased intra-cranial pressure, need not be a prominent symptom in childhood or adolescence (see Case 6–4). Macular changes (particularly a cherry red spot) or pigmentary changes of the retina (retinitis pigmentosa) suggest degenerative neurologic disease (see Chapter 8).

Focal neurologic findings in the psychotic child (such as unilateral hyper-reflexia or weakness) indicate structural involvement of the central nervous system. Whether or not such findings contribute to the psychotic process, they generally merit careful further investigation.

The *mental status examination* is the key to the clinical diagnosis of all childhood psychoses, whether infantile autism, schizophrenia, or other psychosis. Observation of behavior, with minimal interference by the examiner, is the starting point (Bartak and Rutter, 1976; Freeman *et al.*, 1981). Indeed, the mental status examination begins the moment the examiner meets the child and usually overlaps in part with the general description. How does the child react to the circumstances of examination? Is he aloof, withdrawn, hallucinating? What spontaneous activity is he engaged in? Twirling a hair in front of his eyes? Spinning a coin endlessly?

Estimation of overall intelligence should be made, although formal psychometric assessment is usually indicated (*always* in the initial assessment of the autistic child). Intelligence can be estimated by having the child draw a picture of a person with the drawing scored according to Goodenough-Harris norms. Drawing by autistic children may be primitive, reflecting mental retardation, or unusually rich and detailed, constituting an "island of excellence" (see below). The drawings of schizophrenic children may also be rich in detail and often have a bizarre quality.

A pitfall in the use of such drawings can occur in the child with significant motor or perceptual-motor dysfunction. Such impairments can render estimates of intelligence falsely low. Conversely, excessive detail may render the estimate falsely high.

Isolated areas of normal or superior intellectual function are hallmarks of infantile autism. Remarkable mathematic or mnemonic feats among otherwise retarded abilities define idiots savants, most of whom appear to be autistic (Goodman, 1972; Brink, 1980) (see Case 5-1).

Mental status examination should also include testing of orientation, memory, concentration, appearance, affect, and content of speech and language.

Orientation can be assessed in the younger child by asking him to identify parents, doctor, or nurse. The child should be asked why he or she has been brought for evaluation. Standard questions as to knowledge of time and place may not be applicable. In the older child, apparent disorientation (that is, faulty responses to such questions) may be due to confusional state, psychosis, negativism, or a variety of other causes such as hearing impairment or language disorder.

Memory, attention, and concentration are interrelated. Immediate memory, tested by recall of digits presented one second apart, depends upon attention. Short-term memory can be assessed by the child's recall of three or four objects after five to ten minutes. Long-term memory can be examined

CASE 5–1: AUTISTIC SYNDROME IN A 17-YEAR-OLD IDIOT SAVANT (CALENDAR CALCULATOR)

S.N. was the product of a full-term pregnancy complicated only by excessive weight gain. Delivery was unremarkable. The first year of life was described as normal. Language at 2 years consisted of a few single words ("mama," "dada," and "cookie"). Between 2 and 4 years, little speech development occurred. At 4 years, expressive speech was telegraphic. Comprehension was markedly impaired. He referred to himself in the third person. At 5 years, he spent hours reading telephone books and calendars. At 6 years, he was hyperactive, avoidant of human contact, and preoccupied with lights. At 9 years, he continued to be extremely distractable, manifested poor eye contact, and was echolalic.

At 11 years, he was a well-formed child who frequently interjected irrelevant words such as "college" and "grandma" into the conversation and comments such as "The rascal is almost dead." When asked to draw a diamond, he responded, "Club . . . spade." He recalled the examiner's telephone number 45 minutes after hearing it once. Mental arithmetic was unusually good (e.g., multiplication of two-digit numbers). Given a date of the year (e.g., July 20, 1974), he correctly provided the day of the week in 18 of 20 instances. Elemental neurologic examination was normal.

At 15 years, behavior was more impulsive and negativistic. He recalled the examiner's telephone number from four years previously. At 17 years, mental multiplication of two three-digit numbers was carried out with ease. He calculated rapidly and accurately the day of the week of any date (past or future) in the twentieth century. Behavior remained hyperkinetic and attention span limited. Full-scale intelligence on the WAIS was 66 (verbal 66, performance 70). Speech and language function was at the 5-year level.

Comment. This adolescent appeared to have an atypical autistic syndrome. His language function was not definitely abnormal until 4 years of age, although over the next two years he manifested autistic preoccupation with things rather than people, echolalia, and hyperkinesis.

This mentally retarded boy with highly developed skills in circumscribed areas (memory, mental arithmetic, and calendar calculation) can be termed an idiot savant. Such persons, otherwise retarded, may have unusual musical talent, artistic ability, or mathematical skills. A review of reported cases of idiots savants has suggested that most such persons are autistic (Adams *et al.*, 1980). Their unusual skill constitutes an "island" of normal or above-average performance sometimes seen in autism, though not often occurring as strikingly as in this boy. Adams and colleagues have further called attention to the exaggerated ability of idiots savants to concentrate in restricted areas as contrasted with the distractability that otherwise characterizes their behavior.

by questions about birthdays, holidays, or other past events. Concentration can be assessed by having the child count backward from 100 by serial subtraction of threes or sevens.

Appearance will be noteworthy if clothing is bizarre or grooming unkempt. Affect is characteristically flat or bland in autism and childhood schizophrenia. Among autistic children, anxiety may be provoked by relatively trivial circumstances. Abnormalities in content of speech and language may be manifested as illogicality, incoherence, delusions, or hallucinations.

Investigation. A number of investigations and consultations should be considered in the evaluation of the *autistic child*. Formal psychologic testing is essential. Optimally, it should be carried out by a person skilled in assessment of language-impaired and behaviorally disturbed children. Because speech and language disturbance is so prominent in children with autistic syndromes (and because autistic behaviors are frequently encountered among children with a variety of speech and language disorders), formal audiologic testing and speech and language assessment should also be undertaken. Occupational therapy evaluation will provide further information as to skills in activities of daily living. Psychiatric consultation can provide additional information as to emotional and psychosocial aspects and suggestions as to management, including use of psychoactive drugs.

Electroencephalography (in the awake and sleep states) is also generally indicated among autistic children because of the frequency of EEG abnormalities and frank clinical seizures. If the standard EEG tracing has not been revealing and a temporal lobe seizure focus is strongly suspected, a recording with nasopharyngeal leads should be obtained.

Other investigations will depend upon the particular child's clinical picture. With mental retardation, blood studies of chromosomes, amino acids, thyroid hormone, viral antibodies, and lead level may be indicated (see Chapter 18). With a clinical course of behavioral regression, electroencephalogram, lysosomal enzyme determination, and examination of cerebrospinal fluid may be indicated (see Chapter 8).

Plain skull x-rays are rarely valuable in evaluating the autistic child, so they are not indicated routinely. If the head is unusually large or small or if a specific disorder such as tuberous sclerosis is suspected, however, then they should be obtained. Nor is the CT scan indicated on a routine basis because of the frequent need for sedation and the desirability of minimizing radiation exposure. Symptoms and signs of increased intracranial pressure, focal neurologic deficit, or degenerative disorder of the central nervous system would justify a cranial CT scan. CT scanning has rendered pneumoencephalography (PEG) virtually obsolete in the evaluation of an autistic child. PEG should be carried out only when adequate definition of brain structure cannot be achieved by computerized tomography (as may occur with tumors of the third ventricle or temporal lobe) or when a CT scanner is unavailable and other imaging modalities such as arteriography are not appropriate.

With investigation of the autistic child as with any other person, the main criterion for carrying out a study should be, "Would the outcome of this investigation significantly alter the management of the patient?" If the answer is "No" regardless of the result, the need for the investigation should be reconsidered.

Investigation of the child or adolescent with *schizophrenia* or *other psychosis* is directed toward identification of remediable organic causes and elucidation of the basis (or bases) for the disorder. Urine and blood should be analyzed for drugs or other toxic substances (such as lead). Serum glucose level should be measured as well as electrolytes (including calcium and phosphorus), blood urea nitrogen, and thyroxine. If the clinical picture suggests adrenoleukodystrophy, serum cortisol values should be obtained and tests of adrenocortical function carried out. Erythrocyte sedimentation rate and connective tissue studies should be obtained if clinically indicated. When Wilson disease (hepatolenticular degeneration) is being considered, liver function studies (including SGOT, LDH, alkaline phospha-

CASE 5–2: SENSORY DISTURBANCE, DEPRESSION, AND PSYCHOSIS IN A 17-YEAR-OLD GIRL WITH MULTIPLE SCLEROSIS

At the age of 17 years, C.B. complained of a poorly defined "wet" feeling around her lips unassociated with saliva or other liquid. She also described numbness in her left leg and felt that her eyelids were drooping. She lost interest in school and in being with her friends. Nine months after onset of symptoms, she became despondent and was hospitalized with what was described as a "severe depressive catatonic disorder." She was treated with thioridazine (Mellaril), chlorpromazine (Thorazine), and lithium without improvement. Lethargy persisted despite discontinuation of all medication. She became comatose and severely dehydrated, requiring hospitalization.

Neurologic examination revealed a left hemiparesis and bilateral Babinski responses. EEG showed right hemisphere slowing. CT scan and cerebral arteriogram were normal. Cerebrospinal fluid examination showed 12 lymphocytes. Protein level was 56 mg/dl. Dexamethasone was begun, and within 48 hours her mental state had improved. Repeat cerebrospinal fluid examination showed persistent lymphocytosis and elevated protein content. A repeat arteriogram and a pneumoencephalogram indicated a posterior fossa mass. Upon exploratory surgery, only a small cyst of the cerebellum was found.

Over the next three years, she had episodic disturbances of mental function. These have included severe memory impairment and frank psychosis. During one episode in the hospital, she urinated in other patients' beds, smeared lipstick on her face, and sucked on a baby bottle. Treatment with prednisone and haloperidol was associated with a return of normal mental state.

Neurologic examination at the time of one psychotic episode disclosed a swinging flashlight sign (*vide infra*) on the left. On sensory testing, she had patches of decreased touch and pain sensation in all extremities. Deep ten-

tase, and bilirubin) and serum ceruloplasmin levels should be obtained. Slit-lamp examination of the cornea should also be carried out if Wilson disease is suspected. With possible metachromatic leukodystrophy of late onset, arylsulfatase A (a lysosomal enzyme) should be measured.

Examination of cerebrospinal fluid (CSF) should be performed if central nervous system infection (meningitis or encephalitis) is suspected. Appropriate blood samples should also be drawn for viral studies (such as herpes, rubella, and measles antibody levels in acute and convalescent stages of the clinical course). Cerebrospinal fluid immunoglobulin G should be measured when multiple sclerosis, subacute sclerosing panencephalitis, and late rubella panencephalitis are being considered. Visual evoked responses are valuable in assessment of demyelinating diseases such as multiple sclerosis (see Case 5–2).

don reflexes were brisk throughout with an extensor plantar response bilaterally. Tandem gait was ataxic. Follow-up CT scan showed prominent interhemispheric fissure and cortical sulci, evidence of cerebral atrophy. Repeat psychologic testing indicated that significant loss of intellectual function had occurred over the three years since onset of illness.

Comment. The diagnosis of multiple sclerosis is ultimately a clinical one. No single laboratory test establishes the diagnosis with certainty. During relapses, immunoglobulin G (gamma globulin) content of cerebrospinal fluid tends to become elevated to 10 per cent of the total protein content or greater. This test is not, however, definitively diagnostic.

The diagnosis of multiple sclerosis is based upon demonstration of neurologic lesions distributed in place (within the central nervous system) and in time. This young woman's initial symptoms were typical of multiple sclerosis—subjective, transient, and easily mistaken as "nerves" or hysteria. Later clues to diagnosis were objective neurologic findings: a left hemiparesis, bilateral Babinski responses, and an abnormal pupillary response to light.

The swinging flashlight sign implies an afferent defect of the optic nerve. In bringing the flashlight from the "good" eye to the "bad" one (in this case, from the right to the left), the left pupil—which had become smaller because of the consensual light reflex—became larger upon direct exposure to light. The basis for this pupillary escape was demyelination of optic nerve fibers connecting the light-sensitive rods and cones to mesencephalic nuclei mediating pupillary light responses.

The issue of mental changes with multiple sclerosis remains difficult. It appears that changes in alertness, attentiveness, and memory can occur acutely with multiple sclerosis. In some instances the disorder can be associated with loss of intellectual function. In this case, relapses of multiple sclerosis were associated with depressive and psychotic symptoms. This case underscores the importance of approaching apparent "psychiatric disease" with an open mind and examining the course of symptoms over time.

. Electroencephalography should be performed if metabolic encephalopathy, status epilepticus (petit mal or psychomotor), encephalitis, or degenerative disorder is suspected. Computerized tomographic (CT) scan will be of importance in excluding temporal lobe or other cerebral mass or malformation (see Case 5–3).

Psychologic testing—projective as well as psychometric—is valuable in elucidating personality organization, areas of psychopathology, and current levels of intellectual function. Psychometric testing carried out at intervals over several years may reflect a trend of intellectual deterioration that suggests or defines a degenerative neurologic disorder (see Chapter 8).

As with the autistic child, psychiatric assessment can provide important psychosocial and psychodynamic data as well as psychopharmacologic and other treatment recommendations.

Since many, if not most, children who develop psychosis in childhood have had preexisting periods of normal development, the question of degenerative disease of the central nervous system often (appropriately) arises.

CASE 5–3: RECURRENT DEPERSONALIZATION AND AUDITORY HALLUCINOSIS IN A 17-YEAR-OLD GIRL

K.S. was evaluated because of "unusual feelings" she had experienced for two months. She described the sensation as "not knowing who I am or where I am" and said that she felt as if she were in a dream. She acknowledged occasional auditory hallucinations. They were accusatory in nature and consisted of her father yelling at her. She was observed to be quiet and fearful at such times. Past history of pregnancy, birth, and development was unremarkable. School performance had been above average but had declined during the previous two years. She denied drug use.

On examination, she was an intelligent, articulate adolescent who spoke readily of her difficulties. She did not appear to be hallucinating. General physical examination, including visualization of the optic fundi, was normal. Elemental neurologic examination was unremarkable. Investigation included electroencephalography, which showed paroxysmal temporal lobe discharges during sleep. Skull x-rays and brain scan were normal.

Comment. The dreamy, unreal quality that this adolescent girl described suggested temporal lobe dysfunction. The episodic nature of the disturbance implicated seizure or migraine. Migraine was rendered unlikely because of the absence of characteristic vascular headaches and the negative family history. The lack of stereotypy (that is, the variability of the episodes), the absence of behavioral automatisms, and the lack of a confusional state following the episodes argued against seizure. Seizures were not excluded completely, however, for those of temporal lobe origin may be manifested by only an alteration in perception or mood, with little or no other change in mental state.

Other possibilities that merited consideration in this case were illicit use of drugs, affective disorder, and incipient psychosis.

TABLE 5–5. **Differential Diagnosis of Autism**

Deafness
Severe developmental language disturbance
Psychotoxic disorder
Disintegrative psychosis
Childhood schizophrenia
Mental retardation without autism

The evaluation of the child with a syndrome of behavioral regression is presented in Chapter 8.

Differential Diagnosis. In the evaluation of children with infantile autism, schizophrenia, or other psychoses of childhood, several conditions should be borne in mind (see Tables 5–5 and 5–6).

Mental retardation without associated autistic features of behavior should be distinguished from syndromes of autism. Autistic behavior is frequently seen in persons with mental retardation, however, and mental retardation is a usual accompaniment of infantile autism.

Deafness may result in profound language impairment and severe behavioral disturbance. Thus, autism is suggested while the root cause, severe hearing deficit, can be overlooked. Children with congenital deafness typically will have normal language development (cooing and babbling) until 6 to 7 months. Over the next 3 months, however, development ceases and loss of verbal skills ensues.

Aphasia can be a problematic concept in childhood. As used classically in the neurologic sense, aphasia refers to loss of previously acquired, linguistically correct speech. Such loss may occur following head injury, brain tumor, or stroke, for example. The degree of recovery of language function is variable. It may be excellent, or major deficits may persist.

In childhood, significant disturbances in speech and language function (expressive and/or receptive) can occur along with normal development in other spheres of activity such as gross and fine motor development. Such language disturbances may suggest aphasic language disturbances in adults. When children with these aphasic-like language problems develop secondary behavioral disturbances (such as hyperkinesis, tantrums, and impaired interactions), differentiation from autism may be difficult (Sahlmann, 1969).

TABLE 5–6. **Differential Diagnosis of Childhood Schizophrenia**

Night terror
Acute overwhelming anxiety (panic)
Depression
Migraine
Imaginary companions
Normal hallucinations
Schizophreniform or brief reactive psychosis
Drug-related or other organic psychosis

The spontaneous use of gestures for communication may help distinguish "aphasic" from autistic children.

The line between the child with a developmental disorder of speech and language associated with severe behavioral disturbance and a child with infantile autism may be a fine one. In some instances, the two may not be differentiable.

Psychotoxic disorders, such as described by Spitz (1965), include behaviors that are so aberrant that affected children may be considered psychotic. The coprophagia syndrome, for example, which appears to be a severe depressive reaction to emotional deprivation in infancy, involves detached behavior and coprophagia, or the eating of feces.

Degenerative disorders may be associated with a syndrome of disintegrative psychosis suggestive of infantile autism. The clinical course of disintegrative psychosis is marked by behavioral regression—particularly dementia, or loss of intellectual function—and behavioral disturbances of psychotic proportions (Rivinus *et al.,* 1975; Corbett *et al.,* 1977; Evans-Jones and Rosenbloom, 1978).

In considering other psychoses of childhood, one is essentially dealing with *childhood schizophrenia.* Cardinal features of these schizophrenic disorders are hallucinations, delusions, disturbances of thought and affect, and motor abnormalities. These may occur on an unknown basis or secondary to drug effects, among other causes considered below.

Several conditions should be borne in mind in the diagnostic approach to the child with schizophrenia or other psychosis: night terrors, panic attacks, depression, migraine, and imaginary companions.

The *night terror* is a sleep disturbance so dramatic and unsettling for parents that questions of psychosis frequently arise. It is discussed in detail in Chapter 9. The night terror is a paniclike state associated with incomplete arousal. One to two hours after falling asleep, children with night terrors scream as if being chased or attacked, run wildly through the home, fail to recognize their parents, and have no recall of the disturbance the following morning. Nocturnal seizures, toxic delirium, and nightmares are to be differentiated from night terrors.

Acute overwhelming anxiety, a state of panic, may be so severe and disorganizing that acute psychosis is suggested. Panic may result from purely situational events or may occur with use of psychoactive drugs. With LSD, for example, panic may result because the person fears losing his mind (see Chapter 19).

Depression may also suggest psychosis with its associated retardation of motor activities, slowed thinking, and occasionally delusions of a persecutory nature (see Chapter 6).

Migraine presenting as an acute confusional state may also be misinterpreted as acute (toxic) psychosis. Other migraine syndromes may also produce symptomatology characteristic of psychosis such as visual hallucinations, illusions, and feelings of depersonalization or derealization (see Chapter 11).

Imaginary companions are disarming though normal phenomena of early childhood. Children will typically attribute their bad actions to such imaginary companions and converse with them rather than pay attention to their parents. Other *normal hallucinations* of childhood include nightmares, hypnagogic hallucinations, and eidetic ("photographic") images (Egdell and Kolvin, 1972; Morison and Gardner, 1978).

Etiology. Recent decades have seen a marked increase in our understanding of the causes of psychosis in childhood and adolescence (see Table 5–7). Clarification of the biologic basis of development—both normal and abnormal—has occurred at anatomic, biochemical, and physiologic levels. Such a biologic framework can be brought to bear usefully in the psychotic child, particularly one whose psychosocial context is well understood.

Autism provides an example of changes in thinking about "psychiatric" disorders. What had been viewed as a syndrome of a "basically normal child's withdrawal into psychosis" is now considered a severe disorder of development (Rutter, 1977).

Medical Causes. No purely medical causes have been identified as producing the syndrome of early *infantile autism.* The effects of phenylketonuria and prenatal rubella infection are discussed in the section on NEUROLOGIC CAUSES.

Psychoses of later childhood and adolescence including *schizophrenia* can occur with diseases that affect the brain and other organs. These include *thyroid disturbance* (hypo- or hyperthyroidism) (Asher, 1949; Whybrow *et al.,* 1969), *systemic lupus erythematosus* (Johnson and Richardson, 1968;

TABLE 5–7. **Causes of Childhood Psychosis**

Medical	Wilson disease
	Hypo- or hyperthyroidism
	Adrenal insufficiency (Addison disease)
	Systemic lupus erythematosus
	Acute intermittent porphyria
	Homocystinuria
Neurologic	Temporal lobe epilepsy
	Adrenoleukodystrophy
	Metachromatic leukodystrophy
	Herpes simplex encephalitis
	Temporal lobe tumor or abscess
Toxic	Hallucinogens: LSD, mescaline, phencyclidine (PCP), cocaine
	Sympathomimetics: amphetamines, methylphenidate (Ritalin)
	Withdrawal from sedatives: alcohol, barbiturates
Psychologic	"Double bind"
Social-Environmental	Acute and/or chronic stress
Genetic-Constitutional	Inherited susceptibility

Gurland *et al.*, 1972; Brandt *et al.*, 1975), *acute intermittent porphyria* (Stein and Tschudy, 1970; Peters *et al.*, 1974), adrenal insufficiency, and homocystinuria (Freeman *et al.*, 1975). Infections of the central nervous system (such as herpes simplex encephalitis) and progressive disorders such as adrenoleukodystrophy, metachromatic leukodystrophy, and Wilson disease (hepatolenticular degeneration) are considered in the following section. Drug-related psychosis is discussed in the section on TOXIC CAUSES.

With *Addison disease* (*adrenal insufficiency*), an associated encephalopathy may include psychotic features. Other mental status changes can include memory deficit or coma (Bresnan, 1979). The diagnosis may be suggested by the characteristic physical finding of hyperpigmentation and laboratory data demonstrating adrenal failure.

Freeman and colleagues (1975) described a girl with mild mental retardation, without characteristic physical stigmata of *homocystinuria,* whose syndrome of behavioral regression and schizophrenic psychosis responded to oral folic acid. Electroencephalogram showing marked slowing (one cycle per second) in the awake state suggested metabolic disorder. Analysis of blood and urine showed elevated amounts of homocystine. The response to folic acid in this case seems to support a role for methylation in the biochemistry of schizophrenia (see CORRELATION: BIOCHEMICAL ASPECTS).

Neurologic Causes. Several data suggest a neurologic basis for *infantile autism* (see Table 5–8). An increased incidence of prenatal and perinatal complications has been noted in comparison with control groups. Several disorders known to affect the brain adversely such as phenylketonuria (PKU) and prenatal rubella or cytomegalovirus infection can produce an autistic syndrome (Chess, 1971; Stubbs, 1978; Chess *et al.*, 1978). Twenty to 30 per cent of autistic children in some series (60 to 80 per cent in others) have had abnormal electroencephalograms. The incidence of clinical seizures among autistic persons is increased as well (Hauser *et al.*, 1975). A high proportion of autistic children have abnormal neurologic signs, frequently extrapyramidal in nature (Damasio and Maurer, 1978). Diminished nystagmus induced by vestibular stimulation and abnormal eye movements during rapid eye movement (REM) sleep also have been seen disproportionately often among autistic children (Ritvo *et al.*, 1969; Tanguay *et al.*, 1976; Maurer and Damasio, 1979).

The mesolimbic cortex and neostriatum have been singled out by Damasio and Maurer (1978) as the anatomic substrate for autism, susceptible to a wide variety of influences—among them toxic, metabolic, genetic, and in-

TABLE 5–8. **Evidence Suggesting Neurologic Basis for Autism**

Increased incidence of pre- and perinatal complications
Known to occur with a wide variety of disorders associated with brain damage
Increased incidence of abnormal EEG and/or seizures
Increased incidence of abnormal neurologic signs
Increased frequency of nonrighthandedness
Abnormalities of eye movements and vestibular function
Abnormal neuroradiologic studies (PEG, cranial CT scan)

fectious—which may produce an autistic syndrome. These anatomic structures are discussed further in the section on CORRELATION.

The limbic system has also been implicated in autism through radiologic studies. Pneumoencephalography in autistic children has demonstrated underdevelopment or damage to the left cerebral hemisphere, particularly to the left temporal lobe (see Fig. 5–1) (Hauser *et al.*, 1975). This left hemisphere involvement has been evidenced by selective enlargement of the left lateral ventricle or part(s) thereof. In nearly one-third of cases, the right brain appeared abnormal as well (see Case 5–4).

CT scan data also have indicated an abnormal left hemisphere. The right parieto-occipital region has been found larger than the left in a dispropor-

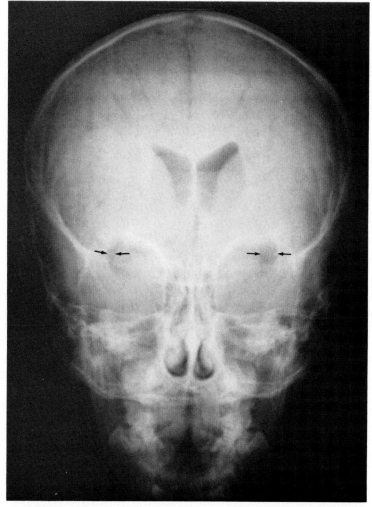

R   L

FIGURE 5–1. Pneumoencephalogram showing enlargement of the left temporal horn in an autistic child. Lateral and medial margins of temporal horns are indicated with arrows.

CASE 5–4: SPEECH DELAY AND AUTISTIC BEHAVIOR IN A 3-YEAR-OLD BOY

A.D. was evaluated because of developmental delay, particularly in speech and language. He had been the full-term product of an uncomplicated pregnancy and delivery. Early development was unremarkable. He sat without support at 6 months, walked at 10 months, and said, "mama" and "bye-bye" at 11 months. Speech development did not progress until 2 years of age. By 3 years, he spoke several three-word combinations. Behavior was notable for fascination with repetitive activities such as switching lights on and off, spinning a bicycle wheel, and watching water run downhill. Past medical history included an illness at 15 months lasting for one week associated with fever, rash, and ataxia (affecting the left side more than the right). Family history was unremarkable.

On examination, the child was a hyperkinetic youngster with a head circumference between the 90th and 98th percentiles. He spoke in brief phrases, poorly articulated. He named several body parts but could identify no colors. He was able to carry out one-step but not two-step commands. Neurologic examination was unremarkable except for an inconsistent response to sound and a right extensor plantar response.

Investigations included normal electroencephalogram, skull x-ray, chromosomes, and amino acids in blood and urine. Pneumoencephalography demonstrated a dilated left ventricular system (see Fig. 5–2). On formal psychologic testing, he performed at age level on nonverbal tasks. Verbal skills were delayed by one year.

This child's educational plan included specific speech and language therapy carried out at first in an aphasia unit in a school for deaf children. Subsequently, instruction was given in a "special needs" classroom for severely

tionate number of autistic children, thereby showing a reversal of the usual cerebral asymmetry (Hier *et al.,* 1978).

On the other hand, Damasio and colleagues (1980) in their review of CT scans of seventeen patients with autistic behavior did not detect a consistent or typical pattern of abnormality. They found neither significant prominence of the left lateral ventricle (or its constituent parts) nor reversal of the usual cerebral hemispheric asymmetry. They noted, however, that discrete enlargement of the temporal horns may not be visualized by computerized tomography.

Postmortem neuropathologic studies of brains of four mentally retarded persons who displayed prominent autistic behavior failed to disclose consistent pathoanatomic findings with autism in these cases (Williams *et al.,* 1980).

All psychoses can be considered ultimately to have their bases in brain function and dysfunction. Hence, *schizophrenia* and *other psychoses* of childhood and adolescence can all be viewed as having a neurologic basis, although precise anatomic, biochemical, and physiologic determinants have not been fully (or in some instances even partially) elucidated. Clues as to

learning-disabled children. Between 3 and 15 years of age, difficulties in receptive and expressive language persisted while visual sequential memory, visual-motor perception, auditory discrimination, and auditory memory improved.

Examined at 15 years, he was sociable, anxious, and somewhat rigid in his interactions. He responded best to brief verbal presentations. Speech was excessive in amount, repetitive, and overly detailed. On psychometric testing, his verbal score was 90—improved over previous verbal scores—and his overall intelligence quotient was 103.

Comment. This child's syndrome of speech delay combined with bizarre, ritualistic behavior overlapped with the syndrome of infantile autism but did not fulfill all diagnostic criteria. He did have significant abnormalities of language development and engaged in spinning and other repetitive activities. He was not, however, as aloof and isolated as classically autistic children tend to be.

This child's language dysfunction can be linked with abnormalities detected upon examination and investigation. The right Babinski sign was consistent with left hemisphere dysfunction. This localization was confirmed by the dilated left ventricular system, suggesting underdevelopment of or injury to the left cerebral hemisphere.

The bearing of the child's illness at 15 months upon subsequent development is unclear. The associated ataxia suggests that he may have suffered encephalitis with developmental deviance the result of brain damage.

The outcome here has been quite good, as it can be in relatively mild cases of autism. He manifested a characteristic social awkwardness and inflexibility along with persisting problems in both expressive and receptive language.

underlying and contributing factors have been provided by diseases affecting the brain. These include herpes simplex encephalitis, temporal lobe disorder (such as epilepsy or other tumor), adrenoleukodystrophy, metachromatic leukodystrophy, and Wilson disease.

Herpes simplex encephalitis is a viral infection of the brain that has a predilection for the temporal lobes. It is marked by changes in mental status: lethargy, memory deterioration, or behavioral changes to the point of psychosis (Bell and McCormick, 1975; Wilson, 1976). The illness may behave as a temporal lobe mass lesion. Diagnosis is based on a characteristic clinical course supported by virologic studies, cerebrospinal fluid analysis (including viral culture), electroencephalogram, CT scan, and (for definitive diagnosis) brain biopsy.

Recurrent episodes of herpes simplex were associated with recurrent episodes of psychosis in a case described by Shearer and Finch (1964). In this instance, the herpetic process, once reactivated, affected the brain rather than the lip or face as it characteristically does with "cold sores."

Temporal lobe disorder has been implicated in many cases of schizo-

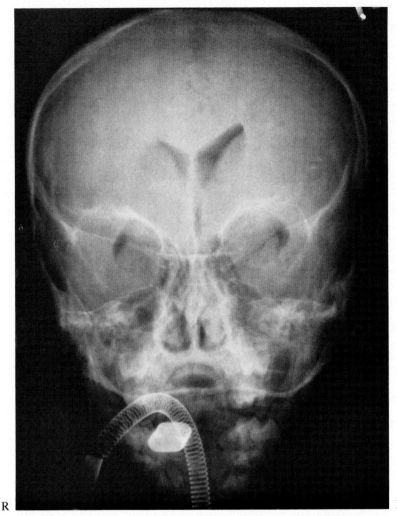

R   L

FIGURE 5–2. Pneumoencephalogram showing enlargement of left frontal and temporal horns in an autistic child (Case 5–4).

phrenic psychosis (Malamud, 1967; Torrey and Peterson, 1974). At times a structural lesion such as destruction of tissue due to tumor or abscess can be identified. In other instances seizures of unknown causes, particularly of temporal lobe origin, can be implicated (Slater and Beard, 1963).

In their long-term studies of children with temporal lobe epilepsy followed into adulthood, Lindsay and colleagues (1979) found that nine of eighty-seven patients (10 per cent) developed a schizophreniform psychosis. Seven of the nine children had a left-sided seizure focus. The other two had bilateral discharges. Lindsay and colleagues concluded that long-standing seizures affecting the left limbic system "potentiate" the development of psychosis. Their data support the evidence of Taylor (1975), Flor-Henry (1976), Demers-Desrosiers *et al.*, (1978), Wexler and Heninger (1979), and Pritchard *et al.*, (1980) in linking seizures of the left hemisphere with psychosis (see Case 5–5).

CASE 5–5: ACUTE PSYCHOSIS WITH TEMPORAL LOBE SEIZURES IN A 7-YEAR-OLD GIRL

K.A., previously well, was brought to the emergency room following the sudden onset of "strange" behavior while playing with friends. They described her taking another child's bicycle, turning it on its side, and stamping on it. Mother found her daughter clawing the air, "acting like she was a monster," and failing to recognize her. She was brought to the emergency room, where she mistook a nurse for her mother and a policeman for her father. During examination, she was incontinent of urine and feces.

Past history was of normal pregnancy, labor, and delivery. Birth weight was 10 pounds. Past history was negative for seizures, head trauma, major illnesses, or exposure to drugs. Development included walking and talking by 1 year of age with toilet-training by $2\frac{1}{2}$ years. Family history was notable for two sisters with grand mal epilepsy.

On examination, the child was subdued and calm. All growth parameters were normal, including head circumference. She had no neurocutaneous findings. Neurologic examination was normal except for mild asymmetry in deep tendon reflexes (slightly accentuated at the right knee) and a right extensor plantar response. Investigations included cerebrospinal fluid examination, analysis of blood and urine for toxic substances, and brain scan. Electroencephalogram showed right temporal lobe spikes (see Fig. 5–3). She was placed on phenytoin, 5 mg/kg/day, and did well until 4 months later. At that time partial complex seizures recurred, apparently due to an unsuspected intercurrent illness (see Case 12–11). Another problem was an episode of phenytoin toxicity (staggering gait and slurred speech) related to an inadequately shaken suspension of the medication.

The child was lost to follow-up for 7 years. During that time, she was seizure-free, and mother discontinued phenytoin at age 10 years. At 15 years of age, she had a normal neurologic examination.

Comment. This child's presenting symptoms of disruptive behavior and hallucinosis suggested not only temporal lobe seizure but drug effects or encephalitis. Laboratory studies (cerebrospinal fluid examination, screen of blood and urine for drugs, and electroencephalogram) helped to exclude these last two possibilities. The family history and focal EEG abnormalities aided in establishing the diagnosis of seizure.

The availability of a chewable 50-mg tablet of phenytoin has made the suspension rarely necessary in school-age children. When the bottle of suspension is insufficiently shaken, the "supernatant" will contain a diminished concentration of medication, leaving increased amounts in the "sediment." As a result, the child may have seizures while taking medication from the first part of the bottle and show evidence of phenytoin toxicity when given the remaining part.

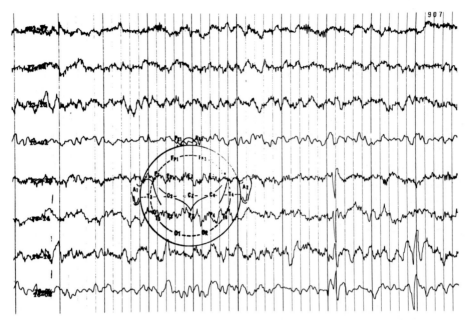

FIGURE 5–3. Electroencephalogram showing right temporal lobe spike discharges (Case 5–5).

Catatonia, which can occur as part of an acute psychotic syndrome, has been reported secondary to apparent psychomotor status epilepticus (Shah and Kaplan, 1980). Other causes include disorders of the basal ganglia and limbic system.

Adrenoleukodystrophy is perhaps better grouped with the disorders of behavioral regression (see Chapter 8). The clinical picture of this dysmyelinating disease is highly variable, however, justifying its inclusion here among neurologic causes for psychosis. As indicated in the section on MEDICAL CAUSES, adrenal insufficiency itself can be associated with a schizophrenic encephalopathy (see Case 5–6).

Metachromatic leukodystrophy may also present with behavioral changes suggesting psychosis (Betts *et al.*, 1968; Manowitz *et al.*, 1978). This disorder characteristically presents in early childhood with an obvious degenerative course. Cases of late onset have been well described, however, beginning in adolescence, young adulthood, or even later adulthood. Intellectual deterioration may dominate the symptomatology, but behavioral changes may be particularly prominent and disabling. Diagnosis can be suggested by a family history of degenerative disorder of the central nervous system in general or metachromatic leukodystrophy in particular. Diagnosis rests ultimately on the demonstration of diminished to absent arylsulfatase A activity (see Chapter 8).

Wilson disease should be considered with onset of psychosis in childhood or adolescence, particularly when it is associated with a movement disorder or liver disease (Cartwright, 1978). The Kayser-Fleischer corneal ring is a pathognomonic sign. Blood studies (serum copper and ceruloplasmin) and measurement of copper in a sample of liver tissue obtained at biopsy are further investigations that can establish the diagnosis.

Toxic Causes.   No toxic causes have been identified as causing *autism,* though brain damage with PKU can be considered to occur on the basis of toxic byproducts of phenylalanine, and lead encephalopathy could conceivably produce an autistic syndrome. One can readily imagine further that—analogous to the effects of prenatal rubella infection—toxic insults during gestation may be identified that are associated with autistic syndromes.

Drugs used illicitly account for the majority of acute *psychoses* in adolescence (see Chapter 19). Most renowned are the hallucinogens such as LSD (lysergic acid diethylamide), mescaline, and psilocybin (Hyde *et al.,* 1978). Nutmeg has also been reported to produce acute psychosis (Faguet and Rowland, 1978). Amphetamines can cause a full-blown picture of paranoid schizophrenia with auditory and sometimes olfactory hallucinations (Snyder, 1973; Angrist, 1978). Marijuana use may be associated with hallucinations and prolonged depersonalization (Szymanski, 1981).

Phencyclidine may also produce a picture of psychosis, particularly catatonic schizophrenia. The hallucinogenic effects of phencyclidine have been linked to the sensory deprivation that seemingly results from use of this drug (see Case 19–1). Tactile, or haptic, hallucinations are characteristic of cocaine intoxication, which also may be associated with a clinical picture of acute psychosis (Snyder, 1977). Such hallucinations typically involve the sensation of ants crawling on or within the skin, so-called formication.

Drug withdrawal may also be associated with psychotic behavior. Alcohol and barbiturate abstinence syndromes are discussed in Chapter 19.

In adults, treatment of myxedema with thyroid replacement may be associated with psychosis. DeGroot and Stanbury (1975) have indicated that this effect may occur at any age without prior history of mental illness.

Rarely, hallucinosis occurs as a side effect of standard "stimulant" medication (such as methylphenidate) used for hyperkinesis or attention deficit disorder (see CORRELATION: BIOCHEMICAL ASPECTS).

Psychologic Causes.   Psychologic factors rarely appear to be of major importance in causing *autism* (see Case 5–7). They are of great relevance, however, in daily life with an autistic child. Although the role of cool, intellectual, "refrigerator parents" in producing an autistic child appears to have been exaggerated, development of normal affective contact and language acquisition requires far more than a biologically sound infant. Indeed, interference with maternal-infant bonding may lead to behavioral syndromes with autistic features (Clancy and McBride, 1975) (see SOCIAL-ENVIRONMENTAL CAUSES).

Among older children and adolescents, psychologic factors (usually intermixed with social, environmental, and genetic influences) frequently play a contributing role, at times a precipitating one, in *psychosis.* One form of chronic stress is the "double-bind" in which the child is subjected to incompatible, stress-producing double messages.

Social-Environmental Causes.   Social and environmental factors are, at all ages and stages of development, closely linked with psychologic ones and frequently contribute to behavioral manifestations of *autism, schizophrenia,*

CASE 5–6: PSYCHOSIS AND BEHAVIORAL REGRESSION IN A 20-YEAR-OLD MAN WITH ADRENOLEUKODYSTROPHY

At 7 years of age, S.X. was evaluated because of seizures and behavioral problems. Behavior problems included disobedience and negativism. On formal psychologic testing, his full-scale intelligence quotient was 120. Past history of pregnancy, birth, and early development was normal. Awkwardness in gross motor skills began at 3 years and slowly worsened. He received above-average grades in first grade. Hyperactivity and inattentiveness occurred the next year, however, and were associated with deterioration in school performance.

Family history included an older brother who died at age 12 years from "Schilder's disease." That child's clinical course began with clumsiness and behavior problems followed by development of seizures, further awkwardness (especially of gait), loss of intellectual function, blindness, and swallowing difficulty. A first cousin had a similar illness and was diagnosed at postmortem examination as having had Schilder's disease.

On examination, the child was a slender, hyperactive, and jocular youngster. General examination was unremarkable. Specifically, no areas of hyperpigmentation involving the skin, gums, or areola were seen. On neurologic examination, visual fields and optic disks were normal. Deep tendon reflexes were symmetrically diminished. Plantar responses were flexor. He showed a mild degree of clumsiness on heel-to-shin testing, heel tapping, and tandem walking. Mental status testing indicated that the child could be insightful and logical. At other times he was tangential and perseverative. He could not (or would not) solve simple calculations such as 4×2.

At 9 years, school performance had deteriorated further. Behavior was described as deviant, antisocial, and aggressive. Psychiatric assessment described "profound regression of psychotic proportion." Investigations included brain scan and pneumoencephalogram, both normal. Cerebrospinal fluid protein was 23 mg/dl, 4 per cent of which was gamma globulin. Urinary 17-hydroxycorticoids and 17-ketosteroids were normal.

Between 10 and 14 years the child attended a residential treatment center, returning home for weekends. Trials of methylphenidate, haloperidol, and primidone were carried out with variable and unsustained improvement.

or *other psychoses*. For example, multiple changes of caretaker can seriously impair attachment, thereby contributing to or causing severe disturbance in personality or behavior. The psychotoxic disorders of Spitz provide examples of the effects of such discontinuity in infancy and early childhood. Analysis of home movies taken during infancy of children later to be diagnosed as psychotic has further suggested the importance of behavioral and interactional factors in some instances of childhood psychosis (Massie, 1978) (see Case 5–8).

Between 14 and 16 years of age, he was hospitalized at a psychiatric facility. Subsequently, he attended a psychiatric day program. Formal psychologic testing at 16 years showed a full-scale intelligence quotient of 77. Cerebrospinal fluid protein level was 32 mg/dl with 5 per cent gamma globulin. CT scan disclosed mildly enlarged lateral ventricles. Baseline levels of cortisol in serum were normal, but an ACTH stimulation test failed to produce a normal elevation in serum cortisol levels. This result suggested insufficient adrenal reserve.

At age 20 years, the young man was completing high school. He had recently received an A in English, B in mathematics, and C in printing. He lost a job at a sheltered workshop because of a temper outburst following criticism. His general physical examination remained normal. On neurologic examination, awkwardness on tandem gait persisted. He still had difficulty with calculations and demonstrated problems with interpretations of proverbs.

Comment. This young man's clinical course, family history, and ACTH stimulation test results suggested strongly the diagnosis of adrenoleukodystrophy. Obviously, he did not have the fulminant form of the disease in which rapid demyelination occurs, resulting in cortical blindness, severe loss of intellectual functions, acute psychosis, and death (see Fig. 5–4).

The relationship between adrenal function and cerebral problems in adrenoleukodystrophy is unclear. In some patients the adrenal problem antedates the cerebral one. The former may be manifested by typical features of adrenal insufficiency such as hyperpigmentation of the skin and salt craving. With systemic stress, adrenocortical insufficiency may be manifested to the point of shock. In other patients, cerebral manifestations predominate and adrenal signs are demonstrable only upon investigation.

In this case specific medical treatment (exogenous steroids) for the adrenal insufficiency was not felt to be necessary under usual circumstances. Should elective surgery be undertaken, however, he would be given exogenous steroids.

The main principles in this young man's treatment have been educational (having him continue his schooling), occupational (attempting to keep him regularly involved in productive and meaningful work), and psychotherapeutic (helping him to deal with his problems of personality and behavior).

As Kagan (1966) has written, "If there are many occasions of discomfort when a caretaker does not arrive, the infant usually discovers responses that attenuate the gnawing discomfort from within. He may bang his head, rock on his knees, pull his hair, or sleep. . . . This infant does not learn to anticipate the arrival of a human agent in time of pain and fear, but learns to stimulate his body or to withdraw from the social environment."

With childhood schizophrenia in particular, social and environmental factors may be sufficiently stressful as to precipitate psychosis. For example,

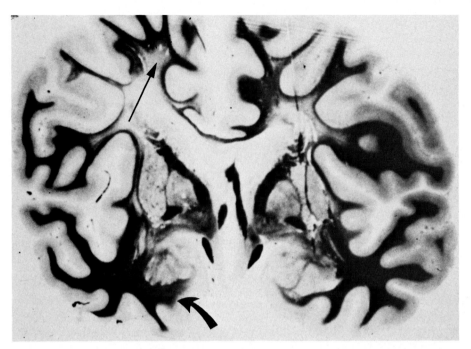

FIGURE 5–4. Section of brain stained for myelin (black) in adrenoleukodystrophy. Compare area of normal myelination (curved, thick arrow) with area of myelin loss (straight, thin arrow).

moving from one community to another carries with it the combined stresses of losing one's established friends, attempting to make new friends, and trying to adjust to a new school.

Genetic-Constitutional Causes.   Though a precise mode of inheritance has not been identified, a study by Folstein and Rutter (1977) suggests that genetic factors influence the development of infantile *autism*.

1. The frequency of autism was increased fiftyfold among siblings of autistic children (to about 2 per cent).
2. A family history of speech delay was found in nearly one-quarter of families with an autistic child.
3. A significantly higher concordance rate for autism was found among monozygotic twins (four of eleven, or 36 per cent) as contrasted with dizygotic twins (zero of eleven, or 0 per cent). Of additional interest is that the concordance for cognitive abnormalities was 82 per cent and 10 per cent, respectively, in monozygotic versus dizygotic twins.

Genetic factors in *schizophrenia* are suggested by the higher concordance rates among identical (monozygotic) twins than fraternal (dizygotic) twins (Kinney and Mathysse, 1978). Adoption studies have further emphasized the importance of genetic factors (Kety *et al.,* 1976).

Although Kety (1978) has expressed that the available data are "compatible with genetic transmission in schizophrenia," he noted that intrauterine factors, birth trauma, early mothering experiences, and perhaps diet and early infection render the genetic data inconclusive. A multifactorial process is suggested, genetic predisposition allowing for the development of schizophrenia under certain circumstances.

Mathysse (1980), noting the diminished intelligence levels found among carriers for ornithine transcarbamylase deficiency, has raised the question (as others have also) as to whether heterozygosity for certain metabolic disorders can predispose to the development of schizophrenia. This intriguing hypothesis remains to be explored more fully.

Developmental Causes. The predominance of males among children with *autism* (about 4:1) suggests that slower neurologic maturation with a prolonged period of vulnerability to various insults may play an etiologic role.

The classic occurrence of *schizophrenia* in adolescence suggests also the influence of developmental and maturational factors. Again, the genetic, hormonal, and experiential influences may be difficult to separate out in an individual case in which any or all may contribute significantly.

TREATMENT AND OUTCOME

Infantile *autism* is a chronic, severely handicapping condition that can be treated and ameliorated, but it is inappropriate to think in terms of a "cure." A multifaceted approach to treatment (as with diagnosis) is essential, the goal being normalization of function at various levels (individual, family, school, and community) insofar as it is possible.

As a general rule one must meet the autistic child at his or her developmental and cognitive level. This level is characteristically delayed significantly if not severely in several areas, not just in the interpersonal and language areas (Wing, 1972). Furthermore, learning is impaired by attentional problems and the autistic child's well-known tendency toward overconcreteness (an inability to abstract).

An additional difficulty in approaching autistic children is that their often-mentioned normal, attractive, composed, and quasi-independent appearance tends to render their associated intellectual deficit usually less than immediately apparent.

An overall goal of therapy is to break through the child's isolation and to seek to establish (or reestablish) affective contact. The dangers of "trying too hard" have been emphasized by Richer and Richards (1975). Progress can be made, generally slowly, built upon interests and activities of the child. Behavior modification is often of value.

Wing (1972) has articulated four principles of fostering the learning process in autistic children:

1. Desirable patterns of behavior should be rewarded.
2. New skills should be broken down into small, simple steps—not presented as a whole.
3. Fairly vigorous prompting should be employed when new activities are introduced. Less urging should subsequently be necessary.
4. New skills should be linked to tasks already familiar and pleasurable to the child.

CASE 5–7: BEHAVIORAL REGRESSION WITH AUTISTIC FEATURES IN A 7-YEAR-OLD GIRL

B.D. was evaluated because of abnormal development and interactive behavior. History of pregnancy and birth was unremarkable. Early development appeared normal until $2\frac{1}{2}$ years of age when she was frightened by a steam shovel being used in her neighborhood. She subsequently became unusually fearful of large and noisy objects. Language development slowed. Speech showed perseveration and echolalia. She sat alone and rocked by herself for hours. She no longer participated in conversation, lost interest in books, and did not show affection as before.

At 5 years, she was withdrawn and spoke in short sentences only. She made clicking noises and clenched her hands about her face. As she played with objects, she spoke to herself, describing what she was doing. She was able to copy a circle and draw a person, though poorly. She recognized colors but not numbers.

At 7 years she was an affectionate, hyperverbal child with a short attention span and diminished eye contact. She identified simple body parts and was able to carry out a three-step command. Echolalia persisted. She was able to complete simple verbal analogies ("If mothers are big, babies are . . ."), but further abstraction was impaired.

General examination was normal, including head circumference and funduscopic visualization. On neurologic examination, motor and sensory functions were intact. Deep tendon reflexes were normal. The left plantar response was extensor.

Investigations included electroencephalography, measurement of thyroid hormone level, analysis of blood and urine for amino acids, CT scan, skull

The long-term outlook for the autistic child will vary with the severity of the disorder, underlying or associated problems, the degree of mental retardation, and to a certain extent the treatment employed (Eisenberg, 1956; Kanner, 1971; DeMyer et al., 1973; Knobloch and Pasamanick, 1975; Rutter, 1977).

In general, the intelligence quotient (IQ) is the best prognostic indicator. A uniformly poor outcome can be anticipated for those autistic children with an IQ below 50 and among those children in whom autism is but one feature of more widespread brain dysfunction (as with a congenital rubella syndrome or phenylketonuria) (Rutter, 1977). When the performance IQ equals or exceeds 70, however, nearly one-half do relatively satisfactorily.

Overall, most autistic children will remain severely impaired, unable to lead an independent life, although many will be able to function in a sheltered setting (Wing, 1972; Rutter, 1977). Ten to 20 per cent have been described as making a "good" social adjustment in terms of holding a job and functioning independently. Social awkwardness, problems in communication, and certain "oddities" of behavior characteristically do remain, however, even in the best of circumstances.

x-rays, audiometry, tympanometry, and lysosomal enzyme determinations. All of these were normal. Assessment of motor skills showed poor balance. On formal speech and language evaluation, articulation was normal. Auditory comprehension was at the $4\frac{1}{2}$-year level. Expressive ability was at the 5- to 6-year level. Figure drawings were scored at an 8-year level. Verbal intelligence quotient was 63, nonverbal 82, with a full-scale score of 72.

The child was placed in a special classroom in which language therapy and behavior modification were emphasized. In addition, she received therapy directed toward improving motor skills.

Comment. This child's language disturbance and interactional difficulties placed her within the category of autism. With onset beyond 30 months, she would fit with cases of later onset. Her intelligence quotient and degree of language development placed her in a relatively favorable prognostic category.

One encounters the history of an apparently significant traumatic event in autistic children sufficiently frequently that it cannot be readily discounted. In this case, the child underwent marked behavioral changes in apparent reaction to a frightening incident at $2\frac{1}{2}$ years of age. One can postulate in such cases a vulnerability of brain such that preexisting or potential pathologies are "uncovered." With this child, her past history was entirely unremarkable, and the only neurologic abnormality was an isolated left Babinski response.

Despite the lack of concrete evidence here, one gets the impression that a neurologic problem (structural, biochemical, or both) underlay her syndrome. One can hope that newer investigative tools will help answer the many questions such children raise.

Language function importantly influences later outcome. Severe comprehension difficulties in childhood or failure to gain useful speech by 5 years of age render a favorable outcome less likely (Rutter, 1977).

The outcome of *schizophrenia* with onset in childhood or adolescence ranges from chronic hospitalization to normalcy. Onset before 10 years of age and persistently disturbed interpersonal relationships are predictive of poor outcome (Steinberg, 1977).

Psychotropic medication is often of great value in the treatment of schizophrenia and other psychotic disorders in children and adolescents. Nonpharmacologic therapies should not be neglected, however, as they can be important in maintaining optimal health and minimizing the likelihood and severity of relapse. It is important from a therapeutic standpoint to keep in mind that schizophrenia appears to be a complex disorder of psychologic development, based on a genetically determined vulnerability acted upon by an unfavorable psychosocial environment (Steinberg, 1977; MacCrimmon *et al.*, 1980).

Several factors have been associated with good prognosis in schizophrenia. These are absence of premorbid personality disturbance, adequate prior

CASE 5–8: AUTISM IN A 4-YEAR-OLD BOY

F.B. was evaluated because of deterioration in language and behavior. He was a 5-pound, 15-ounce product of a full-term pregnancy complicated by mild toxemia. Labor and delivery were unremarkable. Apgar scores were 10 at 1 and 5 minutes. Head circumference at birth was normal (34 cm). Mild jaundice occurred during the neonatal period but did not require phototherapy. Early development was recalled as normal. He walked at 13 months, spoke single words at 12 months, and used phrases by 18 months. He was described as a happy and normally interactive toddler.

Between $2\frac{1}{2}$ and 3 years of age, marked changes occurred. The child became aggressive and less social. Motor coordination and language (receptive as well as expressive) deteriorated markedly. Regression coincided with periods of severe parental discord and numerous changes of caretaker.

On examination, the child was an attractive, well-formed boy with normal growth parameters including head circumference. He paid no attention to strangers and "orbited" around his father. He picked hairs off his father's sweater and twirled them for several minutes at a time. He reacted to loud noises and to his father's request to put an object down. Verbal output consisted of nonsense syllables such as "baw-pwee-thaw" and echoed words. Examination of the skin and optic fundi was unremarkable. Elemental neurologic examination was exquisitely normal, including tone, deep tendon reflexes, and plantar responses.

Investigations included complete blood count, serum thyroxine level, lead level, chromosome analysis, electroencephalogram, cerebrospinal fluid examination, lysosomal enzymes, and CT scan. Formal speech and language assessment demonstrated skills at a 1-year level at best.

Comment. This boy was considered to manifest an atypical autistic syndrome. He fulfilled two of three essential criteria for infantile autism—profound interactional difficulties and severe speech and language impairment—but not the criterion of onset before $2\frac{1}{2}$ years of age. Indeed, his normal development up to nearly three years (as described by his parents) led to active consideration of degenerative neurologic disorders (see Chapter 8).

Despite an extensive evaluation exploring biochemical as well as structural etiologies, the cause or causes of his autism remained a mystery. It did seem that his early upbringing was unusually stressful. But whether these circumstances were in themselves sufficient to produce the profoundly and persistently impaired child described appears doubtful unless one postulates preexisting vulnerability of the child's developing nervous system.

social functioning, precipitating events, abrupt onset, a clinical picture that involves confusion, and a family history of affective disorder.

Medical Management.   No pharmacologic agent or group of agents has been found uniformly effective among children with *autism*. Sleep disturbance is common and can interfere with the autistic child's sleep requirements as well as disrupt the entire family. Chloral hydrate in a dose of

500–1000 mg may be beneficial. When anxiety and emotional outbursts are significant problems, phenothiazines may be of help (see below). With hyperkinesis or attention deficit disorder, standard medication such as dextroamphetamine or methylphenidate can reasonably be tried (see Chapter 14). Megadoses of vitamin B_6 or other vitamins have not been uniformly beneficial among autistic children, but evidence suggests that some children will be helped by such therapy (Rimland *et al.*, 1978). Use of anticonvulsant medication is discussed in NEUROLOGIC MANAGEMENT.

For *schizophrenia* and *other psychoses* of later childhood and adolescence, phenothiazines, butyrophenones, and thioxanthenes are the antipsychotic drugs of choice (see Table 5–9). Because clinical experience with the phenothiazines has been most extensive and their toxic as well as therapeutic effects are well known, they should probably be considered the drugs of first choice.

Whether used for acute or chronic purposes, an antipsychotic drug should be employed with specific target symptoms in mind such as extreme agitation, combativeness, hallucinations, or acute delusions (Kessler and Waletzky, 1981). In treating severe agitation, chlorpromazine can be administered intramuscularly in doses of 0.5–1 mg/kg given every 4 to 6 hours as needed (Winsberg and Yepes, 1978) (see Table 5–10). The child should be observed for sedation, extrapyramidal reaction, and hypotension. Alternatively, haloperidol, 0.3–0.7 mg/kg can be given intramuscularly, although the safety and effectiveness of this drug in children have not been established.

Maintenance treatment is determined by the response to medication in terms of target symptoms and side effects. Among standard agents from the three categories above, none has demonstrated clear antipsychotic superiority over the others. Chlorpromazine is relatively more sedating than tri-

TABLE 5–9. **Antipsychotic Drugs Used in Children**

Drug	Equivalent Dose (mg)	Average Daily Dose (mg/kg)*	Average Total Daily Dose Range (mg)
Phenothiazines			
Chlorpromazine (Thorazine)	100	3–6	75–150
Thioridazine (Mellaril)	100	3–6	75–150
Perphenazine (Trilafon)	8	Not established	4–12
Trifluoperazine (Stelazine)	5	0.25–0.5	6–15
Fluphenazine (Prolixin)	2	0.15–0.3	3–6
Thioxanthene			
Thiothixene (Navane)	4	0.1–0.3	2–6
Butyrophenone			
Haloperidol (Haldol)	2	0.15–0.3	2–6

* Substantially lower dosage should be used for initial therapy.

TABLE 5–10. **Side Effects of Commonly Used Antipsychotic Drugs**[*]

Drug	Side Effect		
	Sedative	Extrapyramidal	Hypotension
Phenothiazines			
Chlorpromazine (Thorazine)	+ + +	+ +	+ +
Thioridazine (Mellaril)	+ + +	+	+ +
Perphenazine (Trilafon)	+ +	+ + +	+
Trifluoperazine (Stelazine)	+	+ + +	+
Fluphenazine (Prolixin)	+	+ + +	+
Thioxanthene			
Thiothixene (Navane)	+	+ +	+ +
Butyrophenone			
Haloperidol (Haldol)	+	+ + +	+

* Adapted from Baldessarini, R. J. Drugs used in the treatment of psychoses. In *The Pharmacological Basis of Therapeutics,* 6th ed. Gilman, A. G.; Goodman, L. S.; and Gilman, A., eds. Macmillan Publishing Co., Inc., New York, 1980.

fluoperazine (another phenothiazine), haloperidol (a butyrophenone), and thiothixene (a thioxanthene) (Baldessarini, 1980). Haloperidol and trifluoperazine are likeliest to produce significant dystonic reactions. These usually occur within 72 hours of beginning therapy. Intramuscular chlorpromazine tends to produce the most marked hypotension among these drugs.

Oral maintenance therapy is begun after side effects of medication are discussed with the family and child (when appropriate). The basic principle is to start with a low dosage (which will often be subtherapeutic) and increase weekly depending upon the clinical response. Two to 3 weeks will usually be required to attain a therapeutic level (Winsberg and Yepes, 1978). Pharmacotherapy of acute psychosis may require only 4 to 6 weeks of medication (Campbell, 1977). Otherwise, medication should be maintained for 3- to 4-month periods, with 1- to 2-week "drug holidays" intervening to allow for assessment of the need for continuing medication and to minimize the risk of developing tardive dyskinesia (see below).

The starting dose for chlorpromazine is 1.5–3 mg/kg/day given in two or three equally divided doses (Winsberg and Yepes, 1978). The average daily therapeutic dose is 3 to 6 mg/kg/day, or 75 to 150 mg. For the adolescent, considerably higher doses (in the adult range: 400 mg or more) may be required (Campbell, 1977). The dosage of thioridazine is comparable to that of chlorpromazine. Haloperidol and thiothixene can be begun in a dosage of 0.025–0.05 mg/kg/day in divided dosage and increased to an average therapeutic dosage of 0.1–0.3 mg/kg/day (2 to 6 mg per day) (Winsberg and Yepes, 1978).

If the initial maintenance drug (for example, chlorpromazine) is ineffective in usual therapeutic doses or if side effects (such as sedation or extrapyramidal reaction) limit its use, one of the other antipsychotic agents can be considered for use.

Because phenothiazines have been implicated in causing an increase in seizures among epileptic patients, antipsychotic drugs among persons with known seizure disorders should be used with caution (Baldessarini, 1980). Thioridazine appears to be less epileptogenic than other phenothiazines and has been reported in some instances to be associated with diminished seizure frequency (Winsberg and Yepes, 1978). For these reasons, some consider thioridazine the phenothiazine of choice in the child or adolescent with a seizure disorder.

Acute dystonic reactions have been described by Winsberg and Yepes (1978) as

> . . . the abrupt contraction of a muscle or group of muscles. Head and neck are more commonly involved, with resulting torticollis (head turned to a side), retrocollis (head turned to back), and jaw pulled to side. There can also be facial grimacing and distortion, tongue protrusion or curling, spasms of throat muscles, with difficulty in speech and swallowing, and occasionally in breathing. Oculogyric crises (fixed upward gaze), opisthotonos (arching of the back), scoliosis, dystonic gait, and shoulder and leg movements have also been described.

Such extrapyramidal side effects will usually respond to diphenhydramine (Benadryl), 25–50 mg, or benztropine mesylate (Cogentin), 1–2 mg, given parenterally. The use of prophylactic anticholinergic medication is controversial and should be avoided if possible.

The late complication of *tardive dyskinesia* is a definite threat in childhood and adolescence for which no uniformly effective treatment (or preventive approach) has been determined (Gaultieri *et al.,* 1980). The following guidelines for the avoidance and management of tardive dyskinesia have been suggested (Baldessarini *et al.,* 1980).

1. The indications for prolonged administration (greater than 6 months) of a phenothiazine or butyrophenone should be carefully assessed with objective evidence of benefit.
2. Alternative therapies should be employed whenever possible.
3. Dosage should be kept to a minimum.
4. "Polypharmacy" (the use of multiple drugs) should be avoided.
5. If antiparkinsonian agents have been needed, they should be discontinued as soon as possible.
6. The risks and benefits of neuroleptic medication should be discussed with parents as well as the child, if appropriate.
7. The patient should be examined regularly for early signs of tardive dyskinesia such as choreoathetosis or oral-lingual dyskinesia.
8. At the first sign of dyskinesia, a lower dosage of medication should be used, a less potent agent chosen, or the drug discontinued altogether, if possible, as long as circumstances permit.
9. Dyskinesia should be treated with relatively benign medications first. These include diazepam, deanol, choline, or lecithin in high doses.
10. Antipsychotic agents themselves should be used only as a last resort to treat the movement disorder at the lowest possible dosage.

Neurologic Management. As noted above, electroencephalographic abnormalities are common among children with *autism*, and an increasing number of autistic children will develop clinical convulsions as they grow older. When EEG abnormalities are found but clinical seizures have not occurred, a several-month trial of anticonvulsant therapy, for example, with phenytoin or carbamazepine, should be considered (Oppenheimer and Rosman, 1979) (see Chapter 12). Diminution in nocturnal enuresis or improved attentiveness by day would suggest beneficial response to anticonvulsant medication. When clinical seizures have occurred, anticonvulsant treatment should be commenced and maintained depending on the subsequent clinical course and EEG.

Phenothiazines should be used with care in *psychotic* children with seizure activity on EEG or with known seizure disorders, as hypersynchronization of cerebral electrical activity may occur and contribute to increased incidence of seizures (Baldessarini, 1980).

Psychotherapy. Individual psychotherapy has not been found significantly helpful for the young child with *autism* (Wing, 1972; Rutter, 1977). In later childhood and adolescence, however, when the less-impaired autistic child becomes increasingly aware of his own differences and handicaps, individual psychotherapy may be beneficial.

Supportive, family-oriented therapy is always indicated. Parents of autistic children often feel responsible for their child's difficulties, and their guilt is frequently compounded by their sense of rejection by the child. Siblings may also bear unspoken feelings of guilt and anger concerning an autistic brother or sister. A discussion of recent findings as to organic factors in childhood autism may be helpful in relieving some of these guilty feelings.

Behavior modification is an important tool in the management and shaping of many aspects of the autistic child's life (Hingtgen *et al.*, 1967; Schopler, 1976). The overall principles are that positive behaviors are reinforced, negative behaviors extinguished. The memory difficulties of the autistic child make it essential that reward be provided immediately. Not responding is one of the ways in which negative behavior may be extinguished.

For the older child or adolescent with *schizophrenia* or *other psychosis,* individual psychotherapy is generally indicated. Family meetings may also be beneficial (Steinberg, 1977).

Social-Environmental Management. This aspect of treatment is of great importance for the *autistic* child and his or her family. The autistic child's lack of usual fears may pose a danger to himself. Hence, access to dangerous portions of the home and its environs such as windows, fire escapes, or swimming pools should be restricted if not actually barred. The name, address, and telephone number of the child should be sewn into his or her clothing in case the child becomes lost (Wing, 1972).

The autistic child's desire for sameness in the environment is commonly associated with ritualized activities or with tantrums if orderliness is not maintained. Anticipating areas of conflict and employing gentle but firm limits are often effective in preventing major tantrums. Play therapy and explanation at the child's affective and cognitive levels of functioning will help to lessen the impact of major changes such as vacations or household moves. The autistic child may nonetheless react to such changes in unusual and upsetting ways.

Not surprisingly, feeding is an area of difficulty for many autistic children. New foods can be gradually mixed with known and accepted ones in order that the diet be broadened and enriched (Clancy *et al.*, 1969). In later childhood and adolescence, sheltered workshops provide enriching and rewarding experiences for many autistic children. With regard to later institutionalization, the degree of mental retardation and behavioral distrubance plus the family's ability to care further for the child will enter importantly into such difficult decisions.

Acute hospitalization of the child or adolescent with *schizophrenia* or *other psychosis* is usually indicated. Whether hospitalization is at a primarily medical or primarily psychiatric facility is not of greatest importance. Rather, it is essential regardless of the setting that the child receive comprehensive diagnostic assessment (medical and neurologic as well as psychiatric) and treatment.

Following acute management, day-hospital treatment, sheltered workshop involvement, and—in some circumstances—family or residential placement should be considered, although most children will be able to return home.

Educational Management. Special education is required for the child with *autism*. Emphasis should be placed first on teaching essential social skills and activities of daily living. These would include feeding, washing, dressing, and toileting. Later, depending on the capabilities of the autistic child, conventional school subjects (both academic and nonacademic) can be pursued.

With the older child or adolescent with *schizophrenia* or *other psychosis,* education is a normalizing activity, keeping the child as much as possible in the mainstream of his or her peers. If academic ground has been lost during hospitalization, tutoring may help the child catch up and perhaps avoid repeating the school year, which in itself might be an additional stress of significance. Care must be taken, of course, that undue academic stress is not placed on the child.

Communication Therapy. "Almost everyone tends to assume that autistic children understand more than they really do" (Wing, 1972). This assumption is fostered by the *autistic child's* appearance of intelligence and thoughtful aloofness, not to mention circumscribed areas of average or better function. It is important to keep in mind that the autistic child's communication problem involves not just language but interpersonal contact in general.

Formal speech and language assessment will have clarified the child's level of function both expressively and receptively, so that the most effective communication program can be instituted. Simplification of communication is important. Short phrases with simple words are to be used. At times, immature (indeed "babyish") grammatical constructions are justified. Whispering into the child's ear, singing, and speaking directly in front of him (without being overwhelmingly close) with hands placed gently on his shoulders can be employed to gain the child's attention. Sign language has been effective with some autistic children.

Communication is an important principle in the treatment of the child or adolescent with *schizophrenia* or *other psychosis*. It is essential that the child be able to share with his or her therapist strange, bizarre, disturbing, or otherwise "crazy" thoughts or feelings. It must be emphasized that not everyone is qualified by training or experience to delve into these areas indiscriminately. Once recognized, these issues should be acknowledged and appropriate referral to a child psychiatrist or psychologist carried out.

Physical Therapy. If spasticity, hemiparesis, or other significant motor problems are present in the child with *autism* or *other psychosis*, physical therapy is indicated. Adaptive physical education will provide not only a chance to develop physical skills but also opportunities for socialization.

Mechanical Therapy. When visual or auditory problems are identified, corrective lenses or a hearing aid should be considered. Individual radio headsets have been used to enhance audio contact with *autistic children*.

CORRELATION

Anatomic Aspects. The varied functions of the temporal lobes are reflected in their anatomic position. Each temporal lobe is directly in contact with the occipital lobe posteriorly and the parietal lobe superiorly. The boundaries between these three lobes are less well defined than that between each frontal and parietal lobe, the central sulcus. The angular gyrus, an important association area, lies at the junction of these three lobes.

Viewed in longitudinal cross-section, the temporal lobe is seen to be connected to other cortical and subcortical structures. Several C-shaped structures involving deep medial portions of the temporal lobe can be recognized (see Fig. 2–11). The hippocampus (part of the temporal lobe), fornix, and mammillary body (part of the hypothalamus) make up one C within each hemisphere. The hippocampus, lying anteriorly and medially within the temporal lobe, makes up part of the medial wall of the temporal horn of the lateral ventricle. Its name, from the Latin word for seahorse, is derived from its anatomic appearance. The fornix arises from the hippocampus. It arches upward and backward, then passes downward to end in the mammillary body on the same side.

Another C is formed by the anterior nucleus of the thalamus, cingulate gyrus, isthmus, parahippocampal gyrus, and uncus. The latter four structures make up the so-called limbic lobe of the brain.

These two C's are connected to each other at both ends. Hypothalamic input reaches the anterior nucleus of the thalamus via the mammillothalamic tract. Fibers connect the parahippocampal gyrus with the adjacent hippocampus. Thus, a circuit is formed that has been postulated as the neural substrate for emotion. As conceptualized by Papez (1937), these pathways allow for connection in both directions between hypothalamus and cerebral cortex, thereby providing for the emotional coloration of perceptual experience and vice versa (that is, enabling cerebral cortical activity to influence hypothalamically mediated emotional events).

This ring of phylogenetically older cortex, in conjunction with certain of the basal ganglia, has been cited by Damasio and Maurer (1978) as the region of the brain most likely to be affected in childhood autism. Thus, implicated are the medially located (or mesial) portions of frontal and temporal lobes (part of the limbic lobe) along with closely connected nuclei of the basal ganglia, principally the caudate and putamen.

Biochemical Aspects. Despite the differences between childhood autism and schizophrenia, they may share important biochemical features. Dopamine has been identified as playing a key role in both.

Regarding autism, the anatomic structures suggested as important by Damasio and Maurer (1978) make up a well-identified neurochemical pathway, the mesolimbic dopamine projection, which connects brainstem nuclei with limbic structures and basal ganglia (Cooper et al., 1978).

Concerning schizophrenia, dopamine has been implicated in several ways (Snyder, 1973 and 1977; Carlsson, 1978; Bacopoulos et al., 1979; Sedvall and Wode-Helgodt, 1980). First, the psychotogenic properties of amphetamines have demonstrated an important role for dopamine. Second, the dopamine-blocking activity of chlorpromazine has been linked clincially to its antipsychotic properties. Third, L-DOPA worsens psychotic symptoms of schizophrenic patients. Fourth, the structural similarity of dopamine and part of the chlorpromazine molecule has suggested the physicochemical basis for chlorpromazine's postsynaptic action, a blocking of dopamine (Snyder, 1973).

Hallucinogenic drugs such as mescaline, LSD, and psilocybin have stimulated much research into biochemical factors that might underlie schizophrenia. Endogenous manufacture of hallucinogenic agents has been postulated to play a role in the production of schizophrenic symptoms (Corbett et al., 1978; Kety, 1978; Benesh and Carl, 1978). For example, dimethyltryptamine, a potent hallucinogenic agent, can be produced by methylation of tryptamine, a widely available amino acid (Saavedra et al., 1973). Mescaline can be produced by methylation of dopamine. Neither substance, however, has been identified naturally in man.

Because of the suggested though not proven role of methylation in producing hallucinogenic effects, clinical trials have been carried out in an attempt to divert methyl groups from such substances as dopamine or tryptamine (Kety, 1978). The results of such trials, employing megadoses of niacin and niacinamide, have been inconclusive.

Also proposed to account for schizophrenia has been failure of breakdown of psychotogenic chemicals. Monoamine oxidase, which plays a role in breaking down dopamine, tryptamine, and related substances, has been found to be lowered in the platelets of paranoid schizophrenics (Potkin et al., 1978). The diagnostic or therapeutic significance of this finding is unclear.

It has been suggested that cholinergic underactivity may underlie some forms of childhood schizophrenia (Cantor et al., 1980). The possible role of endogenous opioids and other peptides in schizophrenia is also currently being investigated (Verebey et al., 1978; Cooper and Martin, 1980; Judd et al., 1981).

Physiologic Aspects. The deep midline portions of the temporal lobes lie in such a way as to reflect their complex integrative functions. They are positioned between cortical centers involved in primary perception (vision and audition) and subcortical centers, chiefly the hypothalamus (involved in emotion and other behaviors). The hypothalamus is the major autonomic center for such instinctual behaviors as eating, drinking, sexual activity, and aggression. It is hardly surprising then that temporal lobe damage produced experimentally in animals or occurring in humans as a result of injury or disease can result in complicated syndromes of disordered behavior, perception, and affect (Malamud, 1967; Betts *et al.,* 1968; Salguero *et al.,* 1969; Darby, 1976).

As mentioned earlier (see NEUROLOGIC CAUSES), the left temporal lobe has been singled out for its role in psychosis largely through studies of persons with temporal lobe epilepsy (Flor-Henry, 1976; Lindsay *et al.,* 1979; Wexler and Heninger, 1979; Pritchard *et al.,* 1980).

The Klüver-Bucy syndrome provides an experimental model of bilateral temporal lobe disease. With surgical removal of both temporal lobes in monkeys, aimless hyperexploratory behavior, hyperorality, and failure to recognize parents result (Shraberg and Weisberg, 1978). In addition, such animals disregard what are customarily fear-provoking situations. Similarities between the Klüver-Bucy syndrome in experimental animals and characteristic behaviors of autistic children underscore the apparent importance of temporal lobe abnormalities in some autistic children (Hauser *et al.,* 1975). The role of the temporal lobe in normal and disordered memory is discussed further in Chapter 16.

SUMMARY

Infantile autism and schizophrenia have become separable as distinct psychotic processes of childhood. Autism is defined by severe disturbances in language and interactive behavior with onset before $2\frac{1}{2}$ years of age. Schizophrenia is defined by characteristic disturbances in thought, affect, motor behavior, and social functioning.

In evaluating the autistic child, several conditions should be recalled as ones that might be mistaken for autism. These include severe deafness, developmental language disturbance without mental retardation, and degenerative neurologic disorder. Causes for autism include phenylketonuria or prenatal rubella infection. Often no specific cause is found.

Schizophrenic psychosis should be distinguished from severe situational reactions, anxiety states, and other affective disorders. Causes of psychosis include drug ingestion, temporal lobe epilepsy, Wilson disease, and adrenoleukodystrophy.

Damage to the temporal lobe(s) and other portions of the mesolimbic cortex has been implicated as underlying childhood autism. The left temporal lobe has been singled out in the pathogenesis of schizophrenia. Dopaminergic pathways appear to play a role not only in autism but in schizophrenia as well. Schizophrenia appears to be rooted in genetic and presumably metabolic vulnerability and to result from superimposed developmental, emotional, social, and possibly other stresses.

Treatment both of autism and schizophrenia is multifaceted. It often will include pharmacologic, psychotherapeutic, and social-environmental management in addition to ongoing educational efforts. Prognosis for the autistic child is usually unfavorable. Only a small minority are able to achieve an independent life. Mental retardation and failure to develop language by 5 years of age are poor prognostic features. The outlook for the child or adolescent with schizophrenia ranges from poor to excellent. Premorbid personality, age at onset of the illness, and abruptness of presenting symptoms are major prognostic factors.

The rapid development of structural, biochemical, and diagnostic tools for study of the central nervous system in autism and schizophrenia is anticipated to bring further insights into these psychotic disorders and to provide further knowledge as to their prevention and treatment.

CITED REFERENCES

Adams, D.; Cummings, J.; Hart, E.; and Rosman, N. P. An idiot savant calendar calculator: case report and review of explanations. *Neurology* (abst.), **30:** 391, 1980.

Angrist, B. M. Toxic manifestations of amphetamine. *Psychiatr. Ann.,* **8:** 443–46, 1978.

Asher, R. Myxoedematous madness. *Br. Med. J.,* **2:** 555–62, 1949.

Bacopoulos, N. C.; Spokes, E. G.; Bird, E. D.; and Roth, R. H. Antipsychotic drug action in schizophrenic patients: effect on cortical dopamine metabolism after long-term treatment. *Science,* **205:** 1405–1407, 1979.

Baldessarini, R. J. Drugs used in the treatment of psychoses. Pp. 395–418 in *The Pharmacological Basis of Therapeutics,* 6th ed. Gilman, A. G.; Goodman, L. S.; and Gilman, A., eds. Macmillan Publishing Co., Inc. New York, 1980.

Baldessarini, R. J.; Cole, J. O.; Davis, J. M.; Simpson, G.; Tarsy, D.; Gardos, G.; and Preskorn, S. H. Tardive dyskinesia: summary of a task force report of the American Psychiatric Association. *Am. J. Psychiatry,* **137:** 1163–72, 1980.

Bartak, L., and Rutter, M. Differences between mentally retarded and normally intelligent autistic children. *J. Autism Child. Schizophr.,* **6:** 109–20, 1976.

Bell, W. E., and McCormick, W. F. Herpesvirus hominis (simplex) infections of the nervous system. Pp. 193–203 in *Neurologic Infections in Children.* Bell, W. E., and McCormick, W. F., W. B. Saunders Company, Philadelphia, 1975.

Benesh, F. C., and Carl, G. F. Methyl biogenesis. *Biol. Psychiatry,* **13:** 465–80, 1978.

Betts, T. A.; Smith, W. T.; and Kelly, R. E. Adult metachromatic leukodystrophy (sulphatide lipidosis) simulating acute schizophrenia. *Neurology,* **18:** 1140–42, 1968.

Brandt, K. D.; Lessell, S.; and Cohen, A. S. Cerebral disorders of vision in systemic lupus erythematosus. *Ann. Intern. Med.,* **83:** 163–69, 1975.

Bresnan, M. J. Case records of the Massachusetts General Hospital. Scully, R. E.; Galdabini, J. J.; and McNeely, B. U., eds. *N. Engl. J. Med.,* **300:** 1037–45, 1979.

Brink, T. L. Idiot savant with unusual mechanical ability: an organic explanation. *Am. J. Psychiatry,* **137:** 250–51, 1980.

Campbell, M. Treatment of childhood and adolescent schizophrenia. Pp. 101–18 in *Psychopharmacology in Childhood and Adolescence.* Wiener, J. M., ed. Basic Books, Inc., New York, 1977.

Campbell, M.; Geller, B.; Small, A. M.; Petti, T. A.; and Ferris, S. H. Minor physical anomalies in young psychotic children. *Am. J. Psychiatry,* **135:** 573–75, 1978.

Cantor, S.; Trevenen, C.; Postuma, R.; Dueck, R.; and Fjeldsted, B. Is childhood schizophrenia a cholinergic disease? I: muscle morphology. *Arch. Gen. Psychiatry,* **37:** 658–67. 1980.

Carlsson, A. Antipsychotic drugs, neurotransmitters, and schizophrenia. *Am. J. Psychiatry,* **135:** 164–73, 1978.

Cartwright, G. E. Diagnosis of treatable Wilson's disease. *N. Engl. J. Med.,* **298:** 1347–50, 1978.

Chess, S. Autism in children with congenital rubella. *J. Autism Child. Schizophr.,* **1:** 33–47, 1971.

Chess, S.; Fernandez, P.; and Korn, S. Behavioral consequences of congenital rubella. *J. Pediatr.,* **93:** 699–703, 1978.

Clancy, H.; Entsch, M.; and Rendle-Short, J. Infantile autism: the correction of feeding abnormalities. *Dev. Med. Child Neurol.,* **11:** 569–78, 1969.

Clancy, H., and McBride, G. The isolation syndrome in childhood. *Dev. Med. Child Neurol.,* **17:** 198–219, 1975.

Cooper, J. R.; Bloom, F. E.; and Roth, R. H. In *The Biochemical Basis of Neuropharmacology,* 3rd ed. Oxford University Press, New York, 1978.

Cooper, P. E., and Martin, J. B. Neuroendocrinology and brain peptides. *Ann. Neurol.,* **8:** 551–57, 1980.

Corbett, J.; Harris, R.; Taylor, E., and Trimble, M. Progressive disintegrative psychosis in childhood. *J. Child Psychol. Psychiatry,* **18:** 211–19, 1977.

Corbett, L.; Christian, S. T.; Morin, R. D.; Bennington, F.; and Smythies, J. R. Hallucinogenic N-methylated indolealkylamines in the cerebrospinal fluid of psychiatric and control populations. *Br. J. Psychiatry,* **132:** 139–44, 1978.

Creak, M. (chairman), *et al.* Schizophrenic syndrome in childhood: further progress of a working party. *Dev. Med. Child Neurol.,* **6:** 530–35, 1964.

Damasio, A. R., and Maurer, R. G. A neurological model for childhood autism. *Arch. Neurol.,* **35:** 777–86, 1978.

Damasio, H.; Maurer, R. G.; Damasio, A. R.; and Chui, H. C. Computerized tomographic scan findings in patients with autistic behavior. *Arch. Neurol.,* **37:** 504–10, 1980.

Darby, J. K. Neuropathologic aspects of psychosis in children. *J. Autism Child. Schizophr.,* **6:** 339–52, 1976.

DeGroot, L. J., and Stanbury, J. B. *The Thyroid and Its Diseases,* 4th ed. John Wiley and Sons, New York, 1975, p. 769.

Demers-Desrosiers, L. A.; Nestoros, J. N.; and Vaillancourt, P. Acute psychosis precipitated by withdrawal of anticonvulsant medication. *Am. J. Psychiatry,* **135:** 981–82, 1978.

DeMyer, M. K.; Barton, S.; DeMyer, W. E.; Norton, J. A.; Allen, J.; and Steele, R. Prognosis in autism: a follow-up study. *J. Autism Child. Schizophr.,* **3:** 199–246, 1973.

Diagnostic and Statistical Manual of Mental Disorders, 3rd ed. American Psychiatric Association, Washington, D.C., 1980, pp. 86–92, 181–203.

Egdell, H. G., and Kolvin, I. Childhood hallucinations. *J. Child Psychol. Psychiatry,* **13:** 279–87, 1972.

Eisenberg, L. The autistic child in adolescence. *Am. J. Psychiatry,* **112:** 607–12, 1956.

Evans-Jones, L. G., and Rosenbloom, L. Disintegrative psychosis in childhood. *Dev. Med. Child Neurol.,* **20:** 462–70, 1978.

Faguet, R. A., and Rowland, K. F. "Spice cabinet" intoxication. *Am. J. Psychiatry,* **135:** 860–61, 1978.

Flor-Henry, P. Lateralized temporal-limbic dysfunction and psychopathology. *Ann. N.Y. Acad. Sci.,* **280:** 777–95, 1976.

Folstein, S., and Rutter, M. Infantile autism: a genetic study of 21 twin pairs. *J. Child Psychol. Psychiatry* **18:** 297–321, 1977.

Freeman, B. J.; Ritvo, E. R.; Schroth, P. C.; Tonick, I.; Guthrie, D.; and Wake, L. Behavioral characteristics of high- and low-IQ autistic children. *Am. J. Psychiatry,* **138:** 25–29, 1981.

Freeman, J. M.; Finkelstein, J. D.; and Mudd, S. H. Folate-responsive homocystinuria and "schizophrenia": a defect in methylation due to deficient 5,10-methylenetetrahydrofolate reductase activity. *N. Engl. J. Med.,* **292:** 491–96, 1975.

Goodman, J. A case study of an "autistic-savant": mental function in the psychotic child with markedly discrepant abilities. *J. Child Psychol. Psychiatry,* **13:** 267–78, 1972.

Gualtieri, C. T.; Barnhill, J.; McGimsey, J.; and Schell, D. Tardive dyskinesia and other movement disorders in children treated with psychotropic drugs. *J. Am. Acad. Child Psychiatry,* **19:** 491–510, 1980.

Gurland, B. J.; Ganz, V. H.; Fleiss, J. L.; and Zubin, J. The study of the psychiatric symptoms of systemic lupus erythematosus. *Psychosom. Med.,* **34:** 199–206, 1972.

Hauser, S. L.; DeLong, G. R.; and Rosman, N. P. Pneumographic findings in the infantile autism syndrome: a correlation with temporal lobe disease. *Brain,* **98:** 667–88, 1975.

Hier, D. B.: Lemay, M.: and Rosenberger, P. B. Autism: association with reversed cerebral asymmetry. *Neurology* (abs.), **28:** 348–49, 1978.

Hingtgen, J. N.; Coulter, S. K.; and Churchill, D. W. Intensive reinforcement of imitative behavior in mute autistic children. *Arch. Gen. Psychiatry,* **17:** 36–43, 1967.

Hyde, C.; Glancy, G.; Omerod, P.; Hall, D.; and Taylor, G. S. Abuse of indigenous psilocybin mushrooms: a new fashion and some psychiatric complications. *Br. J. Psychiatry,* **132:** 602–604, 1978.

Johnson, R. T., and Richardson, E. P. The neurological manifestations of systemic lupus erythematosus. *Medicine,* **47:** 337–69, 1968.

Judd, L. L.; Janowsky, D. S.; Segal, D. S.; Parker, D. C.; and Huey, L. Y. Behavioral effects of methadone in schizophrenic patients. *Am. J. Psychiatry,* **138:** 243–45, 1981.

Kagan, J. Personality, behavior and temperament. In *Human Development.* Falkner, F., ed. W. B. Saunders Company, Philadelphia, 1966, p. 332.

Kanner, L. Autistic disturbances of affective contact. *Nervous Child,* **2:** 217–50, 1943.

Kanner, L. Follow-up study of eleven autistic children originally reported in 1943. *J. Autism Child. Schizophr.* **1:** 119–45, 1971.

Kessler, K. A., and Waletzky, J. P. Clinical use of the antipsychotics. *Am. J. Psychiatry,* **138:** 202–209, 1981.

Kety, S. S. Genetic and biochemical aspects of schizophrenia. Pp. 93–102 in, *The Harvard Guide to Modern Psychiatry.* Nicholi, A. M., Jr., ed. Belknap Press, Cambridge, Mass., 1978.

Kety, S.; Rosenthal, D.; Wender, P. H.; Shulsinger, F.; and Jacobsen, B. Mental illness in the biological and adoptive families of adopted individuals who have become schizophrenic. *Behav. Genetics,* **6:** 219–25, 1976.

Kinney, D. K., and Matthysse, S. Genetic transmission of schizophrenia. *Ann. Rev. Med.*, **29:** 459–73, 1978.

Knobloch, H., and Pasamanick, B. Some etiologic and prognostic factors in early infantile autism and psychosis. *Pediatrics,* **55:** 182–91, 1975.

Kolvin, I.; Ounsted, C.; Humphrey, M.; and McNay, A., II. The phenomenology of childhood psychoses. *Br. J. Psychiatry,* **118:** 385–95, 1971.

Lindsay, J.; Ounsted, C.; and Richards, P. Long-term outcome in children with temporal lobe seizures. III: psychiatric aspects in childhood and adult life. *Dev. Med. Child Neurol.,* **21:** 630–36, 1979.

MacCrimmon, D. J.; Cleghorn, J. M.; Asarnow, R. F.; and Steffy, R. A. Children at risk for schizophrenia. *Arch. Gen. Psychiatry,* **37:** 671–74, 1980.

Malamud, N. Psychiatric disorder with intracranial tumors of limbic system. *Arch. Neurol.,* **17:** 113–23, 1967.

Manowitz, P.; Kling, A.; and Kohn, H. Clinical course of adult metachromatic leukodystrophy presenting as schizophrenia: a report of two living cases in siblings. *J. Nerv. Ment. Dis.,* **166:** 500–506, 1978.

Massie, H. N. The early natural history of childhood psychosis: ten cases studied by analysis of family home movies of the infancies of the children. *J. Am. Acad. Child Psychiatry,* **17:** 29–45, 1978.

Matthysse, S. Genetic detection of cerebral dysfunction. *N. Engl. J. Med.,* **302:** 516–17, 1980.

Maurer, R. G., and Damasio, A. R. Vestibular dysfunction in autistic children. *Dev. Med. Child Neurol.,* **21:** 656–59, 1979.

Morison, P., and Gardner, H. Dragons and dinosaurs: the child's capacity to differentiate fantasy from reality. *Child Dev.,* **49:** 642–48, 1978.

Oppenheimer, E. Y., and Rosman, N. P. Seizures in childhood: an approach to emergency management. *Pediatr. Clin. North Am.,* **26:** 837–55, 1979.

Papez, J. W. A proposed mechanism of emotion. *Arch. Neurol. Psychiatry,* **38:** 725–43, 1937.

Peters, H. A.; Cripps, D. J.; and Reese, H. H. Porphyria: theories of etiology and treatment. *Int. Rev. Neurobiol.,* **16:** 301–55, 1974.

Potkin, S. G.; Cannon, H. E.; Murphy, D. L.; and Wyatt, R. J. Are paranoid schizophrenics biologically different from other schizophrenics? *N. Engl. J. Med.,* **298:** 61–66, 1978.

Pritchard, P. B., III; Lombroso, C. T.; and McIntyre, M. Psychological complications of temporal lobe epilepsy. *Neurology,* **30:** 227–32, 1980.

Richer, J., and Richards, B. Reacting to autistic children: the danger of trying too hard. *Br. J. Psychiatry,* **127:** 526–69, 1975.

Rimland, B.; Callaway, E.; and Dreyfus, P. The effect of high doses of vitamin B_6 on autistic children: a double-blind crossover study. *Am. J. Psychiatry,* **135:** 472–75, 1978.

Ritvo, E. R.; Ornitz, E. M.; Eviatar, A.; Markham, C. H.; Brown, M. B.; and Mason, A. Decreased postrotatory nystagmus in early infantile autism. *Neurology,* **19:** 653–58, 1969.

Rivinus, T. M.; Jamison, D. L.; and Graham, P. J. Childhood organic neurological disease presenting as psychiatric disorder. *Arch. Dis. Child.,* **50:** 115–19, 1975.

Rutter, M. Infantile autism and other child psychoses. Pp. 717–47 in *Child Psychiatry: Modern Approaches.* Rutter, M., and Hersov, L., eds. Blackwell Scientific Publications, Oxford, 1977.

Saavedra, J. M.; Coyle, J. T.; and Axelrod, J. The distribution and properties of the nonspecific N-methyltransferase in brain. *J. Neurochem.,* **20:** 743–52, 1973.

Sahlmann, L. Autism or aphasia? *Dev. Med. Child Neurol.*, **11**: 443–48, 1969.

Salguero, L. F.; Itabashi, H. H.; and Gutierrez, N. B. Childhood multiple sclerosis with psychotic manifestations. *J. Neurol. Neurosurg. Psychiatry*, **32**: 572–79, 1969.

Schopler, E. Toward reducing behavior problems in autistic children. *J. Autism Child. Schizophr.*, **6**: 1–13, 1976.

Schopler, E., and Dalldorf, J. Autism: definition, diagnosis, and management. *Hosp. Pract.*, 64–73, June 1980.

Sedvall, G. C., and Wode-Helgodt, B. Aberrant monoamine metabolite levels in CSF and family history of schizophrenia. *Arch. Gen. Psychiatry*, **37**: 1113–16, 1980.

Shah, P., and Kaplan, S. L. Catatonic symptoms in a child with epilepsy. *Am. J. Psychiatry*, **137**: 738–39, 1980.

Shearer, M. L., and Finch, S. M. Periodic organic psychosis associated with recurrent herpes simplex. *N. Engl. J. Med.*, **271**: 494–97, 1964.

Shraberg, D., and Weisberg, L. The Klüver-Bucy syndrome in man. *J. Nerv. Ment. Dis.*, **166**: 130–34, 1978.

Slater, E., and Beard, A. W. The schizophrenia-like psychoses of epilepsy: i. psychiatric aspects. *Br. J. Psychiatry*, **109**: 95–150, 1963.

Snyder, S. H. Amphetamine psychosis: a "model" schizophrenia mediated by catecholamines. *Am. J. Psychiatry*, **130**: 61–67, 1973.

Snyder, S. H. Biochemical factors in schizophrenia. *Hosp. Pract.* 133–140, October 1977.

Spitz, R. A. *The First Year of Life: A Psychoanalytic Study of Normal and Deviant Development of Object Relations*. International Universities Press, Inc., New York, 1965.

Stein, J. A., and Tschudy, D. P. Acute intermittent porphyria: a clinical and biochemical study of 46 patients. *Medicine*, **49**: 1–16, 1970.

Steinberg, D. Psychotic disorders in adolescence. Pp. 748–70 in *Child Psychiatry: Modern Approaches*. Rutter, M., and Hersov, L., eds. Blackwell Scientific Publications, Oxford, 1977.

Stubbs, E. G. Autistic symptoms in a child with congenital cytomegalovirus infection. *J. Autism Child. Schizophr.* **8**: 37–43, 1978.

Szymanski, H. V. Prolonged depersonalization after marijuana use. *Am. J. Psychiatry*, **138**: 231–33, 1981.

Tanguay, P. E.; Ornitz, E. M.; Forsythe, A. B.; and Ritvo, E. R. Rapid eye movement (REM) activity in normal and autistic children during REM sleep. *J. Autism Child. Schizophr.* **6**: 275–88, 1976.

Taylor, D. C. Factors influencing the occurrence of schizophrenia-like psychosis in patients with temporal lobe epilepsy. *Psychol. Med.*, **5**: 249–54, 1975.

Torrey, E. F., and Peterson, M. R. Schizophrenia and the limbic system. *Lancet*, **2**: 942–46, 1974.

Verebey, K.; Volavka, J.; and Clouet, D. Endorphins in psychiatry: an overview and a hypothesis. *Arch. Gen. Psychiatry*, **35**: 877–88, 1978.

Wexler, B. E., and Heninger, G. R. Alterations in cerebral laterality during acute psychotic illness. *Arch. Gen. Psychiatry*, **36**: 278–84, 1979.

Whybrow, P. C.; Prange, A. J., Jr.; and Treadway, C. R. Mental changes accompanying thyroid gland dysfunction. *Arch. Gen. Psychiatry*, **20**: 48–63, 1969.

Williams, R. S.; Hauser, S. L.; Purpura, D. P.; DeLong, G. R.; and Swisher, C. N. Autism and mental retardation: neuropathologic studies performed in four retarded persons with autistic behavior. *Arch. Neurol.*, **37**: 749–53, 1980.

Wilson, L. G. Viral encephalopathy mimicking functional psychosis. *Am. J. Psychiatry*, **133**: 165–70, 1976.

Wing, L. *Autistic Children: A Guide for Parents.* Brunner/Mazel Publishers, New York, 1972.

Winsberg, B. G., and Yepes, L. E. Antipsychotics (major tranquilizers, neuroleptics). Pp. 234–73 in *Pediatric Psychopharmacology: The Use of Behavior Modifying Drugs In Children.* Werry, J. S., ed. Brunner/Mazel Publishers, New York, 1978.

ADDITIONAL READINGS

Anderson, W. H., and Kuehnle, J. C. Diagnosis and early management of acute psychosis. *N. Engl. J. Med.,* **305:** 1128–30, 1981.

Bergman, P., and Escalona, S. K. Unusual sensitivities in very young children. *Psychoanal. Study Child,* **3,** No. 4: 333–52, 1949.

Deniker, P. Introduction of neuroleptic chemotherapy into psychiatry. Pp. 155–64 in *Discoveries in Biological Psychiatry.* Ayd, F. J., Jr., and Blackwell, B., eds. Lippincott Company, Philadelphia, 1970.

Janssen, P. A. J. The butyrophenone story. Pp. 165–79 in *Discoveries in Biological Psychiatry.* Ayd, F. J., Jr., and Blackwell, B., eds. Lippincott Company, Philadelphia, 1970.

Mahler, M. S. On child psychosis and schizophrenia. *Psychoanal. Study Child,* **7:** 286–305, 1952.

Manschreck, T. C. Schizophrenic disorders. *N. Engl. J. Med.,* **305:** 1628–32, 1981.

North, C., and Cadoret, R. Diagnostic discrepancy in personal accounts of patients with "schizophrenia." *Arch. Gen. Psychiatry,* **38:** 133–37, 1981.

Park, C. C. *The Siege: The First Eight Years of an Autistic Child.* Little, Brown and Co., Boston, 1967.

Simon, N. Kaspar Hauser's recovery and autopsy: a perspective on neurological and sociological requirements for language development. *J. Autism Child. Schizophr.* **8:** 209–17, 1978.

Whitley, R. Diagnosis and treatment of herpes simplex encephalitis. *Ann. Rev. Med.,* **32:** 335–40, 1981.

Wing, L., ed. *Early Childhood Autism.* 2nd ed. Pergamon Press, Oxford, 1976.

Zimbardo, P. G.; Andersen, S. M.; and Kabat, L. G. Induced hearing deficit generates experimental paranoia. *Science,* **212:** 1529–31, 1981.

6 Depression

Depression is a normal part of life. It usually occurs in reaction to life experiences and typically is self-limited. Depression—the *syndrome* rather than just the *symptom*—is pathologic when the intensity of the emotional state is overwhelming, the degree of depression is out of proportion to the precipitating circumstances, or it persists.

Depression in childhood occurs at all ages. As children change markedly from infancy to adolescence, the symptomatology of depression will vary from one age to another. Characteristic manifestations of adult depression can be seen at any age, however, though associated problems may at times mask depressive symptoms.

This chapter will define depression, describe its clinical aspects, discuss conditions that might be mistaken for depression, analyze its causes, and discuss its treatment. Relevant anatomic, biochemical, and physiologic aspects of depression will be presented.

Among the questions that will be addressed are the following:

What forms does depression take in childhood?
What conditions must be differentiated from childhood depression?
What are the causes of depression?
How should the child who appears depressed be evaluated?
How should depression in childhood be managed?
What is the role of drugs?
What is the outlook for the depressed child?

DEPRESSION

DEFINITION

Before looking specifically at depression, it will be pertinent to consider the definitions of emotion, affect, mood, and emotional disorder. An *emotion* is a feeling state. Common examples from everyday life are sadness,

111

TABLE 6–1. **Definitions Related to Emotional State**

Emotion	Feeling state
Affect	Observed emotion
Mood	Pervasive and sustained emotion

joy, anger, and love. *Affect* is observed emotion. *Mood* is the pervasive and sustained emotion that colors the person's world and experiences. Affect is to mood as weather is to climate (*DSM*-III, 1980) (see Table 6–1). *Emotional disorder* is present when the feeling state significantly interferes with personal, familial, academic, or occupational spheres of activity.

Depression may be viewed as the child's reaction to loss. Perhaps this statement is an oversimplification, but nonetheless it provides a useful point of reference. The loss may be concrete or conceptual. Examples might be a loved person (due to death or separation), a valued object (misplaced, broken, or stolen), bodily integrity (due to disease or trauma), self-esteem (due to failure) or self-control (due to panic, weakness, lack of planning, or powerlessness).

The reaction to loss can be manifested through changes in several areas: affect, motor function, vegetative function, and state of arousal or attentiveness. A typical syndrome of depression thus involves subjective and objective sadness (affect), diminished activity (motor function), changes in sleeping and eating (vegetative functions), and difficulty in concentrating (attentiveness).

The *DSM*-III criteria for depressive disorder in school-age children include (1) dysphoric mood (depression, anxiety, or anger) or loss of interest or pleasure in (nearly) all usual activities and (2) several of the following:

   a. Significant change (increase or decrease) in appetite or weight,
   b. Sleep disturbance (hypersomnia or insomnia)
   c. Psychomotor retardation or agitation (hypoactivity or hyperactivity)
   d. Lack of energy
   e. Lowered self-esteem
   f. Excessive or inappropriate guilt
   g. Impaired thinking or concentration
   h. Suicidal thoughts or actions

Use of *DSM*-III criteria for diagnosis of depression in childhood has demonstrated their apparent validity (Cytryn *et al.*, 1980; Carlson and Cantwell, 1980). Application of these criteria has also shown that symptoms of so-called masked depression such as physical complaints, school avoidance, delinquency, and enuresis are often associated features of depressive syndromes. If the basic criteria for a depressive syndrome are sought in the presence of such symptoms, they often are met.

Depressive illness is one form of unipolar affective disorder. The other is manic disorder. The latter is defined (*DSM*-III, 1980) by periods lasting at least 1 week of elevated, expansive, or irritable mood, plus several of the following:

a. Increased activity or restlessness
b. Increased talkativeness
c. Flight of ideas or racing of thoughts
d. Grandiosity or inflated self-esteem
e. Diminished requirement for sleep
f. Increased distractability
g. Impulsive behavior

The overlap of manic disorder with syndromes of attention deficit disorder is obvious and important (see Chapter 14). Bipolar affective disorder, or manic-depressive disorder, includes periods of both mania and depression.

DIAGNOSIS

In considering the diagnosis of depression in childhood and adolescence, it is essential to keep in mind that depression is a descriptive diagnosis, not an etiologic diagnosis. As with problems such as seizure or headache, specific causes must be sought so that the most appropriate treatment plan can be made.

Clinical Process. *History.* A child rarely complains of depression. It is likely that the evaluation has been initiated by someone else. The teacher may have noted apathetic behavior, sleeping in class, or deterioration in school performance. The parents may be concerned about withdrawal from usual activities, irritability, and a general unhappiness. Court officers may have cited fighting and stealing.

As noted above, dysphoric mood is an important diagnostic criterion for a major depressive episode. The pervasive emotional state may be depression, anxiety, or anger typically associated with loss of interest or pleasure in usual activities. Other features of depression, also noted earlier, may include weight change (not related to dieting), sleep disturbance, altered activity level, easy fatiguability, self-deprecatory ideation, feelings of guilt, difficulties in concentration, suicidal thoughts, or somatic complaints such as headache or abdominal pain.

The degree of interference with the child's life should be determined. Has the child gotten along well with parents, other family members, and friends? Has he enjoyed school as much as usual and maintained previous levels of academic performance? Has he continued to pursue hobbies, afterschool sports, part-time jobs, and weekend activities?

It is important to learn what experiences may have precipitated or contributed to the depressive syndrome. Specific incidents may be identifiable such as the death of a grandparent, a parent's hospitalization, or a move to a new city. Medical problems such as asthma, migraine, and ulcerative colitis also may be significant. Medication history should be obtained.

If previous depressive episodes have occurred, their symptomatology and periodicity should be defined. What was their nature? How long did they last? What was the time interval between episodes? What diagnostic or therapeutic intervention was pursued? What appeared to help? Was intervening behavior normal, hyperactive, irritable, or aggressive?

Family history should include inquiry as to depressive illness in siblings, parents, aunts, uncles, and grandparents. Have family members been treated with psychoactive medication or electroconvulsive therapy? Have any been hospitalized for depression? Has any family member attempted or committed suicide? If so, when and by what means?

Review of systems should include questioning as to headaches, changes in coordination, urinary incontinence, visual disturbance, hallucinations, seizures, drug use, skin rashes, and constipation.

Examination. The *general description* of the depressed child should convey important features of the child's appearance. Sadness may be apparent as flattened facial contours, diminished expression, and absence of smiling (see Fig. 6–1). Posture may be bent as if in defeat or turned away in anger. Activity level may be diminished or exaggerated with fidgeting and glancing frequently around the room. Ordinary lines of questioning may produce tears or yield only stony silence.

Depression often has an "infectious" quality not unlike other affective states such as joy or hilarity. For that reason, the examiner's own feelings of sadness or depression provide objective data as to the child's mood.

The *general physical examination* should begin as usual with vital signs and measurement of growth parameters. The pulse may be slowed with hypothyroidism, temperature elevated with infection. Height, weight, and head circumference should be recorded and plotted on standard growth curves. Increase or decrease in weight should be noted. Examination of the skin should include inspection for self-inflicted wounds such as scars across the wrist or needle puncture marks. Truncal obesity and purplish-red abdominal striae would suggest Cushing syndrome.

Neurologic examination must include visualization of the optic fundi. Blurring of disk margins with increased intracranial pressure (papilledema)

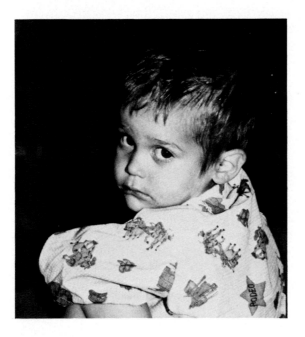

FIGURE 6–1. Sad child.

can occur without obvious headache (see Fig. 6–2). Cranial nerve examination should include attention to facial symmetry at rest, with voluntary effort
(such as retracting the corners of the mouth or wrinkling the forehead), and
with involuntary emotional actions (smiling or crying). When laughing or
crying are exaggerated or occur with minimal provocation, the concurrent
emotional state should be determined.

Changes in deep tendon reflexes may be seen with hypothyroidism (associated with slowed contraction and relaxation phases), multiple sclerosis (in
which reflexes may be exaggerated and asymmetric), and brain tumor or
other cause of increased intracranial pressure (in which reflexes are often
symmetrically increased with extensor plantar responses). It sometimes will
be valuable in conducting the *mental status examination* to interview the
child and the parent(s) separately. This separation may facilitate the child's
sharing of difficult, troubling, and personal information. The parents, too,
may be better able to provide information, particularly as to previous periods of depression or other behavioral disturbance.

When speaking with the child, further exploration of fantasies, fears, feelings about oneself, delusions, hallucinations, dreams, or suicidal thoughts
and actions (perhaps unknown to parents) can be carried out. Cytryn (1977)
has found that depressed children are likelier to have dreams in which they

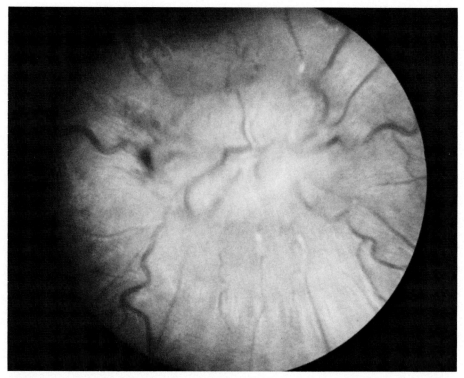

FIGURE 6–2. Marked elevation of optic disk and blurring of disk margins from increased intracranial pressure (papilledema).

are killed or injured than are children who are not depressed, who tend to escape or be rescued (see Case 6–1).

Suicide should be discussed in a straightforward, though not blunt, manner when appropriate. Acknowledging the child's depressed state, the examiner can ask, "Have you thought of harming yourself in any way?" "Have you made plans to injure or to kill yourself?" "Have you attempted to do so?"

In approaching the potentially suicidal child, assessment is directed toward understanding the child's distress, assessing his or her willingness to accept help, and evaluating the degree of suicide risk (Curran, 1979). At one end of the spectrum is a child who says, "I'll kill myself if I can't go to the movies tonight." At the other end is a child who has survived self-hanging only because of inadvertent discovery. Such information will influence importantly decisions as to whether hospitalization is required.

CASE 6–1: DEPRESSIVE SYNDROME WITH ATTENTION DEFICIT DISORDER IN A 10-YEAR-OLD BOY

C.D., a fifth-grade student, was evaluated because of behavioral problems. As the boy himself indicated: "I fight a lot." His mother described him as a loner, finding it difficult to establish or maintain friendships. "He craves friends, but doesn't know how to make or keep them," she said. In school, he performed at grade level despite attentional problems that had been noted since first grade. He did his best academically in a one-to-one situation. Past history was unremarkable—negative for seizures, significant head trauma, major medical problems, or frequent accidents. The family history included an uncle hospitalized for depression. No family members had committed suicide.

On examination, the child was a pleasant youngster, not overtly depressed, who was fidgety though attentive. He could repeat six digits forward. He told of a recurrent nightmare that involved his head being placed in a guillotine, the blade dropping, and his head being chopped off. He denied suicidal ideation or actions. The general physical and neurologic examinations were normal.

Comment. This youngster presented with an attention deficit disorder on a constitutional-developmental basis manifested by hyperkinesis, impulsivity, mood disturbance, attentional difficulties, and impaired social interactions. Although depression was not apparent in the office setting, his long-standing problems reflected a chronic affective disturbance. The significance of depressive components was reflected in the family history of significant depression and the child's dream in which a violent act was consummated. Psychiatric evaluation was recommended to identify psychosocial issues and consider the possible role of medication.

Although not found here, excessive risk-taking and frequent accidents would raise concerns as to "unintentional" self-destructive behavior.

Investigation. Investigations to be considered in evaluation of the child with depression are summarized in Table 6–2. Not every depressed child need undergo investigation. When intercurrent illness appears to be involved, relevant investigations should be undertaken. When the cause of depression is not evident, measurement of serum thyroxine, cortisol, electrolytes, and calcium levels may be worthwhile. For the child on anticonvulsant therapy, quantitation of blood levels may disclose toxic amounts. Analysis of urine and blood for toxic substances may be indicated at any age. Skull x-rays or computerized tomographic scan of the cranium should be carried out when structural intracranial pathology is suspected.

The dexamethasone suppression test and measurement of urinary MHPG (3-methoxy-4-hydroxyphenylglycol) are promising techniques in the evaluation of depression. With the dexamethasone suppression test, baseline values of serum cortisol are obtained in the morning, and 1 or 2 mg of dexamethasone are given that evening. The serum cortisol level is measured the next morning. Normally, the morning cortisol level is suppressed by dexamethasone. Some groups of depressed patients, however, fail to show such suppression (Sachar *et al.,* 1980).

Measurement of urinary MHPG may be useful in predicting responsiveness to one tricyclic antidepressant drug versus another (Cytryn *et al.,* 1974; Spiker *et al.,* 1980). MHPG, a major metabolite of norepinephrine, has been found in some studies to be low in concentration in the urine of persons who respond to imipramine. Elevated MHPG levels, by contrast, have been found in some patients responding to amitriptyline. It has been suggested that this latter group constitutes a different biochemical subtype, with dysfunction in the serotonergic rather than the catecholaminergic system.

Differential Diagnosis. In evaluating the child or adolescent who appears to have a depressive syndrome, it is important to keep in mind other conditions that may be mistaken for depression (see Table 6–3).

Misdiagnosis can occur when a child appears depressed but does not feel depressed. *Depressed appearance without emotional depression* often occurs when neuromuscular disease affects the muscles of facial expression (see Fig. 6–3). Facioscapulohumeral muscular dystrophy, myotonic dystrophy, and the Moebius syndrome typically produce a bland, sad-looking,

TABLE 6–2. **Investigations to Be Considered in the Depressed Child**

Thyroid function tests
Serum calcium
Serum electrolytes
Serum cortisol
Anticonvulsant blood levels
Toxic screen (urine, blood)
Skull x-rays
Cranial CT scan
Dexamethasone suppression test
Urinary MHPG levels

TABLE 6–3. **Differential Diagnosis of Depression**

Myopathic facial appearance
Pseudobulbar affect
Drug effect
Degenerative disease of central nervous system
Depressive reaction in examiner
Attention deficit disorder
Hypersomnia

myopathic facial appearance. A smile takes on a transverse (or even "snarling") configuration instead of the characteristic U-shape. A relatively expressionless face may also occur as a *drug effect*. Such changes can be seen with phenothiazines, butyrophenones, and methylphenidate.

Degenerative disease of the nervous system with manifestations of psychomotor slowing may be misperceived as depression. Parkinsonism provides an illustration from adulthood, Hallervorden-Spatz disease from childhood (see Case 8–4). Both disorders affect the basal ganglia and are associated with diminished facial expression that mimics a depressed appearance. In persons with Down syndrome, a premature dementia of Alzheimer type can occur (see Case 6–2).

CASE 6–2: DEPRESSIVE SYNDROME IN A 36-YEAR-OLD MAN WITH DOWN SYNDROME

I.B. was referred for evaluation because he was "continually losing weight and seemed unhappy," according to his mother. He had lost 15 pounds over one year without diarrhea, vomiting, or other gastrointestinal disturbance. His appetite even for ice cream, his favorite food, had diminished. He had lost no previously acquired skills and had manifested no deterioration in memory. He was taking no medications. He had experienced no trauma or major infections within the year. The only recent significant stress was the death 2 years previously of a relative with whom he had lived.

He had been the 6-pound, 8-ounce product of an uncomplicated full-term pregnancy, born to a 24-year-old woman with two normal children. Down syndrome was recognized at birth. He walked at 3 years, used single words at 4 years, and spoke in sentences at 7 years. Currently, he recognized some letters and words and worked in a sheltered workshop.

On examination, he was a subdued, slender, well-dressed man with characteristic features of Down syndrome. These included upward slant of the eyes, Brushfield spots of the irides, broad skull, and prominent tongue. He spoke in a low voice, showed little facial animation, and appeared sad. He did not express depressed thoughts. Head circumference was small (52.4 cm). General examination showed no evidence for hepatitis, thyroid disease, or other systemic disorder. Funduscopic examination was normal. Neurologic examination was unremarkable except for his gait. He walked slowly, bent forward slightly at the waist, with arms held stiffly alongside his

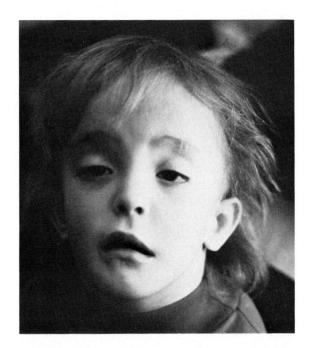

FIGURE 6–3. Sad facial appearance in girl with muscle disease.

legs. Gait was not festinating, and arising from a chair was not performed *en bloc*. Tone was normal.

Investigation included liver enzymes, serum electrolytes, thyroid function studies, and complete blood count. All were normal. CT scan of the head showed a mild degree of cortical atrophy diffusely. EEG in the awake state was normal.

Comment. This man certainly appeared depressed. Because of his mask-like facial appearance, bent posture, and diminished arm movements with walking, pseudodepression was considered, perhaps on the basis of basal ganglia disease. Parkinsonism was suggested by certain aspects of his examination, but cogwheel rigidity, festinating (accelerating) gait, and a tendency to get up from the seated position *en bloc* were absent.

Another condition that could produce psychomotor and affective depression is hypothyroidism, found with increased frequency among persons with Down syndrome. It was excluded in this case by normal thyroid function tests.

Dementia was an important diagnostic consideration in this man, since it tends to occur prematurely in persons with Down syndrome, during the third and fourth decades of life. By history, however, his memory and other intellectual functions had not deteriorated.

Depression due to unidentified psychosocial reasons remained the leading etiologic choice. Perhaps he was still suffering from the loss of his uncle 2 years previously. Further evaluation was recommended, as well as neurologic follow-up to exclude the possibility of dementing illness.

Pseudobulbar palsy is characterized by exaggerated or inappropriate affective display. Affect is inappropriate when it does not correspond to the subjective feeling state (for example, a person laughing hilariously though feeling sad). Such "emotional incontinence" results from loss of supranuclear input to brainstem nuclei that ultimately provide innervation to the facial muscles that express affect. As a result, fine modulation of expression is lost, and minimal emotional stimuli may set off a full-blown affective display.

Pseudobulbar palsy can occur with multiple sclerosis (see Chapter 13) or vascular injury to the brainstem. Such patients may, indeed, be depressed because of their neurologic illness and its associated disability. Recognition of their pseudobulbar state of affective disturbance will allow for more accurate perception of their true emotional state.

The *examiner's depressive reaction* to a child's illness or injury may contaminate his or her perception of the patient and lead to a misdiagnosis of depression.

Syndromes of *hypersomnia* and *attention deficit disorder* overlap with depression sufficiently so that they should be considered as alternative or additional diagnoses (see Chapters 9 and 14) (see Case 6–3).

Etiology.   Causes of depression are summarized in Table 6–4. Most depression in childhood is reactive, resulting from losses of various kinds. As discussed earlier in the section DEFINITION, the losses may be concrete or perceived. Illness itself is often cause for depression because of the loss of normal function it usually involves. Metabolic and structural causes of depression can be identified only infrequently, but depending upon the child's clinical picture they generally should be considered.

Medical Causes.   Medical illness, particularly chronic systemic illness, is an important cause of depression in childhood and adolescence. Asthma, ulcerative colitis, cystic fibrosis, and collagen vascular disease, such as systemic lupus erythematosus, are examples of systemic illness that may be chronically incapacitating, recurrently troubling, and depressing. Lupus (and its treatment) may also have more direct effects upon the brain.

Specific medical conditions associated with depression include hyperparathyroidism, Cushing syndrome, adrenal insufficiency, and hypothyroidism.

With *hyperparathyroidism,* a syndrome of fatigue, memory disturbance, psychomotor retardation, and affective disturbance may occur (Petersen, 1968; Smith *et al.,* 1972). Associated symptoms may include anorexia, constipation, headaches, and excessive thirst. Serum calcium levels are elevated (usually greater than 12 mg/dl) often with phosphorus levels below 4 mg/dl. Elevation in parathyroid hormone level is usually secondary to excessive secretion by a parathyroid gland adenoma. Serum calcium can also be significantly elevated with *vitamin D overdosage,* resulting in the same behavioral and emotional effects as noted with hyperparathyroidism.

Cushing syndrome may be associated with a variety of mental changes, including depression, euphoria, and psychosis (Smith *et al.,* 1972; Martin *et al.,* 1977; Ling *et al.,* 1981). The syndrome can be on a hypothalamic, pituitary, adrenal, or iatrogenic basis. It can be recognized by classic features of

CASE 6-3: DEPRESSION, AGGRESSIVE BEHAVIOR, AND ENCOPRESIS IN A 15-YEAR-OLD ADOLESCENT

F.G. was referred for evaluation because of temper tantrums, headache, and encopresis. He had been described since early childhood as moody, unhappy, withdrawn, and inclined to pull away when approached. Nocturnal enuresis had occurred until 9 years of age. The child tended to hold back his bowel movements, bowel-training was difficult, and fecal soiling had been a long-standing problem.

Since the age of 10 years, temper outbursts had occurred with increasing frequency. Precipitating events tended to be relatively trivial, such as a minor criticism or a refusal. The child had grabbed his mother in a bear hug, knocked his father down, and punched his fist through a wall. He was fully aware of his actions. Outbursts occurred only at home. Episodes were unaccompanied by pallor, rhythmic movements, or sweating.

Past history was notable for normal pregnancy, birth, and development except for mild clumsiness. Academic performance had been at grade level. Review of systems was notable for bifrontal supraorbital aching and pounding headaches, occurring up to twice weekly, brought on by anxiety and relieved by aspirin and rest. Headaches occurred without an aura and were unassociated with nausea or vomiting.

Upon examination, the child was a large, well-developed, unhappy-looking teenager. He minimized his problems and felt he could work them out himself. The only problem he volunteered was his headaches. He did not bring up the encopresis. He acknowledged readily that he had a "temper" but felt that it was under control. The general physical and neurologic examinations were normal. Investigations were unrevealing. They included a glucose tolerance test, which showed an asymptomatic dip in blood sugar to 51 mg/dl at 4 hours.

Comment. This youngster was clearly having difficulty in several areas, though he had been able to make adequate academic and social progress. His relationship with his parents continued to be disturbed, and individual and family psychotherapy was recommended.

The question arose in his evaluation as to whether his temper outbursts were ictal in nature. The specific features of the episodes, however, effectively excluded seizure. The tantrums involved purposeful, not automatic, behavior. He was fully aware of his outbursts and did not have symptoms of lethargy, tongue-biting, or urinary incontinence. A person who has had a seizure may, in fact, be somewhat aggressive during a postictal confusional state. Such behavior would not, however, be recalled fully if at all (see Chapter 12).

Because this child's symptoms of impulsive behavior and long-standing dysphoria overlapped with those of attention deficit disorder, a trial of dextroamphetamine (Dexedrine), methylphenidate (Ritalin), or imipramine (Tofranil)—in conjunction with psychotherapy and medical treatment for encopresis (see Chapter 10)—merited consideration.

TABLE 6–4. **Causes of Depression**

Medical	Chronic illness
	Hypothyroidism
	Cushing syndrome
	Adrenal insufficiency
	Hyperparathyroidism, hypercalcemia, vitamin D poisoning
Neurologic	Brain tumor or other cause of increased intracranial pressure
	Seizure disorder
	Migraine
	Degenerative neurologic disorder
Toxic	Sedatives (including barbiturates, alcohol)
	Stimulants (such as dextroamphetamine [Dexedrine] or methylphenidate [Ritalin] used with attention deficit disorder or with rebound following Dexedrine abuse)
	Anticonvulsants (such as phenobarbital, primidone [Mysoline])
	Antidepressants (including imipramine [Tofranil])
Psychologic	Reaction to loss or change
Social-Environmental	Situational events
Genetic-Constitutional	Unipolar or bipolar affective disorder
Developmental	Age-related stresses

moon-shaped facies, truncal obesity, abdominal striae, proximal muscle weakness, and demineralization of bone on x-ray.

Adrenal insufficiency, or *Addison disease,* has also been associated with mental disturbances that include depression and psychosis (Smith *et al.,* 1972; Sachar, 1974). Diagnosis is suggested on history by anorexia, weight loss, salt craving, and poor resilience with minor infections. On examination, hyperpigmentation of skin folds, gums, and areolae is a classic finding, but it may be subtle or absent.

Hypothyroidism characteristically presents with a picture of psychomotor retardation of insidious onset and slow progression. Depressed mood can be a prominent part of the behavioral syndrome (Whybrow *et al.,* 1969; Smith *et al.,* 1972; Martin *et al.,* 1977, Gold *et al.,* 1981). Diagnosis is suggested by overall slowing in physical and mental activities (the child often becoming unusually "agreeable") fall-off in height, dry skin, and abnormal deep tendon reflexes. Reflexes are "hung-up"; that is, the contraction and relaxation phases are prolonged. Thyroid function studies should confirm the diagnosis.

Neurologic Causes. Hemispheric differences in affective function have been recognized for decades. A striking example is the difference in affect in adults who have suffered left versus right middle cerebral artery strokes associated with a contralateral hemiparesis. Persons with left-sided lesions typically have a severe depressive response, at least initially. Those with a right-sided lesion are characteristically indifferent or even jocular.

In studies of persons with temporal lobe epilepsy, Flor-Henry (1976) found affective disorder more common among those with right rather than left hemisphere seizure foci. Other electrophysiologic and neurophysiologic investigations have led to somewhat conflicting data as to laterality and specificity within each hemisphere (Tucker *et al.*, 1981).

When the frontal or temporal lobes are involved by a *brain tumor*, affective disturbances such as depression, irritability, or apathy may result. Tumors produce their effects in such cases by direct invasion of brain tissue, by compression of vascular supply, and by causing cerebral edema. On the other hand, brain tumors in childhood may produce a depressive syndrome due to elevation of intracranial pressure alone. Symptoms of irritability, difficulty in concentrating, and worsening school performance are often of subtle onset and progression, and headache need not dominate the clinical picture (see Cases 6–4 and 11–3).

Seizures and *migraine* are often associated with recurrent affective changes that suggest depression. An ictal aura may be emotional in nature, experienced by the person as fear, gloom, or sadness. Such auras, in themselves focal seizures, need not progress to a generalized seizure. Hence, a child might experience recurrent episodes of dysphoria whose convulsive nature escapes notice.

Migraine auras, like those of epilepsy, can exist independent of the headache. Irritability, anger, and tearfulness commonly occur before or during a migraine attack. These are often associated with vegetative signs such as lethargy, fatigue, or change in appetite (Sacks, 1970). The diagnosis of migraine is suggested by pounding headaches, characteristic aura, autonomic symptoms including gastrointestinal upset, and a positive family history (see Chapter 11).

In addition to being a cause of depressive symptoms, however, migraines (and other headaches as well) are often a result of affective disorder (Ling *et al.*, 1970).

A *chronic neurologic disease* like a chronic medical illness, particularly if it is a degenerative disorder, can itself cause a depressive reaction (see Chapters 8 and 21). An inexorable downhill course, combined with lack of specific treatment, can create gloom that envelops a family and child. Further, if the family withdraws from the affected child in anticipation of death, the child's depression may be vastly worsened.

Toxic Causes. Both prescribed and illicitly used drugs can cause or contribute to depression. They may complicate the clinical picture further when ingested for suicidal purposes (see Case 6–5).

Anticonvulsant medication may cause psychomotor retardation when taken in excess. Addition of a second anticonvulsant medication may influence metabolism of the first drug, rendering a previous anticonvulsant dos-

CASE 6–4: IRRITABILITY AND WORSENED SCHOOL PERFORMANCE IN AN 11-YEAR-OLD GIRL WITH A BRAIN TUMOR

L.C. was evaluated because of headaches and behavior disturbance occurring over 12 to 18 months. Headaches were bifrontal and pounding in quality. They had increased gradually to a maximum of two to three times per week, lasting from 1 to several hours. The headaches were occasionally associated with nausea, rarely with vomiting. Pain was not increased with shaking of the head nor with coughing. Episodes of visual obscuration had not occurred.

Over the preceding 2 years, school performance had deteriorated and interactions with peers and siblings worsened, apparently due to irritability. She had been involved in weekly psychotherapy for a year and a half for treatment of apparent emotional problems at the time of evaluation. Two episodes of "rubbery-leggedness" had led to her being sent home from school and to her mother's insistence on neurologic evaluation.

On examination, the child was alert, subdued, and cooperative. She did not appear at all anxious or depressed. Indeed, she demonstrated an appropriate sense of humor during the "lighter sides" of the interview. General physical examination was normal. Neurologic examination was remarkable for advanced papilledema bilaterally on funduscopic examination. The remainder of the neurologic examination was strikingly normal, although reflexes were generally increased, and she had mild difficulties in coordinative tasks involving her legs.

Investigations confirmed the clinical impression of increased intracranial

age intolerable. Sodium valproate (Depakene), for example, tends to elevate blood levels of phenobarbital. Quantitation of blood levels will confirm or identify this problem.

In addition to these dose-related effects, some children have idiosyncratic reactions to anticonvulsant medication. With phenobarbital and primidone (Mysoline), for example, moodiness, irritability, and hyperactivity may be associated (Stores, 1975).

Some children treated with dextroamphetamine or methylphenidate for attention deficit disorder develop a depressive syndrome. Characteristic symptoms are sadness, listlessness, weepiness, mournfulness, and hopelessness (Cantwell, 1977). The basis for this effect is unclear.

Other drugs used for therapeutic purposes that may also be associated with depressive syndromes include imipramine and corticosteroids (see Case 6–6).

Psychologic Causes.   Depression on a reactive basis is the commonest cause for childhood depression, both the symptom and the disorder. As described above, depression appears to occur as a psychophysiologic response to loss. A depressive reaction to illness, injury, or significant psychosocial

pressure. Plain skull x-rays demonstrated splitting of cranial sutures and erosion of the sella turcica (see Fig. 6–4). CT scan showed moderately severe hydrocephalus including part of the fourth ventricle, where a mass was evident.

She underwent ventriculoperitoneal shunting for hydrocephalus and 2 days later had a posterior fossa exploration, which disclosed an infiltrative mass (a medulloblastoma) that could be removed only subtotally. She received radiation therapy and chemotherapy over the following weeks but succumbed to her illness several months later.

Comment. This case is troubling in several respects. Unlike most headache syndromes in childhood, this one did not declare itself by history alone. Indeed, the pounding character of the headache would suggest migraine, and the lack of persistence of the headache (occurring with a maximum frequency of three times weekly) might lead one away from increased intracranial pressure.

This case emphasizes that symptoms of brain tumor in childhood may develop gradually and insidiously. Symptoms tend not to be manifested as seizures or focal deficits, as in adults, but rather as nonspecific changes in personality (irritability in this instance) and school performance (perhaps related to concentration problems). The reason for this presentation is based on the characteristic location of brain tumors in childhood—in the posterior fossa, often near to the midline. As a result, hydrocephalus can develop gradually with minimal signs or symptoms of motor dysfunction.

This case underscores the importance of funduscopic evaluation in the child with academic and behavioral deterioration, whether headaches are present or not.

stress (such as divorce) is so predictable that it can be assumed. It should be treated according to its severity (see Case 6–7).

In psychodynamic terms, depression may result from anger directed against the self. For example, angry thoughts or actions toward a sibling may cause anxiety, guilt, and ultimately depression in the child.

Social-Environmental Causes. Social and environmental events normally provide stresses of varying degrees in everyone's life. Moving to a new city, changing schools, experiencing a death in the family or the birth of a sibling all demand adjustment and change. Several of these events occurring at once may be particularly stressful for family and child and cause or contribute to a depressive syndrome.

Genetic-Constitutional Causes. Genetic factors in affective illness are suggested by increased risk among first-degree relatives and by the more than doubled concordance among monozygotic as opposed to dizygotic twins: 43 per cent versus 19 per cent for unipolar illness, 74 per cent versus 17 per cent for bipolar (Schlesser *et al.,* 1980; Waters and Marchenko-Bouer, 1980; Weitkamp *et al.,* 1980). Such data suggest a multifactorial

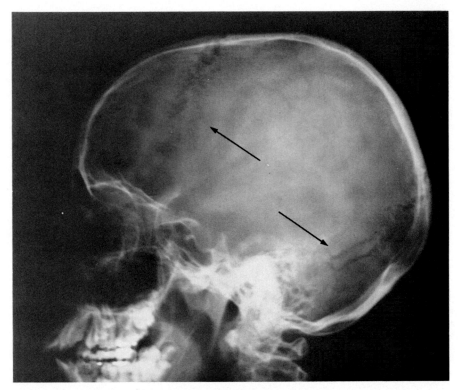

FIGURE 6–4. Lateral radiograph of skull showing splitting of cranial sutures (coronal and lambdoid indicated with arrows) (Case 6–4).

mode of inheritance and patterns of heritability that may differ among familial subgroups.

In the adult population, the prevalence of major depressive disorder among women is double that in men. The figures in childhood and adolescence have not been determined. In the series of Weinberg and colleagues (1973) involving forty-two children, the ratio was three girls to five boys.

Developmental Causes. Normal development carries with it readily identifiable periods of stress that may contribute to a depressive syndrome. These periods of change include going off to kindergarten, advancing to junior high school, entering puberty, being graduated from high school, and beginning college (Committee on Adolescence, 1980). These developmental stresses may be combined with others, as described above in SOCIAL-ENVIRONMENTAL CAUSES.

The degree to which early experiences cause or predispose to later depression has not been determined (Arieti and Bemporad, 1980). The concept of "learned helplessness" has been proposed to account for later depression in some persons. Others have suggested that early parenting experiences (for example, mothering that is variably adequate because of physical illness, affective disorder, or drug abuse) may lead to an infant's alternation in emotional state between complete satisfaction and helpless rage, providing a prototype for later mood swings.

CASE 6–5: INTENTIONAL ANTICONVULSANT OVERDOSAGE IN A 6-YEAR-OLD BOY

A.I. was brought to the emergency room by his mother because he had "trouble walking." He went to bed as usual the evening prior to hospitalization, awakened during the night, and crawled into his mother's bed. In the morning he was more difficult to arouse than usual, complained of being drowsy, and was unable to walk.

In the emergency room, the child was lethargic but responded to verbal stimulation. When not engaged in conversation, he drifted off to sleep. General examination was normal. Neurologic examination showed horizontal nystagmus that was gaze-evoked. Speech was dysarthric. Coordination was impaired in general. He was unable to walk without assistance. Past history was notable for seizures of unknown cause that began at 3 years of age. The child had been treated with phenobarbital, which made him intolerably hyperactive, so he was placed on phenytoin (Dilantin). Early development was delayed. He walked at 18 to 24 months and spoke in sentences at 5 years. The parents had been separated for 2 years. The child had recently been furious with his mother because of the separation. Although he denied intending to kill himself, he took extra phenytoin tablets in an angry, impulsive gesture.

Comment. Transiently altered mental status and impaired coordination in a child with a seizure disorder would ordinarily suggest that the child was postictal, having just had a seizure. In this instance, however, the persistence of slurred speech, incoordination, drowsiness, and exaggerated nystagmus suggested phenytoin toxicity. This diagnosis was confirmed by a blood level of 3.8 mg/dl, double the usual upper therapeutic limit.

Although overdosage of medication is classically associated with adolescence, self-destructive thoughts and actions are probably more frequent at younger ages than is commonly recognized. In this case, an angry, immature, and depressed child acted out his feelings to produce the syndrome described above. Acute psychiatric consultation was followed by outpatient psychotherapy, and the child did well over at least the next 2 years.

TREATMENT AND OUTCOME

Although syndromes of depression are usually self-limited (the child eventually, it is said, "gets over it"), treatment should be directed toward diminishing the intensity and duration of suffering and interference with normal activity. Psychotherapy is a cornerstone of treatment. It can help the child understand what he or she is feeling and what has caused the depression, and can suggest ways to deal with it now and in the future. If contributing medical or neurologic factors are identified, they should be treated specifically. In some instances use of antidepressant medication will be helpful.

Medical Management. Treatment of systemic illness should be undertaken to reverse the depressive spiral of fatigue, apathy, and curtailment of

CASE 6–6: DEPRESSIVE SYNDROME IN A 12-YEAR-OLD BOY TREATED WITH IMIPRAMINE FOR MIGRAINE

F.V. was begun on imipramine, 25 mg three times daily, for treatment of a migraine syndrome characterized by throbbing headaches associated with nausea that had been unresponsive to standard pain medications. Approximately one week later his mother noted him to be easily provoked to crying. No stressful events of significance could be identified within the preceding weeks to months.

On examination, the boy appeared mildly depressed and acknowledged feeling sad. Most striking was his response to even minimally stressful questions such as, ''How has school gone for you this year?'' He became red in the face and burst into tears five times within half an hour. He indicated that he felt sad during these crying episodes. The remainder of the examination was normal.

Imipramine was discontinued over 3 days. Within a week, lability of mood had cleared completely and behavior returned to normal. Headaches did not recur.

Comment. It is ironic that imipramine, an antidepressant medication, should produce a depressive syndrome in this child. The mechanism for this apparent effect is obscure, but it may have resulted from drug-related sleep disturbance (see Chapter 9).

The extraordinary lability of the child's emotional display suggested a pseudobulbar state. His neurologic examination did not, however, support that possibility.

Among illicitly used drugs, barbiturates and alcohol depress the central nervous system and may produce affective depression as well. The use of amphetamines, central nervous system stimulants, is typically followed by a ''down'' period, which may be manifested by hypersomnolence, inattentiveness, and affective depression. In approaching the child or adolescent abusing such drugs, one should keep in mind that these drugs may be used to ward off depression or other intolerable emotion.

usual pursuits and to restore the child to a more normal sense of well-being and activity. With asthma, for example, therapy might involve adequate rest, hydration, and nutrition, combined with bronchodilators and antibiotics. Should the child have cystic fibrosis (or other progressive chronic disease), then long-range issues of survival and quality of life can contribute significantly to the child's depressive syndrome (see Chapter 21).

Antidepressant medication in childhood and adolescence should be used only after careful consideration. It should never be the sole mode of therapy. Medications commonly employed, the tricyclic compounds imipramine (Tofranil) and amitriptyline (Elavil), have significant side effects and serious toxicity in overdosage. For that reason and because most children will respond to other therapeutic measures, it is recommended that antidepressant

CASE 6–7: HEADACHES AND DEPRESSION IN A 9-YEAR-OLD BOY

L.B. missed 3 weeks of school because of "needlelike" frontal headaches of sudden onset unaccompanied by nausea, vomiting, or lethargy. During this period, he gained 10 pounds, stayed at home, and watched television or read. Coordination and sleep patterns were unchanged. He had not sustained recent head trauma. He was next to youngest in a sibship of five. His father was a businessman whose work kept him busy every day of the week and many evenings as well. Mother was active in local politics and a regular tennis player.

On examination, the boy was a sad-appearing child who manifested a poverty of spontaneous movement. He acknowledged his state of unhappiness and noted that he complained of headache and ate impulsively when angry. The general physical and neurologic examinations were normal.

This child's headaches appeared to be part of a depressive syndrome. Psychosocial history suggested chronic "emotional malnutrition," but the reasons for the several-week deterioration in function were not established. Pharmacologic treatment was begun with amitriptyline. A structured activity program (including return to school) was established for the child, and the family was referred for psychiatric assessment and therapy.

Comment. The diagnosis of depressive syndrome in this case was established by inclusion, as well as exclusion. Other causes for persistent headache, such as sinusitis or increased intracranial pressure, were not borne out by history or examination. The diagnosis of depression was based upon dysphoric mood, somatic complaints (headaches), vegetative disturbance (weight gain), and interference with normal functioning (school attendance). Antidepressant medication was employed because of the intensity of affective disturbance and the associated disruption of normal activity.

medication not be employed unless (1) the severity of the depressive illness warrants such a trial, (2) the clinical situation can be monitored adequately as to improvement and side effects, and (3) the risk of overdosage (suicidal or otherwise) to the patient or others is not prohibitive (see Table 6–5). Childproof containers or individually wrapped pills should be specified by prescription.

Imipramine (Tofranil) can be used in daily dosages of 10 to 60 mg in younger children, 50 to 150 mg in older children and adolescents, divided into two or three portions (Lucas, 1978). Side effects include dry mouth and other anticholinergic effects, appetite disturbance, tremulousness, tachycardia, other arrhythmias, orthostatic hypotension, lowered seizure threshold, and dermatitis (Rapoport and Mikkelsen, 1978). Glaucoma and cardiac disorders usually contraindicate use of tricyclic antidepressant compounds. Beneficial clinical response should be evident days to weeks after initiation of therapy.

Definite indications for the use of monoamine oxidase (MAO) inhibitors in the treatment of childhood depression have not been established, although

TABLE 6–5. **Antidepressant Drugs**

	Usual Daily Dose (mg)	Main Side Effects
Tricyclics		
Imipramine (Tofranil)	10–60 (younger children) 50–150 (older children)	Blurred vision, dry mouth, dizziness, constipation, urinary retention, tachycardia, orthostatic hypotension, cardiac arrhythmia, fatigue, weakness, manic excite-ment, delirium
Amitriptyline (Elavil)	75–200*	
Nortriptyline (Aventyl)	75–150*	
Doxepin (Sinequan)	75–150*	
Protriptyline (Vivactyl)	15–40*	
Monoamine oxidase inhibitors		
Isocarboxazid (Marplan)	10–30*	Orthostatic hypotension, hepatotoxicity, tremor, insomnia, hyperhydrosis, constipation, hyper-tensive crises
Phenelzine (Nardil)	15–30*	
Tranylcypromine (Parnate)	20–30*	
Lithium salts		
Lithium carbonate (Eskalith)	450–1,200	Polyuria, polydipsia, thyroid gland enlarge-ment, vomiting, diarrhea, abdominal pain, tremor, ataxia, lethargy, coma, cardiac arrhythmias, hypo-tension, renal abnormalities

* Usual adult dosage. Standard therapeutic dosages for children have not been established.

several of these have been employed in pediatric trials (Lucas, 1978; Rapo-port and Mikkelsen, 1978). This class of drugs includes phenelzine (Nardil), tranylcypromine (Parnate), and isocarboxazid (Marplan).

The interaction of a monoamine oxidase inhibitor with certain foods or other drugs constitutes a serious risk in persons taking medication of this kind. Severe hypertensive crises can result from the combination of a mon-oamine oxidase inhibitor and foods with high tyramine content such as cer-tain beers, wines, and cheeses, pickled herring, chicken liver, and coffee. Blood pressure elevation occurs because of the norepinephrine-releasing ef-fect of tyramine, whose breakdown is opposed by the MAO inhibitor. Ad-verse reactions also can occur when MAO inhibitors are combined with other drugs, including another MAO inhibitor, amphetamines, or other sym-pathomimetic agents (Lucas, 1978; Weiner, 1980).

Lithium, extensively used in adults for treatment of major affective disor-ders, has been less widely employed in children and adolescents. Accordingly, its clinical effects, both therapeutic and toxic, remain to be determined more definitively within the pediatric age range (see Case 15–4). In adults, lithium is used for treatment of acute manic episodes and for prophylactic maintenance therapy in bipolar affective disorders.

Reviews of lithium use in children and adolescents have suggested criteria that make a beneficial response more likely (Lucas, 1978; Youngerman and Canino, 1978; DeLong, 1978). These include a clinical course of bipolar (manic-depressive) disease, a history of this disorder within the family (particularly if lithium-responsive), or the symptom complex of excitement, explosiveness, impulsiveness, aggressiveness, and hyperactivity. The usual therapeutic dosage of lithium carbonate ranges from 450 to 1200 mg daily. Blood levels should be maintained generally within a range of 0.5–1.2 mEq/L. Renal and thyroid function studies should be obtained periodically because of potential side effects.

Side effects of lithium use include polyuria and polydipsia (constituting a form of diabetes insipidus), nausea, diarrhea, weakness, tremor, and blurred vision. Overdosage is marked by lethargy, vomiting, and coma.

Carbamazepine (Tegretol) has appeared to benefit some adults with manic-depressive syndromes, particularly those with abnormal electroencephalograms (Ballenger and Post, 1980). The usefulness of this drug in treating affective disorders in childhood and adolescence has not yet been determined.

Dietary treatment of depression in adults is being actively explored. Studies have indicated a beneficial response to tryptophan (a serotonin precursor) in some adults and to tyrosine (a precursor of norepinephrine) in others (Møller et al., 1980; Gelenberg et al., 1980). The effects of dietary therapy in children have not been reported.

Endocrine disorders associated with depression will be specifically amenable to treatment. Hypothyroidism is treated with replacement thyroid hormone, adrenal insufficiency with glucocorticoids and mineralocorticoids. Hyperparathyroidism occurring secondary to parathyroid adenoma is treated surgically, as may be several of the forms of Cushing syndrome.

When depressive syndromes occur secondary to drug effects (as with dextroamphetamine, methylphenidate, imipramine, phenobarbital, or primidone), these medications should be withdrawn carefully.

Neurologic Management. The treatment of headache is frequently a component of the management of depressive syndromes of childhood and adolescence. If headache is recognized as part of a depressive syndrome, a more comprehensive approach to the problem can be made and escalating doses of increasingly potent analgesics can be avoided. Pain medication of mild-to-moderate strength, in conjunction with other modes of therapy, should suffice with most headache syndromes (see Chapter 11).

The treatment of brain tumors and seizures is discussed in Chapters 11 and 12. With chronic neurologic disease of any kind (such as spinal cord injury or Huntington disease), the depressive syndrome can be managed according to the principles suggested in this section and in Chapter 21.

Surgical Management. As mentioned above, hyperparathyroidism may be treated surgically. As the calcium metabolic disturbance is corrected, the affective state may return entirely to normal (Smith et al., 1972).

With Cushing syndrome caused by a pituitary tumor, removal by a transphenoidal approach (through the nasopharynx) may be carried out with or without radiation therapy. In other forms of Cushing syndrome, adrenal surgery is performed.

With other brain tumors, surgical therapy may include ventriculoperitoneal shunting to relieve obstructive hydrocephalus and definitive removal of the tumor insofar as it is possible.

Psychotherapy.   Individual and family-centered psychotherapy is often valuable in treating childhood depression. Treating depression is far more difficult than treating a streptococcal pharyngitis. When depression is of moderate severity or greater, psychotherapy should be carried out by an experienced mental health professional.

Supportive therapy can provide encouragement, hope, optimism, and suggestions for constructive activity. Family sessions can enhance understanding of the causes of the problem and can establish guidelines for participation of family members in overall management. Insight-oriented psychotherapy, when appropriate, should be undertaken cautiously and gently.

For the depressed child who may have unexpressed suicide potential, channels of communication must be established. The child must understand that he or she is not isolated and that help is available virtually immediately in person or by telephone. It is important for the depressed child to learn that, with time and with therapy, recovery is an achievable goal.

Social-Environmental Management.   Hospitalization is a potentially lifesaving aspect of treatment with the severely depressed child or adolescent, especially when suicidal (Eisenberg, 1980). Clear indications for hospitalization of the depressed child include (1) a significant suicide attempt, (2) an uncommunicative child, (3) psychosis, (4) rejecting, unconcerned, or unavailable parents, (5) major vegetative disturbance (such as inanition or dehydration), or (6) other significant intercurrent medical problems.

Inpatient management of the acutely suicidal patient generally requires the continuous presence of an attendant who is skilled in the care of children potentially dangerous to themselves or others. If the child is not admitted to a room on the ground floor, windows must be made inaccessible. Matches, knives, drugs, and other potentially harmful items also must be made unavailable.

For outpatient management, firearms and other dangerous weapons should be removed from the home and unused medications thrown away. Drugs that are currently being taken should be kept in small amounts only, unavailable, in childproof containers. Scheduled activities can help depressed children and adolescents become more involved in daily life. Thus, progressive inertia, apathy, brooding, and sadness can be counteracted or minimized.

A beneficial response to partial deprivation of total sleep and rapid eye movement sleep has been described in depressed adults (Vogel *et al.*, 1980; Schilgen and Tölle, 1980). These modes of therapy have not been reported in children.

Physical Therapy.   Physical therapy has long been recognized to offset depression. This effect appears to be mediated through time-structuring and distraction, as well as by neurochemical changes currently under investigation. The role of regular physical activity such as jogging in treating depression in childhood has not been established.

Mechanical Therapy. Electroconvulsive therapy has played a useful, though oftentimes controversial, role in the treatment of depressive disorders in adults (Fink, 1978; Paul *et al.*, 1981). It is occasionally used in children with severe depression refractory to pharmacologic and other modes of therapy (de la Fuente and Rosenbaum, 1980). No clear indications for its use in children have been determined, however.

CORRELATION

Anatomic Aspects. The hypothalamus is intimately involved in essential autonomic vegetative functions of the human organism. It has major input into eating, sleeping, and sexual functions. It influences pulse and blood pressure as part of the classic "fight or flight" reaction. It contributes to emotional states such as rage, anxiety, and depression. The hypothalamus influences a wide variety of organ systems, themselves distributed widely. It does this through neuroanatomic connections to nearby structures and through neurohumoral connections to more distant structures via the bloodstream and cerebrospinal fluid pathways (Martin *et al.*, 1977; Tepperman, 1980).

The pituitary gland, lying immediately below the hypothalamus, is a major target organ (see Fig. 6–5). It receives "direction" from the hypothalamus by both neuroanatomic and neurohumoral means. Nerve cells within the hypothalamus manufacture antidiuretic hormone (or vasopressin) and oxytocin. These hormones travel within nerve fibers through the infundibular stalk to enter the posterior pituitary or neurohypophysis, from which they are released into the bloodstream.

Hormones of the anterior pituitary, or adenohypophysis, are synthesized there. These consist of thyrotropin (thyroid-stimulating hormone, or TSH), corticotropin (or adrenocorticotropic hormone, ACTH), luteinizing hormone (LH), follicle-stimulating hormone (FSH), growth hormone (GH), prolactin, melanocyte-stimulating hormone (MSH), and beta-lipotropin.

The delivery of these hormones to the systemic circulation is controlled through releasing substances produced in the hypothalamus and sent "downstream" to the pituitary gland via the hypothalamic-hypophysial portal system of blood vessels. These hypothalamic substances include thyrotropin-releasing hormone (TRH), corticotropin-releasing factor (CRF), luteinizing hormone-releasing hormone (LHRH), growth hormone release-inhibiting hormone (GIH, or somatostatin), and prolactin release-inhibiting factor (PIF).

CRF, then, of hypothalamic origin, reaches the anterior pituitary via the hypothalamic-hypophysial portal system to cause liberation of ACTH. ACTH travels by way of the systemic bloodstream to the adrenal gland where it stimulates production of adrenocortical hormones.

Biochemical Aspects. Although the biochemical basis of depression has not been fully elucidated, several important points have been established.

Both the toxic and the therapeutic effects of certain drugs clarify the im-

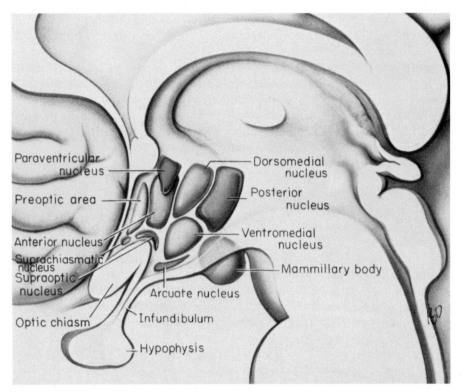

FIGURE 6–5. Hypothalamic nuclei in relation to the hypophysis (pituitary gland) and neighboring structures. (From Carpenter, M. B. *Core Text of Neuroanatomy,* 2nd ed. © 1978, The Williams & Wilkins Company, Baltimore.)

portance of monoamines. The chronic use of reserpine, an antihypertensive agent, has been well recognized to cause a prolonged and severe depressive syndrome in adults. This effect apparently occurs because reserpine interferes with storage of norepinephrine and serotonin in granules in presynaptic neurons where these neurotransmitters are made (Cooper *et al.*, 1978). As a result, less monoaminergic neurotransmitter is available to act at postsynaptic membranes.

The effectiveness of monoamine oxidase-inhibiting drugs in treating depression in adults further underscores the importance of monoamines in depressive disorders. Although the primary means of inactivation of norepinephrine and serotonin is reuptake from the synaptic cleft, further inactivation occurs when these transmitter substances are broken down within the presynaptic neuron (following reuptake) by monoamine oxidase. By counteracting this catabolic effect, monoamine oxidase inhibitors increase amounts of norepinephrine and serotonin available in the presynaptic neuron, thus causing pharmacologic and clinical effects opposite those of reserpine.

Lithium, by contrast, appears to act by inhibiting release of norepinephrine and serotonin, as well as by facilitating reuptake of norepinephrine. The mood-altering effects (if any) of lithium upon nonneural membranes remain to be clarified (Tosteson, 1981).

Physiologic Aspects. The hypothalamic-pituitary-adrenal (HPA) system appears to play a significant role in depression as suggested by several data. Baseline levels of serum cortisol are elevated in some persons with depression. The diurnal variation in cortisol levels (normally high in the morning, low in the evening) is not seen. Cortisol is not suppressed with administration of dexamethasone, a synthetic corticosteroid (see INVESTIGATION). The significance of these changes, their applicability to persons of different ages and categories of depression, and therapeutic implications remain to be established.

Ordinarily the administration of dexamethasone will mimic an endogenous increase in corticosteroids and inhibit the body's own production of cortisol. Corticosteroid production is under feedback control, which provides for relatively stable blood levels of hormone. Control of corticosteroid secretion is mediated through the hypothalamic-pituitary portion of the HPA axis. ACTH production is inhibited directly by an increased blood level of corticosteroid or through diminished activity of CRF (corticotropin-releasing factor). It has been suggested that norepinephrine may exert an inhibitory influence upon CRF (Sachar et al., 1980). Thus, were norepinephrine to be depleted or otherwise unavailable, CRF, ACTH, and serum cortisol would increase.

Clinically, it has been observed that persons with Cushing syndrome on a hypothalamic or pituitary basis (in which levels of ACTH are elevated) are likely to manifest a depressive syndrome, whereas persons with Cushing syndrome on an adrenal or iatrogenic basis (when ACTH levels are low) tend to be euphoric (Sachar, 1974; Martin et al., 1977). Depression is also characteristic of Addison disease, in which ACTH levels may be greatly elevated.

SUMMARY

Depression, a symptom and a syndrome, can be considered a disorder if severe or prolonged. Depressive disorder in childhood and adolescence has essentially the same features as that in adulthood, though its recognition may be masked by prominent coexisting scholastic and behavioral disturbances. Essential diagnostic criteria for depressive disorder include dysphoria (depression, anxiety, or anger), vegetative disturbance (disordered sleep, altered activity level, or fatigue), lowered self-esteem, and suicidal thoughts or actions. Depression in childhood, as well as in adulthood, can occur as part of a unipolar or bipolar affective disorder.

Depressive disorder must be distinguished from conditions such as uncomplicated bereavement, depressed facial expression due to neuromuscular disorder, intoxication due to prescribed or illicitly used drugs, pseudobulbar lability or exaggeration of affect, sleep disorder, and hyperkinetic syndrome.

Causes and contributors to depression include chronic illness, metabolic disorder (such as hypothyroidism, Cushing syndrome, hyperparathyroidism, or adrenal insufficiency), social-environmental stresses, and genetic-familial influences.

Evaluation of the depressed child or adolescent should characterize the disorder in terms of impairment of function, duration, periodicity, and etiologic factors. The potential for suicide must be considered. Examination should seek evidence of chronic systemic illness. It should always include funduscopic inspection, since increased intracranial pressure (due to brain tumor or other cause) may be insidious in onset and progression. Therapy should be individualized. It will usually be multifaceted, combining psychotherapeutic measures, treatment of identified medical or neurologic problems, social-environmental measures, and, at times, the use of antidepressant medication such as imipramine (Tofranil). Hospitalization may be necessary for the severely depressed or suicidal child.

Abnormal results of investigation of hypothalamic-pituitary-adrenal (HPA) function (elevation of baseline serum cortisol and nonsuppression of cortisol following dexamethasone administration) have pointed to the importance of this axis in the pathogenesis of depression. The link between alterations in central norepinephrine and serotonin pathways and dysfunction of the HPA axis remains to be determined definitively. Norepinephrine depletion may lead to disinhibition of corticotropin-releasing factor (CRF), with consequent elevation of ACTH and cortisol.

CITED REFERENCES

Arieti, S., and Bemporad, J. R. The psychological organization of depression. *Am. J. Psychiatry,* **137:** 1360–65; 1980.

Ballenger, J. C., and Post, R. M. Carbamazepine in manic-depressive illness: a new treatment. *Am. J. Psychiatry,* **137:** 782–90, 1980.

Cantwell, D. P. Psychopharmacological treatment of the minimal brain dysfunction syndrome. P. 129 in *Psychopharmacology in Childhood and Adolescence.* Wiener, J. M., ed. Basic Books, Inc., New York, 1977.

Carlson, G. A., and Cantwell, D. P. Unmasking masked depression in children and adolescents. *Am. J. Psychiatry,* **137:** 445–49, 1980.

Committee on Adolescence, American Academy of Pediatrics (Cohen, M. I., chairperson). Teenage suicide. *Pediatrics,* **66:** 144–46, 1980.

Cooper, J. R.; Bloom, F. E.; and Roth, R. H. *The Biochemical Basis of Neuropharmacology,* 3rd ed. Oxford University Press, New York, 1978, pp. 180, 218.

Curran, B. E. Suicide. *Pediatr. Clin. North Am.,* **26:** 737–46, 1979.

Cytryn, L. Discussion of Dr. Malmquist's chapter. Pp. 64–68 in *Depression in Childhood: Diagnosis, Treatment, and Conceptual Models.* Schulterbrandt, J. G., and Raskin, A., eds. Raven Press, New York, 1977.

Cytryn, L.; McKnew, D. H., Jr.; Logue, M.; and Desai, R. B. Biochemical correlates of affective disorders in children. *Arch. Gen. Psychiatry,* **31:** 659–61, 1974.

Cytryn, L.; McKnew, D. H., Jr.; and Bunney, W. E., Jr. Diagnosis of depression in children: a reassessment. *Am. J. Psychiatry,* **137:** 22–25, 1980.

de la Fuente, J. R., and Rosenbaum, A. H. Neuroendocrine dysfunction and blood levels of tricyclic antidepressants. *Am. J. Psychiatry,* **137:** 1260–61, 1980.

DeLong, G. R. Lithium carbonate treatment of select behavior disorders in children suggesting manic-depressive illness. *J. Pediatr.,* **93:** 689–94, 1978.

Diagnostic and Statistical Manual of Mental Disorders, 3rd ed. Affective disorders, pp. 205–24. American Psychiatric Association, Washington, D.C., 1980.

Eisenberg, L. Adolescent suicide: on taking arms against a sea of troubles. *Pediatrics,* **66:** 315–20, 1980.

Fink, M. Electroshock therapy: myths and realities. *Hosp. Pract., pp. 77–82,* November 1978.

Flor-Henry, P. Lateralized temporal-limbic dysfunction and psychopathology. *Ann. N.Y. Acad. Sci.,* **280:** 777–97, 1976.

Gelenberg, A. J.; Wojcik, J. D.; Growdon, J. H.; Sved, A. F.; and Wurtman, R. J. Tryosine for the treatment of depression. *Am. J. Psychiatry,* **137:** 622–23, 1980.

Gold, M. S.; Pottash, A. C.; Mueller, E. A., III; and Extein, I. Grades of thyroid failure in 100 depressed and anergic psychiatric inpatients. *Am. J. Psychiatry,* **138:** 253–55, 1981.

Ling, M. H. M.; Perry, P. J.; and Tsuang, M. T. Side effects of corticosteroid therapy: psychiatric aspects. *Arch. Gen. Psychiatry,* **38:** 471–77, 1981.

Ling, W.; Oftedal, G.; and Weinberg, W. Depressive illness in childhood presenting as severe headache. *Am. J. Dis. Child.,* **120:** 122–24, 1970.

Lucas, A. R. Treatment of depressive states. Pp. 149–68 in *Psychopharmacology in Childhood and Adolescence.* Wiener, J. M., ed. Basic Books, Inc., New York, 1978.

Martin, J. B.; Reichlin, S.; and Brown, G. M. Psychologic disturbance in endocrine disease. Pp. 279–83 in *Clinical Neuroendocrinology.* F. A. Davis Co., Philadelphia, 1977.

Møller, S. E.; Kirk, L.; and Honoré, P. Relationship between plasma ratio of tryptophan to competing amino acids and the response to L-tryptophan treatment in endogenously depressed patients. *J. Affective Disord.,* **2:** 47–59, 1980.

Paul, S. M.; Extein, I.; Calil, H. M.; Potter, W. Z.; Chodoff, P.; and Goodwin, F. K. Use of ECT with treatment-resistant depressed patients at the National Institute of Mental Health. *Am. J. Psychiatry,* **138:** 486–89, 1981.

Petersen, P. Psychiatric disorders in primary hyperparathyroidism. *J. Clin. Endocrinol.,* **28:** 1491–95, 1968.

Rapoport, J. L., and Mikkelsen, E. J. Antidepressants. Pp. 208–33 in *Pediatric Psychopharmacology: The Use of Behavior Modifying Drugs in Children.* Werry, J. S., ed. Brunner/Mazel, Inc., New York, 1978.

Sachar, E. J. Psychiatric disturbances in endocrine disease: some issues for research. Pp. 239–51 in *Brain Dysfunction in Metabolic Disorders.* Plum, F., ed. *Res. Publ. Assoc. Nerv. Ment. Dis.,* Vol. **53.** Raven Press, New York, 1974.

Sachar, E. J.; Asnis, G.; Nathan, R. S.; Halbreich, U.; Tabrizi, M. A.; and Halpern, F. S. Dextroamphetamine and cortisol in depression. *Arch. Gen. Psychiatry,* **37:** 755–57, 1980.

Sacks, O. W. *Migraine: Evolution of a Common Disorder.* University of California Press, Berkeley, 1970.

Schilgen, B., and Tölle, R. Partial sleep deprivation as therapy for depression. *Arch. Gen. Psychiatry,* **37:** 267–71, 1980.

Schlesser, M. A.; Winokur, G.; and Sherman, B. M. Hypothalamic-pituitary-adrenal axis activity in depressive illness. *Arch. Gen. Psychiatry,* **37:** 737–43, 1980.

Smith, C. K.; Barish, J.; Correa, J.; and Williams R. H. Psychiatric disturbance in endocrinologic disease. *Psychosom. Med.,* **34:** 69–86, 1972.

Spiker, D. G.; Edwards, D.; Hanin, I.; Neil, J. F.; and Kupfer, D. J. Urinary MHPG and clinical response to amitriptyline in depressed patients. *Am. J. Psychiatry,* **137:** 1183–87, 1980.

Stores, G. Behavioural effects of anti-epileptic drugs. *Dev. Med. Child Neurol.,* **17:** 647–58, 1975.

Tepperman, J. *Metabolic and Endocrine Physiology: An Introductory Text,* 4th ed. Year Book Medical Publishers, Inc., Chicago, 1980, pp. 51–86.

Tosteson, D. C. Lithium and mania. *Sci. Am.,* **244:** 164–74, 186, April 1981.

Tucker, D. M.; Stenslie, C. E.; Roth, R. S.; and Shearer, S. L. Right frontal lobe activation and right hemisphere performance: decrement during a depressed mood. *Arch. Gen. Psychiatry,* **38:** 169–74, 1981.

Vogel, G. W.; Vogel, F.; McAbee, R. S.; and Thurmond, A. J. Improvement of depression by REM sleep deprivation. *Arch. Gen. Psychiatry,* **37:** 247–53, 1980.

Waters, B. G. H., and Marchenko-Bouer, I. Psychiatric illness in the adult offspring of bipolar manic-depressives. *J. Affective Disord.,* **2:** 119–26, 1980.

Weinberg, W. A.; Rutman, J.; Sullivan, L.; Penick, E. C.; and Dietz, S. G. Depression in children referred to an educational diagnostic center: diagnosis and treatment. *J. Pediatr.,* **83:** 1065–72, 1973.

Weiner, N. Norepinephrine, epinephrine, and the sympathomimetic amines. P. 159 in *The Pharmacological Basis of Therapeutics,* 6th ed. Gilman, A. G.; Goodman, L. S.; and Gilman, A., eds. Macmillan Publishing Co., Inc., New York, 1980.

Weitkamp, L. R.: Pardue, L. H.; and Huntzinger, R. S. Genetic marker studies in a family with unipolar depression. *Arch. Gen. Psychiatry,* **37:** 1187–92, 1980.

Whybrow, P. C.; Prange, A. J., Jr.; and Treadway, C. R. Mental changes accompanying thyroid gland dysfunction. *Arch. Gen. Psychiatry,* **20:** 48–63, 1969.

Youngerman, J., and Canino, I. A. Lithium carbonate use in children and adolescents: a survey of the literature. *Arch. Gen. Psychiatry,* **35:** 216–24, 1978.

ADDITIONAL READINGS

Cade, J. F. J. The story of lithium. Pp. 218–29 in *Discoveries in Biological Psychiatry.* Ayd, F. J., Jr., and Blackwell, B., eds. J. B. Lippincott Co., Philadelphia, 1970.

Chiles, J. A.; Miller, M. L.; and Cox, G. B. Depression in an adolescent delinquent population. *Arch. Gen. Psychiatry,* **37:** 1179–84, 1980.

de la Fuente, J. R., and Rosenbaum, A. H. Psychoendocrinology. *Mayo Clin. Proc.,* **54:** 109–18, 1979.

Guillemin, R. Peptides in the brain: the new endocrinology of the neuron. *Science,* **202:** 390–402, 1978.

Kashani, J. H.; Husain, A.; Shekim, W. O.; Hodges, K. K.; Cytryn, L.; and McKnew, D. H. Current perspectives on childhood depression: an overview. *Am. J. Psychiatry,* **138:** 143–53, 1981.

Kuhn, R. The imipramine story. Pp. 205–17 in *Discoveries in Biological Psychiatry.* Ayd, F. J., Jr., and Blackwell, B., eds. J. B. Lippincott Co., Philadelphia, 1970.

Pfeffer, C. R. Suicidal behavior of children: a review with implications for research and practice. *Am. J. Psychiatry,* **138:** 154–59, 1981.

Sato, T.; Funahashi, T.; Mukai, M.; Uchigata, Y.; Okuda, N.; and Ichizen, T. Periodic ACTH discharge. *J. Pediatr.,* **97:** 221–25, 1980.

Schachter, S., and Singer, J. E. Cognitive, social, and physiological determinants of emotional state. *Psychol. Rev.,* **69:** 379–99, 1962.

Whitlock, F. A., and Siskind, M. M. Depression as a major symptom of multiple sclerosis. *J. Neurol. Neurosurg. Psychiatry,* **43:** 861–65, 1980.

7 Hysteria

Hysteria did not disappear with the end of the nineteenth century. Indeed, it appears to be quite common still, though often unrecognized, particularly in childhood. Hysteria has undergone several changes of name. Conversion, conversion reaction, conversion hysteria, and hysterical neurosis, conversion type all are used equivalently. They are to be distinguished from hysterical personality and Briquet's hysteria, discussed below in the section on DEFINITION.

Several questions will be addressed:

What is the definition of hysteria?
Is it a diagnosis of exclusion or inclusion?
What organic conditions should be considered in evaluating the child whose symptoms appear to be hysterical?
What are the causes of hysteria?
How should it be treated?
What is its prognosis?

HYSTERIA

DEFINITION

Hysteria, as used nowadays, refers to one of three clinical entities. These are Briquet's hysteria, hysterical personality, and conversion hysteria.

Briquet's hysteria, or somatoform disorder, is a disorder of adulthood manifested by symptoms suggesting physical illness in the absence of objective signs of such disorder. The person with Briquet's hysteria usually has undergone multiple operations and may manifest symptoms related to these surgeries.

Hysterical personality refers to a style of behavior incorporating histrionic personality characteristics (Torgersen, 1980). Typical features include the "four G's": garb, gab, gaze, and gait. These refer to the person's

139

sometimes flamboyant and often attractive manner of dressing, speaking, looking, and walking.

The third syndrome of hysteria, conversion disorder, is the focus of this chapter. Conversion is a syndrome of motor, sensory, or other disturbance of function whose features cannot be accounted for by known structural or metabolic cause. The dominant symptom typically involves absence (or impairment) of function (such as blindness, deafness, mutism, incoordination, or paralysis). Excessive activity (as with a "seizure") may also occur.

Hysteria is used in this book, unless otherwise specified, to indicate conversion disorder (or its *DSM*-III equivalent: hysterical neurosis, conversion type). Hysteria by definition occurs on an involuntary basis. It is to be distinguished from malingering and factitious illness, which are under voluntary control.

DIAGNOSIS

It is essential to keep in mind that the person with a hysterical paralysis of the arm does indeed have a useless limb. The child may appear unconcerned about the deficit and the problem may obviously be psychogenic in nature; but the personal and social disability involved should emphasize the seriousness of the situation and the need for prompt, definitive diagnosis and treatment.

With hysteria, as with any other illness of childhood, its pathogenesis should be sought. This task involves understanding the meaning of the hysterical symptom within the context in which it has arisen. As the diagnostic process is begun and an alliance with the child and family established, treatment will be under way; anger, misunderstanding, and feelings of mutual manipulation can be minimized or avoided altogether. As a result, the child can return to normal function as soon as possible.

Clinical Process.   The diagnosis of hysteria is by inclusion, not just by exclusion. In a child with severe gait disorder, for example, it will be important to consider and exclude by appropriate means such disorders as spinal cord disease, muscular dystrophy, and peripheral neuropathy. By contrast, the delineation of neurologic findings in a nonanatomic distribution (such as a tourniquet pattern of sensory loss affecting a single extremity) or the lack of demonstrable neurologic signs will support, by inclusion, the diagnosis of hysteria.

History.   The child's chief complaint should be recorded exactly: "I can't move my left arm." "My right eye is blind." "I can't seem to walk in a straight line."

A complete history of the presenting problem should be obtained. When did the problem begin? What was the first thing you noticed? Has it gotten worse, better, or stayed about the same? What evaluation and treatment have been undertaken? Has anything helped? What do you think is causing the problem?

It is important to determine the medicial and psychosocial context in which the problem has arisen. What specifically were the circumstances at the onset of symptoms? Was the child healthy or recovering from illness? If the child had been ill, what were the symptoms, their duration, and asso-

CASE 7–1: HYSTERICAL BLINDNESS IN A 5-YEAR-OLD GIRL

B.N. was referred for neurologic evaluation because of a several-week history that she "can't see well" in her right eye. For 6 weeks the child had complained of bifrontal headaches that occurred nearly daily. They were unassociated with nausea, vomiting, lethargy, diplopia, seizure, incoordination, or personality change. Sleeping and eating behavior had been undisturbed. Psychosocial history revealed numerous major stresses during the preceding year. The girl's parents had separated. Mother and daughter had moved several times, most recently to the home of a friend whose 4-year-old son had lost his right eye because of retinoblastoma.

On examination the child was a pleasant, intelligent, and articulate girl who appeared entirely at ease. She did not express any concern about her visual problem. At one point she asked her mother which eye was bothering her. General physical examination was normal. Specifically, there were no neurocutaneous lesions. On neurologic examination, the optic disks, pupillary reactions, and color vision all were normal. Visual acuity was 20/30 in the left eye, 20/100 in the right. Upon the suggestion that she clap her hands before reading the eye chart, vision in the right eye was restored to normal. The remainder of the neurologic examination was unremarkable.

Comment. The diagnosis of hysterical syndrome was made in this case not merely by exclusion but by inclusion as well. Other diagnostic possibilities included eye tumor, hydrocephalus, toxoplasmosis, vascular episode, trauma, foreign body, and demyelinating disease. The diagnosis of hysteria was established by specific aspects of the examination (uncertainty as to the affected eye; normalization of visual function with suggestion) and the history (chronic stress, recent exposure to a child who was blind in the same eye).

The family was referred for social service consultation. The child was reassured that the eye problem was not serious and was expected to get better and stay better within the next several days. Should the problem have persisted or other difficulties arisen, psychiatric evaluation would be recommended. Treatment of headaches was to consist of rest, local massage, and mild analgesic agents if needed.

ciated disability? What was happening at home, in school, on the job? Were there family moves, loss of a boyfriend, or other significant changes? The role of disability benefits or legal action should be considered. Has there been an automobile accident or an alleged injury at work? Is litigation involved?

Past history should include inquiry about previous similar problems in addition to the standard parts of the comprehensive data base such as hospitalizations and operations. Inconsistencies in the child's account often suggest the diagnosis of conversion hysteria. For example, the child who complains of blurred vision when looking at the classroom blackboard may be able to pick out exquisite details on a distant scoreboard at a sporting event.

Examination. The *general physical examination,* usually normal with hysteria, should be carried out nonetheless to exclude contributing medical illness.

The *neurologic examination* is often crucial in establishing the diagnosis of hysteria. A complete examination should be carried out regardless of the complaint and its apparent nature. Selected aspects of the examination are included here.

Hysteria in childhood frequently involves *visual complaints* (Rada *et al.*, 1978) (see Case 7–1).

Double vision (diplopia) can be assessed by having the child count objects (such as fingers or pencils) with one or both eyes. Usually organically determined diplopia disappears when one eye is covered, though occasionally uniocular diplopia can occur on an organic basis (as with a dislocated lens).

Tunnel vision, or constriction of visual fields, may also be encountered. Assessment should include testing of peripheral vision by confrontation (checking the child's ability to detect movements of the examiner's hands or fingers) and use of a tangent screen whenever possible. With a tangent screen, visual fields can be mapped out more definitively. Constancy in size of the visual field, regardless of the child's distance from the screen ("tubular vision") is a characteristic finding with hysteria.

With blindness in one eye, the use of a colored lens may be diagnostic. A red lens is placed over the "good" eye and the child is asked to read a series of words, some of which are written in red ink, some in black. The red ink will normally be invisible to the eye looking through the red lens, though black letters will readily be evident. If red letters or words are seen, it is the "blind" eye that sees them.

With total blindness due to hysteria, elicitation of optokinetic nystagmus is objective evidence that the visual system from the retina to parieto-occipital cortex is intact. An optokinetic drum or striped tape can be used.

Normal pupillary reaction to light by no means excludes organically based visual loss (see DIFFERENTIAL DIAGNOSIS).

Hysterical deafness may be suggested by a child's apparent lack of concern, or even awareness, of the problem. A deaf person will usually scan the environment visually, paying close attention to the faces of persons who are attempting to communicate with him or her. The person with hysterical deafness, by contrast, may appear oblivious to efforts of others to communicate. Overly skillful lip-reading, too, may suggest hysteria; some words ("mutton" and "button," "most" and "post," "no" and "toe") are very difficult to distinguish by lip-reading alone (DeJong, 1979).

Sometimes the person with hysterical deafness will turn his head or otherwise react to a disparaging comment or to mention of unpleasant tests being considered. Such techniques should not be used since they can seriously damage the diagnostic-therapeutic relationship.

Motor dysfunction, particularly gait disturbance, is a common manifestation of hysteria in childhood (see Chapter 13). One form of gait disturbance is astasia-abasia. The person is unable to stand or walk but may demonstrate extraordinary balancing skills, such as skittering across the room on one leg without falling. Though swaying unsteadily from the waist, he does not

CASE 7–2: HYSTERICAL PARALYSIS AND SENSORY DISTURBANCE IN A 16-YEAR-OLD ADOLESCENT

I.L. was brought to the emergency room because her left arm was "paralyzed." The problem began immediately after she had allegedly experienced an electric shock while working at a factory. She complained of numbness affecting her entire left arm and was completely unable to use the limb. Family members indicated that 1 year previously, following a head injury, she had suffered paralysis of the right arm and leg that resolved following psychotherapy. Past history was also noteworthy for "nerve spells" described by the patient as involving hyperventilation and carpal spasms.

On examination, the patient was an alert, well-dressed, composed young woman whose left arm hung limply at her side. She was aware of her disability, though expressed only mild concern about it. General physical examination showed no contracture or wasting. Neurologic examination disclosed loss over the entire left arm of all modalities of sensation except for deep pain, which she acknowledged she felt slightly. The sensory deficit began as a tourniquet at the shoulder. Tone was normal in all extremities. With walking, the left arm remained close to the body with diminished swinging movements. Deep tendon reflexes were normally active and symmetric throughout. Upon arising from a seated position on the floor, she did not use her left arm at all.

She was treated as an outpatient with psychotherapy and physical therapy. Eight days later, her examination was entirely unchanged. She returned to her home in another city, and it was learned by telephone 2 weeks later that her status remained the same.

Comment. This case illustrates dramatically how useless, how truly paralyzed, this girl's left arm was. Although the physicians and therapists working with her were focused on her left arm, she clearly was not. Indeed, to her it seemed not to exist, as evidenced by her extraordinary insensitivity to pain and her arising from the floor without "forgetting" and using the arm.

With her profound and persistent paralysis, this young woman was at significant risk for sustaining secondary changes in the affected arm such as contracture and disuse atrophy. Unfortunately, her move to another city made it impossible to provide continuing care.

In this case, the diagnosis of hysteria was based upon the nonneurologic distribution of her sensory deficit and the past history of similar paralysis. Compensation from her place of employment did not appear to play a significant role here, though such aspects should always be considered.

widen the distance between his legs to establish a broader base. Gradual withdrawal of physical assistance by the examiner may further support the diagnosis of hysteria.

The quality of one or both feet being "glued to the floor" in attempting to walk, run, or skip also characterizes hysterical gait disturbance (Dubowitz and Hersov, 1976). Once the feet become "unstuck," the gait should be ob-

CASE 7–3: PSEUDOSEIZURES AND CARDIAC DISORDER IN AN 11-YEAR-OLD BOY

V.K. was hospitalized for evaluation of six episodes of "dizziness and fainting" that had occurred during the 3 months prior to admission. He described the dizziness as lightheadedness, which then progressed to vertigo ("everything spins"). Several episodes included loss of consciousness. After one such episode he was found submerged in a bathtub for an undetermined period of time. Neither tongue-biting nor incontinence was reported.

Past history was unremarkable. He weighed 10 pounds, 8 ounces at birth, but experienced no perinatal difficulties. Growth, development, and school performance were normal. Family history was positive for diabetes mellitus, negative for seizures, migraine, deafness, or sudden death.

On examination the child was a somewhat silly and immature boy who appeared entirely healthy. On general physical examination, postural hypotension was not found. Neurologic examination was likewise unremarkable. Investigations included a normal electroencephalogram in the sleep and awake states with nasopharyngeal electrodes used. Glucose tolerance test was normal. A 24-hour recording of his electrocardiogram revealed a prolonged Q-T interval.

He was treated with propranolol, which appeared to diminish the frequency of syncopal episodes. Over the next 6 months, however, the boy had several generalized pseudoseizures, which were followed by periods of markedly diminished responsiveness. Psychiatric evaluation elucidated a tightly knit family with major concerns shared as to the mother's chronically

served for signs of spastic diplegia (scissoring with toe-walking), muscular dystrophy (waddling, often with toe-walking also), hemiparesis (circumduction of the leg with flexion of the arm on the affected side), and other signs of physical disorder.

Distraction, encouragement, and suggestion may be employed diagnostically to enable the child with hysterical disability of motor function to perform better during the examination. Rhythmic clapping, chanting, or singing by the child or examiner may be employed.

With hysterical paralysis of a limb, several measures can be used to establish the diagnosis. Having the child sit on the floor and then stand up may bring a "paralyzed" arm into play. With hysterical paralysis of one leg, voluntary elevation of the "good" leg will usually result in a palpable downward push of the purportedly paralyzed limb.

Contracture and wasting (atrophy) can result from hysterical paralysis, particularly when associated with a fixed posture: tightly fisted fingers, rigid hyperextension of the toes, or plantar flexion at the ankles (Gold, 1965). Trophic changes—cyanosis and coolness of affected limbs, swelling and scaling of the skin, and brittleness of the nails—may be seen. These changes signify an urgent need for prompt, definitive diagnosis and treatment.

poor health. During the next several months conversion symptoms (pseudo-seizures) gave way to aggressive acting-out behavior.

Comment. The complaint of "dizziness" in a child always merits clarification. Differentiation should be made between vertigo and lightheadedness. Vertigo is associated with a sense of motion. Either the person or the surroundings spin. Lightheadedness involves a sensation of floating or of being on the verge of passing out.

The history did not suggest the specific nature of the dizzy spells but did suggest several areas of concern. One of these was temporal lobe epilepsy. Since the child was large at birth and was delivered vaginally, one might be suspicious that difficulties at delivery resulted in temporal lobe damage with subsequent development of a seizure focus. The child's electroencephalogram was, however, fully normal, including recording with nasopharyngeal leads. This latter technique picks up electrical activity of the brain much closer to its undersurface than does conventional scalp recording (see Chapter 12).

In this case the 24-hour electrocardiogram appeared to solve the diagnostic problem. It demonstrated a prolonged Q-T interval that predisposed to stretches of longer arrhythmias that could be associated with "dizzy" episodes or even lead to death. Several long Q-T syndromes have been recognized, often marked by a history of sudden death at an early age. One syndrome is distinguished by a family history of sensorineural deafness.

The child's pseudoseizures further complicated an already complex situation. This case is one of an infrequent number that require the collaboration of pediatrician, neurologist, psychiatrist, *and* cardiologist.

Sensory disturbance with hysteria may take the form of absent sensation (anesthesia—loss of touch; analgesia—loss of pain), diminished sensation (hypesthesia or hypalgesia), or altered sensation (dysesthesia). Dysesthesia includes causalgia (burning discomfort) and paresthesia (a "pins and needles" sensation). Hysterical analgesia may be extraordinarily profound.

Hysteria is suggested by sensory findings that do not conform to an anatomic distribution. An example is a strictly "stocking-and-glove" distribution of deficit cut off precisely at wrists and ankles. This kind of deficit must, of course, be distinguished from sensory loss occurring with peripheral neuropathy. In the latter instance, the deficit characteristically extends farther up the legs than the arms, a difference apparently related to the length of the affected nerves.

Other nonneurologic patterns of sensory deficit may involve an individual limb or half the body. With a tourniquet-like distribution of loss, all modalities of sensation are absent distally from a point encircling the limb (see Case 7–2).

When sensory loss affects one-half of the body, a line of demarcation that runs precisely through the midline of the sternum or skull on testing of vibratory sensation should always suggest conversion because of the normal transmissibility of vibration through bone.

Hysterical seizures, or *pseudoseizures,* occur relatively frequently in childhood (Schneider and Rice, 1979; Finlayson and Lucas, 1979; Ramani *et al.,* 1980; Holmes *et al.,* 1980) (see Case 7–3).

Pseudoseizures should be differentiated from seizures that are feigned and from epileptic seizures, which the child may also experience (see Chapter 12). In contrast to epileptic seizures, pseudoseizures are not characteristically associated with incontinence, postictal drowsiness, or EEG abnormalities. (It must be acknowledged, however, that even with "true" seizures, none of these criteria need be met. Furthermore, EEG abnormalities *may* occur when the child has a coexisting seizure disorder.) Pseudoseizures may involve combative behavior, whereas epileptic seizures themselves do not involve directed violence (Holmes *et al.,* 1980). Other hallmarks of pseudoseizures are sustained opisthotonic posturing and thrashing from side to side.

Hysterical coma may present a difficult diagnostic problem. Postictal state, drug overdosage, and catatonic state must be considered as additional causes of unresponsiveness.

The diagnosis of hysterical coma is suggested by several neuro-ophthalmologic signs. Though the eyes are closed, they may be seen to blink periodically. The lids may be held forcibly shut at rest or upon attempt to examine pupils or optic fundi. The oculocephalic ("doll's head") maneuver may show the eyes to be fixed forward in the absence of other brainstem findings. Caloric stimulation of the vestibular apparatus will produce a rapid, cortically based nystagmus inconsistent with structural or metabolic causes of coma.

The *mental status examination* should note particularly the child's perception of his or her problem and the associated affect. An apparent lack of concern is illustrated in Cases 7–1 and 7–2.

Investigation.   Extensive investigation of the child in whom the diagnosis of hysteria has been based on solid historical data and clinical examination is not indicated. Indeed, it may be detrimental to the child, reinforcing the sick role (Dubowitz and Hersov, 1976).

On the other hand, investigation such as electroencephalogram, cerebrospinal fluid examination, or computerized tomographic scan may be warranted at times to exclude specific organic disorder. Hospitalizing the child may itself constitute a form of investigation, allowing for close observation and supervision. In evaluating children with pseudoseizures, telemetered electroencephalography with simultaneous video recording has proved valuable (Holmes *et al.,* 1980; Binnie *et al.,* 1981). Auditory and visual evoked responses may be useful in the evaluation of the child with a specific sensory deficit. Ophthalmologic consultation with charting of visual fields is often worthwhile in assessing the child with visual problems. The use of interview after barbiturate (sodium amytal) infusion is occasionally helpful.

Differential Diagnosis.   Several questions should be addressed by the person evaluating the child with hysteria. What organic disorder could account for this symptomatology? What else, in addition to hysteria, might be going

TABLE 7–1. **Differential Diagnosis of Hysteria**

Movement disorders	Dystonia musculorum deformans
	Sydenham chorea
	Wilson disease
	Tourette syndrome
	Drug-related (phenothiazine, butyrophenone)
Spinal cord disorder	Multiple sclerosis
	Spinal tumor (cyst, neoplasm)
Brainstem tumor	Pontine glioma
Infection	Botulism
Migraine	Paresthetic, confusional
Seizure disorder	Partial complex or petit mal seizures (including status epilepticus)
Head trauma	Posttraumatic cortical blindness
	Posttraumatic memory deficit
Metabolic disorder	Hypocalcemia
	Hypoglycemia (as with insulinoma)
Induced illness	By child
	By parent or other caretaker

on? This section will deal with conditions that might be mistaken for hysteria, hence must be differentiated from it (see Table 7–1).

Movement disorders of childhood and adolescence are notorious for being mistaken as hysteria (Lesser and Fahn, 1978) (see Chapter 13). Worsening of the movement disorder with stress and absence of abnormal movements during sleep (though characteristic of organic movement disorders) may incorrectly be taken to support the diagnosis of conversion hysteria. Movement disorders particularly likely to be misinterpreted as hysterical are those that affect the basal ganglia, those that are drug-related, and those that involve the spinal cord or brainstem.

Among disorders of the basal ganglia, *dystonia musculorum deformans*—with its postural changes and bizarre gait—is renowned for being misperceived as hysterical (Cooper, 1973; Rivinus *et al.*, 1975). *Sydenham chorea*, a late complication of streptococcal infection, may also be viewed as emotionally based with its associated lability of mood and symptomatic worsening with stress (Weissberg and Friedrich, 1978; Nausieda *et al.*, 1980). *Wilson disease* (hepatolenticular degeneration) can be manifested not only by movement disorder and liver disease, but by behavioral and emotional problems as well (Roueché, 1979). *Tourette syndrome* is often considered to be purely psychogenic in origin.

Drug-related dyskinesias can occur after phenothiazine, butyrophenone, antihistamine, or "stimulant" drug administration. Dystonic reactions, particularly those involving writhing movements of the head and neck, may suggest hysteria (see Case 19–2). Careful history-taking, analysis of urine and blood for drugs, and a therapeutic trial of diphenhydramine or an anticholinergic agent should establish the diagnosis.

Carpal spasm associated with hyperventilation or hypocalcemia should be distinguished from hysterical posturing (see Fig. 7–1).

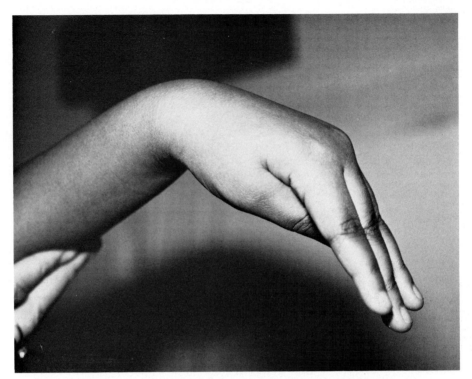

FIGURE 7–1. Carpal spasm associated with hypocalcemia.

Spinal cord disorders may develop in an insidious manner with fluctuating motor or sensory symptoms suggesting conversion. *Multiple sclerosis,* which can affect adolescents or even younger children, may be manifested by peculiar, hard-to-characterize waxing and waning sensory disturbances. The diagnosis of multiple sclerosis is established clinically by determination of neurologic deficits disseminated in time and location (within the central nervous system). These may include visual disturbance, other sensory deficits, ataxia of gait, unclear speech, and urinary incontinence (which should always suggest organic disease). Analysis of cerebrospinal fluid and studies of visual-evoked responses may help further to establish the diagnosis.

Intraspinal tumors may themselves suggest multiple sclerosis or hysteria when they are associated with vague, intermittent, or peculiar symptoms (Rivinus *et al.,* 1975; Herskowitz *et al.,* 1978). Diagnosis is established definitively by radiographic studies (which may include plain spine x-rays, myelography, or computerized tomography) in conjunction with characteristic clinical features of history and examination. *Brainstem tumor,* especially a slowly growing pontine glioma, may also suggest hysteria by causing nonspecific symptoms such as vomiting and dysphagia (Hinman, 1958).

Botulism, with clinical features of mutism and swallowing difficulty, may readily be misdiagnosed as conversion (Goldfrank *et al.,* 1981).

Childhood migraine may also be mistaken as hysteria because of its often peculiar manifestations of self-limited sensory, motor, language, or perceptual disturbance occurring with or without headache. Recurrent symptoms of visual disturbance, paresthesia (affecting face, tongue, or limbs), aphasia, unilateral weakness, or confusion in a child with a normal neurologic examination should suggest a diagnosis of childhood migraine even if headache is lacking (see Chapter 11).

Seizures, especially those of temporal lobe origin, may also suggest hysterical disorder (see Chapter 12). Staring spells, visual hallucinations, perceptual distortions, and behavioral automatisms resulting from temporal lobe seizures may suggest drug abuse, psychosis, or hysteria. The diagnosis of seizures is suggested by stereotyped, involuntary behavioral episodes. Electroencephalography is usually confirmatory, but it can be entirely normal in a child with well-defined epilepsy.

Transient blindness and memory deficit following head trauma may also suggest hysteria. Post-traumatic cortical blindness lasting from several minutes to a few hours may occur immediately following or soon after apparently uncomplicated head trauma (without loss of consciousness or focal neurologic deficit (Griffith and Dodge, 1968; Kaye and Herskowitz, 1980). Normal pupillary reactions to light indicate the intactness of anterior visual pathways.

Similarly, a transient posttraumatic memory deficit may follow cerebral concussion or even less severe head trauma. The affected child is able to recall past events but is unable to acquire new information (that is, lay down new memories) for up to several hours. Consequently, the child continues to repeat the same question even though it has been answered many times (see Chapter 16).

The pathophysiologic basis for these disturbances is unclear. Dysfunction of occipital lobes (with blindness) and temporal lobes (with memory deficit) is suggested by the nature of the particular loss.

Metabolic disorders such as hypocalcemia or hypoglycemia may be associated with nonspecific behavioral irregularities that suggest hysteria. With hypocalcemia, the child may complain of tightness and difficulty in using the hands, which can assume unusual involuntary postures (carpal spasm) (see Fig. 7–1). Hypocalcemia is suggested further on neurologic examination by generalized exaggeration of deep tendon reflexes. Hypoglycemia may be manifested by irritability, anxiety, sweating, lightheadedness, syncope, or seizures. Insulinoma (an insulin-producing tumor of the pancreas) is among the causes for hypoglycemia.

Induced illness may also merit consideration. In contrast to malingering, in which symptoms are voluntarily created and the examination is essentially normal, induced illness involves objective abnormalities on examination, and often on investigation as well. An example is injection with insulin to cause symptoms of hypoglycemia. When a child's illness is induced by a parent or other adult (e.g., by administration of a sedative drug), the problem becomes one of child abuse as well (see Case 20–4).

Etiology. Hysteria is ultimately emotional in nature. An intolerable feeling state, which may be associated with intrapsychic conflict, is converted into a symptom that provides a partial solution to the problem. For example, the teenager enraged at his father develops a paralysis of the arm that renders attack impossible but leaves him with a useless limb. Hysterical symp-

CASE 7–4: HYSTERICAL GAIT DISTURBANCE FOLLOWING BRAIN INJURY IN AN 18-YEAR-OLD MALE

O.B. sought neurologic consultation because of "spasms" of the right leg that had made it increasingly difficult for him to walk over the preceding 3 months. He had sustained trauma to the left side of the head 4 years previously, which rendered him comatose for a week. A right hemiparesis resolved nearly fully over the next several months. Recently he had experienced a sensation of tightness of the right leg when he tried to walk. This feeling was reduced after drinking alcoholic beverages. While his gait disturbance progressed, he withdrew increasingly from social contacts. His relationship with his mother, however, became closer as she was drawn away from a man whom the son did not like.

On examination, the boy expressed concern about his disability and said that he wished it to get better. Concerns about his mother readily surfaced. Neurologic examination showed unequivocal abnormalities affecting the right arm and leg. Deep tendon reflexes were increased (3+) on the right, normally active (2+) on the left. The right plantar response was extensor. Examination of gait disclosed a peculiar, variable limp. There were a delay in flexion of the right hip, tilting of the pelvis, placement of the right leg in an equinovarus position, and a rhythmic tentativeness in putting the right foot to the floor. Strength of arms and legs was normal and symmetric. Investigations included a CT scan, which showed generalized ventricular enlargement; the left lateral ventricle was slightly larger than the right (see Fig. 7–2). EEG showed left frontal slowing.

Comment. This young man appeared to have made an excellent recovery from major head injury associated with brain damage. Why, then, did he present with a gait problem several years later? The answer appeared to be primarily psychologic rather than neurologic. His close relationship with his mother was furthered by his disability. Furthermore, his physical problems made it seemingly impossible for him to become involved in educational or occupational pursuits that would be normal for his age.

Treatment in this case involved the collaboration of neurologist, psychiatrist, physical therapist, and social worker. Several medications, including carbamazepine and haloperidol, were tried without beneficial response. Alcohol abuse remained a significant problem. Attempts to involve the teenager in hypnotherapy were likewise unsuccessful. A year later the young man had made little or no progress and was admitted to another hospital for an extended period of time for further evaluation and treatment.

toms may also arise as a prolongation of, or superimposition upon, a child's organically based illness (Dubowitz and Hersov, 1976) (see Case 7–4).

Medical Causes. As indicated above, a preexisting or coexisting medical or neurologic illness may give rise to a hysterical syndrome. Dubowitz and Hersov (1976) described five children with hysterical disturbance of gait that

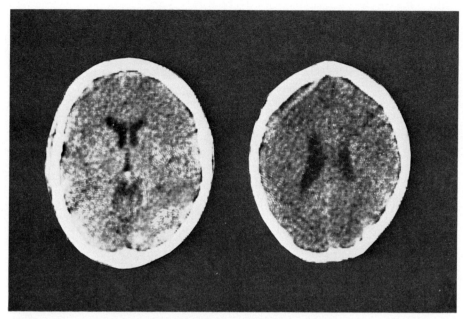

FIGURE 7–2. Computerized tomographic (CT) scan of the head showing generalized ventricular enlargement, left greater than right (Case 7–4).

developed after an organic illness, for example, a flulike syndrome associated with myositis.

Neurologic Causes. No strictly neurologic causes of hysteria have been identified, although neurologic factors doubtless play a role in hysterical symptomatology (see CORRELATION: PHYSIOLOGIC ASPECTS). A child who has witnessed a seizure may utilize this event as a model for his or her own pseudoseizures.

Toxic Causes. Toxic substances do not cause hysteria but may complicate a clinical picture in which hysteria is suspected. For example, when a boy with known seizures and pseudoseizures presented with an ataxic gait disturbance thought likeliest to be hysterical, his blood level of phenobarbital proved to be markedly elevated.

Psychologic Causes. As indicated above, a hysterical symptom appears to be a compromise solution, a defense against anger, anxiety, depression, or other intolerable emotion (see Case 7–5).

Hysteria has also been described as a form of nonverbal communication (''body language'') employed particularly when verbal skills are deficient (Chodoff, 1974).

Social-Environmental Causes. Since children do not have the same capability of altering their environment as adults and since they often do not have the necessary language skills or emotional maturity to deal with certain of the complicated life situations in which they find themselves, conversion (speaking through the body) may result. For example, Stevens (1968) cited

CASE 7–5: HYSTERICAL NARCOLEPSY IN AN 18-YEAR-OLD MALE

I.G. came to the emergency room following an episode of "total body paralysis" that occurred during a school examination earlier that day. The problem had its onset 2 years previously with an "attack" that began with paresthesias in the hands, arms, and face, followed by a sudden loss of body tone lasting 20 to 90 minutes. During that and subsequent episodes, which were not associated with loss or alteration of consciousness, only eyelid and finger movements were possible. Attacks were not precipitated by acute emotional stress. Sleep paralysis, hypnagogic hallucinations, seizures, and sleep attacks were denied (see Chapter 9). Prior treatment had included phenytoin (Dilantin), ethosuximide (Zarontin), and diazepam (Valium). Most recently he had been taking imipramine (Tofranil) and methylphenidate (Ritalin) for treatment of narcolepsy. Family history was negative for seizures, sleep disorder, or periodic paralysis.

Initial examination disclosed an intelligent, relaxed, articulate young man whose general physical and neurologic examinations were exquisitely normal. Investigation included serum glucose and electrolytes (all normal) and cervical spine x-rays, which showed an anatomic variation of no pathologic significance. EEG in the awake and sleep states also was normal.

On follow-up examination 2 weeks later, he suddenly began to blink his eyes rapidly and slumped to the floor. He did not appear to lose consciousness. Approached in a gentle and supportive manner, he was able to walk within 5 minutes by following the suggestion that strength would be restored as he pressed his legs together. He was referred for psychiatric consultation. It was learned that his attacks had begun 3 months after the sudden death of his mother due to a ruptured cerebral aneurysm. The current year, when he was away from home in his first year of college, had been particularly difficult, and numerous episodes had occurred.

Comment. This young man's episodes did, indeed, suggest a narcoleptic syndrome in which the major symptoms appeared to be a combination of cataplexy and daytime sleep paralysis. The diagnosis of hysterical narcolepsy was established only by direct observation of a typical episode. It involved rapid eye blinking (uncharacteristic of narcolepsy) and symptom removal through suggestion. As this young man appeared to be experiencing an unresolved grief reaction, psychotherapy was recommended and medication was discontinued.

the case of a "paraplegic" girl whose symptoms protected her from further sexual assault and led to her being brought to medical attention.

Epidemics of hysteria occurring in schools illustrate the potential situational and environmental influences upon conversion (Benaim *et al.*, 1973).

Developmental Causes. Maturational difference between adults and children that appear to contribute to hysterical symptom formation are cited above.

TREATMENT AND OUTCOME

Treatment of the child with hysteria (summarized in Table 7–2) should be symptomatic and supportive. The short-term outcome is generally good, though resolution may take several weeks to months, and there may be recurrences. The long-term outcome of hysteria in childhood is uncertain.

A team approach to therapy is often best because of the mixture of psychologic, social, and medical components to the problem. A mental health professional, social worker, physical therapist, and pediatrician thus might constitute a nuclear therapeutic group.

The treatment plan should include scheduled follow-up examination. Such examination is to ensure that medical or neurologic illness has not, in fact, caused or contributed to the presumably hysterical syndrome.

Medical Management. When medical aspects of a hysterical syndrome are identified, they should receive further diagnostic and therapeutic attention commensurate with their contribution to overall disability. Just as continuing investigation may promote the sick role, so may further administration of medicines such as analgesic drugs that have been determined to be unnecessary.

Neurologic Management. Seizures, if they occur, should be treated by standard means (see Chapter 12). Pseudoseizures should also be treated—by psychologic and behavioral means (see below).

Psychotherapy. Psychotherapy involving the child and family is a necessary part of overall management. In many instances gentle, firm, and regular encouragement by a concerned and caring pediatrician or neurologist will be sufficient. In other cases a child psychiatrist experienced with medical and psychosomatic problems can play an especially valuable role in what can be a difficult management problem (Maloney, 1980).

The meaning of the symptom to the child and an understanding of its significance within the family need to be determined. The child should not be disrobed of the hysterical symptom without allowing psychologic, social, environmental, and other therapeutic adjustments to take place. These may take several weeks or even longer.

Suggestion can play a valuable therapeutic role. For example, when a medical or neurologic problem has given rise to the conversion syndrome, the child and family can be informed that the prognosis is good, that resolution of the medical problem is well under way, and that full resolution of that illness can be anticipated (Dubowitz and Hersov, 1976). Hypnotherapy may also be of benefit (Olness and Gardner, 1978).

TABLE 7–2. **Management of Hysteria**

Therapy of intercurrent illness (if any)
Discontinuation of medical therapy if medical problems are resolved
Psychologic support (explanation, reassurance)
Suggestion (including hypnosis)
Behavior modification
Physical therapy
Follow-up examination

In the treatment of pseudoseizures, understanding the child's perception of a seizure—its causes, its manifestations, and its cures—is a valuable place to begin. Individual counseling may also provide useful insights in identifying stresses that trigger episodes.

Behavior modification techniques have been effectively employed in treating pseudoseizures (Williams *et al.,* 1978). For example, an allowance system may be established in which the child is rewarded for each day that the number of episodes is diminished.

Social-Environmental Management.   In reestablishing the child's normal participation in activity, scheduling of activities over a several-week span should be undertaken. Such a program, which might be organized with the assistance of a social worker, may include regularly increasing activity and gradual reentry into school. Not only parents but siblings as well should understand the treatment plan so that its effectiveness can be maximized.

Physical Therapy.   Physical therapy will often be an integral part of treatment. Graduated physical activity (using a bicycle or treadmill, for example) allows the child to build confidence and strength. It also provides the child a face-saving "out" as he employs a physical exercise program to overcome his "physical" disability.

When joint contracture complicates hysteria, physical therapy is essential in order to reverse or prevent further disability.

CORRELATION

Anatomic Aspects.   Testing of motor functions through examination of muscle bulk, tone, strength, posture, movement, and reflexes provides a relatively objective assessment of such functions. Sensory testing, on the other hand, is ultimately subjective. The examiner necessarily relies on the understanding, attentiveness, cooperation, and communicativeness of the child. As a consequence, organically based sensory disturbance (as with multiple sclerosis or spinal cord mass) may be interpreted as psychogenic and vice versa.

Despite its subjective nature, the sensory examination often provides objective data upon which to base the diagnosis of hysteria. As mentioned above, the diagnosis is suggested by findings that cannot be accounted for on an anatomic or physiologic basis (see Fig. 7–3). A "tourniquet" distribution of multimodal sensory loss affecting an entire limb is one such pattern. Sensation to the arm is mediated by nerves derived from cervical and thoracic roots, which make up the brachial plexus. For sensation of the entire arm to be lost without motor deficit, sensory roots from the midcervical to upper thoracic regions would have to be injured. If that could be accomplished, the sensory deficit would extend beyond the arm onto the shoulder, trunk, and neck, approaching the midline. Nor would more distal injury to the major nerves of the arm produce an exclusively sensory pattern of deficit in a tourniquet configuration. The diagnosis of hysteria is thus supported on objective grounds.

Biochemical Aspects.   The tolerance of pain seen among some hysterical patients is striking. A stimulus barely noted by a person with hysterical anesthesia (e.g., pressure upon a fingernail) might normally bring tears to a per-

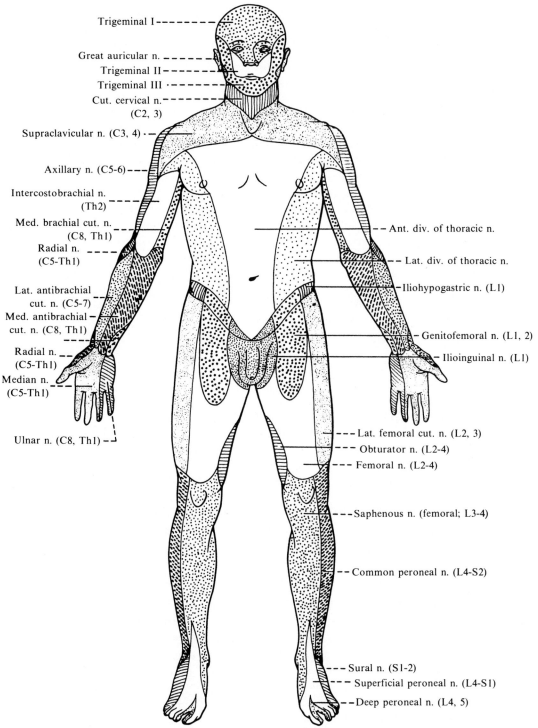

FIGURE 7–3. Areas of distribution of peripheral sensory nerves. (From DeJong, R. N. *The Neurologic Examination,* 4th ed. Harper and Row, Publishers, Hagerstown, Md., 1979.)

son's eyes. This tolerance of painful stimuli is reminiscent of that induced by hypnosis or achieved by champion athletes (for example, runners or swimmers). Evidence suggests that alterations in endogenous opioids may modify the perception of pain (Jaffe and Martin, 1980; Willer *et al.*, 1981) (see Chapter 19: CORRELATION). An alternative, or additional, explanation is that hysteria (including apparent indifference to pain) can be accounted for by attentional mechanisms (see below).

Physiologic Aspects.   Attention has long been a crucial aspect of hysteria. Because everyone else is focused on the hysterical symptom, it is generally assumed that the affected person is also. Actually, the opposite appears to be occurring. Rather than being attended to, a particular function or body part is, in fact, being ignored. (Perhaps this form of attentional neglect accounts for the absence of affect, the "la belle indifference" state that is a classic, though not commonly encountered, finding in hysteria.)

Hemispheric influences upon attention are evident in persons who have suffered right middle cerebral artery strokes (Mesulam *et al.*, 1976). Affected persons show a striking lack of emotional response to their left-sided paralysis, which they neglect or fail to pay attention to. When they are tested by double simultaneous stimulation, extinction of left-sided stimuli occurs, even though primary sensory perception is preserved.

It has been suggested that the basis for this neglect lies in hemispheric asymmetry of cerebral function. Heilman and Van Den Abell (1980) have investigated attentional functions through specialized electroencephalographic techniques measuring desynchronization of alpha rhythm as an index of attention. Their results indicate that the right parietal lobe functions bilaterally in attentional processes, whereas the left parietal lobe acts primarily contralaterally. With right hemisphere injury, left-sided stimuli then would not be processed by the right parietal lobe, hence would be neglected.

The applicability of such studies to hysteria in childhood and adolescence remains to be determined. Perhaps dynamic functional studies such as measurement of somatosensory evoked potentials, brain electrical activity mapping (BEAM), and positron emission tomography (PET) will shed further light upon this matter.

SUMMARY

Conversion hysteria in childhood is to be distinguished from Briquet's hysteria and hysterical (or histrionic) personality, both of which occur essentially only in adulthood. A hysterical symptom may arise *de novo* as a psychologic compromise or may represent a prolongation of a preexisting organic illness. Hysteria, an involuntary disorder, must be distinguished from malingering, in which disability is feigned, and from organic disorders such as multiple sclerosis or complex partial seizures, which may suggest hysteria by their symptoms.

The diagnosis of hysteria should not be made by exclusion alone but should be established primarily by history and by demonstration of findings that cannot be accounted for on an anatomic-physiologic basis. Investigations should be carried out only when clearly indicated, never out of annoyance or anger.

Treatment should be multifaceted and will often involve a team that includes a psychotherapist, primary physician, social worker, and physical therapist. Coexisting medical or neurologic illness should be treated without undue emphasis that might support an ongoing sick role. Individual and family counseling, behavior modification, social-environmental planning, and physical therapy are other aspects of treatment.

The prognosis of hysteria in childhood is variable. It may range from complete resolution of the problem to permanent physical (and psychologic) disability. Follow-up reexamination is important in determining the child's current status and in assuring that organic disorder does not cause or contribute to the hysterical syndrome.

CITED REFERENCES

Benaim, S.; Horder, J.; and Anderson, J. Hysterical epidemic in a classroom. *Psychol. Med., 3:* 366–73, 1973.

Binnie, C. D.; Rowan, A. J.; Overweg, J.; Meinardi, H.; Wisman, T.; Kamp, A.; and Lopes da Silva, F. Telemetric EEG and video monitoring in epilepsy. *Neurology,* **31:** 298–303, 1981.

Chodoff, P. The diagnosis of hysteria: an overview. *Am. J. Psychiatry,* **131:** 1073–78, 1974.

Cooper, I. S. *The Victim Is Always the Same.* Harper and Row, Publishers, New York, 1973.

DeJong, R. N. Examination in cases of suspected hysteria and malingering. Pp. 721–39 in *The Neurologic Examination,* 4th ed. By DeJong, R. N., Harper and Row, Publishers, Hagerstown, Md., 1979.

Diagnostic and Statistical Manual of Mental Disorders. 3rd ed. American Psychiatric Association, Washington, D.C., 1980.

Dubowitz, V., and Hersov, L. Management of children with non-organic (hysterical) disorders of motor function. *Dev. Med. Child Neurol.,* **18:** 358–68, 1976.

Finlayson, R. E., and Lucas, A. R. Pseudoepileptic seizures in children and adolescents. *Mayo Clin. Proc.,* **54:** 83–87, 1979.

Gold, S. Diagnosis and management of hysterical contracture in children. *Br. Med. J.,* **1:** 21–23, 1965.

Goldfrank, L.; Flomenbaum, N.; and Weisman, R. S. Hysteria or botulism: a fatal misdiagnosis. *Hosp. Physician,* **17:** 38–49, 1981.

Griffith, J. F., and Dodge, P. R. Transient blindness following head injury in children. *N. Engl. J. Med.,* **278:** 648–51, 1968.

Heilman, K. M., and Van Den Abell, T. V. Right hemisphere dominance for attention: the mechanism underlying hemispheric asymmetries of inattention (neglect). *Neurology* (Minneapolis), **30:** 327–30, 1980.

Herskowitz, J.; Bielawski, M. A.; Venna, N.; and Sabin, T. D. Anterior cervical arachnoid cyst simulating syringomyelia: a case with preceding posterior arachnoid cysts. *Arch. Neurol.* **35:** 57–58, 1978.

Hinman, A. Conversion hysteria in childhood. *Am. J. Dis. Child.,* **95:** 42–45, 1958.

Holmes, G. L.; Sackellares, J. C.; McKiernan, J.; Ragland, M.; and Dreifuss, F. E. Evaluation of childhood pseudoseizures using EEG telemetry and video tape monitoring. *J. Pediatr.,* **97:** 554–58, 1980.

Jaffe, J. H., and Martin, W. R. Opioid analgesics and antagonists. Pp. 494–534 in *The*

Pharmacological Basis of Therapeutics, 6th ed. Gilman, A. G.; Goodman, L. S.; and Gilman, A., eds. Macmillan Publishing Co., Inc., New York, 1980.

Kaye, E. M., and Herskowitz, J. Posttraumatic cortical blindness: clinical and CT studies. *Neurology* (abst.), **30:** 417, 1980.

Lesser, R. P., and Fahn, S. Dystonia: a disorder often misdiagnosed as a conversion reaction. *Am. J. Psychiatry,* **135:** 349–52, 1978.

Maloney, M. J. Diagnosing hysterical conversion reactions in children. *J. Pediatr.,* **97:** 1016–20, 1980.

Mesulam, M.-M.; Waxman, S. G.; Geschwind, N.; and Sabin, T. D. Acute confusional states with right middle cerebral artery infarctions. *J. Neurol. Neurosurg. Psychiatry,* **39:** 84–89, 1976.

Nausieda, P. A.; Grossman, B. J.; Koller, W. C.; Weiner, W. J.; and Klawans, H. L. Sydenham chorea: an update. *Neurology,* **30:** 331–34, 1980.

Olness, K., and Gardner, G. G. Some guidelines for uses of hypnotherapy in pediatrics. *Pediatrics,* **62:** 228–33, 1978.

Rada, R. T.; Meyer, G. G.; and Kellner, R. Visual conversion reaction in children and adults. *J. Nerv. Ment. Dis.,* **166:** 580–87, 1978.

Ramani, S. V.; Quesney, L. F.; Olson, D.; and Gumnit, R. J. Diagnosis of hysterical seizures in epileptic patients. *Am. J. Psychiatry,* **137:** 705–709, 1980.

Rivinus, T. M.; Jamison, D. L.; and Graham, P. J. Childhood organic neurological disease presenting as psychiatric disorder. *Arch. Dis. Child.,* **50:** 115–19, 1975.

Roueché, B. Live and let live. *The New Yorker,* July 16, 1979, pp. 82–87. Reprinted in *The Medical Detectives,* Roueché, B., New York Times Book Co., Inc., 1980. pp. 345–60.

Schneider, S., and Rice, D. R. Neurologic manifestations of childhood hysteria. *J. Pediatr.,* **94:** 153–56, 1979.

Stevens, H. Conversion hysteria. *Mayo Clin. Proc.,* **43:** 54–64, 1968.

Torgersen, S. The oral, obsessive, and hysterical personality syndromes. *Arch. Gen. Psychiatry,* **37:** 1272–77, 1980.

Weissberg, M. P., and Friedrich, E. V. Sydenham's chorea: case report of a diagnostic dilemma. *Am. J. Psychiatry,* **135:** 607–9, 1978.

Willer, J. C.; Dehen, H.; and Cambier, J. Stress-induced analgesia in humans: endogenous opioids and naloxone-reversible depression of pain reflexes. *Science,* **212:** 689–91, 1981.

Williams, D. T.; Spiegel, H.; and Mostofsky, D. I. Neurogenic and hysterical seizures in children and adolescents: differential diagnostic and therapeutic considerations. *Am. J. Psychiatry,* **135:** 82–86, 1978.

ADDITIONAL READINGS

Black, C. Pupils become ill in Norwood school. *Boston Globe,* May 22, 1979.

Glaser, G. H. Epilepsy, hysteria, and "possession": a historical essay. *J. Nerv. Ment. Dis.,* **166:** 268–74, 1978.

Heilman, K. M., and Howell, G. J. Seizure-induced neglect. *J. Neurol. Neurosurg. Psychiatry,* **43:** 1035–40, 1980.

Horvath, T.; Friedman, J.; and Meares, R. Attention in hysteria: a study of Janet's hypothesis by means of habituation and arousal measures. *Am. J. Psychiatry,* **137:** 217–20, 1980.

Mai, F. M., and Merskey, H. Briquet's *Treatise on Hysteria:* a synopsis and commentary. *Arch. Gen. Psychiatry,* **37:** 1401–1405, 1980.

Nardi, T. J., and Di Scipio, W. J. The Ganser syndrome in an adolescent Hispanic-black female. *Am. J. Psychiatry,* **134:** 453–54, 1977.

8 Behavioral Regression

The spectrum of behavioral regression is broad. The loss of abilities once acquired may merely be a transient, self-limited deflection in the curve of development. Or it may be the beginning of an ominous and inexorable decline, the manifestation of a degenerative or progressive disease of the central nervous system. In children the former is relatively common, the latter rare. In between these extremes lie many clinical situations of different causes.

This chapter will look broadly at the problem of behavioral regression, discuss conditions that might be mistaken for it, and present relevant aspects of diagnosis, treatment, and prognosis.

Several questions will be addressed specifically:

What constitutes behavioral regression?
What are its causes?
What investigations are indicated when behavioral regression is being considered or once it has been established?
Are disorders of behavioral regression treatable? If so, by what means?
What structural and metabolic factors underlie behavioral regression?

BEHAVIORAL REGRESSION

DEFINITION

The loss of milestones in a young child or deterioration in intelligence in an older child defines some syndromes of *behavioral regression*. A clear loss of skills does not always occur, however; a fall-off in rate of development can itself signify a disorder of behavioral regression.

Aberrant development fitting the pattern of behavioral regression may describe three curves: loss of skills, failure to acquire new skills, or acquisition of new skills at a rate slower than that previously seen. *Dementia* refers to loss of previously acquired intellectual function. (*Mental retardation,* on the other hand, applies to failure to learn.) Dementia is a term more commonly used to describe loss of intellectual function in adults rather than in children; but it can be applied to any age group. The first sign of dementia is often memory loss, resulting in an impaired ability to retain new information and to learn from experience. Loss of social skills and change in personality may follow, with motor deterioration and loss of bowel or bladder control occurring later.

Included within the spectrum of behavioral regression is *disintegrative psychosis*. It is characterized by essentially normal development for the first several years of life, followed by deterioration in social skills, language, and behavior often suggesting organic disturbance (Malamud, 1959; Creak, 1963; Corbett *et al.*, 1977; Evans-Jones and Rosenbloom, 1978). Behavioral manifestations typically include stereotyped mannerisms suggesting autism (see Chapter 5). Disintegrative psychosis is included in the category of dementia in the *DSM*-III (1980).

DIAGNOSIS

Clinical Process.   With problems suggesting behavioral regression, the history is crucial. Characteristically, a period of normal development has given way to one of the aberrant patterns described above. The examination is important not just in identifying and clarifying etiologic factors but also for recording pertinent data as to growth and development. Combined with information obtained at other times, these data can be used to determine the tempo of the process. In contrast to clinical problems such as headache, in which the history and examination alone may provide a specific diagnosis, investigation of behavioral regression will usually be necessary and will relatively frequently provide a specific diagnosis where one had not been arrived at previously.

History.   Information should be derived from several sources whenever possible: parent, child, psychologist, and teacher. Parents may complain: "Our daughter is losing ground in her development instead of gaining." "She seems to be doing much more poorly in school than in the past." The child may be aware of changes also: "I can't seem to remember things as well as I used to." "My coordination is off."

Each area of difficulty should be identified and characterized as to onset, rate of change, and current status. Bed-wetting may occur years after the child has been toilet trained. Coordinational problems may have become so severe that the child is afraid to walk up or down stairs. Loss of mathematical abilities may have rendered it impossible for the child to purchase groceries at the corner market.

Establishing that a disorder is, indeed, one of behavioral regression is of primary importance. Information derived from detailed history-taking, past medical records, and previous psychologic assessment should resolve this issue.

Family history is important, particularly in establishing a diagnosis of degenerative disease of the central nervous system. It may indeed suggest the specific diagnosis (Juberg, 1977). An example would be Huntington disease, which is transmitted as an autosomal dominant. With autosomal recessive disorders, consanguinity will enhance the likelihood of having an affected child. With recessive disorders such as Tay-Sachs disease, the child may not be the product of a strictly consanguineous union, but parents may be of the same ethnic background, in this instance Ashkenazi Jews, among whom the gene frequency is high.

School information may be useful not merely in terms of academic scores or results of standardized tests but also because of teachers' observations of behavioral change. Memory problems, staring spells, hyperactivity, incontinence of urine or feces, or withdrawn behavior may have been noted.

Review of systems should include inquiry as to systemic illness such as fever, skin rash, fatigue, or weight loss. Endocrine dysfunction can be manifested by lassitude, cold intolerance, exaggerated salt intake, excessive fluid ingestion, increased urination, or vegetative dysfunction (e.g., sleep disturbance, orthostatic hypotension, or symptoms of vasomotor instability). Inquiry should also be made about seizures, headaches, abdominal pain, visual difficulty, auditory function, and drug use.

Examination. The *general description* should include features of the child's appearance and behavior that are most striking upon observation and interaction. Is the child mute and withdrawn? Does he appear chronically ill or healthy? Are abnormal movements such as myoclonic jerks readily apparent?

General physical examination should include measurement and recording of vital signs and growth parameters (height, weight, and head circumference). Growth data should be plotted as to percentile and compared with previous measurements. Such comparison may disclose loss of weight, failure to grow in stature, or excessive head growth, for example. Examination of the skin should include search for characteristic signs of tuberous sclerosis: white macules, adenoma sebaceum, and shagreen patches. Examination of the eyes may show jaundice of the sclera or a Kayser-Fleischer corneal ring with Wilson disease (see CORRELATION: ANATOMIC ASPECTS). A slit-lamp examination may be necessary to visualize this greenish-brown discoloration of the margin of the cornea. Fundus examination may disclose a cherry red macula with Tay-Sachs disease or other storage disorders (see Fig. 8–1). It may also disclose papilledema secondary to hydrocephalus, retinal degeneration with subacute sclerosing panencephalitis, or optic atrophy (see Fig. 8–2). Optic atrophy is signified by a pale or chalky white disk with a diminished number of vessels that are smaller than usual. It can occur with optic nerve tumor, certain toxic agents, and degenerative neurologic disorders such as the ceroid lipofuscinoses. Peripheral portions of the retina may show pigmentary degeneration (retinitis pigmentosa).

Evidence for a systemic illness such as hypothyroidism, diabetes mellitus, or urinary tract infection should be sought. Examination should include assessment of lymph glands, spleen, and liver. Involvement of these organs might suggest diseases ranging from infectious mononucleosis or acute leukemia to hepatitis.

On *neurologic examination,* pupillary reactions to light may be abnormal with multiple sclerosis or other causes of optic neuropathy. A "swinging flashlight" sign may be evident (see CORRELATION: ANATOMIC ASPECTS). Vi-

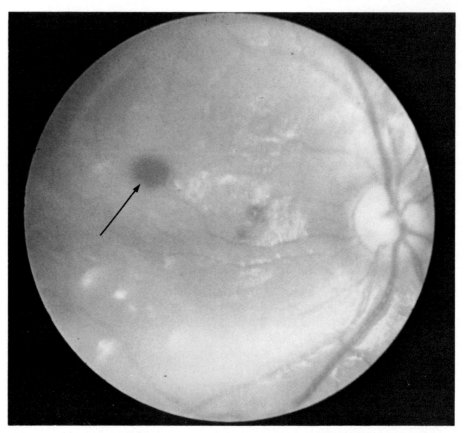

FIGURE 8–1. Fundus photograph showing cherry red macula (arrow) in Tay-Sachs disease.

sual fields, extraocular movements, and acuity should also be examined. Cortical blindness should be looked for when adrenoleukodystrophy is being considered.

Motor examination should include description of posture, spontaneous movement, tone, strength, and gait. Rigidity and paucity of spontaneous movement are characteristic of juvenile Huntington disease. Myoclonus may be seen in subacute sclerosing panencephalitis (SSPE), marked tremulousness with Wilson disease. Spasticity may be found with hydrocephalus or diseases affecting cerebral white matter (leukodystrophies). Coordination may be impaired in multiple sclerosis. Deep tendon reflexes are often exaggerated in demyelinating disease, though diminished in polyneuropathies.

The *mental status examination* should note the child's degree of alertness, orientation, attention, and cooperation with the examiner. Affect, memory, cognition, and awareness of the presenting problems should also be noted.

Investigation. Investigation of the child with behavioral regression may be definitively diagnostic. Studies may range from the mundane (urinalysis) to the esoteric (brain biopsy with electron microscopic analysis). Complete

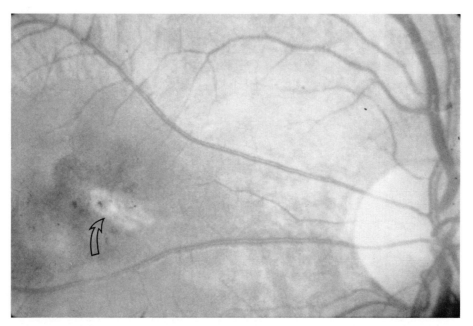

FIGURE 8–2. Fundus photograph showing retinal degeneration (curved arrow) in subacute sclerosing panencephalitis (SSPE).

blood count and urinalysis provide the starting point for investigation. They may suggest urinary tract infection or hematologic disorder such as anemia or leukemia. Thyroid function studies, lead level, and measurement of serum cortisol level may also be indicated. More specialized blood studies might include lysosomal enzyme determinations in serum. Diminished or absent enzyme activity underlies several storage disorders such as Tay-Sachs disease, in which hexosaminidase A is deficient, and metachromatic leukodystrophy, characterized by deficiency of arylsulfatase A. Serum ceruloplasmin is usually markedly depressed in Wilson disease. Serum measles titers may be markedly elevated in subacute sclerosing panencephalitis.

Cerebrospinal fluid characteristically shows increased protein level in metachromatic leukodystrophy, increased IgG in multiple sclerosis and subacute sclerosing panencephalitis, and measurable measles antibody titers in subacute sclerosing panencephalitis. The electroencephalogram typically shows reduced voltage in hypothyroidism and burst-suppression complexes in subacute sclerosing panencephalitis. Nerve conduction velocities tend to be markedly slowed in the peripheral neuropathy of metachromatic leukodystrophy or Krabbe leukodystrophy (see CORRELATION: PHYSIOLOGIC ASPECTS). Liver biopsy with measurement of copper content may establish the diagnosis of Wilson disease. With suspected or apparent storage disorders, biopsy of skin, rectum, conjunctiva, or brain may also merit consideration (see Fig. 8–3) (MacGregor *et al.,* 1978; Arsenio-Nunes *et al.,* 1981).

Computerized tomography (CT) of the brain should be carried out when hydrocephalus or other cause for increased intracranial pressure is sus-

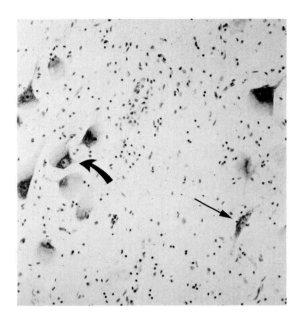

FIGURE 8–3. Neuronal storage in Farber lipogranulomatosis. Contrast normal neuron (straight arrow) with those distended with storage material (curved arrow).

pected. Sequential CT scans taken months to years apart may demonstrate progressive cerebral atrophy.

Formal psychometric or developmental testing is often indicated. Ophthalmologic consultation is frequently valuable because of the common occurrence of eye abnormalities in progressive neurologic disorders.

Differential Diagnosis.   Several conditions must be differentiated from behavioral regression. These include normal development, mental retardation, infantile autism, and "pseudodeterioration" of intelligence due to testing techniques.

Normal development itself, though a continuing process, is not always continuously apparent, nor does it proceed at a constant rate. Spurts and plateaus in development do occur, with occasional self-limited setbacks in reaction to identifiable events (such as the birth of a sibling) or without identifiable cause.

Mental retardation may suggest behavioral regression because of its developmental course. For example, with Down syndrome the tempo of development more nearly approximates normal during infancy than in subsequent years. True dementia can, however, take place prematurely in persons with Down syndrome. It characteristically occurs in the third or fourth decade of life and is associated neuropathologically with features of Alzheimer disease (senile plaques and neurofibrillary tangles) (Wisniewski *et al.*, 1978; Ropper and Williams, 1980).

Infantile autism is typified by abnormalities in behavior present since earliest life. In some instances, however, seemingly normal development has occurred for 1 or 2 years with subsequent deterioration to an autistic state. Under these latter circumstances, the autistic syndrome would fall within the category of behavioral regression, as well as childhood psychosis (see Chapter 5).

"Pseudodeterioration" *of intelligence* in children may result from use of different forms of the same intelligence test. Barkley and Murphy (1978) described children of school age who were referred for neurologic evaluation because of decline in intelligence scores of 11 to 30 points over a several-year period. They linked this apparent decline in follow-up testing to use of the WISC-R (Wechsler Intelligence Scale for Children—Revised), noting that children generally score from 7 to 20 points higher on the previous standard WISC than on the newer version (WISC–R). Continued use of the WISC-R should obviate this problem.

Etiology.   Causes of behavioral regression are summarized in Table 8–1.

Medical Causes.   Chronic Illness such as diabetes mellitus, cystic fibrosis, ulcerative colitis, or malignancy may interfere with the child's energy level and educational involvement to such a degree that a leveling off of development or even loss of skills may result. Depression may further interfere with progress, accentuating the clinical picture of behavioral regression.

Acute lymphoblastic *leukemia,* often converted nowadays into a chronic illness, deserves special mention, because behavioral regression may occur for several reasons. These include the child's emotional reaction to hospitalization (involving multiple procedures such as venipuncture, bone marrow

TABLE 8–1. **Causes of Behavioral Regression**

Medical	Hypo- or hyperthyroidism
	Leukemia or other malignancy
	Chronic illness
Neurologic	Progressive viral infection (subacute sclerosing panencephalitis, progressive rubella panencephalitis)
	Demyelinating disease (multiple sclerosis, adrenoleukodystrophy)
	Leukodystrophy (Krabbe or metachromatic)
	Neuronal storage disease (Tay-Sachs disease, ceroid lipofuscinosis)
	Neurocutaneous disorder (tuberous sclerosis)
	Progressive extrapyramidal disorder (Huntington disease, Hallervorden-Spatz disease)
	Brain tumor with or without hydrocephalus
	Seizures
	Other metabolic disorders
Toxic	Anticonvulsants (phenytoin [Dilantin], phenobarbital)
Psychologic	Depression
Social-Environmental	Multiple caretakers
	Child abuse or neglect
Genetic-Constitutional	See Neurologic causes

aspiration, and lumbar puncture) and the family's gloom as to the diagnosis (see Chapter 21).

The central nervous system may itself be affected by the leukemia, as well as by its treatment. Leukemic infiltration of the meninges, progressive multifocal leukoencephalopathy (a complicating viral infection), cerebral abscess (involving opportunistic organisms), intracranial hemorrhage (rendered more likely with blastic crises and thrombocytopenia), or central pontine myelinolysis can occur. Irradiation to the brain, with or without intrathecal administration of neoplastic agents, may cause somnolence and lassitude lasting up to several weeks and has been implicated in producing a leukoencephalopathy (McIntosh and Aspnes, 1973; Price and Jamieson, 1975; DeVivo et al., 1977; Ch'ien et al., 1980). Cerebral atrophy has been demonstrated by computerized tomography in some children being treated for acute lymphoblastic leukemia (Peylan-Ramu et al., 1978). The clinical correlation and precise cause of this finding are unclear.

Hypothyroidism or *hyperthyroidism* in the school-age child may present a picture of behavioral regression. With hypothyroidism, slowness pervades the child's behavior, and schoolwork may suffer. With hyperthyroidism, attentional problems may interfere with memory, neatness, and behavior (see Case 16–1).

Neurologic Causes.   Several categories of neurologic disease involve loss of intellectual function as part of a syndrome of behavioral regression. Disorders that primarily involve the motor system (such as dystonia musculorum deformans) are discussed in Chapter 13. This section will consider the following categories: progressive viral infection, demyelinating disease, leukodystrophy, neuronal storage disorder, neurocutaneous disorder, extrapyramidal degenerative disorder, motor neuron disease, brain tumor, seizures, and other metabolic disorders.

Progressive viral infection of the central nervous system, also called slow virus infection, is exemplified by *subacute sclerosing panencephalitis* (SSPE). SSPE appears to result from progressive measles (rubeola) infection of the brain (see Case 8–1).

Routine measles immunization appears to have reduced the number of cases of SSPE, now a rare disease in the United States. A registry of cases has been established in this country to pool data as to diagnosis and treatment, which, at this point, has been ineffective in altering significantly the course of this disorder.

The disease has been divided into four clinical stages (Jabbour et al., 1969) (see Table 8–2). During the first, school performance declines as memory is impaired (see Chapter 16). Personality change ranges from withdrawal to unusual degrees of affection. The next phase is marked by more obvious neurologic signs and symptoms. Seizures, typically myoclonic in type, and visual loss are often seen. The third stage involves increasing dementia, spasticity, and blindness. It culminates in a vegetative state leading to death within several months to years.

SSPE generally affects children of school age, though it has been reported within the first year of life (Bhettay et al., 1976). Children who have had natural measles infection in early childhood (within the first one to two years of

CASE 8–1: SUBACUTE SCLEROSING PANENCEPHALITIS IN AN 11-YEAR-OLD BOY

K.E. was brought for evaluation because, as he said, "the vision in my left eye is pooping out." For several weeks his coordination had been "off," according to his mother. He stumbled, had difficulty in turning around, and dropped things frequently. During this time his mother noted a change in his personality. He acted giddy and silly, more like a 7-year-old child. His memory seemed altered as well. He would begin a task and not complete it, having forgotten what he had started out to do. He got lost attempting to carry out a neighborhood errand. He wet his bed for the first time in years. He became much more affectionate than previously, kissing and hugging his mother more than in the past. His visual complaint led to evaluation.

On examination, the child was a jocular, cooperative youngster who acted several years younger than his chronologic age. He was disoriented to the date. Though easily distracted, he recalled three of three objects after 5 minutes. Neurologic examination disclosed numerous abnormalities. Visual acuity was 20/400 in the left eye, 20/100 in the right. Funduscopic examination showed macular pigmentary defects bilaterally, more prominent on the left. Visual field testing revealed a left homonymous hemianopia. Left-sided weakness of the face, arm, and leg was detected. Deep tendon reflexes were exaggerated symmetrically in the legs. Plantar responses were extensor. Stereognosis, graphesthesia, and double simultaneous stimulation were impaired on the left.

Investigations included an electroencephalogram (showing bursts of high-amplitude slow wave activity; see Fig. 8–4), a pneumoencephalogram (demonstrating enlarged lateral ventricles suggesting loss of white matter), and a lumbar puncture (yielding cerebrospinal fluid under normal pressure containing 90 mg/dl of protein, 12 per cent of which was IgG). Measles antibody titer in serum was 1:64, in CSF 1:8.

Within 3 weeks of hospital admission, the child began having myoclonic jerks of the trunk and legs. Over the next 2 months, he experienced further mental and motor deterioration. His behavior became even more immature, like that of a 5-year-old child. He became unable to walk without assistance. Further deterioration led to biopsy of the right parietal lobe, which yielded results upon microscopic examination consistent with SSPE. He tolerated the surgery satisfactorily but declined further over the next several months to attain a spastic, bedridden state in which he was variably alert but did not appear to recognize his surroundings. He died 3 years after the onset of his illness due to respiratory causes.

Comment. This child's clinical course presented a somewhat confusing picture initially, with personality change, memory problems, and a constellation of neurologic signs that suggested cortical as well as white matter involvement. Adrenoleukodystrophy, ceroid lipofuscinosis, brain tumor, and SSPE were considered the likeliest diagnostic possibilities. The funduscopic findings, EEG abnormalities, myoclonic seizures, and elevated measles antibody titers in serum and cerebrospinal fluid, in conjunction with the clinical progression, all helped to establish the diagnosis of SSPE.

TABLE 8–2. **Clinical Stages of SSPE***

STAGE 1: Personality Change and Behavioral Signs

Affectionate displays
Drooling
Forgetfulness
Indifference
Irritability
Lethargy
Regressive language
Slurred speech
Withdrawal

STAGE 2: Motor and Convulsive Signs

Dyskinesia—choreoathetoid postures, movements, tremors
Incoordination of trunk and limbs
Myoclonus

STAGE 3: Coma, Opisthotonos

Decerebrate rigidity
Extensor hypertonus
Irregular, stertorous respiration
Unresponsiveness to stimulation

STAGE 4: Mutism and Loss of Cerebral Cortical Function

Flexion of all limbs
Hypotonia
Occasional myoclonus
Pathologic laughter or crying
Startle by noise
Turning of head to one side
Wandering of eyes

* Adapted from Jabbour, J. T., *et al*. Subacute sclerosing panencephalitis: a multidisciplinary study of eight cases. *JAMA*, **207:** 2248–54, 1969. Copyright 1969, American Medical Association.

life) have an increased incidence of SSPE. It has been suggested that this increased incidence results from persisting maternal antibodies to measles passed through the placenta, which interfere with the child's immunologic response and allow the virus to persist. Alternatively, the child's immunologic response may itself be abnormal.

The increased frequency of SSPE in boys versus girls (a 3:1 ratio) and the predominance of cases reported from rural areas have not been explained. The latter has been attributed to exposure to farm animals harboring organisms that interact with measles virus to produce the disease. This hypothesis remains speculative.

Live measles vaccine has itself been reported to cause SSPE. This complication is, however, extremely rare; and morbidity and mortality asso-

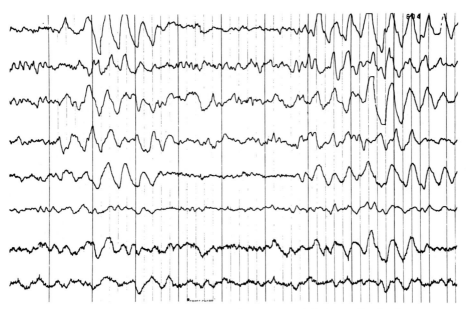

FIGURE 8–4. Electroencephalogram showing bursts of high-amplitude slow-wave activity (Case 8–1).

ciated with natural measles infection, which includes measles meningoencephalitis as well as SSPE, support the continued general use of live measles vaccine.

An SSPE-like syndrome, progressive rubella panencephalitis, has been reported following congenital rubella infection or the naturally acquired childhood infection (Weil *et al.*, 1975; Townsend *et al.*, 1975; Wolinsky *et al.*, 1976; Jan *et al.*, 1979; Coyle and Wolinsky, 1981). Intellectual decline, ataxia, and seizures characteristically inaugurate the syndrome of progressive deterioration (see Case 8–2).

Demyelinating diseases include multiple sclerosis and adrenoleukodystrophy (Addison-Schilder disease). *Multiple sclerosis* is generally regarded as a disease of young adulthood, although cases in childhood are well recognized. Its characteristic symptoms and central nervous system lesions are disseminated in time and in location. In other words the disease tends to pursue an intermittent course with exacerbation and remission of symptoms involving visual, motor, sensory, and other functions. These symptoms result from breakdown of myelin, which occurs for unknown reasons in areas scattered throughout the central nervous system. Viral infection and immunologic factors have been implicated in the pathogenesis of multiple sclerosis (Nathanson and Miller, 1978; Cook and Dowling, 1980; Lisak, 1980). Remyelination and gliotic scarring follow, accounting for the descriptive term "sclerosis."

Complete visual loss in one or both eyes may occur in multiple sclerosis, as may diplopia or impairment of color vision (see Fig. 8–5) (Hoeppner and Lolas, 1978). Other manifestations include ataxia of gait, slurred speech, paresthesias of the extremities, difficulties with bladder and bowel control,

CASE 8–2: BEHAVIORAL DETERIORATION IN A 15-YEAR-OLD BOY WITH A CONGENITAL RUBELLA SYNDROME

C.S. was referred for neurologic evaluation because of aggressive behavior, worsening of memory, and deterioration of school performance over a 6- to 9-month period. He was the 5-pound, 12-ounce product of a pregnancy complicated by mother's exposure to rubella during the first trimester. She developed a characteristic rash without other symptoms. No problems were recognized in the newborn nursery. At 3 weeks of age, the child was hospitalized because of congestive heart failure and was treated with digoxin. At 4 months, he underwent surgical closure of a patent ductus arteriosus. Early growth and development were normal. Sensorineural hearing loss in one ear and "salt and pepper" retinopathy led to the diagnosis of congenital rubella syndrome at age 3 years. Prior to recent difficulties, school and social progress had been unremarkable. He was known to have smoked marijuana.

Examination disclosed an alert, pleasant, somewhat immature teenager of low-normal intelligence. Digit span and recall of objects after 15 minutes both were normal. Head circumference was 52 cm (below the third percentile for age). Funduscopic inspection revealed rubella retinopathy. Visual acuity was 20/20 bilaterally. No cataracts were evident. Hearing in the left ear was diminished to whisper. Deep tendon reflexes, gait, and coordination all were normal.

Investigations included EEG (normal) and formal psychologic testing, which showed no deterioration when compared with results from 7 years earlier. The child's behavioral deterioration was linked to developmental stresses of adolescence, issues of parental separation, and drug experimentation. A plan of individual and family psychotherapy was arranged.

Comment. Personality change and memory disturbance in this teenager with recognized prenatal rubella infection struck an ominous chord, for it has been recognized recently that children with a congenital rubella syndrome, even if relatively mild, can develop a panencephalitis 6 to 10 years after birth, manifested by dementia, ataxia, and seizures. Ongoing rubella infection has been implicated in producing this disorder, as with measles (rubeola) infection in SSPE.

In this case, progressive rubella panencephalitis was excluded by neurologic examination (showing no motor abnormalities), psychologic testing (which demonstrated no loss of intellectual function), and electroencephalography. If it were necessary to pursue further the diagnosis of ongoing rubella infection, measurement of CSF protein, immunoglobulins, and antibody titers to measles and rubella would have been carried out and, perhaps, brain biopsy performed.

and "electric" sensations shooting through the extremities when the neck is flexed (Lhermitte's sign). This last sign has been linked to sclerotic plaques in the posterior columns of the cervical spinal cord.

Multiple sclerosis in childhood appears to take one of two forms. The first

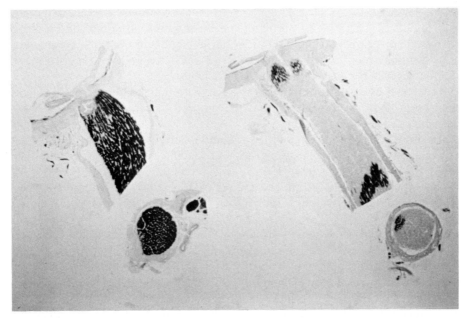

FIGURE 8–5. Longitudinal and cross-sections of optic nerves stained for myelin (black). Contrast the demyelinated nerve (right) of multiple sclerosis with a normal one.

is essentially the same as that described above, an intermittent course as typically seen in young adults. The other, termed acute multiple sclerosis, presents a fulminant clinical picture leading to death within weeks to months (Picard, 1965). In some instances definitive diagnosis may be established only upon postmortem examination.

Specific behavioral and emotional effects of multiple sclerosis have been suggested but have been difficult to establish with certainty. Loss of intellectual function sometimes occurs, as documented by deterioration in school performance or decline in measured intelligence quotient. This deterioration may be associated with cerebral atrophy as demonstrated by CT scan. At times, however, the decline in school function may be part of a depressive reaction to relapse, which may itself occur in association with emotional stress, intercurrent illness, warm bathing, or no identifiable cause. Multiple sclerosis may also present with symptoms of acute psychosis (Salguero *et al.,* 1969) (see Case 5–2).

Adrenoleukodystrophy (ALD, or Addison-Schilder disease) is a disorder typically affecting boys of school age. Symptoms at onset of ALD range from subtle personality change to frank psychosis. Cortical blindness is a typical finding. The course may be fulminant, leading to death within weeks to months; or it may be chronic, manifested primarily by behavioral irregularities (Hoefnagel *et al.,* 1962; Bresnan, 1979) (see case 5–6). It may be difficult to differentiate ALD clinically from SSPE.

The clinical manifestations of ALD are linked with demyelination, often massive, which generally proceeds from occipital to frontal portions of brain. The disorder is of X-linked inheritance, so only males are affected, with females as carriers. Hyperpigmentation of gums, skin folds, and areolae is variable but may be prominent. This darkening occurs because of melanocyte-stimulating effects of adrenocorticotropic hormone (ACTH) produced in great excess because of adrenal insufficiency.

Investigation of adrenal function by injection of synthetic ACTH and measurement of serum cortisol may be required to demonstrate adrenal insufficiency. Diagnosis is supported radiologically by characteristic changes upon computed tomography of the head and positive radioisotope brain scan (Valenstein *et al.*, 1971). Demonstration of specific cytoplasmic inclusions in brain and other organs have suggested a metabolic basis for the disorder (Schaumburg *et al.*, 1974). Moser and colleagues (1981) have implicated defective metabolism of very long chain fatty acids in the pathogenesis of ALD.

Leukodystrophies typically affect children below 3 years of age. *Krabbe* (or *globoid cell*) *leukodystrophy* usually presents at 4 to 6 months of age with symptoms of irritability and loss of motor skills. Later manifestations include seizures, temperature instability, and flaccidity. *Metachromatic leukodystrophy* (*MLD*) characteristically presents somewhat later than Krabbe leukodystrophy, with deterioration in walking at around 18 months to 2 years followed by dementia and death within several years. Onset in later childhood has been recognized with both forms of leukodystrophy. Manifestations of late-onset MLD include dementia and psychosis (Betts *et al.*, 1968; Percy and Kaback, 1971; Manowitz *et al.*, 1978; Farrell *et al.*, 1979).

In both forms of leukodystrophy, the protein content of cerebrospinal fluid is increased, and nerve conduction velocities are slowed. Sulfatide is excreted in the urine of children with MLD, which is definitively diagnosed by demonstration of absent arylsulfatase A activity in blood. The defective enzyme in Krabbe leukodystrophy is galactocerebroside beta-galactosidase. Both conditions are transmitted as autosomal recessive disorders.

Neuronal storage disease is typified by Tay-Sachs disease. This disorder, invariably fatal, stems from profound deficiency or complete absence of the enzyme hexosaminidase A. As a result, ganglioside GM_2 accumulates within neurons of brain and retinal ganglion cells. An affected child, normal at birth, suffers progressive impairment of intellectual, motor, and visual functions beginning at about 6 months. Failure to acquire further motor and language milestones, exaggerated startle response (often mistaken as "hyperacusis"), progressive visual loss, and myoclonic seizures are characteristic symptoms. Ganglioside storage eventually results in an enlarged head due to a large brain (megalencephaly) rather than hydrocephalus.

Accumulation of ganglioside in retinal ganglion cells produces a so-called cherry red spot. This characteristic macular lesion of *Tay-Sachs disease* results from the normally red macula being surrounded by pale, ganglioside-laden retinal ganglion cells. Cherry red spots may also be seen with Niemann-Pick disease, generalized gangliosidosis, infantile Gaucher disease, Sandhoff disease, and mucolipidosis I.

Diagnosis of Tay-Sachs disease is established by assay of the lysosomal enzyme hexosaminidase A. This enzyme can also be measured in fetal amniotic fluid; hence the diagnosis can be established *in utero*. Tay-Sachs disease is inherited in an autosomal recessive manner. Since 2 to 3 per cent of Ashkenazi Jews are carriers for Tay-Sachs disease, this group has been targeted for preventive screening programs.

Ceroid lipofuscinosis is a family of disorders with storage of the waxy pigments ceroid and lipofuscin. Diagnosis is made by a characteristic clinical course (*vide infra*), ophthalmologic findings (by funduscopy or electroretinogram), and biopsy of skin, rectum, or brain. Electron micrography of skin biopsy specimens has been especially valuable in identifying characteristic inclusions. A precise metabolic defect has not been identified.

Several clinical forms of the ceroid lipofuscinoses are recognized. An infantile form leads to profound dementia and death by 10 years. The late infantile variant (Jansky-Bielschowsky form) has its onset between the ages of 2 and 4 years and follows a course similar to the infantile form. Seizures are prominent in both of these variants.

The juvenile variant (Batten disease, or Spielmeyer-Vogt disease) begins in the school-age child with visual impairment, behavioral change (which may include hyperactivity), and fall-off in school performance (associated with intellectual decline) (Rivinus *et al.*, 1975; Barlow, 1978). Seizures, ataxia, dystonia, and dementia are later features of the disease, with progressive disability and death by the late teens or early twenties (Rapin, 1976). Kufs disease, a chronic adult variant, presents during the second decade of life or later, primarily with motor disturbance involving cerebellar, pyramidal, and extrapyramidal systems. Blindness is not characteristic, and dementia is relatively mild in degree (Dyken, 1975).

Rivinus and colleagues (1975) described a school-age child initially considered to have a psychiatric disorder with aggressive and "excitable behavior." He also had difficulty in seeing the blackboard. When vision deteriorated further, the child was reevaluated and was found, on neurologic examination, to have abnormal retinal pigmentation, optic atrophy, and impaired acuity. The diagnosis of Batten disease was made subsequently. Progressive mental deterioration occurred, and institutionalization was eventually required.

Among the most common *neurocutaneous disorders* (neurofibromatosis, tuberous sclerosis, and Sturge-Weber syndrome), *tuberous sclerosis* is likeliest to manifest a syndrome of behavioral regression. With tuberous sclerosis, intellectual and motor deterioration can occur in several ways. Disruption of cerebral cortical organization is associated with seizures that tend to be multifocal in origin, often become increasingly difficult to control, and may interfere with further development and learning. In addition, anticonvulsant medications may cause sedation or behavioral changes that limit optimal performance (see Case 8–3).

The diagnosis of tuberous sclerosis is generally based upon seizures, mental retardation, and characteristic skin findings (hypopigmented macules, adenoma sebaceum, and shagreen patches) (see Fig. 4–2). Plain skull x-rays and CT scan may establish or confirm the diagnosis (see Fig. 12–3).

Progressive extrapyramidal disorders include Huntington disease, Wilson disease, and Hallervorden-Spatz disease. Although *Huntington disease* is usually considered a disorder of adulthood, with initial symptoms in the late twenties or thirties, onset may be within the first decade of life (Jervis, 1963; Markham and Knox, 1965: Hansotia *et al.,* 1968). Dementia, seizures, and rigidity (rather than chorea) characterize the disorder in childhood. It is inherited as an autosomal dominant with complete penetrance. All persons affected manifest a relatively complete and severe form of the disease. Death usually occurs within 10 years. Diagnosis is based upon the clinical course, positive family history, and demonstration of caudate atrophy by CT scan or upon postmortem examination.

Wilson disease, or hepatolenticular degeneration, is a familial disorder of autosomal recessive inheritance in which copper accumulation is found in brain, liver, and cornea. Initial manifestations commonly become evident in the child of school age and reflect involvement of liver (hepatitis, cirrhosis) or brain. A wide variety of behavioral changes have been described, including impulsivity, temper outbursts, bizarre behavior, and loss of intellectual function (Scheinberg *et al.,* 1968; Davis and Goldstein, 1974). Other mani-

CASE 8–3: BEHAVIORAL REGRESSION AND REFRACTORY SEIZURES IN A 13-YEAR-OLD BOY WITH TUBEROUS SCLEROSIS

S.D. was hospitalized because of worsened seizure control despite attempts to adjust his anticonvulsant medication as an outpatient. Global developmental delay had been recognized within the first 2 years of life in association with generalized and partial seizures. The diagnosis of tuberous sclerosis was established on the basis of seizures, developmental delay, and characteristic skin findings: hypopigmented macules and adenoma sebaceum (the latter evident by $3\frac{1}{2}$ years of age). Family history was negative for tuberous sclerosis. His highest developmental achievements were attained by 3 years of age, when he spoke several single words and could walk briefly without assistance. Over the next 5 years he lost these skills, as he developed several additional seizure types that were not consistently responsive to anticonvulsant therapy.

On examination, the child was a wheelchair-bound youngster in early stages of puberty with frequent staring and lip-smacking episodes lasting 5–15 seconds. He seemed to have some awareness of his surroundings but did not initiate any contact with the examiner. On general physical examination he had adenoma sebaceum of the cheeks and hypopigmented macules of the trunk (see Fig. 8–6). No evidence for intercurrent infection was found. Neurologic examination disclosed generalized hyperreflexia, extensor plantar responses, and normal optic disks and retinal background.

Past investigations had shown intracranial calcifications on plain skull x-ray and "candle guttering" on pneumoencephalography. Current studies revealed a mild increase in ventricular size bilaterally on computerized tomography of the cranium with prominent periventricular calcifications. Electro-encephalogram showed frequent clinical and subclinical seizure discharges

festations may include tremor, chorea, rigidity, drooling, and dysarthria (Cartwright, 1978).

Diagnosis is suggested by a characteristic clinical course and sometimes by a positive family history. It is established definitively by recognition of a Kayser-Fleischer corneal ring, diminution in serum ceruloplasmin level, increased copper excretion in the urine, and increased copper content in liver tissue obtained at biopsy. Ceruloplasmin is a protein that binds copper and carries it throughout the circulation (Dobyns *et al.*, 1979).

Hallervorden-Spatz disease is illustrated by Case 8–4.

Other disorders affecting the *motor system* may spare intellectual functions (see Case 8–5).

Brain tumor may cause behavioral regression in several ways. Increased intracranial pressure from the tumor mass, from associated brain edema, or from complicating hydrocephalus can lead to personality change, visual disturbance, and headache (which need not, however, be a prominent symptom) (Platt and Rosman, 1972) (see Case 6–4). By contrast, brainstem

of multifocal origin. Levels of phenytoin, phenobarbital, and sodium valproate in blood all were within the usual therapeutic range.

Comment. Although the underlying diagnosis (tuberous sclerosis) was not in doubt during this hospitalization, the cause of the child's worsened state was not clear. One possibility for his recent deterioration was inadequate levels of anticonvulsant medication (due to weight gain or other cause) (see Chapter 12). Another possibility was excessive anticonvulsant medication, which can worsen seizure control because of drowsiness that potentiates abnormal electrical activity of brain. Anticonvulsant blood levels did not support either of these possibilities, nor did intercurrent illness appear to account for his worsened clinical state.

Hydrocephalus or malignant brain tumor may complicate tuberous sclerosis. The wartlike lesions within the ventricles that produce the characteristic candle-dripping appearance on pneumoencephalography may grow to obstruct the cerebrospinal fluid pathways and produce hydrocephalus. In fact, dilatation of a single frontal horn of the lateral ventricle (due to obstruction of a foramen of Monro) is almost pathognomonic of tuberous sclerosis. Furthermore, these lesions, subependymal giant cell astrocytomas, may undergo malignant change and behave as more aggressive tumors. The CT scan excluded these possibilities in this case. Primarily by exclusion, the likeliest cause for this child's deterioration was a worsening in his seizure control due to his entering adolescence.

In approaching complicated problems such as this one, the neurologist must always bear in mind the trade-off between seizure control and drug effects. "Perfect" seizure control may be achievable only in the highly sedated child whose behavior is then compromised as much by the treatment as by the disease.

glioma typically causes personality alteration, behavioral changes, and multiple cranial nerve signs without producing hydrocephalus (Bray *et al.*, 1958; Panitch and Berg, 1970).

Frequent *seizures* themselves may be responsible for behavioral regression (see Chapter 12).

Other *metabolic disorders* that may produce a picture of behavioral regression are homocystinuria, Leigh disease, and acute intermittent porphyria. *Homocystinuria* is an autosomal recessive condition usually resulting from deficiency of cystathionine synthase. Typical features are a tall, slender habitus suggestive of Marfan syndrome, dislocation of the ocular lenses, multiple thromboembolic episodes, and mental retardation. The thromboembolic episodes ("strokes") may be due to structural deficiencies of blood vessel walls or hypercoagulability of blood.

It has been suggested that the associated mental retardation results from repeated episodes of thromboembolism, many escaping clinical detection (while others might cause hemiplegia or seizure). Alternatively, the brain dysfunction may be secondary to the metabolic (amino acid) abnormalities that are present. Behavioral regression with psychotic features has been re-

CASE 8–4: DEGENERATIVE DISEASE AFFECTING MOTOR AND INTELLECTUAL FUNCTIONS IN A 20-YEAR-OLD MAN

I.S. was hospitalized for evaluation of slowly progressive loss of intellectual and motor functions over the preceding 8 to 10 years. Pregnancy, birth, and early development were normal. He rode a bicycle at 4 years, a horse at 6 years, and a motorbike at 8 years. He was an A student in second grade. At 10 years, deterioration in school performance was noted, perhaps related to attentional problems. He repeated the fourth grade and required special classes by age 12. Motor problems also had become apparent by that time. Gait was shuffling. Speech was slurred and increasingly difficult to understand. Between ages 14 and 20, motor skills declined further, and it became necessary for him to give up previous activities such as swimming and playing basketball. At the time of hospitalization, activities consisted essentially of eating, standing, sitting, and watching television. No seizures had been noted. Family history was negative for degenerative disease or other neurologic disorder. The parents were not consanguineous.

On examination, the young man was alert, oriented, and cooperative, sitting in a wheelchair. He had a bland, expressionless facial appearance. Affect ranged from sullen to jovial and changed rapidly. Digit span was reduced. Intellectual functions were at an 8-year level. General physical examination was unremarkable. Specifically, Kayser-Fleischer corneal rings were absent. On neurologic examination, speech was markedly dysarthric. Motor examination was notable for rigidity in all extremities. Tone was of a paratonic, "lead pipe" character. His arms were kept in adduction with hands tightly clenched. Little spontaneous movement of body or face was evident, except for frequent blinking. Purposeful movements were carried

ported in patients with homocystinuria who lack the typical stigmata of that disorder (Freeman *et al.*, 1975) (see Chapter 5).

Leigh disease (subacute necrotizing encephalomyelopathy) is classically seen in infancy or early childhood. It is manifested by feeding difficulties, intermittent vomiting, incoordination, weakness, seizures, behavioral regression, and intellectual decline. Death due to respiratory compromise usually ensues within a few years. Leigh disease can also become manifest in adolescence, in which case it is characterized by less florid progression (Sipe, 1973; Gordon *et al.*, 1974; Plaitakis *et al.*, 1980).

Neuropathologically, Leigh disease shows scattered areas of necrosis and myelin breakdown affecting chiefly the brainstem. This picture is similar (but not identical) to that occurring with Wernicke-Korsakoff syndrome, a sequel of thiamine deficiency classically seen in nutritionally deprived chronic alcoholics.

Thiamine metabolism has been implicated in the pathophysiology of Leigh disease. It appears that an active form of thiamine, thiamine triphosphate, cannot be made due to the presence of an inhibitory substance in blood, cerebrospinal fluid, and urine. Detection of this inhibitory material in

out slowly and awkwardly. Arising from a chair required a rocking movement. Gait was widely based and festinating. Muscle strength was normal. Deep tendon reflexes were exaggerated bilaterally with ankle clonus and extensor plantar responses.

Investigations included normal liver enzymes, serum copper, ceruloplasmin, thyroid hormones, amino acids, lysosomal enzymes, serum protein electrophoresis, skin fibroblast studies, bone marrow examination, and electron microscopic examination of peripheral lymphocytes. Cerebrospinal fluid protein was mildly elevated (56 mg/dl, 14 per cent of which was IgG). Viral antibody studies in CSF were negative. EEG showed generalized slowing and left hemisphere spike discharges. CT scans over a 3-year period demonstrated progressive enlargement of the lateral ventricles at the level of the caudate nuclei with progressive gyral atrophy (see Fig. 8–7).

Comment.   Although the nature of this young man's problems was initially unclear, it declared itself within several years to be a progressive degenerative disorder of the central nervous system affecting motor and intellectual functions. His disturbances in posture and tone suggested that the disease affected the basal ganglia. Among this family of disorders, the best clinical match was Hallervorden-Spatz disease (Dooling *et al.*, 1974; Vakili *et al.*, 1977). It is characterized neuropathologically by accumulations of iron-containing pigment within the basal ganglia. Treatment is symptomatic.

Other important considerations in the school-age male with progressive deterioration of this sort would include subacute sclerosing panencephalitis (SSPE), adrenoleukodystrophy (ALD), seizure disorder (or overtreatment thereof), and ceroid lipofuscinosis.

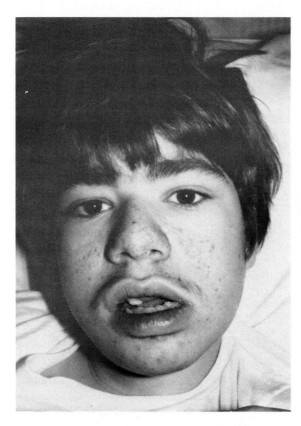

FIGURE 8–6. Adenoma sebaceum of the cheeks in tuberous sclerosis (Case 8–3).

urine strongly supports the diagnosis of subacute necrotizing encephalomyelopathy in a living patient. Disturbance in lactate, pyruvate, and alanine metabolism in some children with a Leigh-like illness has suggested that deficiency of pyruvate carboxylase may play a role in this disorder (Tang *et al.*, 1972).

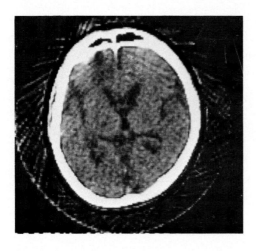

FIGURE 8–7. Plain computerized tomographic (CT) scan of the head demonstrating generalized ventricular enlargement and cortical atrophy (Case 8–4).

CASE 8–5: PROGRESSIVE MOTOR NEURON DISEASE IN A 13-YEAR-OLD BOY

L.O. was referred for evaluation because of progressive right arm weakness. Past history was notable for mild language delay and ataxia in early childhood associated with tremulousness, hyperreflexia, and extensor plantar responses. For 3 months prior to assessment, progressive loss of strength in the right arm had been noted. Weakness progressed so rapidly that it soon became difficult for the boy to brush his teeth or comb his hair. No pain or other sensory disturbance was associated; nor had the child experienced headache, neck pain, vomiting, diplopia, speech difficulty, or swallowing problems. Trauma, immunizations, and infection had not been associated with development of neurologic symptoms.

On examination, the boy was alert, cooperative, friendly, and cheerful. Wasting of the right shoulder, chest, and arm was evident. The left arm and shoulder were also diminished in bulk, though to a lesser degree. Fasciculations were seen upon inspection of the shoulder girdle, pectoralis, and paraspinal muscles. Deep tendon reflexes were brisk throughout, though decreased in the right arm, which was also hypotonic. Plantar responses were flexor. Testing of coordination revealed dysmetria of all limbs. The boy could walk only a few steps without assistance. Sensation and cranial nerves were normal.

Investigations included serum "muscle enzymes," myelography, cerebrospinal fluid examination, analysis of urine for toxic substances, and viral studies. All were normal. Electromyography confirmed the clinical picture of denervation. Nerve conduction velocities were normal. Muscle biopsy showed characteristic changes of denervation.

Over the next several months further deterioration of motor function occurred. Despite progressive difficulties in walking and later with swallowing, the child's spirits never flagged. He insisted on continuing to attend school as long as possible. With the close cooperation of parents, physicians, and teachers, this goal was accomplished. Within a year of onset of right arm weakness, the child died of respiratory causes despite tracheostomy and use of suctioning equipment to assist in handling of oral secretions.

Comment. This tragic case illustrates a rapidly progressive neurologic disease leading to death in which intellect did not decline. He appeared to have a juvenile form of spinal muscular atrophy, juvenile amyotrophic lateral sclerosis (ALS, or "Lou Gehrig disease") (see Fig. 8–8). The reason for the aggressive course of the illness in this boy was obscure but perhaps was related to the child's earlier neurologic difficulties (ataxic cerebral palsy).

His disorder was also reminiscent of infantile spinal muscular atrophy, Werdnig-Hoffmann disease, in which affected children characteristically remain bright and alert while their motor functions deteriorate inexorably toward a respiratory death.

In either case, medical and neurologic management is essentially symptomatic. Supportive psychotherapy is essential. It is often best provided by a person who is not involved directly in medical or neurologic treatment, someone without diagnostic or therapeutic needles.

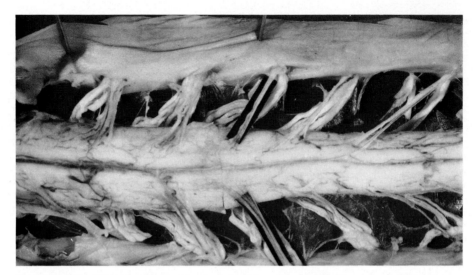

FIGURE 8–8. Ventral surface of spinal cord in amyotrophic lateral sclerosis showing atrophic ventral (motor) roots.

Acute intermittent porphyria is an autosomal dominant condition rarely seen in childhood. It may, however, present in adolescence with impaired school performance, personality disturbance, or psychosis. It is most commonly manifested by abdominal pain, seizures, and polyneuritis. Abdominal pain may be so severe that surgical exploration is considered (or actually carried out). Polyneuritis may pose a threat to life when acute demyelination of intercostal nerves results in respiratory failure.

Episodes of acute intermittent porphyria may be spontaneous or triggered by barbiturates, sulfonamides, and griseofulvin, among other medications. Alcohol and intercurrent illness are other potentially provocative agents (Barclay, 1974). Deficiency of uroporphyrinogen I synthetase appears to underlie acute intermittent porphyria. The diagnosis is established by assay of this enzyme in blood and measurement of urinary porphobilinogen. Urine exposed to sunlight characteristically takes on the color of red wine.

Toxic Causes. Phenytoin intoxication can produce a picture of behavioral regression even in standard doses that previously were well tolerated. Logan and Freeman (1969) described four patients (ages 17 months to 19 years) in whom the classic triad of ataxia, nystagmus, and dysarthria did not occur. Rather, a loss of previously acquired skills was seen. Serum levels of phenytoin were elevated in only two of these cases.

Other anticonvulsant medications may cause behavioral deterioration when blood levels are excessive. Drug interactions may influence such levels significantly. For example, sodium valproate added to an anticonvulsant regimen that includes phenobarbital can elevate the concentration of phenobarbital in blood to a toxic level, with resulting irritability, drowsiness, and ataxia of gait.

Lead poisoning can exert effects on the central nervous system acutely or chronically. Acute lead poisoning can cause a life-threatening encephalopathy marked by generalized seizures and dangerously elevated intracranial pressure. Death and severe neurologic deficit are usual outcomes. Chronic plumbism can result in less severe intellectual deficit or hyperactivity (Needleman et al., 1979).

Particularly among children between 1 and 4 years of age, lead poisoning should always be considered as a cause of behavioral regression, because lead ingestion is frequently unobserved, and the effects of chronic lead poisoning are insidious.

Psychologic Causes. Depression due to a variety of causes may be associated with behavioral regression (see Chapter 6). Psychomotor retardation, failure to participate in usual activities, impaired concentration, memory decline, and a fall-off in school performance commonly occur in depressive syndromes.

Behavioral regression secondary to major psychosocial events is another potential psychologic cause. For example, adverse reaction to the birth of a sibling may be benign and self-limited or it may require professional intervention. A new baby's entry into the family may be accompanied by the older child's increased desire to be held and "babied." The older child may return to wetting and wish to take milk from bottle or breast. With parental understanding, support, and guidance, such behavior usually disappears within several weeks. When the pattern of regressive behavior becomes relatively fixed (for example, with loss of previously acquired bladder control and continued baby talk), psychiatric intervention would be indicated.

Social-Environmental Causes. Behavioral regression can result from social and environmental causes in several ways. In the younger child, multiple changes of primary caretaker can lead to detached, aloof behavior, suggesting a depressive syndrome. With child abuse or neglect involving single or repeated injuries to the brain, behavioral deterioration, including loss of intellectual and motor function, can occur (see Chapter 20). Strangulation may be associated with late onset of behavioral and intellectual decline, with deterioration manifested several weeks after an apparently uneventful recovery from the initial injury (Dooling and Richardson, 1976; Feldman and Simms, 1980) (see Case 20–3).

Genetic-Constitutional Causes. Many conditions associated with behavioral regression have a genetic-metabolic basis. Different patterns of inheritance are exemplified by Wilson disease (autosomal recessive), acute intermittent porphyria (autosomal dominant), and adrenoleukodystrophy (X-linked recessive) (see Table 8–3).

Developmental Causes. As mentioned above (see DIFFERENTIAL DIAGNOSIS), normal development includes transient periods of leveling off in development that may suggest behavioral regression. For example, a 5-month-old child who had produced many speech sounds by $2\frac{1}{2}$ months uttered few new sounds over the next $2\frac{1}{2}$ months. This period was accompanied, however, by a marked increase in ability to manipulate objects and localize sounds. Within the next 2 months, speech and language development advanced briskly.

TABLE 8–3. **Patterns of Inheritance in Selected Disorders of Behavioral Regression**

Autosomal recessive	Wilson disease
	Metachromatic leukodystrophy
	Tay-Sachs disease
	Homocystinuria
Autosomal dominant	Tuberous sclerosis
	Huntington disease
	Acute intermittent porphyria
X-linked recessive	Adrenoleukodystrophy

TREATMENT AND OUTCOME

Therapy and prognosis are not uniformly gloomy aspects of syndromes of behavioral regression. Certainly, the management of a child with SSPE or other progressive disorder leading to death is a most difficult undertaking. By contrast, specific treatment is available for children with Wilson disease, and the outcome can be highly favorable with improvement in hepatic, neurologic, and psychologic functions.

Medical Management. Treatment of systemic illness such as diabetes mellitus or acute lymphoblastic leukemia will generally be accompanied by acceleration in development and improvement in learning, presumably by counteracting associated loss of energy and fatigue. The therapy of these disorders may, however, cause self-limited setbacks in behavior and development. Hospitalization, for example, involving separation from family and often requiring multiple procedures, can exert a depressing influence. Radiation and chemotherapy often cause fatigue, nausea, and other systemic effects. These problems are treated symptomatically and usually last only a few weeks or months. On the other hand, complications such as leukoencephalopathy and intracranial hemorrhage can produce permanent loss of intellectual function.

Hypothyroidism is treated with replacement thyroid hormone. Overall slowness in movement and mentation improve with such therapy, and some gains in intelligence as measured by psychologic testing can result (Money, 1975).

Drug overdosage with anticonvulsant medication will usually respond to withholding medication for several days, then reinstituting it at a lower dosage level. The influence of drug interactions (such as those involving sodium valproate and phenobarbital mentioned above) should be considered.

The treatment of *lead poisoning* will vary with the degree of symptomatology. Acute central nervous system intoxication constitutes a medical emergency, for increased intracranial pressure poses an immediate threat to life. Intracranial hypertension in such circumstances should be treated with passive hyperventilation and an intravenous osmotic agent such as mannitol (Rosman, 1982). Seizures should be treated with standard anticonvulsant agents and chelation accomplished through use of BAL and calcium EDTA.

Acute lead encephalopathy is a grave illness that usually results in severe, permanent intellectual disability or death. Fortunately, nationwide lead screening and lead removal programs in conjunction with legislation limiting the use of lead-based paint have reduced greatly the frequency of this serious complication. Chronic lead poisoning can affect the central nervous system also, giving rise to hyperactivity and intellectual impairment (see Chapter 14) (Needleman *et al.*, 1979). Levels of blood lead and free erythrocyte protoporphyrin in urine guide the therapy along with the child's symptoms, if any (Center for Disease Control, 1978). Treatment usually involves calcium EDTA given intramuscularly and permanent removal from the leaded environment. With marked elevation in lead levels or in the symptomatic child, BAL is added to the regimen. Penicillamine has been used effectively on an outpatient basis when a lead-free environment has been assured.

Neurologic Management. Treatment of neurologic conditions associated with behavioral regression generally involves a combination of symptomatic, supportive, and (when available) specific therapies. With Wilson disease, for example, management would include dietary measures, penicillamine use, and often psychotherapy.

Subacute sclerosing panencephalitis is an almost invariably fatal disease, proceeding to death within a few months to years after onset. Therapy is symptomatic: controlling seizures, treating hyperpyrexia, and providing for adequate nutrition. Treatment with anti-inflammatory or antiviral agents has not been successful to date.

Multiple sclerosis usually consists of episodes of neurologic dysfunction lasting days, weeks, or months that usually remit spontaneously. The subsequent level of function may be fully normal, mildly impaired, or very significantly impaired.

Prednisone, ACTH, and other immunosupressive agents have been used with apparent effectiveness in some children and adolescents with multiple sclerosis, although efficacy has not been demonstrated convincingly by controlled clinical studies (Ellison and Myers, 1980; Dowling *et al.*, 1980) (see Chapter 14). The side effects of prednisone and ACTH must be kept in mind when either drug is being considered for use (see Case 21–1). These include weight gain, proximal muscle weakness, peptic ulcer, and osteoporosis.

Adrenoleukodystrophy may be treated with steroid replacement depending upon the degree of adrenocortical insufficiency. ACTH has been used in an attempt to halt rapidly progressive demyelination in the more fulminant cases, but without definite clinical effect.

The course of *Krabbe leukodystrophy, metachromatic leukodystrophy* (MLD), and *Tay-Sachs disease* in their classic early childhood forms has not been significantly altered by therapy. With the later-onset, more slowly progressive forms of MLD, symptomatic treatment with antipsychotic or antianxiety drugs can be employed if circumstances warrant. Treatment of the *ceroid lipofuscinoses* is also essentially symptomatic, directed toward the problems of seizures, visual deficit, and intellectual decline. High doses of vitamin E have been used with encouraging results in several children (Zeman and Dyken, 1969).

Management of *tuberous sclerosis* is focused upon certain of the central nervous system manifestations of the disorder (seizures, hydrocephalus, and tumors), as well as on other organ systems that may be involved (including the heart, kidneys, and lungs). Seizure control is frequently difficult because of multiple seizure foci. Thus, one is often forced to use several anticonvulsant medications in dosages as high as possible without producing intolerable side effects such as sedation or ataxia. Subependymal lesions adjacent to the ventricular system may produce hydrocephalus amenable to shunting or may develop into malignant tumors that may be resectable surgically.

The dementia of *Huntington disease* has not responded to pharmacologic management. Seizures are treated with standard anticonvulsant agents. The movement disorder, whose suggested pathophysiologic basis is cholinergic underactivity or dopaminergic overactivity, has been treated with variable success with cholinergic and dopamine-blocking agents. An attempt to increase brain content of gamma aminobutyric acid (GABA) (an inhibitory neurotransmitter suggested to be deficient in the brains of persons with Huntington disease) through the administration of amino oxyacetic acid did not produce beneficial effects (Perry *et al.*, 1980).

Treatment of *Wilson disease* is directed toward reducing the body's "copper burden" in liver, brain, and other organs. D-Penicillamine, a chelating agent, is used orally in conjunction with limitation of foods rich in copper (Rapin, 1976). These include chocolate, nuts, mushrooms, liver, and shellfish. Potassium disulfide has been used to bind copper in the stomach. With early detection and prompt institution of treatment, hepatic and central nervous system effects can be minimized (Berry *et al.*, 1974). Under these circumstances, prognosis is good to excellent, whereas the untreated child cannot be expected to survive beyond 5 years (Swaiman, 1975).

The course of *brainstem glioma* is variable and consistent with survival for several years, sometimes longer. Operative removal is usually not possible. Radiotherapy is frequently employed. When hydrocephalus is a complicating feature, ventriculoperitoneal shunting can be carried out.

Treatment of seizures is presented in Chapter 12.

Homocystinuria is treated with a low-methionine diet and with high doses of vitamins (pyridoxine, folic acid, or vitamin B_{12}, depending upon the form of the disorder). Associated behavioral disturbances have been reversed by such vitamin and dietary therapy (Freeman *et al.*, 1975). Early detection of affected children through newborn screening programs for amino acid disorders has led to early therapy and apparent prevention of mental retardation.

Leigh disease has, in some instances, been treated successfully with high doses of thiamine (Pincus, 1972; Plaitakis *et al.*, 1980). More often, however, the disease pursues a progressively downhill course that is not significantly influenced by any therapy.

The cornerstone of management in *acute intermittent porphyria* is prevention. Affected persons must avoid exposure to offending agents such as phenobarbital, sulfa drugs, griseofulvin, and alcohol. Relatives of affected persons should be screened for the disorder by assay of uroporphyrinogen I synthetase in blood. When seizures occur, they must not be treated with phenobarbital. Likewise, with severe abdominal pain, phenobarbital should not be used for sedation. Rather, use of a phenothiazine is recommended. A medical identification bracelet indicating sensitivity to phenobarbital and sulfa drugs will help to minimize the danger of inadvertent administration of these offending agents. When acute demyelination severely compromises respiratory function, ventilatory support may be required.

Surgical Management. Surgery plays a relatively minor role in the treatment of syndromes of behavioral regression. As indicated above, ventriculoperitoneal shunting may be carried out to relieve increased intracranial pressure due to hydrocephalus.

Psychotherapy. The following statement, though pertaining specifically to Wilson disease, can be applied to other syndromes of behavioral regression as well: "Really significant improvement in emotional health can only be brought about if removal of copper and appropriate psychotherapy are simultaneously employed" (Scheinberg, 1975).

This statement acknowledges the multiple levels (chemical, psychologic, and social) that Wilson disease characteristically affects and pleads, in effect, for more comprehensive treatment than mere administration of penicillamine. Scheinberg has described how individual psychotherapy provided a young man with Wilson disease insights into his illness and his own behavior.

In most instances therapy involving the child and family will be primarily supportive, particularly when the illness produces a chronic downhill course (Shoulson and Fahn, 1979) (see Chapter 21). When a child is withdrawn and depressed, several sessions may be necessary to establish a therapeutic relationship. It may then be possible for the child to talk about difficult issues of death and dying.

Social-Environmental Management. When a disturbed and discontinuous social setting has produced a syndrome of depression or behavioral regression, appropriate foster care, pending stabilization of the home environment, or a support system involving the family of origin should be effected.

Physical Therapy. Physical therapy is often an integral part of symptomatic and supportive care. Children with degenerative neurologic disorders may acquire contractures secondary to limitation of voluntary movement and develop pneumonia because of difficulty in handling oral secretions. Not only can physical therapy help the child maximize motor and pulmonary functions, but it provides meaningful interpersonal contact in illnesses that can be marked by increasing isolation of the child.

Mechanical Therapy. Crutches, braces, elevators, wheelchairs, and specially equipped vans are mechanical modes of therapy that can help the motorically handicapped child and his or her family.

CORRELATION

Anatomic Aspects. Examination of the eyes is an essential part of the general physical and neurologic examinations. It will often provide valuable diagnostic information in the evaluation of the child with behavioral regression.

A Kayser-Fleischer ring at the outer margin (or limbus) of the cornea is a diagnostic hallmark of Wilson disease, though it need not be present for the diagnosis to be established. It is a brownish or greenish ring, 3 to 4 mm wide, resulting from deposition of copper within the cornea. Slit-lamp examination may be necessary for its visualization. The ring may disappear during the course of dietary and pharmocologic treatment.

Extraocular movements are often abnormal in conditions causing behavioral regression that affect the brainstem. These include multiple sclerosis, Leigh disease, and brainstem glioma. With multiple sclerosis, a common complaint is diplopia (double vision) resulting from a disturbance in conjugate lateral gaze.

Conjugate lateral gaze depends upon an intact sixth nerve nucleus (abducens) of one side connected to the third cranial nerve nucleus (oculomotor) of the opposite side by the medial longitudinal fasciculus (MLF) (see Fig. 8–9). Movements of eyes conjugately to the right thus involve the right abducens nucleus, the left oculomotor nucleus, and the interconnecting MLF. Cortical input for lateral gaze reaches the right sixth nerve nucleus from the left frontal lobe cortex through centers for conjugate lateral gaze lying adjacent to each abducens nucleus, to which they are connected. These centers

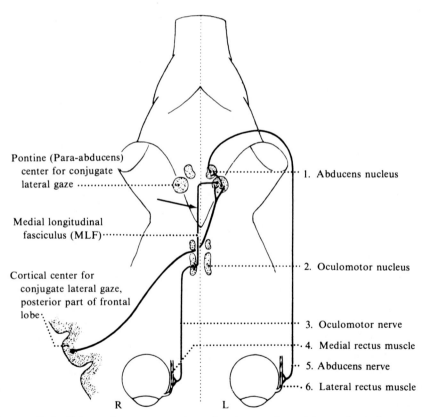

FIGURE 8–9. Schematic representation of pathways for conjugate lateral gaze. (From DeMyer, W. *Technique of the Neurologic Examination,* 3rd ed. Copyright © 1980, McGraw-Hill Book Company. Used with the permission of McGraw-Hill Book Company.)

are not connected directly to the oculomotor nuclei. Interruption of the MLF on the left (e.g., as a result of demyelination) will not influence abduction on the right but will interfere with adduction of the left eye. On attempted lateral gaze to the right, therefore, the affected person will see double.

Altered pupillary reactions to light also may be seen with multiple sclerosis. Demyelination of optic nerve fibers (with or without subsequent remyelination) is often associated with pupillary "escape" (a so-called Marcus Gunn pupil). Prompt constriction (usually partial) occurs on the affected side, but it cannot be sustained for longer than a few seconds.

The swinging flashlight sign also provides evidence of afferent pupillary dysfunction. It involves demonstrating that the pupil of the affected eye constricts normally upon consensual stimulation, that is, when light is shined in the normal eye. When the light is brought across the bridge of the nose to the abnormal eye (without startling the child, which can cause pupillary dilation as part of a fear reaction), the previously constricted pupil dilates despite direct exposure to light.

Funduscopic inspection is an essential part of the examination of the child with behavioral regression. The macula, optic disk, and retinal background each may provide valuable information (see Fig. 2–15). The macula may show degeneration in SSPE or a cherry red appearance in storage disorders such as Tay-Sachs disease, Sandhoff disease, Niemann-Pick disease, generalized gangliosidosis, and mucolipidosis I. In fact, the macula itself is normally colored. The surrounding retina, however, appears pale yellow because ganglion cells are engorged with storage material, GM_2 ganglioside in Tay-Sachs disease.

Optic atrophy is often seen with metachromatic leukodystrophy, Krabbe leukodystrophy, Tay-Sachs disease, and the ceroid lipofuscinoses. The disk is pale or chalky white rather than pink in color. Arterial vessels are attenuated and often diminished in number. Visual acuity is often reduced.

Visualization of the retinal background may disclose evidence of pigmentary degeneration of the retina (retinitis pigmentosa). Black pigment may appear as tiny chunks of coal. Fibroadenomatous lesions (retinal phakomas) may be evident in the child with tuberous sclerosis.

Examination of the optic disks may disclose elevation of the nerve heads and blurring of the disk margins. These changes are characteristically seen with increased intracranial pressure (as might result from a brain tumor) or optic papillitis (as with multiple sclerosis).

Biochemical Aspects. Myelin, distributed widely throughout the nervous system, functions as an electrical insulator allowing efficient communication between parts of the body (Morrell and Norton, 1980). Myelin is made by oligodendroglial cells within the central nervous system and by Schwann cells within the peripheral nervous system.

Some 70 per cent of the dry weight of myelin within the central nervous system is lipid material. Among the lipids are cholesterol, phospholipids, and glycolipids. The major glycolipid of brain is cerebroside, which is virtually restricted to myelin sheaths and constitutes nearly 6 per cent of the dry weight of the entire brain. Cerebroside consists of ceramide and a hex-

TABLE 8–4. **Important Lipids of Brain**

Ceramide	=	Sphingosine	+	Fatty acid
Cerebroside	=	Ceramide	+	Hexose
Sulfatide	=	Cerebroside	+	Sulfate

ose, either glucose or galactose. Ceramide, in turn, consists of sphingosine (a lipid) combined with a fatty acid (see Table 8–4).

The cerebroside containing galactose, galactocerebroside, is broken down into ceramide and galactose by the enzyme galactocerebrosidase. When this enzyme is deficient, as in Krabbe leukodystrophy, ceramide-galactose (or galactocerebroside) accumulates (see Table 8–5).

The addition of sulfate to galactocerebroside produces sulfatide. Breakdown of sulfatide into galactocerebroside and sulfate is catalyzed by the enzyme arylsulfatase A. With metachromatic leukodystrophy (MLD, or sulfatide lipidosis), arylsulfatase A is deficient and sulfatide accumulates in many tissues (see Table 8–5). These include brain, kidney, gallbladder, and peripheral nerve. In MLD, renal tubules may shed epithelial cells that contain sulfatide granules into the urine. Because these granules are stained orange-brown with cresyl-violet dye instead of blue, they are termed metachromatic. Older diagnostic tests were based upon this metachromatic staining. Availability of assay of the enzyme arylsulfatase A, however, has rendered diagnosis of MLD by analysis of urine rarely necessary. Storage of sulfatide also accounts for nonvisualization of the gallbladder by cholecystogram (an older diagnostic method) and slowing of peripheral nerve conduction velocity (still a valuable sign of the disorder).

Physiologic Aspects.   Special investigations can serve to elucidate areas of impaired function in several of the syndromes of behavioral regression. These include measurement of nerve conduction velocities and determination of visual evoked responses.

Measurement of nerve conduction velocity is accomplished by simulating the normal physiologic process of neuromuscular transmission by electrically stimulating a nerve to produce muscular contraction (see Fig. 8–10). For example, a mild electrical stimulus is delivered to the peroneal nerve at the knee, and the time it takes for the extensor digitorum brevis to contract

TABLE 8–5. **Metabolism of Sulfatide and Galactocerebroside**

	Metachromatic Leukodystrophy	*Krabbe Leukodystrophy*
Reaction	Ceramide-galactose sulfate → ceramide-galactose	Ceramide-galactose → ceramide
Necessary Enzyme	Arylsulfatase A	Galactocerebrosidase
Material Accumulated Because of Enzyme Deficiency	Sulfatide (ceramide-galactose-sulfate)	Galactocerebroside (ceramide-galactose)

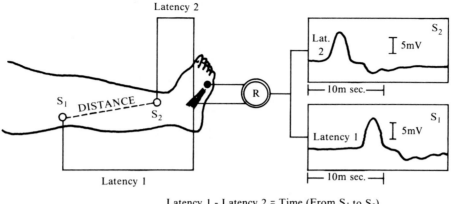

Latency 1 - Latency 2 = Time (From S_1 to S_2)

$$\frac{\text{Distance}}{\text{Time}} = \text{Velocity}$$

FIGURE 8–10. Schematic representation of method of determining nerve conduction velocity. S_1 and S_2 are points of stimulation, with muscle contraction recorded at R. (From Wright, F. S. Electrodiagnosis of neuromuscular diseases. In *The Practice of Pediatric Neurology*. Swaiman, K. F., and Wright, F. S., eds. C. V. Mosby Company, Saint Louis, 1975.)

is recorded. This process is repeated more distally with stimulation of the nerve just above the ankle. The measured distance between the two points of stimulation is divided by the difference in times obtained to give the nerve conduction velocity. The mean conduction velocity for the peroneal nerve in a 5-year-old child is 58 meters per second (Wright, 1975).

Nerve conduction velocities are characteristically slowed in metachromatic leukodystrophy, Krabbe leukodystrophy, and acute intermittent porphyria. The clinical correlate of slowed nerve conduction is absence or diminution of deep tendon reflexes.

The measurement of visual evoked responses is useful in assessing involvement of the visual pathways in multiple sclerosis. The test involves presentation of bursts of light or patterns (e.g., a checkerboard) and recording resultant electrical responses over the occipital cortex. Undesired electrical activity is averaged out through the use of a computer. Cortical evoked responses thus become apparent as characteristic wave patterns. Delay in appearance of an evoked response or abnormal configuration confirms a problem affecting the visual system and provides localizing information. With multiple sclerosis affecting the visual pathway by demyelination of optic nerve fibers (with or without subsequent remyelination), delayed conduction through the optic nerve and diminished amplitude of evoked responses are seen.

The clinical analog of altered conduction through the optic nerve is the so-called Pulfrich phenomenon. A pendulum swung in front of an affected person in side-to-side fashion will appear to move in an elliptoid course, traveling closer to and farther from the person, rather than simply back and forth (Wist *et al.*, 1978).

SUMMARY

Syndromes of behavioral regression in childhood range from benign, self-limited episodes to relentlessly progressive degenerative disorders. Behavioral regression may be described by a pattern of loss of previously gained skills, failure to acquire new skills, or acquisition of new skills at a slower pace than before.

Causes of behavioral regression range widely. Among the medical causes are systemic illness such as hypothyroidism and malignancy. Neurologic causes include storage disorders, demyelinating diseases, leukodystrophies, progressive viral disease, neurocutaneous disorders, brain tumor, metabolic disorders, and hydrocephalus. Social and psychologic trauma may also produce syndromes of behavioral regression, as may toxic agents such as lead and drugs, including anticonvulsants.

Medical and neurologic management will depend upon the particular disorder. Supportive therapy is always indicated for family and child. Genetic counseling will often be beneficial in assisting family planning.

CITED REFERENCES

Arsenio-Nunes, M. L.; Goutières, F.; and Aicardi, J. An ultramicroscopic study of skin and conjunctival biopsies in chronic neurological disorders of childhood. *Ann. Neurol.*, **9:** 163–73, 1981.

Barclay, N. Acute intermittent porphyria in childhood. *Arch. Dis. Child.*, **49:** 404–406, 1974.

Barkley, R. A., and Murphy, J. V. Pseudodeterioration of intelligence in children. *Ann. Neurol.*, **4:** 388, 1978.

Barlow, C. F. Case records of the Massachusetts General Hospital (Case 29–1978) *N. Engl. J. Med.*, **299:** 189–94, 1978.

Berry, W. R.; Aronson, A. E.; Darley, F. L.; and Goldstein, N. P. Effects of penicillamine therapy and low-copper diet on dysarthria in Wilson's disease (hepatolenticular degeneration). *Mayo Clin. Proc.*, **49:** 405–408, 1974.

Betts, T. A.; Smith, W. T.; and Kelly, R. E. Adult metachromatic leukodystrophy (sulphatide lipidosis) simulating acute schizophrenia. *Neurology*, **18:** 1140–42, 1968.

Bhettay, E.; Kipps, A.; and McDonald, R. Early onset of subacute sclerosing panencephalitis. *J. Pediatr.*, **89:** 271–72, 1976.

Bray, P. F.; Carter, S.; and Taveras, J. M. Brainstem tumors in children. *Neurology*, **8:** 1–7, 1958.

Bresnan, M. J. Case records of the Massachusetts General Hospital (Case 18–1979) *N. Engl. J. Med.*, **300:** 1037–45, 1979.

Cartwright, G. E. Diagnosis of treatable Wilson's disease. *N. Engl. J. Med.*, **298:** 1347–50, 1978.

Center for Disease Control. Preventing lead poisoning in young children. *J. Pediatr.*, **93:** 709–20, 1978.

Ch'ien, L. T.; Aur, R. J. A.; Stagner, S.; Cavallo, K.; Wood, A.; Goff, J.; Pitner, S.; Hustu, H. O.; Seifert, M. J.; and Simone, J. V. Long-term neurological implications of somnolence syndrome in children with acute lymphocytic leukemia. *Ann. Neurol.*, **8:** 273–77, 1980.

Cook, S. D., and Dowling, P. C. Multiple sclerosis and viruses: an overview. *Neurology*, **30:** 80–91, 1980.

Corbett, J.; Harris, R.; Taylor, E.; and Trimble, M. Progressive disintegrative psychosis of childhood. *J. Child Psychol. Psychiatry,* **18:** 211–19, 1977.

Coyle, P. K., and Wolinsky, J. S. Characterization of immune complexes in progressive rubella panencephalitis. *Ann. Neurol.,* **9:** 557–62, 1981.

Creak, E. M. Childhood psychosis: a review of 100 cases. *Br. J. Psychiatry,* **109:** 84–89, 1963.

Davis, L. J., and Goldstein, N. P. Psychologic investigation of Wilson's disease. *Mayo Clin. Proc.,* **49:** 409–11, 1974.

DeVivo, D. C.; Malas, D.; Nelson, J. S.; and Land, V. J. Leukoencephalopathy in childhood leukemia. *Neurology,* **27:** 609–13, 1977.

Dobyns, W. B.; Goldstein, N. P.; and Gordon, H. Clinical spectrum of Wilson's disease (hepatolenticular degeneration). *Mayo Clin. Proc.,* **54:** 35–42, 1979.

Dooling, E. C., and Richardson, E. P., Jr. Delayed encephalopathy after strangling. *Arch. Neurol.,* **33:** 196–99, 1976.

Dooling, E. C.; Schoene, W. C. and Richardson, E. P., Jr. Hallervorden-Spatz syndrome. *Arch. Neurol.,* **30:** 70–83, 1974.

Dowling, P. C.; Bosch, V. V.; and Cook, S. D. Possible beneficial effect of high-dose intravenous steroid therapy in acute demyelinating disease and transverse myelitis. *Neurology,* **30:** 33–36, 1980.

Dyken, P. Ceroid-lipofuscinoses. Pp. 735–39 in *The Practice of Pediatric Neurology.* Swaiman, K. F., and Wright, F. S., eds. C. V. Mosby Company, Saint Louis, 1975.

Ellison, G. W., and Myers, L. W. Immunosuppressive drugs in multiple sclerosis: pro and con. *Neurology,* **30:** 28–32, 1980.

Evans-Jones, L. G., and Rosenbloom, L. Disintegrative psychosis in childhood. *Dev. Med. Child Neurol.,* **20:** 462–70, 1978.

Farrell, D. F.; MacMartin, M. P.; and Clark, A. F. Multiple molecular forms of arylsulfatase A in different forms of metachromatic leukodystrophy (MLD). *Neurology,* **29:** 16–20, 1979.

Feldman, K. W., and Simms, R. J. Strangulation in childhood: epidemiology and clinical course. *Pediatrics,* **65:** 1079–85, 1980.

Freeman, J. M.; Finkelstein, J. D.; and Mudd, S. H. Folate-responsive homocystinuria and "schizophrenia": a defect in methylation due to deficient 5,10-methylenetetrahydrofolate reductase activity. *N. Engl. J. Med.,* **292:** 491–96, 1975.

Gordon, N.; Marsden, H. B., and Lewis, D. M. Subacute necrotising encephalomyelopathy in three siblings. *Dev. Med. Child Neurol.,* **16:** 64–78, 1974.

Hansotia, P.; Cleeland, C. S., and Chun, R. W. M. Juvenile Huntington's chorea. *Neurology,* **18:** 217–24, 1968.

Hoefnagel, D.; van den Noort, S., and Ingbar, S. H. Diffuse cerebral sclerosis with endocrine abnormalities in young males. *Brain,* **85:** 553–68, 1962.

Hoeppner, T., and Lolas, F. Visual evoked responses and visual symptoms in multiple sclerosis. *J. Neurol. Neurosurg. Psychiatry,* **41:** 493–98, 1978.

Jabbour, J. T.; Garcia, J. H.: Lemmi, H.; Ragland, J.; Duenas, D. A.; and Sever, J. L. Subacute sclerosing panencephalitis: a multidisciplinary study of eight cases. *JAMA,* **207:** 2248–54, 1969.

Jan, J. E.; Tingle, A. J.; Donald, G.; Kettyls, M.; Buckler, W. S. J.; and Dolman, C. L. Progressive rubella panencephalitis: clinical course and response to isoprinosine. *Dev. Med. Child Neurol.,* **21:** 648, 1979.

Jervis, G. A. Huntington's chorea in childhood. *Arch. Neurol.,* **9:** 244–57. 1963.

Juberg, R. C. . . . but the family history was negative. *J. Pediatr.,* **91:** 693–94, 1977.

Lisak, R. P. Multiple sclerosis: evidence for immunopathogenesis, *Neurology,* **30:** 99–104, 1980.

Logan, W. J., and Freeman, J. M. Pseudodegenerative disease due to diphenylhydan-toin intoxication. *Arch. Neurol.,* **21:** 631–37, 1969.

Malamud, N. Heller's disease and childhood schizophrenia. *Am. J. Psychiatry,* **116:** 215–18, 1959.

MacGregor, D. L.; Humphrey, R. P.; Armstrong, D. L.; and Becker, L. E. Brain biopsies for neurodegenerative disease in children. *J. Pediatr.,* **92:** 903–905, 1978.

Manowitz, P.; Kling, A.; and Kohn, H. Clinical course of adult metachromatic leuko-dystrophy presenting as schizophrenia. *J. Nerv. Ment. Dis.,* **166:** 500–506, 1978.

Markham, C. H., and Knox, J. W. Observations on Huntington's chorea in child-hood. *J. Pediatr.,* **67:** 46–57, 1965.

McIntosh, S., and Aspnes, G. T. Encephalopathy following CNS prophylaxis in childhood lymphoblastic leukemia. *Pediatrics,* **52:** 612–15, 1973.

Money, J. Intellectual functioning in childhood endocrinopathies and related cyto-genic disorders. Pp. 1207–10 in *Endocrine and Genetic Diseases of Childhood and Adolescence,* 2nd ed. Gardner, L. I., ed. W. B. Saunders Company, Philadelphia, 1975.

Morell, P., and Norton, W. T. Myelin. *Sci. Am.,* **198:** 88–114, 1980.

Moser, H. W.; Moser, A. E.; Frayer, K. K.; Chen, W.; Schulman, J. D.; O'Neill, B. P.; and Kishimoto, Y. Adrenoleukodystrophy: increased plasma content of sat-urated very long chain fatty acids. *Neurology,* **31:** 1241–49, 1981.

Nathanson, N., and Miller, A. Epidemiology of multiple sclerosis: critique of the evi-dence for a viral etiology. *Am. J. Epidemiology,* **107:** 451–61, 1978.

Needleman, H. L.; Gunnoe, C.; Leviton, A.; Reed, R.; Peresie, H.; Maher, C.; and Barrett, P. Deficits in psychologic and classroom performance of children with ele-vated dentine lead levels. *N. Engl. J. Med.,* **300:** 689–95, 1979.

Panitch, H. S., and Berg, B. O. Brain stem tumors of childhood and adolescence. *Am. J. Dis. Child.,* **119:** 465–72, 1970.

Percy, A. K., and Kaback, M. M. Infantile and adult-onset metachromatic leukodys-trophy: biochemical comparisons and predictive diagnosis. *N. Engl. J. Med.,* **285:** 785–87, 1971.

Perry, T. L.; Wright, J. M.; Hansen, S.; Allan, B. M.; Baird, P. A.; and MacLeod, P. M. Failure of aminooxyacetic acid therapy in Huntington disease, *Neurology,* **30:** 772–75, 1980.

Peylan-Ramu, N.; Poplack, D. G.; Pizzo, P. A.; Adornato, B. T., and Di Chiro, G. Abnormal CT scans of the brain in asymptomatic children with acute lymphocytic leukemia after prophylactic treatment of the central nervous system with radiation and intrathecal chemotherapy. *N. Engl. J. Med.,* **298:** 815–18, 1978.

Price, R. A., and Jamieson, P. A. The central nervous system in childhood leukemia: II. subacute leukoencephalopathy. *Cancer,* **35:** 306–18, 1975.

Picard, E. H. Case records of the Massachusetts General Hospital (Case 43–1965). *N. Engl. J. Med.,* **273:** 760–67, 1965.

Pincus, J. H. Subacute necrotizing encephalomyelopathy (Leigh's disease): a consid-eration of clinical features and etiology. *Dev. Med. Child Neurol.,* **14:** 87–101, 1972.

Plaitakis, A.; Whetsell, W. O., Jr.; Cooper, J. R.; and Yahr, M. D. Chronic Leigh disease: a genetic and biochemical study. *Ann. Neurol.,* **7:** 304–10, 1980.

Platt, M., and Rosman, N. P. Choroid plexus papilloma mimicking degenerative brain disease in childhood. *J. Pediatr.,* **80:** 483–84, 1972.

Rapin, I. Progressive genetic-metabolic diseases of the central nervous system in chil-dren. *Pediatr. Ann.,* **5:** 313–49, 1976.

Rivinus, T. M.; Jamison, D. L.; and Graham, P. J. Childhood organic neurological disease presenting as a psychiatric disorder. *Arch. Dis. Child.,* **50:** 115–19, 1975.

Ropper, A. H., and Williams, R. S. Relationship between plaques, tangles, and dementia in Down syndrome. *Neurology,* **30:** 639–44, 1980.

Rosman, N. P. Elevated intracranial pressure. In *The Practice of Pediatric Neurology,* 2nd ed. Swaiman, K. F., and Wright, F. S., eds. C. V. Mosby Company, Saint Louis, 1982.

Salguero, L. F.; Itabashi, H. H.; and Gutierrez, N. B. Childhood multiple sclerosis with psychotic manifestations. *J. Neurol. Neurosurg. Psychiatry,* **32:** 572–79, 1969.

Schaumburg, H. H.; Powers, J. M.; Suzuki, K.; and Raine, C. S. Adreno-leukodystrophy (sex-linked Schilder disease). *Arch. Neurol.,* **31:** 210–13, 1974.

Scheinberg, I. H. A psychogenetic anecdote. *Psychosom. Med.,* **37:** 368–71, 1975.

Scheinberg, I. H.; Sternlieb, I.; and Richman, J. Psychiatric manifestations in patients with Wilson's disease. Birth Defects Original Article Series, Vol. 4, No. 2, pp. 85–87, 1968.

Shoulson, I., and Fahn, S. Huntington disease: clinical care and evaluation. *Neurology,* **29:** 1–3, 1979.

Sipe, J. C. Leigh's syndrome: the adult form of subacute necrotizing encephalomyelopathy with predilection for the brainstem. *Neurology,* **23:** 1030–38, 1973.

Swaiman, K. F. Lipid diseases of the central nervous system. Pp. 397–412 in *The Practice of Pediatric Neurology.* Swaiman, K. F., and Wright, F. S., eds. C. V. Mosby Co., Saint Louis, 1975.

Tang, T. T.; Good, T. A.; Dyken, P. R.; Johnsen, S. D.; McCreadie, S. R.; Sy, S. T.; Lardy, H. A.; and Rudolph, F. B. Pathogenesis of Leigh's encephalomyelopathy. *J. Pediatr.,* **81:** 189–90, 1972.

Townsend, J. J.; Baringer, J. R.; Wolinsky, J. S.; Malamud, N.; Mednick, J. P.; Panitch, H. S.; Scott, R. A. T.; Oshiro, L. S.; and Cremer, N. E. Progressive rubella panencephalitis: late onset after congenital rubella. *N. Engl. J. Med.,* **292:** 990–93, 1975.

Vakili, S.; Drew, A. L.; Von Schuching, S.; Becker, D.; and Zeman, W. Hallervorden-Spatz syndrome. *Arch. Neurol.,* **34:** 729–38, 1977.

Valenstein, E.; Rosman, N. P., and Carter, A. P. Schilder's disease. Positive brain scan. *JAMA,* **217:** 1699–1700, 1971.

Weil, M. L.; Itabashi, H. H.; Cremer, N. E.; Oshiro, L. S.; Lennette, E. H.; and Carnay, L. Chronic progressive panencephalitis due to rubella virus simulating subacute sclerosing panencephalitis. *N. Engl. J. Med.,* **292:** 994–98, 1975.

Whitley, R. J.; Soong, S.-J.; Dolin, R.; Galasso, G. J.; Ch'ien, L. T.; Alford, C. A.; and the Collaborative Study Group. Adenine arabinoside therapy of biopsy-proved herpes simplex encephalitis. *N. Engl. J. Med.,* **297:** 289–94, 1977.

Wisniewski, K.; Howe, J.; Williams, D. G.; and Wisniewski, H. M. Precocious aging and dementia in patients with Down's syndrome. *Biol. Psychiatry,* **13:** 619–27, 1978.

Wist, E. R.; Hennerici, M.; and Dichgans, J. The Pulfrich spatial frequency phenomenon: a psychophysical method competitive to visual evoked potentials in the diagnosis of multiple sclerosis. *J. Neurol. Neurosurg. Psychiatry,* **41:** 1069–77, 1978.

Wolinsky, J. S.; Berg, B. O.; and Maitland, C. J. Progressive rubella panencephalitis. *Arch. Neurol.,* **33:** 722–23, 1976.

Wright, F. S. Electrodiagnosis of neuromuscular diseases. Pp. 57–64 in *The Practice of Pediatric Neurology.* Swaiman, K. F., and Wright, F. S., eds. C. V. Mosby Company, Saint Louis, 1975.

Zeman, W., and Dyken, P. Neuronal ceroid-lipofuscinosis (Batten's disease): relationship to amaurotic family idiocy? *Pediatrics.* **44:** 570–83, 1969.

ADDITIONAL READINGS

Choppin, P. W. Measles virus and chronic neurological diseases. *Ann. Neurol.,* **9:** 17–20, 1981.

Gajdusek, D. C., and Zigas, V. Kuru. *Am. J. Med.,* **26:** 442–69, 1959.

Heller, T. About dementia infantilis. *J. Nerv. Ment. Dis.,* **119:** 472–77, 1954.

Rosenberg, R. N. Biochemical genetics of neurologic disease. *N. Engl. J. Med.,* **305:** 1181–93, 1981.

9 Sleep Disorders: Nightmares, Night Terrors, and Hypersomnias

Disorders of sleep in childhood frequently present diagnostic and therapeutic puzzles to pediatricians, neurologists, or psychiatrists called upon by distressed parents to solve them. Fortunately, the last three decades have seen a tremendous increase in our understanding of normal sleep and its disorders, and further elucidation is anticipated. Progress has been based upon both simple observations of sleeping persons and the use of sophisticated sleep laboratories, both of which will be reviewed in this chapter.

Two areas of sleep disturbance in childhood will be focused upon. The first will comprise nightmares and night terrors, among the commonest and most dramatic sleep problems. The second will be the hypersomnias, a group of disorders in which sleep is inappropriate in time of occurrence or excessive in amount. These problems will be characterized in terms of distinct syndromes, with emphasis upon important historical points, characteristic features of examination, appropriate investigation, and therapy.

A number of questions will be addressed:

What is the definition of sleep?
What is a "night terror" and how can it be distinguished from a "nightmare"?
What investigation, if any, should be undertaken in the child with nightmares? Night terrors?
Is simple reassurance enough, or should drugs be employed in treatment of these problems?
Does narcolepsy occur in childhood?
What other causes for hypersomnia occur among children?
How should they be evaluated and treated?
What are the anatomic, biochemical, and physiologic correlates of sleep?

195

NIGHTMARES AND NIGHT TERRORS

DEFINITION

Despite its familiarity, sleep is somewhat difficult to define. The *Oxford English Dictionary* (1971) calls it "the unconscious state or condition regularly and naturally assumed by man and animals during which the activity of the central nervous system is almost entirely suspended and recuperation of its powers takes place." Oswald (1971) termed it "a recurrent, healthy state of inertia and unresponsiveness."

Both definitions, most would agree, include important features of sleep but are not in themselves complete. Unconsciousness does indeed occur, in that the sleeping person is unaware of self. On the other hand, the sleeping person is at least somewhat responsive. For example, a limb will be withdrawn from painful stimulation, and a sleeping mother may be very attentive to the stirrings of her infant. Nor does inertia describe fully accurately the motor state of the sleeping person, as limb, trunk, and eye movements variously occur during sleep.

A particular difficulty in the definition of sleep is that it is not a single state but rather a succession of states, indeed a process, as studies of sleeping persons have demonstrated (Aserinsky and Kleitman, 1955; Dement and Kleitman, 1957). Dement and Kleitman (1957) investigated sleep in adults in a sleep laboratory and found through continuous electroencephalographic recording with monitoring of pulse, respiration, and muscle activity an orderly periodicity to the process.

Sleep is made up of a succession of cycles, each lasting some 90 minutes and consisting of two relatively distinct phases. During "orthodox" sleep, heart rate and respirations are regular; some skeletal muscle tone is maintained; and slow, drifting eye movements occur. "Paradoxical" sleep derives its name from the associated electroencephalographic pattern, which resembles that of the awake state more than that of orthodox sleep. Pulse and respiration are relatively irregular, and the body appears virtually paralyzed save for occasional flickering movements of the extremities occurring distally.

A most striking feature of paradoxical sleep is the occurrence of rapid eye movements. This phase of sleep is thus usually called *rapid eye movement* (or *REM*) sleep. Orthodox sleep is accordingly called *non-rapid eye movement (non-REM, or NREM) sleep.*

A night's sleep generally consists of four to six sleep cycles of about 90 minutes each. The non-REM phase makes up nearly three-quarters of each sleep cycle and is followed by REM periods lasting between 10 and 30 minutes. Dreaming appears to occur primarily during REM sleep as determined by studies of dream recall involving persons awakened at different stages of the sleep cycle (see Table 9–1) (Fisher *et al.,* 1973). Additional aspects of REM versus non-REM sleep are discussed in the section on CORRELATION: PHYSIOLOGIC ASPECTS.

The *night terror* is probably the most dramatic and upsetting sleep disturbance of childhood. An important though ironic feature of the night terror is that the child is usually quite oblivious to the uproar created, while parents are often shaken by what they have just experienced.

TABLE 9–1. **The Two Phases of Sleep**

	Non-REM ("orthodox")	REM ("paradoxical")
Proportion of sleep cycle	$\frac{3}{4}$	$\frac{1}{4}$
Body movement and tone	Some	Little
Pulse and respirations	Regular	Irregular
Eye movements	Slow, roving	Rapid bursts
Duration	60–80 minutes	10–30 minutes
EEG	Sleep spindles, slow waves	Low-amplitude, relatively fast activity
Dreaming	Usually absent	Typically present

The following account typifies the night terror. An hour or two after the child has fallen asleep, the parents hear a terrified scream coming from the child's bedroom. Upon entering the room, they see him sitting upright in bed, obviously panic-stricken and not recognizing them. His heart is racing, his skin is warm to the touch, and he is not calmed by their efforts to console him. The parents may otherwise have been alerted by the child's yelling and running through the house, knocking over objects in his rampage. After 5 to 15 minutes, the episode usually ceases spontaneously. When the child, now fully alert, is asked what he was afraid of, he responds only in vague and general terms. He then returns to sleep readily and has no recall of the event whatsoever the next morning.

The *nightmare*, by contrast, is usually over by the time the parents know about it. Typically, the child walks into their bedroom crying that monsters have attacked him, threatening to chop off his head; but he has managed to escape just in time. Though worried, he is not panic-stricken. With reassurance from his parents, he returns to his bedroom, where the door is left open a bit wider than usual so the hallway light can shine in. Perhaps with some difficulty, he falls back to sleep. The next morning the child recalls having had a "bad dream."

These two descriptions illustrate fundamental differences between the night terror and the nightmare (see Table 9–2). In summary, these are the child's state of alertness (incomplete versus complete arousal), degree of dream content (limited versus rich), affective state (panic versus mild-to-moderate anxiety), difficulty in getting to sleep afterward (none versus a variable degree), and recollection of the event the following day (none versus at least partial recall). Evaluation of the child with nightmares or night terrors should be undertaken when the sleep disturbance interferes significantly with sleep or appears linked with changes in behavior or affect during the day.

DIAGNOSIS

Clinical Process.   The history provides the most crucial diagnostic information when evaluating the child with a nightmare or night terror. Examination and investigation generally play less important roles, though the sleep laboratory (when available) may be definitively diagnostic.

TABLE 9–2. **Differentiation Between Nightmares and Night Terrors**

	Nightmares	*Night Terrors*
State of alertness	Asleep	Incomplete arousal
Ease of arousal to full alertness	Relatively easy	Difficult
Degree of autonomic activation	Mild to moderate	Marked
Automatic behavior (including sleepwalking)	Absent	Typical
Associated dream content	Rich	Little if any
Difficulty in returning to sleep	Often	Not usually
Amnesia for episode	No	Usually
Phase of sleep	During REM sleep	Arises from slow-wave portion of non-REM sleep
EEG pattern	Typical of REM sleep	Resembling wakefulness

History.   The child's description of the problem is especially important with sleep disturbances. For, as discussed above, nightmares and night terrors are differentiable in part by the child's recall of the episode. Thus, the chief complaint may be a shrug of the shoulders and "I don't know." This response would suggest a night terror. On the other hand, the child may say "I've been having nightmares." Such a statement should be recorded but not necessarily taken at face value, however, because the parents may have labeled a night terror incorrectly as a nightmare and the child may be following their example.

The history of the presenting problem should characterize the episodes in terms of onset, frequency, and specific features. When did they begin? How often do they occur? Have precipitating causes been identified? How soon after going to sleep do the episodes begin? How do parents become aware of the sleep disturbance? What is the child's state of arousal and agitation? What have the parents tried in order to bring the situation under control? How long do the episodes last? Are involuntary movements or incontinence associated? Once the episode has ended, what does the child recall—a bad dream in detail or poorly defined feelings of dread and terror? Does the child have difficulty in returning to sleep? What does he or she remember of the sleep disturbance the next morning?

Additional history should clarify the psychosocial and family setting in which the episodes have taken place. Current and past medical illnesses (particularly psychophysiologic disorders such as asthma, eczema, and ulcerative colitis) should be noted. Seizures or conditions predisposing to seizures, such as head trauma or perinatal difficulties, should be sought. History of recent drug habits, including discontinuation of barbiturates or alcohol, also should be noted.

Examination.   The child's perception of the problem, including recall of the episodes, is part not only of the history but of the *mental status examina-*

CASE 9–1: NIGHT TERRORS AND ABNORMAL EEG IN A 9-YEAR-OLD GIRL

L.O. was referred for evaluation because of episodes of sleep disturbance for several weeks. Two hours after falling asleep, she jumped out of bed and ran "screeching" into the parlor, where she pawed at the walls in fright. She failed to recognize her mother, who said she had to "slap" her to arouse her from her wide-eyed state of panic, of which she had no recall. The family was disrupted for several consecutive nights by similar disturbances until the parents took the child for evaluation later that week.

Past history was notable for episodes of sleepwalking beginning at age 2 years (one of which was associated with enuresis), "nightmares" first noted at 4 years, and poorly defined staring spells at 6 years. She was a 4-pound, 4-ounce (small for gestational age) product of a 43-week pregnancy. Family history included a maternal uncle with a grand mal seizure disorder beginning in adolescence.

The child was entirely normal on examination. Electroencephalogram in the awake state showed bursts of generalized spike-and-slow-wave discharges made more frequent with hyperventilation and photic stimulation (see Fig. 9–1). Placed on phenytoin (Dilantin), she developed an erythematous macular rash. On phenobarbital, she became unusually hyperactive. She was then treated with mephobarbital (Mebaral), 150 mg daily, which eliminated night terrors within 3 days, although she continued to have occasional nightmares and episodes of sleepwalking.

Comment. This child presented a picture typical for night terrors with incomplete arousal from sleep to a state of panic and with amnesia for the episodes. An EEG was obtained because of the frequency of night terrors and the possibility of seizure disorder as suggested by the episode of sleepwalking with enuresis and the history of staring spells. Although the EEG was markedly abnormal and the child responded to treatment with anticonvulsant medication, the episodes themselves are night terrors, not seizures. One can infer that spike-and-wave discharges disrupted her sleep cycle to produce the night terrors.

Management in this case was complicated by a coexisting attention deficit disorder manifested by hyperactivity, impulsivity, easy distractability, and dysphoria. Her treatment has been multifaceted with medical, psychiatric, and neurologic management coordinated by the family pediatrician. Treatment has included environmental measures to ensure the child's safety, individual and family psychotherapy, and use of dextroamphetamine in addition to mephobarbital. Her parents were advised not to shake or slap the child to arouse her because of the danger of causing a whiplash injury.

tion as well. Evidence of anxiety or depression should be noted. The *general physical examination* should include particular attention to evidence of psychophysiologic disorder such as eczema or asthma that might play a contri-

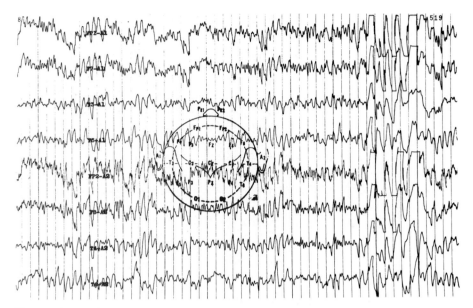

FIGURE 9–1. Electroencephalogram showing generalized bursts of spike-and-slow-wave discharges in the awake state (Case 9–1).

buting role. Both the general examination and the *neurologic examination* usually will be normal in children with nightmares or night terrors.

Investigation. The child with well-defined nightmares ("bad dreams") need undergo no investigation. With night terrors, however, the situation may be more complicated (see Table 9–3). In general, frequent episodes (arbitrarily, more than one a week) occurring after 3 or 4 years of age, atypical features suggesting seizure (such as stereotyped movements or incontinence), or abnormal signs on neurologic examination are indications for electroencephalography carried out in the awake and sleep states (see Case 9–1). When seizures of temporal lobe origin are suspected, use of nasopharyngeal leads for EEG recording should be considered, especially when a standard EEG has been unrevealing.

An all-night electroencephalographic recording that includes monitoring of pulse, respirations, and eye and limb movements may be of great diagnostic value. Other investigations such as skull x-rays or CT scan should be obtained as the clinical situation warrants.

TABLE 9–3. **Investigations to Be Considered in the Child with Night Terrors**

EEG (in awake and sleep states)
EEG with nasopharyngeal recording
All-night EEG with monitoring of eye movements, pulse, respirations, and other
  physiologic functions
Skull x-rays
Cranial CT scan

TABLE 9–4. **Differential Diagnosis of Night Terror**

Nightmare
Sleepwalking
Temporal lobe seizure
Febrile delirium

Differential Diagnosis (see Table 9–4).   Nightmares and night terrors can be differentiated from each other by clinical criteria presented earlier.

Sleepwalking (somnambulism) shares many clinical features with night terrors. Most prominent among these are the state of incomplete arousal and the child's lack of recall for the event. Sleepwalking, however, is not associated with a state of panic.

Temporal lobe (*partial complex*) *seizures* may occur at night, manifested by hallucinosis, incomplete arousal, fear, and automatic behavior. Seizures can generally be distinguished from night terrors by the lesser degree of autonomic activation and by clinical features of seizure disorder such as incontinence or characteristic skin markings, for example, hypopigmented macules (see Chapter 12) (see Case 9–2).

Febrile delirium may closely resemble a night terror. By definition, fever is demonstrable, whereas with a night terror the child might feel warm but temperature is not elevated.

Etiology (see Table 9–5).   The pathophysiologic basis of nightmares and night terrors can be approached usefully by considering the stages of the sleep

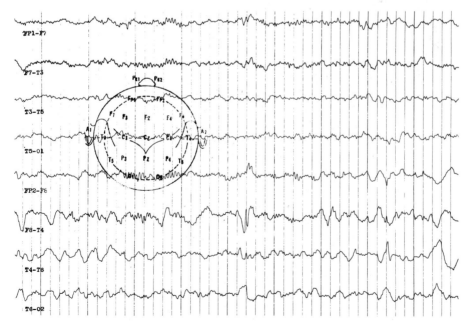

FIGURE 9–2. Electroencephalogram showing spikes and sharp waves in right frontal and temporal regions (Case 9–2).

CASE 9–2: ACUTE HALLUCINOSIS, TEMPORAL LOBE SEIZURES, AND SLEEP DISTURBANCE IN A 10-YEAR-OLD BOY

B.C. was referred for neurologic evaluation because of "nightmares" over a 2-month period. Episodes usually began 1½ hours after onset of sleep and consisted of heavy breathing followed by speaking such phrases as, "Oh, my God! Oh, my God!" After 30 seconds, he would return to sleep. At other times he sat up in bed and rocked. He did not recall any of these episodes the next morning.

At school on several occasions he had suddenly left his chair, clutched his throat, and breathed heavily. These episodes appeared to end when he was asked to stop them. One day he interrupted class by running to the window and exclaiming that there was "blood all over." While traveling in the car with his family, he declared every 15 minutes or so, "There's a brain following us." The evening prior to hospitalization, he told his parents that spiders were all over him. On the day of admission, he complained of headache and was noted to be lethargic. Past history was unremarkable, although delivery was described as precipitous.

On examination, the child had several episodes lasting 15 to 30 seconds of mouthing and chewing movements associated with rapid blinking of the eyelids. He sat up abruptly during these episodes and appeared panic-stricken. The general physical examination was remarkable only for a single hypopigmented macule. On neurologic examination a left Babinski sign was found. Optic disks were not elevated, nor were margins blurred. On mental status testing, the child was alert, disoriented to time, and able to repeat only three digits forward. Investigations included CT scan with contrast and cerebro-

cycle during which they occur. Like other dreams, nightmares ("bad dreams") take place during rapid eye movement sleep. The purpose of dreams, bad or otherwise, is obscure. Freud (1900) described dreams as providing hallucinatory wish-fulfillment and acting to guard (i.e., maintain) sleep, particularly when dreams contain elements that would be unacceptable to the awake person. From a neurologic standpoint, limbic structures (particularly the temporal lobes) have been implicated in dreaming because of highly charged emotional content and visual hallucinations that are so prominent. The occurrence of penile erection during REM sleep and the sexual nature of many dreams further support a limbic origin (Oswald, 1971).

Night terrors, by contrast, arise out of the non-REM phase of sleep in a state whose EEG pattern, unlike that usual in non-REM sleep, resembles wakefulness (Broughton, 1968). As observed in the sleep laboratory, episodes of night terror are characterized by six features: disorientation, automatic behavior, diminished responsiveness to external stimuli, difficulty in being aroused to full alertness, amnesia for events during the episode, and minimal (or no) recall of dreams.

In studies involving children without night terrors, Broughton found that

spinal fluid examination, both of which were normal. EEG showed spikes and sharp waves in the right frontal and temporal regions (see Fig. 9–2).

He was treated on the evening of admission with phenytoin, 700 mg, given by slow intravenous infusion. Within 5 minutes seizures ceased and mental status became normal. Maintained on 300 mg per day of phenytoin, he has had no further seizures, nightmares, visual hallucinations, or headaches.

Comment. This boy's behavioral change, lethargy, and headache combined with seizures suggested a progressive neurologic process, very likely a mass lesion. The CT scan, obtained on an emergency basis, excluded brain tumor. The dramatic response to phenytoin and the negative cerebrospinal fluid examination helped rule out herpes simplex encephalitis, which can behave as a mass lesion.

The etiology of this boy's seizure disorder was not specifically determined. His precipitous delivery could be implicated in producing temporal lobe damage by causing transient temporal lobe herniation compressing vascular structures, the brain itself, or both. The CT scan did not, however, disclose evidence for cerebral injury such as lateral ventricular enlargement.

This child's sleep disturbance did not fit clearly into the category of nightmares or night terrors, though his episodes showed several features of the latter: frightened appearance, lack of dream content, and amnesia. In view of its frequency and response to medication, the sleep disturbance was probably the result of temporal lobe seizures accounting for the visual imagery and related emotional content with discharge into diencephalic structures resulting in autonomic arousal.

forced arousal from non-REM sleep produced essentially the same six features as noted above but without the intense autonomic activation typical of night terrors. These findings in normal children reflect the experience of par-

TABLE 9–5. **Causes of Nightmares and Night Terrors**

Medical	Psychophysiologic disorder
Neurologic	Seizure
Toxic	Drug withdrawal
Psychologic	Stress-related
Social-Environmental	Precipitated by noise
Genetic-Constitutional	Familial influences
Developmental	Often around ages 3 to 5 years

CASE 9–3: NIGHTTIME HALLUCINOSIS IN A 3-YEAR-OLD GIRL WITH ECZEMA

C.Q. awakened her parents around midnight screaming, "The bugs are on me!" They found her sitting in bed panic-stricken, rubbing her arms in an apparent attempt to crush the bugs she felt were on her. She did not respond to her parents' attempts to comfort her and continued in an extremely agitated state for half an hour. Recognizing that the crushing motions were like scratching, her mother forced her to take two teaspoons of hydroxyzine (Atarax), which had been used in the treatment of her daughter's eczema earlier in life. Within half an hour she was asleep. She awakened the following morning without agitation but complained that the bugs were still there. She was seen by her pediatrician, who hospitalized her. Evaluation included lumbar puncture, analysis of urine for toxic substances, and electroencephalogram, all of which were normal. The hallucinosis abated spontaneously over 48 hours.

Past history was noteworthy for severe eczema between the ages of 1 and 2 years that had apparently been highly stressful. Her mother recalled her crawling along the carpet until her limbs were raw and bleeding. She was constantly being told not to do exactly what her body demanded her to do, namely, scratch. As a result, she would run from her mother to rub herself against an armchair. The eczema improved spontaneously at around 2 years and thereafter required only occasional topical therapy.

On the day of the sleep disturbance she had wandered across a busy street to the home of people rumored to be infested with lice. When her worried

ents who awaken a child to go to the bathroom during the night and learn in the morning that the child has no recollection of being awakened or of walking to the bathroom. Sleepwalking, too, shares these same features of automaticity and amnesia. It likewise arises from non-REM sleep.

Broughton concluded that partial arousal from non-REM sleep caused night terrors. This conclusion has been supported by the work in the sleep laboratory of Fisher and colleagues (1973), in which typical night terrors were produced in susceptible persons by a buzzer sounded during certain portions of non-REM sleep. By contrast, sounding of the buzzer during REM sleep led neither to night terrors nor to nightmares.

Medical Causes. Following hospitalization for medical or surgical problems, a child may experience nightmares for several nights upon returning home—a cause which is as much psychologic as it is medical.

The influence of psychophysiologic disorders upon night terrors is not clear. Case 9–3 illustrates a child with eczema in whom acute psychosocial stresses produced a syndrome of hallucinosis with features of night terror.

Neurologic Causes. Abnormal arousal from sleep to produce night terrors appears to be secondary to seizure activity in some children, even though clinical seizures may never have been observed (see Case 9–1). Ab-

mother located her, she was severely reprimanded. Her older siblings admonished her further because of their worries that lice would be brought into the home.

During the 2 weeks following hospitalization, she complained sporadically about "the bugs" and asked for "the medicine," which appeared to allay her anxiety. Because of issues that surfaced during the psychosocial evaluation of the family—particularly mother's intense unresolved guilt as to her handling of the infantile eczema—further psychiatric involvement was recommended.

Comment. This case shows several features of "classical" night terrors, yet it has several atypical aspects. The extreme agitation, difficulty in being fully aroused, hallucinosis, and ease of returning to sleep (aided by mother's serendipitous pharmacologic choice) are quite characteristic. On the other hand, the duration of the initial episode was much longer than is usual in night terrors of childhood, even though children's night terrors tend to be longer than the 1- to 3-minute episodes typical in adults.

The return of the hallucinosis is decidedly unusual. It suggests that recurrent night terrors can be a form of traumatic neurosis as postulated by Sperling (1971). Fisher and colleagues (1973) cited as an example a 40-year-old concentration camp survivor who for 25 years reexperienced scenes of persecution in his night terrors. In our case the severe infantile eczema provided the emotional and somatic backdrop for the child's sleep disturbance, which seems to have been precipitated by acute anxiety-producing events.

normal electrical activity of brain presumably interrupts the orderly progression of the sleep cycle, which is then manifested as a night terror.

Toxic Causes. Abrupt withdrawal from barbiturates can be associated with severe nightmares. The mechanism for this effect may be REM rebound, a period of increased REM activity and associated dreaming (often unpleasant) that occurs following discontinuation of drugs such as alcohol, barbiturates, and imipramine that diminish the amount of REM sleep.

Psychologic Causes. The link between emotionally upsetting events and nightmares is well recognized. A link between traumatic experiences and night terrors is less clear. As Fisher and colleagues (1973) have described, night terrors may persist into adulthood after unusually stressful circumstances, as noted above. Some children will react to relatively minor stresses with night terrors (see Case 9–4).

Social-Environmental Causes. As mentioned above, the work of Fisher and co-workers (1973) conducted in a sleep laboratory suggests that environmental noise may, in susceptible persons, precipitate night terrors. Such a circumstance occurring naturally has not been reported but seems possible.

Genetic-Constitutional Causes. Nightmares appear to be a universal phenomenon. In that sense, they might be considered constitutional.

CASE 9–4: RECURRENT NIGHT TERRORS IN A 6-YEAR-OLD GIRL

I.F. was referred for evaluation because of an episodic sleep disturbance that began at $2\frac{1}{2}$ years of age. A typical episode was described as follows. The child goes to bed at 7:30 and awakens at 10:30 crying. Her mother finds her sitting in bed cross-legged, "crying without tears." She appears frightened and, though staring about the room, does not seem aware of her mother's presence. She walks around her room but does not break anything or injure herself. The episode lasts about 15 minutes and is terminated by the parents with difficulty. Afterward, when asked if she has had a nightmare, she replies, "I don't know." She has no recall of the episode the following morning. This sleep disturbance has tended to occur two or three nights in a row, then to be absent for several weeks.

Both parents feel that emotional stresses during the day will trigger night-time sleep disturbance. For example, if the child has been disciplined even mildly before going to bed, an episode is virtually certain. A typical night terror occurred (as predicted) the day she was reprimanded by her father for creating a disturbance on the school bus. At the time of neurologic evaluation, the family was in the process of moving. This period was associated with an increase in the frequency of night terrors. Past history was negative for seizures, significant head trauma, or enuresis.

On examination, the child was a pleasant, cooperative youngster, not at all anxious or depressed. Head circumference and optic fundi were normal. School achievement was at grade level. The remainder of the examination was likewise unremarkable. Investigation was limited to an electroencephalogram, which was normal. For several months following the evaluation, she had no further night terrors.

Comment. There was nothing distinctive about these night terrors except for their frequency and their apparent link with emotional stresses during the day. The diagnosis of night terror was made on the basis of episodes of incomplete arousal associated with agitation, lack of rich dream content, and amnesia for the event.

Persistence of night terrors is uncommon, and the impressive association with even relatively trivial situational stresses as seen here is distinctly unusual. The basis for this association is obscure. It is reminiscent of the susceptibility of some persons to external noise (such as the sounding of a buzzer in a sleep laboratory), which can provoke a typical night terror.

Upon being reassured of the essentially benign nature of their child's night terrors, her parents were better able to set limits for her and enforce discipline without worrying that they were damaging her emotionally or physically.

With night terrors, family history is often positive for night terrors or sleepwalking (Kales, Kales *et al.*, 1980).

CASE 9–5: SITUATIONAL SLEEP DISTURBANCE IN A
4-YEAR-OLD GIRL

On the day of her sleep disturbance, L.N. had traveled alone by airplane to visit relatives. She awakened her aunt by rummaging through her closet in the middle of the night worriedly crying for her mother. Although she did not respond to her aunt's presence, she was easily awakened and expressed concerns as to her mother's whereabouts and safety. She had difficulty in returning to sleep that night but was reassured by speaking with her mother by telephone the following day. Subsequent sleep was unremarkable except for occasional episodes of sleepwalking and "bad dreams" of mild intensity over the next few days before returning home.

Past history was notable for hospitalization at 3 months of age for viral meningitis without apparent sequelae. She was an only child who was intensely rivalrous with her mother for her father's attention. Her mother described her as "very grown up" for her age: "4 going on 24."

Comment. This child's sleep disturbance showed several features of both night terrors and nightmares. She was neither fully awake nor asleep, and behavior was semiautomatic (sleepwalking and sleeptalking)—both of which are characteristic of night terrors. On the other hand, she was relatively easy to arouse and had difficulty getting back to sleep, which are features more typical of nightmares.

The difficulties in classification notwithstanding, her evaluation (limited to history, examination, and EEG) confirmed the diagnosis of a sleep disturbance based on acute separation anxiety against a background of intense competition with her mother. Though the sleep disturbance was self-limited, the child was referred for psychiatric consultation because of daytime behavioral problems that included frequent temper tantrums.

Developmental Causes. Nightmares are part of normal experience and often appear to stem from everyday activities and relationships. Only when they occur with notable frequency or intensity should they be considered pathologic (see Case 9–5).

Many children between the ages of 3 and 5 years experience one or a few night terrors, which never recur. This developmental pattern has, it seems, led many professionals to do little more than provide reassurance whenever the problem of night terror arises. Clearly, this approach may be insufficient when medical, neurologic, psychologic, and social influences act in addition to (or instead of) developmental factors.

TREATMENT AND OUTCOME

Night terrors may pursue a benign, self-limited, developmentally related course. Or they may recur during later childhood, adolescence, and even adulthood, in which case they are associated with increased degrees of psychopathology (Kales, Kales *et al.*, 1980). Nightmares recur transiently and generally resolve without professional intervention. When nightmares continue into adulthood, they too have been found associated with characteristic patterns of psychologic and personality disturbance (Kales, Soldatos *et al.*, 1980).

The acute treatment of a night terror is directed to terminating the episode by attempting to bring the child to a full state of alertness. This can usually be accomplished by turning the lights on, speaking loudly to the child, patting the face gently with a cold washcloth, or rubbing the back over the spine with one's knuckles somewhat noxiously but not injuriously (see Table 9–6). The child should never be shaken or slapped because of injuries that might result. These include subdural hemorrhage associated with whiplash injury (see Chapter 20). The acute treatment of nightmares is primarily psychologic support, along with an attempt to identify the stresses that might have contributed to the "bad dreams."

Medical Management.   When contributing or intercurrent problems such as eczema occur, they should be treated in a standard manner.

Diazepam (Valium) has benefited some adults with night terrors. This drug diminishes the amount of non-REM sleep (specifically stage 4), an effect that appears to underlie or contribute to its efficacy (see CORRELATION: PHYSIOLOGIC ASPECTS). Imipramine (Tofranil), diphenhydramine (Benadryl), and hydroxyzine (Atarax) each have been used with apparent efficacy in treatment of night terrors in childhood (see Case 9–3). Pharmacotherapy is usually not needed.

Neurologic Management.   When abnormal electrical activity of brain is implicated in causing night terrors, a trial of anticonvulsant therapy may be worthwhile, particularly if episodes are frequent.

Psychotherapy.   The child with nightmares should receive reassurance, comfort, and explanation. Under most circumstances, these can be provided by the parents, and professional involvement is not necessary. Nightmares often occur against a background of changing family events such as the birth of a sibling or an anticipated move. When sources of stress are suspected but

TABLE 9–6. **Treatment of Nightmares and Night Terrors**

Medical	Treatment of intercurrent illness Pharmacotherapy: diazepam (Valium), imipramine (Tofranil), diphenhydramine (Benadryl), hydroxyzine (Atarax) for night terrors
Neurologic	Anticonvulsant therapy (as indicated)
Psychologic	Explanation Reassurance Treatment of any associated emotional disturbance
Social-Environmental	Arousal of child to alert state for night terrors "Accident-proofing" bedroom and other parts of home

not clearly identified, consultation with a child psychiatrist, psychologist, or psychiatric social worker to explore the matter further will often be of value.

With night terrors, the parents rather than the affected child will benefit from explanation and reassurance. When emotional stress appears to play a role in precipitating night terrors, involvement of a mental health professional may be indicated.

Social-Environmental Management. With night terrors, specific measures should be undertaken to ensure the safety of the child. Appropriate doors and windows should be locked, and sharp or breakable objects should be removed from the child's bedroom. A ground-floor bedroom may be advisable (Kales and Kales, 1974). The environment should be quiet and free of irregular noises that might trigger a night terror.

With nightmares, anxiety may be lessened by a night light, leaving the bedroom door open, or having the child share a room with an older sibling.

HYPERSOMNIAS

DEFINITION

Hypersomnia is a descriptive term referring to an increase in amount of sleep, the occurrence of sleep at inappropriate times, or both. For example, sleep may have increased from 9 or 10 hours a day to 14 or 15 hours. It may be occurring not only at night but at uncharacteristic times of the day as well, such as during classroom activities or lunch.

What constitutes a normal amount of sleep per day for a child is not clearly defined. It varies greatly from one individual to another and, for a given individual, from one developmental stage to another. Usually the amount of sleep diminishes progressively from infancy to adulthood, with a temporary increase during adolescence. For the school-age child, sleeping 11 hours a night should be considered marginally excessive; 12 hours or more a night would be unequivocally excessive.

DIAGNOSIS

In assessing the child with hypersomnia, one should keep in mind several disorders (described below) with which it is typically associated. These include systemic illness, narcolepsy, sleep apnea, depression, drug effects, seizure disorder, and the Kleine-Levin syndrome. In addition, several disorders that might be mistaken as hypersomnia should also be borne in mind. These include normal sleep, periodic paralysis, and hysteria (see DIFFERENTIAL DIAGNOSIS).

Clinical Process. *History.* The chief complaint should be recorded, as usual, in the words of the child whenever possible: "I feel like sleeping all day." "I've been falling asleep when I don't really want to." "I can't seem to get enough sleep."

The history of the presenting problem should seek to characterize the sleep disturbance in terms of onset and progression of symptoms, associated features, past evaluation, and therapy, if any. When did the problem begin? Is it getting better, getting worse, or staying about the same? How many hours a day does the child sleep? Does sleep occur just at night, or does it include daytime naps? Is he refreshed when he gets up? Does he snore? Do unusual pauses in breathing occur? Is the child enuretic? Have any drugs been prescribed, or might they have been taken illicitly? How have mood and general health been recently?

When episodes occur during the day, the following questions pertaining specifically to narcolepsy should be asked. Does dreaming occur? Have there been episodes of paralysis of the limbs during which awareness has been maintained? Have emotional stimuli such as anger or exultation led to falls associated with sudden loss of body tone? What evaluation has been carried out? What therapy undertaken? With what effect?

Past history should include previous medical problems, hospitalizations, and operations. The family history should seek similar sleep disorders among relatives. Psychosocial data should include educational history, career interests, living situation, and recent stresses. Review of systems should include attention to seizures, headaches, visual impairment, coordinational change, personality alteration, appetite change (increased or decreased), temperature intolerance, and weight loss or gain.

Examination. The *general description* should note how the child strikes the examiner. Does he appear healthy, chronically ill, cheerful, euphoric, depressed, anxious, or bored? Is he sleepy? Did he actually fall asleep during the examination?

The *general physical examination* should seek systemic factors that might cause or contribute to hypersomnia. Evidence of systemic illness such as asthma, regional enteritis, or cystic fibrosis should be noted. Palpation of the neck for the thyroid gland should be carried out, texture of the skin noted, and pulse rate and temperature determined. Examination of the pharynx should specifically include visualization of the tonsils. The occurrence and degree of obesity should be noted. *Neurologic examination* should seek lateralizing signs and evidence of increased intracranial pressure, especially altered state of alertness. The *mental status examination* should include particular attention to affect (primarily depression or anxiety) and behavior (e.g., hyperactivity, impulsivity, distractability).

Investigation. Investigation will depend upon the clinical syndrome suggested by the history and examination (see Table 9–7). Studies might include thyroid hormone determination, anticonvulsant blood level(s), anal-

---

TABLE 9–7. **Investigations to Be Considered in the Child with Hypersomnia**

Thyroid function tests
Anticonvulsant blood levels
Analysis of blood and urine for other drugs
EEG (in awake and sleep states)
All-night polygraphic EEG
Arterial blood gases
Pulmonary function tests
Cranial CT scan
Cervical spine x-rays

TABLE 9–8. **Differential Diagnosis of Hypersomnia**

Normal sleep
Periodic paralysis
Feigned sleep
Hysteria
Cervical spine disorder (subluxable odontoid process)

ysis of blood and urine for drugs, cervical spine x-rays with views of the odontoid process, lateral radiographs of the neck, pulmonary function tests, arterial blood gas determinations, electroencephalogram, all-night polygraphic sleep study, or CT scan.

Differential Diagnosis. Several disorders should be differentiated from the hypersomnias (see Table 9–8). *Normal sleep* may be misinterpreted as being excessive. Although no rigid guidelines can be drawn, the older school-age child who sleeps more than 12 hours a night would be considered to manifest hypersomnia, particularly if this amount represented an increase over previous levels.

The *periodic paralyses* are a group of disorders associated with episodes of loss of voluntary movement of the extremities. These may be misinterpreted as episodes of sleep paralysis, a feature of the narcolepsy syndrome (see below). Family history, serum potassium level (increased, decreased, or normal), and associated clinical features such as myotonia and relationship to diet or exercise will help to differentiate periodic paralysis from narcolepsy.

Feigned sleep may occur in the bored or manipulative child (see Chapter 7).

Hysteria may take the form of a hypersomnia or even coma.

Cervical spine disorder, particularly a subluxable odontoid process, may lead to periodic loss or alteration in consciousness.

Etiology (see Table 9–9). The possibility of multifactorial cause for a syndrome of hypersomnia should be kept in mind. For example, a depressed person may take barbiturates in an attempt to make an emotional state more tolerable, thereby compounding an associated sleep disturbance. In some instances (e.g., narcolepsy), the underlying cause of hypersomnia has not been determined.

Medical Causes. *Chronic illness* such as asthma, ulcerative colitis, and cystic fibrosis may exhaust the child sufficiently for increased amounts of sleep to be necessary. In addition the child may experience a depressive reaction to illness that intensifies the desire to sleep.

The *obesity-hypoventilation (Pickwickian) syndrome* is associated with impaired respiratory function due to excessive adiposity (Spier and Karelitz, 1960; Simpser *et al.,* 1977). Underventilation leads to carbon dioxide retention and cerebral vasodilation, resulting in hypersomnolence, headache, and other signs of increased intracranial pressure.

Metabolic disorders (*hypoglycemia, hypothyroidism,* and *hypercalcemia*) can be associated with lethargy, hypersomnolence, or even coma. Seizures can also occur with hypoglycemia.

TABLE 9–9. **Causes of Hypersomnia**

Medical	Chronic illness
	Obesity-hypoventilation (''Pickwickian'') syndrome
	Hypoglycemia
	Hypothyroidism
	Hypercalcemia
Neurologic	Narcolepsy
	Seizures
	Brainstem disorder (such as encephalitis, neoplasm, Leigh disease)
	Periodic hypersomnia (such as Kleine-Levin syndrome)
	Hypothalamic tumor
	Sleep apnea syndrome (obstructive vs. central)
Toxic	Anticonvulsant drug excess
	Illicit drug use (sedatives, amphetamines, narcotics)
	Environmental toxins (carbon monoxide)
Psychologic	Depression
	Chronic psychologic stress
Social-Environmental	Understimulation
	Overstimulation
Genetic-Constitutional	Familial
Developmental	Age-related

Neurologic Causes. *Narcolepsy* (or the *narcoleptic syndrome*) consists essentially of sleep attacks, which may be associated with any or all of the following three symptoms: cataplexy, hypnagogic hallucinations, or sleep paralysis.

The *sleep attack* is the hallmark of narcolepsy. The person experiences a nearly irresistible desire to sleep, regardless of the circumstances and surroundings. Sleep can usually be delayed by several minutes to an hour or so. A typical episode lasts about 15 minutes and is usually accompanied by dreaming. The person awakens refreshed. A sleep attack is generally followed by a refractory period of 1 to 5 hours (Kales and Kales, 1974).

So-called micro-sleep episodes may precede overt napping in some persons with narcolepsy (Anders *et al.,* 1980). Such episodes, lasting from 5 to 15 seconds, are associated with staring (''glassy eyes'') and altered consciousness (lack of full awareness). This clinical picture should be distinguished from petit mal and psychomotor seizures.

Cataplexy is the sudden loss of muscle tone, partial or complete, following certain emotional stimuli. For example, a father reported suddenly falling limp when he angrily prepared to spank his child. Another person slumped to the tennis court following his exultation after a winning shot.

Hypnagogic hallucinations are vivid, usually unpleasant, dreamlike visual and/or auditory episodes that occur normally upon going to sleep. With narcolepsy, however, such hallucinations may occur independently of sleep with the result that the person, in effect, dreams while awake. The combination of hypnagogic hallucination and sleep paralysis may be especially terrifying.

Sleep paralysis is manifested by inability to move the limbs for periods of several minutes to hours. Full awareness is maintained during an episode that begins in the drowsy or awake state. Paralysis remits spontaneously or is "broken" immediately once the person is touched.

About 10 per cent of persons with a narcoleptic syndrome experience all four symptoms, while nearly 70 per cent have both sleep attacks and cataplexy (Kales and Kales, 1974). Sleep paralysis alone occurs in less than 5 per cent of affected persons.

Narcolepsy typically has its onset in adolescence or young adulthood. Kales and Kales (1974) reported that 80 per cent of cases begin before 30 years of age. Zarcone (1973) noted that approximately 5 per cent of cases began before age 10 years. An example of the latter is an 8-year-old girl described by Weech in 1926. One-third of adults with narcolepsy had experienced learning and behavior problems (typically hyperactivity) in childhood and adolescence that were associated with daytime sleepiness (Anders *et al.*, 1980).

In view of these figures, it is suprising that narcolepsy is recognized so infrequently in the pediatric age group. Perhaps the diagnosis is being overlooked, or affected children are not being brought for evaluation.

The sleep of the person with narcolepsy is remarkable for direct entry into REM sleep rather than first proceeding through the non-REM phases of sleep (see CORRELATION: PHYSIOLOGIC ASPECTS). Only in the newborn does this pattern of direct entry from the awake state into REM sleep occur normally. In the narcoleptic this progression is correlated clinically with the rapid onset of dreaming during sleep attacks.

Zarcone (1973) has summarized the symptoms of narcolepsy by relating them to normal REM sleep. Cataplexy and sleep paralysis can be considered manifestations of the motor inhibitory process, hypnagogic hallucinations as dream phenomena. A narcoleptic syndrome thus represents a dissociated form of REM sleep.

Not all narcoleptic syndromes fit neatly into this model, however. Roth and colleagues (1969) have described persons whose sleep attacks did not occur in a REM state. Their syndrome was further atypical in that affected persons were drowsy in between attacks and associated symptoms of sleep paralysis, cataplexy, and hypnagogic hallucinations were absent.

Seizure disorder may produce a clinical picture of periodic hypersomnia. The child who sleeps unusually late several days a month may, in fact, have had a seizure before awakening followed by a postical state of lethargy. In other children, hypersomnia itself seems to be an ictal manifestation (see Case 9–6).

Brainstem encephalitis can cause hypersomnia (or other disorder of the sleep-wake cycle) due to involvement of the reticular activating system.

CASE 9–6: HYPERSOMNOLENCE AND ABNORMAL EEG IN A 4-YEAR-OLD BOY

A.A. was evaluated for episodes of falling asleep. He always slept a great deal, his mother said. Daytime naps usually lasted 4 hours, and the child slept 11 hours a night. During the day he often fell asleep at unusual times or places, for example, while sitting in a dentist's chair or while playing with friends. Such naps lasted from a half hour to a few hours. He was awakened with difficulty and did not appear refreshed upon arousal. Incontinence was not associated. No episodes of cataplexy, sleep paralysis, or hypnagogic hallucinations were described. Pregnancy, birth history, and development were unremarkable. Family history was negative for sleep disturbance. A sister had a seizure disorder.

On examination, the child was an alert, pleasant, cooperative, and healthy-appearing youngster whose head circumference (53.5 cm) was greater than two standard deviations above the mean. Examination of the skin disclosed no neurocutaneous markings. Optic disks, visual fields, and extraocular movements were normal. The remainder of the examination, including deep tendon reflexes and plantar responses, was normal.

Investigations included an abnormal electroencephalogram with spike and polyspike activity arising from central regions during drowsiness and sleep (see Fig. 9–3). CT scan showed mild dilatation of the right lateral ventricle. A trial of dextroamphetamine (in a dosage of up to 25 mg per day) carried out over a 2-month period was associated with some improvement in lethargy and reduction in the number of naps. A later trial of anticonvulsant medication (without dextroamphetamine) resulted in still fewer sleep episodes.

Comment. Daytime sleep episodes should suggest interference with nighttime sleep as in a sleep apnea syndrome. This child did not, however, snore, sleep fitfully, or have prolonged respiratory pauses at night. Nor did he appear to have a narcoleptic syndrome associated with cataplexy, hypnagogic hallucinations, or sleep paralysis.

His daytime sleepiness appeared to be on the basis of chronic underarousal associated with a markedly abnormal EEG. Because he had not had clinical seizures, dextroamphetamine was tried first with some benefit. Because of the incomplete response to stimulant therapy and the EEG findings, anticonvulsant therapy with phenytoin was then pursued with further symptomatic gains.

Leigh disease (subacute necrotizing encephalomyelopathy) is another pathologic process that can affect the brainstem to cause sleep disturbances. *Microglioma of the midbrain* has been reported to produce a narcoleptic syndrome manifested by cataplexy and sleep attacks (Anderson and Salmon, 1977).

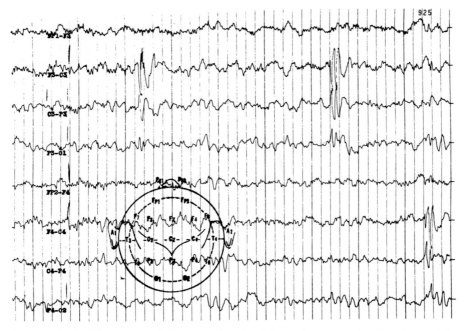

FIGURE 9–3. Electroencephalogram showing bilateral spike and polyspike activity arising frontocentrally (Case 9–6).

The *Kleine-Levin syndrome* is a rare disorder involving *periodic hypersomnia* and hyperphagia (Billiard *et al.*, 1975; Powers and Gunderman, 1978). It is presumed to occur on the basis of hypothalamic dysfunction because of disturbance in autonomic vegetative functions including sleeping and eating. Atypical syndromes occur, for example, without excessive eating (see Case 9–7).

Hypothalamic tumor is another cause of hypersomnia (see Fig. 9–4) (see Case 10–2).

A *sleep apnea syndrome* may consist of a constellation of behavioral symptoms of irritability, inattentiveness, and hyperkinesis alternating with unscheduled naps. Interference with nighttime sleep appears to cause this daytime behavior. Inspiratory snoring and prolonged respiratory pauses are valuable clinical indicators of some sleep apnea syndromes.

Two kinds of obstructive patterns have been identified: peripheral (frequently involving excessive adenoidal tissue) and central (secondary to "floppy" respiratory passages) (see Fig. 9–5) (Guilleminault *et al.*, 1976). Abnormal function of the genioglossus muscles of the tongue (failing to maintain adequate pharyngeal patency during sleep) has also been implicated as playing an obstructive role in some persons (Strohl *et al.*, 1978; Turino and Goldring, 1978). In other children, central nervous system irregularities (perhaps defective chemoregulation) appear to underly apneic episodes (Cherniack, 1981). Cessation of breathing for 20 seconds or more can occur dozens or even hundreds of times during nighttime sleep in an affected

CASE 9–7: PERIODIC HYPERSOMNIA AND DEREALIZATION IN AN 11-YEAR-OLD GIRL

J.C. was referred for evaluation because of episodes lasting 10 to 14 days of regressive behavior and excessive daytime sleep that had occurred intermittently for 3 years. Episodes began without consistent medical or emotional precipitants. After a transitional period of moodiness, irritability, and loss of interest in her usual activities, she would withdraw to her bedroom and sleep for 16 to 20 hours. She arose to use the bathroom. Appetite was diminished, and she ate little. The day the episode ended, she had difficulty falling asleep at night. The following day she was ready to resume her normal activities. Episodes occurred irregularly with intervening periods of up to several months. A variety of medications had been employed without benefit. Past history and family history were unremarkable.

On examination during a typical episode, the child was a normally developed girl in early stages of adolescence who was strikingly anxious and wished to be left alone. When she was not being "bothered," she went to sleep, from which she was easily aroused. Otherwise the general physical and neurologic examinations were normal. Investigations—including EEG, thyroid function studies, and serum electrolytes—were unremarkable.

Examined after an episode had ended, she was an articulate and intelligent girl who acted her chronologic age if not older. She described her episodes as ushered in by a sense that things became "blurry . . . unreal." This feeling pervaded the entire episode. Excessive sleep appeared to result not from an overwhelming urge to sleep but from a desire to be left alone.

Comment. This girl's syndrome of hypersomnia and derealization appears related to, but different from, the periodic hypersomnia syndrome of Kleine and Levin. With the Kleine-Levin syndrome, megaphagia (excessive eating) is an integral feature; whereas in this case, eating behavior was the opposite. The recurrent, highly stereotyped nature of the episodes suggests, nonethless, kinship with the Kleine-Levin syndrome.

They also share the common feature of being of unknown etiology. Because of the change in mental status (derealization) that inaugurates the episodes, one might implicate the temporal lobe as playing an etiologic role. It might then influence the adjacent hypothalamus. The nature of the pathologic process is obscure. A seizure disorder of temporal lobe origin, though considered, would not be associated with spells of up to 2 weeks. Thus far, efforts to abort or shorten the episodes have been unrewarding. Supportive psychotherapy has continued, and consideration has been given to a trial of dextroamphetamine early in the episode to try to stave off a full-blown attack.

person, as documented by polygraphic sleep recordings (Guilleminault *et al.*, 1976).

Toxic Causes. Drugs can contribute to sleep disturbance in several

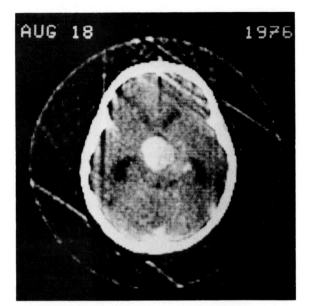

FIGURE 9–4. Computerized tomographic (CT) scan demonstrating hypothalamic tumor in a 5-year-old child.

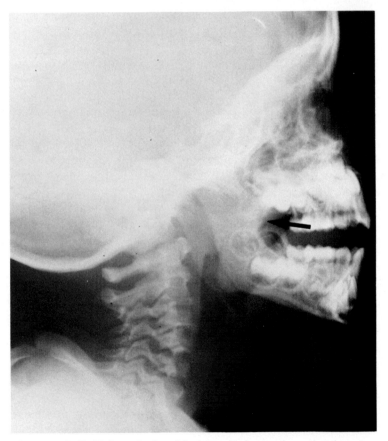

FIGURE 9–5. Enlarged adenoids (arrow) obstructing nasopharynx.

ways. Hypersomnia is well-recognized complication of anticonvulsant medication overdosage. Errors in prescribing, dispensing, shaking, or taking the medicine may underlie the overdosage problem. The addition of sodium valproate to an anticonvulsant regimen that includes phenobarbital will often cause sedation, as sodium valproate tends to elevate blood levels of phenobarbital. Determination of anticonvulsant blood levels will readily define the problem.

Illict drug usage with sedatives ("downers") such as barbiturates ("reds"), glutethimide (Doriden), or methaqualone (Quaalude) may be associated with excessive sleep. When overdosage involves these drugs or opiates such as morphine or heroin, the problem can be one of stupor or coma rather than merely hypersomnia. Excessive sleepiness can also be seen following an amphetamine "jag" (see Chapter 19).

Environmental toxins such as carbon monoxide can also cause hypersomnia. Carbon monoxide poisoning is often insidious in its presentation. Diagnosis is suggested by symptoms of irritability, distractability, and lethargy, particularly if occurring in several members of a household. The skin may assume a peculiar reddish hue. Determination of carboxyhemoglobin should establish the diagnosis.

Psychologic Causes.   Increase in amount of sleep may be part of a depressive syndrome. Symptoms may be intensified by simultaneous drug use involving sedative agents such as alcohol, barbiturates, or diazepam (Valium) (see Chapter 6).

A learning-disabled child whose difficulty has been unrecognized or undertreated may be so exhausted from his day's work that he forgoes customary after-school activities to take a nap (see Chapter 17). Such chronic psychologic stress may be evident in other children through the psychophysiologic channels of headache or stomach ache.

Social-Environmental Causes.   Understimulation (boredom) or overstimulation (stimulus overload) may lead to sleep. It has been suggested that some children with attention deficit disorders are chronically overstimulated and respond by excessive daytime napping.

The physical conditions in which a child sleeps can significantly affect the quality of nighttime sleep. Cold surroundings due to inadequate heat or bedding, worries as to roaches or rodents, and excessive noise due to automobiles, trains, family members, or neighbors may interfere with nighttime sleep and contribute to daytime somnolence.

Genetic-Constitutional Causes.   A familial element appears to play a role in some cases of narcolepsy. It has been reported in identical twins (Imlah, 1961), and an autosomal dominant pattern of inheritance has been noted by Daly and Yoss (1959) in a family with three generations involved. In general, however, a multifactorial mode of transmission with variable penetrance has been found (Anders et al., 1980).

Developmental Causes.   The increased sleep needs of infants, young children, and adolescents have been noted earlier. The increase at adolescence has been linked with as yet unidentified maturational changes associated with pubescence (Anders et al., 1980). Poor time management in integrating academic, social, and athletic activities in adolescence often leads to chronic sleep deprivation that worsens daytime hypersomnia.

TREATMENT AND OUTCOME

The hypersomnias are treated by a variety of measures. The benefits of a multifaceted approach to management is epitomized by the treatment of narcolepsy (see Table 9–10). Drugs should not be the exclusive focus of therapy since medications may not help, side effects are not infrequent, and amphetamines in particular may be abused.

When the cause of daytime hypersomnia is impairment of nighttime sleep, identifying the cause(s) of interference (such as airway obstruction, noisy environment, or drug use) will allow for specific treatment. At times the only therapy necessary is simply sleep.

Medical Management.   The drugs usually employed in the treatment of narcolepsy are dextroamphetamine (Dexedrine) and methylphenidate (Ritalin). Though often effective, these medications may not be of long-lasting benefit and can interfere with nighttime sleep, which can lead to a worsening of daytime spells. Monoamine oxidase inhibitors and tricyclic compounds have also been used in treating narcolepsy. Of the tricyclics, imipramine (Tofranil) has been particularly effective in managing cataplexy (Kales and Kales, 1974). Sleep attacks are less responsive to this drug. The combination of imipramine and methylphenidate has been of benefit in some patients with both cataplexy and sleep attacks (Dement and Guilleminault, 1973). This combination must be used with caution, however, as effects of excessive catecholamines, including hypertension, may result. The basis for this potential complication is methylphenidate's effect of promoting release of norepinephrine and imipramine's effect in blocking its reuptake. Thus the amount of norepinephrine available postsynaptically can become elevated at times to dangerous levels.

Improvement in nighttime sleep in adults with narcolepsy may be accomplished with the use of diazepam (Valium) or flurazepam (Dalmane) in conjunction with environmental measures. Other medical treatments for hyper-

TABLE 9–10. **Treatment of Narcolepsy**

Medical	Treatment of associated medical illness
	Symptomatic pharmacotherapy (dextroamphetamine [Dexedrine], methylphenidate [Ritalin], imipramine [Tofranil] for narcoleptic symptoms; diazepam [Valium], flurazepam [Dalmane] for improvement of nighttime sleep)
Psychologic	Psychotherapy
Social-Environmental	Scheduled naps
	Appropriate choice of work, recreation, transportation
	Measures to improve nighttime sleep

somnia include thyroid hormone replacement (for hypothyroidism), progesterone (in some cases of the Pickwickian or obesity-hypoventilation syndrome), and weight reduction (also for the latter) (Simpser et al., 1977; Orenstein et al., 1977).

Amphetamines have been successfully used in treating (that is, terminating) episodes of the Kleine-Levin syndrome (Powers and Gunderman, 1978).

Systemic illness causing or contributing to hypersomnia should be treated specifically as well as symptomatically.

Neurologic Management. Seizures should be treated with anticonvulsant medication. Blood levels should be monitored periodically to ensure therapeutic efficacy without overdosage (see Chapter 12) (see Case 9–6).

Surgical Management. A sleep apnea syndrome caused by peripheral obstruction may respond well to removal of hypertrophied tonsils and adenoids. With some forms of sleep apnea, nighttime ventilatory assistance, sometimes facilitated by tracheostomy, may be required. Benefit may be dramatic (Guilleminault et al., 1976).

Psychotherapy. Treatment of depression is discussed in Chapter 6.

Social-Environmental Management. The person with narcolepsy should learn about his sleep disorder and understand its implications for home, school, and work place. Naps should be taken on a scheduled basis. Work should be chosen so that a sleep attack does not present a danger to the affected person or others. Transportation arrangements must also take the narcolepsy into consideration.

The adolescent with a developmentally based increase in sleep needs should have adequate time to sleep so that daytime drowsiness does not interfere with academic and social functioning. The adolescent should plan school, athletic, and social activities to ensure proper amounts of sleep during the week as well as on weekends.

With morbidly obese persons, social and environmental planning is an essential part of overall behavior management (see Chapter 10).

Mechanical Therapy. As mentioned above, a ventilator may be used at night in the treatment of some sleep apnea syndromes.

CORRELATION

Anatomic Aspects. Two areas of the brain appear to play particularly important roles in sleep and wakefulness: the hypothalamus and the midbrain (Bremer, 1977). Plum and Van Uitert (1978) term the posterior hypothalamus a "wake center" and note that stimulation of this structure in animals has been known for nearly 40 years to evoke arousal. The anterior hypothalamus, on the other hand, acts as a "sleep center."

The normal functioning of these centers appears to depend on an intact brainstem, specifically the reticular activating system of the midbrain. As with other neurologic conditions, stimulation of brain typically causes effects opposite to those of destruction. Accordingly, a state of diminished level of consciousness (sleep, hypersomnia, or coma) will result from stimulation of the anterior hypothalamus, destruction of the posterior hypothalamus, or destruction of the midbrain reticular formation. Correspondingly, a state of arousal (including insomnia) will result from destruction of anterior

TABLE 9–11. **Anatomic Aspects of Sleep and Wakefulness**

	Stimulation	Destruction
Anterior hypothalamus	Sleep, hypersomnia, or coma	Arousal, insomnia
Posterior hypothalamus	Arousal, insomnia	Sleep, hypersomnia, or coma
Upper brainstem	Arousal, insomnia	Sleep, hypersomnia, or coma

hypothalamus or from stimulation of posterior hypothalamus or midbrain (see Table 9–11).

Biochemical Aspects. Recent research has shed further light on biochemical aspects of sleep (Pappenheimer, 1976; Krueger *et al.*, 1978; Pappenheimer, 1979). Pappenheimer (1976) has studied an apparent "sleep factor" obtained from the cerebrospinal fluid (CSF) of sleep-deprived goats. He infused this CSF into the cisterna magna of cats, causing them to fall asleep. The cats did not fall asleep immediately, however. Sleep episodes of longer duration than usual began some 2 to 3 hours after the infusion. This time lag may be due to the time required for diffusion of the sleep factor from the cisternal subarachnoid space to its site of action, perhaps the hypothalamus. The origin of this sleep-promoting factor has been suggested by work demonstrating that a neurohumoral substance mediating sleep is released into venous blood during electrical stimulation of the diencephalon (Pappenheimer, 1976).

The site of action of such sleep factors is not known but may involve not only the hypothalamus but nuclear groups in the brainstem as well. Dahlstrom and Fuxe (1964) have linked sleep with "chemical factories" in the brainstem. Through the use of fluorescent staining techniques, they demonstrated that the midline raphé nuclei of the pons and midbrain are rich in serotonin (5-hydroxytryptamine). When synthesis of serotonin was blocked in experimental animals, brain serotonin was reduced and animals experienced several days of insomnia. Conversely, human studies have demonstrated that ingestion of tryptophan, a serotonin precursor, can shorten the time of onset of sleep and increase the duration of its non-REM component (Growdon, 1979).

Lying lateral to serotonin-containing nuclei in the pons are cell bodies of the locus coeruleus, which have been found to be rich in norepinephrine. The importance of norepinepherine in REM sleep has been demonstrated in experimental work in animals with lesions of the locus coeruleus in whom REM sleep has been diminished (Dahlstrom and Fuxe, 1964). Dement and Guilleminault (1973) have likened REM sleep to a seizure discharge of the brainstem that presumably links the locus coeruleus with nearby conjugate eye movement centers of the pons.

In summary, though not all experimental data support these associations, orthodox or non-REM sleep appears to be closely associated with serotonin, whereas paradoxical or REM sleep appears to be linked with norepinephrine.

Physostigmine, a cholinergic drug, may also have a significant role in REM sleep. Normal human volunteers given this anticholinesterase agent intravenously during non-REM sleep were induced to enter REM sleep, with which dreaming was associated as is characteristic (Sitaram *et al.,* 1978).

Physiologic Aspects.   The two phases of sleep, orthodox (non-REM) and paradoxical (REM), have been further characterized through the use of the electroencephalogram, often in conjunction with monitoring of eye movements, pulse rate, respirations, and other muscle activity.

Orthodox sleep has been divided into four stages by EEG criteria (Oswald, 1971). Stage 1 is marked by loss of alpha rhythm, the 8- to 10-cycle-per-second activity which characterizes the quiet awake state, and by the establishment of a theta rhythm, 4 to 6 cycles per second. In stage 2, sleep spindles, 12- to 16-cycle-per-second complexes, appear along with brief runs of high-voltage slow waves. Stages 3 and 4 are often called slow wave sleep because of their characteristic high amplitude delta rhythm, 1 to 3 cycles per second. Stage 4 is differentiated from stage 3 by the absence of spindles and by further slowing of rhythm (see Fig. 9–6).

Paradoxical sleep is not conventionally subdivided. Its EEG pattern resembles the awake state more than slow wave sleep. It is low in amplitude and irregular in rhythm, what Dement and Guilleminault (1973) have cited as evidence of "tumultuous brain activity" presumably associated with dreaming.

In view of these electroencephalographic patterns, the sleep cycle can be

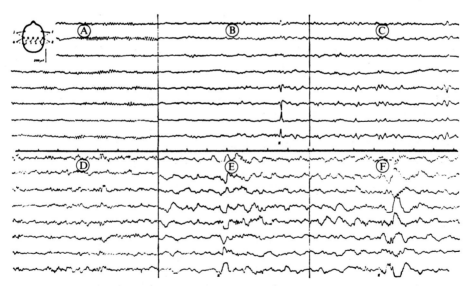

FIGURE 9–6. Progressive stages of drowsiness and sleep in a normal adult. (*A*) Widespread alpha rhythm in drowsiness. (*B*) Diminution in amplitude with further drowsiness. Response to sound at *X*. (*C*) Light sleep with prominent theta rhythm. (*D*)–(*F*) Increasing delta activity (1–3 Hz) as sleep deepens. (From Kiloh, L. G., *et al. Clinical Electroencephalography,* 3rd ed. Butterworth Publishers, Inc., Woburn, Mass., 1972.)

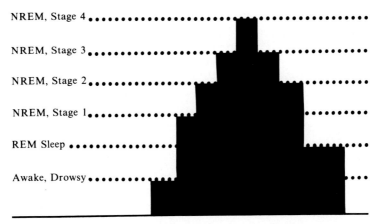

NREM, Stage 4
NREM, Stage 3
NREM, Stage 2
NREM, Stage 1
REM Sleep
Awake, Drowsy

FIGURE 9–7. Schematic illustration of a night's first sleep cycle. Note that REM sleep is not entered directly from the awake state but only after NREM sleep.

characterized further. After alert and drowsy states, sleep begins with stage 1 of the non-REM phase and moves through stages 2, 3, and 4. REM sleep does not occur at this point, however. The cycle returns to stage 2 (often through stage 3) and only then proceeds to the REM phase (see Fig. 9–7) (Kales and Kales, 1974). Each cycle lasts about 90 minutes, approximately one-quarter of which is REM sleep. Periods of REM sleep become progressively longer during the night.

SUMMARY

This chapter focuses upon nightmares, night terrors, and the hypersomnias. The nightmare is essentially a "bad dream" occurring in rapid eye movement (REM) sleep. The night terror is a disorder of arousal, arising from the non-REM phase of sleep. Night terrors are dissociative, confusional states that occur in susceptible persons whose sleep cycle is interrupted during non-REM sleep by internal or external factors. Seizure discharges may occasionally be seen on EEG, and rarely clinical seizures coexist. Emotional factors and a background of psychophysiologic illness may also contribute to night terrors. Treatment of night terrors includes environmental precautions and specific therapy suggested through the child's assessment. Diazepam, imipramine, or hydroxyzine may be of symptomatic benefit. Explanation combined with environmental measures will usually suffice in the treatment of nightmares, although psychologic evaluation may be indicated with severe cases.

The hypersomnias present a mixed picture of etiologies and management. Narcolepsy is a nonepileptic disorder which may begin in childhood or adolescence that has, as its cardinal feature, sleep attacks which may be associated with cataplexy, hypnagogic hallucinations, and sleep paralysis. A person with narcolepsy enters REM sleep immediately from the awake state.

Treatment of narcolepsy is multifaceted, with drugs playing as limited a role as possible. Narcolepsy must be differentiated from other hypersomnias. These include the Kleine-Levin and Pickwickian syndromes, seizure disorders, hypothyroidism, sleep apnea syndromes, and depression. Treatment will depend upon the cause of the specific hypersomnia syndrome.

The brainstem and hypothalamus play the major anatomic roles in the sleep-wake cycle. Norepinephrine and serotonin appear to play key biochemical roles in sleep, corresponding to its REM and non-REM phases, respectively. An important cholinergic contribution to REM sleep has also emerged. Physiologically, the electroencephalogram combined with simultaneous monitoring of other body functions in the sleep laboratory has vastly enhanced our understanding of sleep and its disorders, supplementing important observations made at the bedside with the unaided eye.

CITED REFERENCES

Anders, T. F.; Carskadon, M. A.; and Dement, W. C. Sleep and sleepiness in children and adolescents. *Pediatr. Clin. North Am.,* **27:** 29–43, 1980.

Anderson, M., and Salmon, M. V. Symptomatic cataplexy. *J. Neurol. Neurosurg. Psychiatry,* **40:** 186–91, 1977.

Aserinsky, E., and Kleitman, N. Two types of ocular motility occurring in sleep. *J. Appl. Physiol.,* **8:** 1–10, 1955.

Billiard, M.; Guilleminault, C.; and Dement, W. C. A menstruation-linked periodic hypersomnia: Kleine-Levin syndrome or new clinical entity? *Neurology,* **25:** 436–43, 1975.

Bremer, F. Cerebral hypnogenic centers. *Ann. Neurol.,* **2:** 1–6, 1977.

Broughton, R. J. Sleep disorders: disorders of arousal? *Science,* **159:** 1070–78, 1968.

Cherniack, N. S. Respiratory dysrhythmias during sleep. *N. Engl. J. Med.,* **305:** 325–30, 1981.

Dahlstrom, A., and Fuxe, K. Evidence for the existence of monoamine-containing neurons in the central nervous system. I. Demonstration of monoamines in the cell bodies of brain stem neurons. *Acta Physiol. Scand. Suppl.,* **232:** 1–55, 1964.

Daly, D. D., and Yoss, R. E. A family with narcolepsy. *Staff Meetings Mayo Clin.,* **34:** 313–19, 1959.

Dement, W. C., and Guilleminault, C. Sleep disorders: the state of the art. *Hosp. Pract.,* **8:** 57–71, November 1973.

Dement, W., and Kleitman, N. Cyclic variations in EEG during sleep and their relation to eye movements, body motility, and dreaming. *Electroencephalogr. Clin. Neurophysiol.,* **9:** 673–90, 1957.

Fisher, C.; Kahn, E.; Edwards, A.; and Davis, D. M. A psychophysiological study of nightmares and night terrors. I. Physiological aspects of the stage 4 night terror. *J. Nerv. Ment. Dis.,* **157:** 75–98, 1973.

Freud, S. *The Interpretation of Dreams.* Brill, A. A., trans. Random House, New York, 1950. Originally published 1900.

Growdon, J. H. Neurotransmitter precursors in the diet: their use in the treatment of brain disease. Pp. 117–81 in *Nutrition and the Brain,* vol. 3. Wurtman, R. J., and Wurtman, J. J., eds. Raven Press, New York, 1979.

Guilleminault, C.; Eldridge, F. L.; Simmons, F. B.; and Dement, W. C. Sleep apnea in eight children. *Pediatrics,* **58:** 23–31, 1976.

Imlah, N. W. Narcolepsy in identical twins. *J. Neurol. Neurosurg. Psychiatry,* **24:** 158–60, 1961.

Kales, A., and Kales, J. D. Sleep disorders: recent findings in the diagnosis and treatment of disturbed sleep. *N. Engl. J. Med.,* **290,** 487–99, 1974.

Kales, J. D.; Kales, A.; Soldatos, C. R.; Caldwell, A. B.; Charney, D. S.; and Martin, E. D. Night terrors: clinical characteristics and personality patterns. *Arch. Gen. Psychiatry,* **37:** 1413–17, 1980.

Kales, A.; Soldatos, C. R.; Caldwell, A. B.; Charney, D. S.; Kales, J. D.; Markel, D.; and Cadieux, R. Nightmares: clinical characteristics and personality patterns. *Am. J. Psychiatry,* **137:** 1197–1201, 1980.

Krueger, J. M.; Pappenheimer, J. R.; and Karnovsky, M. L. Sleep-promoting factor S: purification and properties. *Proc. Nat. Acad. Sci. USA,* **75:** 5235–38, 1978.

Orenstein, D. M.; Boat, T. F.; Stern, R. C.; Doershuk, C. F.; and Light, M. S. Progesterone treatment of the obesity hypoventilation syndrome in a child. *J. Pediatr.,* **90:** 477–79, 1977.

Oswald, I. Sleeping and dreaming. Pp. 193–221 in *Modern Perspectives in World Psychiatry.* Howells, J. G., ed., Brunner/Mazel Publishers, New York, 1971.

Oxford English Dictionary. Compact ed. Oxford University Press, Glasgow, 1971.

Pappenheimer, J. R. The sleep factor. *Sci. Am.,* **235:** 24–29, August 1976.

Pappenheimer, J. R. "Nature's soft nurse": a sleep-promoting factor isolated from brain. *Johns Hopkins Med. J.,* **145:** 49–56, 1979.

Plum, F., and Van Uitert, R. Nonendocrine diseases and disorders of the hypothalamus. In *The Hypothalamus.* Reichlin, S.; Baldessarini, R. J.; and Martin, J. B., eds. Raven Press, New York, 1978.

Powers, P. S., and Gunderman, R. Kleine-Levin syndrome associated with fire setting. *Am. J. Dis. Child.,* **132:** 786–89, 1978.

Roth, D.; Brůhová, S.; and Lehovský, M. REM sleep and NREM sleep in narcolepsy and hypersomnia. *Electroencephalogr. Clin. Neurophysiol.,* **26:** 176–82, 1969.

Simpser, M. D.; Strieder, D. J.; Wohl, M. E.; Rosenthal, A.; and Rockenmacher, S. Sleep apnea in a child with the Pickwickian syndrome. *Pediatrics,* **60:** 290–93, 1977.

Sitaram, N.; Moore, A. M.; and Gillin, J. C. The effect of physostigmine on normal human sleep and dreaming. *Arch. Gen. Psychiatry,* **35:** 1239–43, 1978.

Sperling, M. Sleep disturbances in children. Pp. 418-54 in *Modern Perspectives in International Child Psychiatry.* Howells, J. G., ed. Brunner/Mazel Publishers, New York, 1971.

Spier, N., and Karelitz, S. The Pickwickian syndrome: case in a child. Am. J. Dis. Child., **99:** 822–27, 1960.

Strohl, K. P.; Saunders, N. A.; Feldman, N. T.; and Hallett, M. Obstructive sleep apnea in family members. *N. Engl. J. Med.,* **299:** 969–73, 1978.

Turino, G. M., and Goldring, R. M. Sleeping and breathing. *N. Engl. J. Med.,* **299:** 1009–11, 1978.

Weech, A. A. Narcolepsy—a symptom complex: report of a case in a child. *Am. J. Dis. Child.,* **32:** 672–81, 1926.

Zarcone, V. Narcolepsy. *N. Engl. J. Med.,* **288:** 1156–66, 1973.

ADDITIONAL READINGS

Dement, W. C. *Some Must Watch While Some Must Sleep.* San Francisco Book Co., San Francisco, 1976.

Hobson, J. A., and McCarley, R. W. The brain as a dream state generator: an activation-synthesis hypothesis of the dream process. *Am. J. Psychiatry,* **134:** 1335–48, 1977.

Kales, A.; Soldatos, C. R.; Caldwell, A. B.; Kales, J. D.; Humphrey, F. J., II; Charney, D. S.; and Schweitzer, P. K. Somnambulism: clinical characteristics and personality patterns. *Arch. Gen. Psychiatry,* **37:** 1406–10, 1980.

Vogel, G. W. A review of REM sleep deprivation. *Arch. Gen. Psychiatry,* **32:** 749–61, 1975.

10 Disorders of Eating and Elimination: Anorexia Nervosa, Obesity, Enuresis, and Encopresis

Eating and elimination are major vegetative functions throughout life. They are involved in maintaining the well-being of the human organism through voluntary and involuntary means. For example, the process of eating begins with conscious and willed activity: the preparation, cutting, chewing, and swallowing of food. Most of the digestive process, however, is unconscious and automatic: the movement of food along the alimentary tract and the enzymatic degradation of foodstuffs. The interaction between the involuntary biologic necessities of urination and defecation and the learned, volitional processes of control is well known. It follows, then, that disorders of eating or elimination can stem from or involve problems of voluntary behavior, involuntary behavior, or both.

This chapter will focus upon four major areas of concern in childhood and adolescence: anorexia nervosa, obesity, enuresis, and encopresis. Each of these problems will be considered from the standpoint of definition, diagnosis (including investigation), differential diagnosis, etiology, treatment, and outcome. Selected anatomic, biochemical, and physiologic aspects of these problems also will be presented.

ANOREXIA NERVOSA

Anorexia nervosa is a striking disorder of eating that, like infantile autism, has caught the public eye because of its dramatic symptomatology: self-inflicted starvation typically seen in adolescent girls, who often are highly intelligent. This section will address several questions pertaining to anorexia nervosa:

How does anorexia nervosa differ from anorexia?
What features define the syndrome of anorexia nervosa?
Are there biologic causes for the problem, or is it purely psychogenic in origin?

227

What organic disturbances are associated with anorexia nervosa?
Is psychotherapy by itself sufficient?
What is the role of behavior modification?
What is the outcome of persons who have had anorexia nervosa?

DEFINITION

Anorexia itself refers to loss of appetite. It frequently is associated with loss of interest in food, diminished food intake, and ultimately loss of weight. As such, it often results from systemic illness such as hepatitis and commonly accompanies emotional disorder such as depression.

Anorexia nervosa is an eating disturbance characterized by elective restriction of food intake associated with disturbed body image, fear of becoming obese, and intense denial of the real body image leading to weight loss of 25 or more pounds or 25 per cent or more of original body weight (Martin *et al.*, 1977; *DSM*-III, 1980) (see Table 10–1). The weight gain anticipated with normal growth in childhood and adolescence but not found in a person with possible anorexia nervosa can be added to the overall weight loss figure in order to determine if the criteria for the diagnosis of anorexia nervosa are met. It has been found to affect about one out of 100 girls between 16 and 18 years of age (Crisp *et al.*, 1976).

Confusion in the use of the terms "anorexia" and "anorexia nervosa" arises when the former is used as an abbreviation for the latter. Lack of clarity may be compounded by use of the descriptive terms "anorectic" or "anorexic" to refer either to the specific syndrome of anorexia nervosa or to a state of appetite loss. It is ironic that appetite loss is frequently absent even with typical anorexia nervosa until relatively late in the course of the disorder.

DIAGNOSIS

The criteria for necessary weight loss to establish the diagnosis of anorexia nervosa are presented above. Characteristic associated features may assist in making the diagnosis. The disorder typically has its onset during pubescence (ages 12 through 18 years), affects girls much more often than boys (fifteen to twenty times), and is associated with amenorrhea (primary or secondary) (Rollins and Piazza, 1978). Hypothermia, bradycardia, hypotension, and lanugo (soft, fine hair characteristically seen in newborns) may be found.

Behavior has been described as a "relentless pursuit of thinness" associated with "a frantic fear of being or becoming fat" (Bruch, 1979). In an effort to lose weight or to keep it at a minimum, self-induced vomiting

TABLE 10–1. **Diagnostic Criteria for Anorexia Nervosa**

Elective restriction of food intake
Disturbed body image
Fear of becoming obese
Weight loss of 25 or more pounds (or at least 25 per
    cent of previous or anticipated body weight)

(which may occur after binges of eating), laxative use, and extreme hyperactivity (such as running outdoors, up stairs, or in place) are often resorted to. In boys, hyperactivity may occur in an athletic context (e.g., running or wrestling) in which weight reduction often is advantageous (Smith, 1980).

Bruch (1979) has articulated three major areas of disordered psychologic functioning: (1) disturbed body image (an almost delusional belief that skeletal emaciation is "just right"), (2) misperception or misinterpretation of bodily sensations (for example, hunger transformed into a pleasurable feeling), and (3) a pervasive sense of ineffectiveness (paralyzing passivity against a background of earlier overconformity).

Atypical forms of anorexia nervosa occur in which weight loss is accompanied by fatigue and indolence rather than overactivity. The obsession with slimness is absent. Indeed, the patient may complain of weight loss, and true anorexia may be present.

Clinical Process. The diagnosis of anorexia nervosa is essentially clinical, based upon the history and examination.

History. The chief complaint will often reflect the mental status of the patient: "They say I'm not eating enough." "I'm too fat." "They don't want me to lose more weight." These statements typify the failure to recognize the emaciated state as being abnormal, and they further reflect the passivity characteristically seen in such patients.

The amount of weight lost and the time over which it has occurred should be documented. The kinds and amounts of food eaten should be determined as well as the patterns of intake, including binges. Increase or decrease in appetite should be sought. The episode of anorexia nervosa that led to evaluation may have been an extension of a period of dieting begun because of real or imagined chubbiness. Menstrual history should be obtained and onset of menstruation, irregularity, or cessation of periods noted. Activity level, athletic participation, and exercise pattern should be established upon interviewing parents as well as child. They should also be questioned about self-induced vomiting and use of enemas, laxatives, diuretics, or diet drinks to lose weight.

Review of systems should include inquiry as to intercurrent illness (particularly hepatitis or other gastrointestinal disorder), headache, visual disturbance, changes in sleep habits, preference of cold versus warm weather, and changes in urinary habits such as enuresis or nocturia.

Examination. The *general description* should note the most striking aspects of the child's appearance and behavior. Persons affected with anorexia nervosa typically look like a skeleton clad in skin. Lack of facial fat allows the skull to become virtually apparent. Loss of bodily fat causes loss of normal contours of breasts and buttocks, making an adolescent girl look like a "beanpole."

The *general physical examination* should include recording of present and past heights and weights on standard growth charts. Not only may weight loss be evident, but an adolescent's typically rapid rise in height may be blunted. Vital signs should be recorded. Blood pressure (normally lower in children than in adults) and temperature may be abnormally low. Nearly three-quarters of children in the series of Rollins and Piazza (1978) had temperatures below 98 degrees Fahrenheit. Bradycardia (with a pulse rate of below 60) may also be found. The skin should be examined for mottling, edema, dehydration, self-induced injuries, and lanugo. Evidence for systemic disease such as hepatitis, ulcerative colitis, regional enteritis (Crohn disease), or malignancy should be sought.

A complete *neurologic examination* should be carried out with particular attention to neuro-ophthalmologic function. It should include careful inspection of the optic fundi to exclude papilledema and optic atrophy. Blurring of disk margins and elevation of optic nerve heads can occur due to increased intracranial pressure. With prolonged elevation in intracranial pressure (secondary to a slowly growing, deep midline mass, for example), optic atrophy can result. Visual fields should be tested not only by finger movements but with a small (4–5 mm) white-headed pin. Optimally, a tangent screen should be used. A temporal field deficit should specifically be sought. This may be quadrantic or hemianopic with lesions of the hypothalamus or nearby structures.

Testing of other cranial nerves should focus on the olfactory, facial, glossopharyngeal, and vagus nerves. Loss of sense of smell may occur with tumors of the frontal lobe. They are classically also associated with apathy and indifference such as may be seen in atypical syndromes of anorexia nervosa. Taste can be impaired with lesions of the facial or glossopharyngeal nerves. Testing of the ninth and tenth cranial nerves should include assessment of swallowing function, since swallowing difficulty may be a complaint in atypical syndromes with hysterical features, with malignancy of the nasopharynx, or with brainstem gliomas (see Chapter 7).

The *mental status examination* should include assessment of mood and affect. The child's perception of the problem should be explored as well as fantasies (of oral impregnation, for example) and fears (such as insatiable appetite). The child's body image should be determined through conversation and projective techniques such as drawings of self and others. The meaning of food for the child should also be examined.

Investigation (see Table 10–2).   Several investigations should be included on a routine basis in evaluating the child with anorexia nervosa.

TABLE 10–2. **Investigations to Be Considered in the Child with Anorexia Nervosa**

CBC
Urinalysis, including measurement of specific gravity
Blood urea nitrogen, serum electrolytes, including calcium
Liver function tests, including serum proteins
Serologic tests for infectious mononucleosis
Thyroid function tests
Electrocardiogram
Skull x-rays, standard views
Special radiologic studies: sellar tomography, views of optic canals, cranial CT
    scan, pneumoencephalography (PEG)
Neuro-ophthalmologic testing, including visual fields
Luteinizing hormone (LH) level and other neuroendocrinologic studies
Urinary MHPG levels

These include complete blood count (hemoglobin, hematocrit, estimation or quantitation of platelets, white blood cell count and differential), urinalysis (including microscopic examination and measurement of specific gravity), and plain skull x-rays (with lateral views to visualize the pituitary fossa) (see Fig. 10–1). If these x-rays are abnormal or if hypothalamic-pituitary disorder is otherwise implicated, other radiographic studies may be pursued. These might include tomograms of the sella turcica, films of the optic canals, computerized tomography (CT) of the cranium, or pneumoencephalography, which remains an effective way of gathering information about deep midline structures difficult to visualize well by CT scan.

Evidence of brain atrophy on CT scan manifested by cortical atrophy, ventricular dilatation, or both was found in seven of fourteen patients with anorexia nervosa reported by Nussbaum and colleagues (1980). Abnormality of CT scan was correlated with higher rates of weight loss (5.2 pounds per month versus 2.5). In two patients restudied by this means, the scan remained abnormal (though improved in one) following weight gain.

Hematologic studies should include serum electrolytes, blood urea nitrogen, liver function tests (including bilirubin, SGOT, alkaline phosphatase, and LDH), serum proteins, thyroxine (T_4), triiodothyronine (T_3) uptake, thyroid index, and thyroid-stimulating hormone (TSH). A serologic test for infectious mononucleosis should be considered. With electolyte disturbance (especially hypokalemia or hypocalcemia) or with evidence of cardiac disturbance (such as bradycardia), electrocardiogram should be obtained.

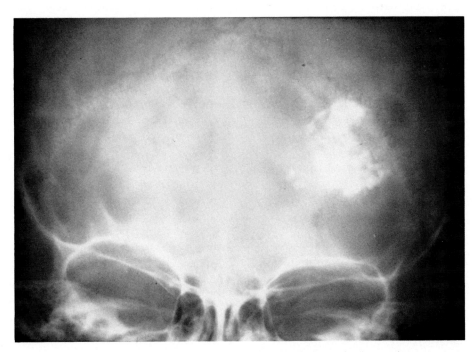

FIGURE 10–1. Plain skull x-ray showing calcified craniopharyngioma.

TABLE 10–3. **Conditions to Be Differentiated from Anorexia Nervosa**

Systemic illness (causing anorexia and weight loss)
Hyperthyroidism (causing weight loss without anorexia)
Diabetes mellitus (causing weight loss without anorexia)
Hypothalamic or pituitary tumor
Drug abuse
Depression
Hysteria
Schizophrenia
Degenerative disorder of the nervous system
Normal adolescence

Several endocrine studies have been found typically abnormal in anorexia nervosa. These include diminished T_3 (triiodothyronine) and LH (luteinizing hormone) levels. These effects, which revert to normal after weight gain, have been attributed to starvation (Boyar, 1978; Halmi, 1978; Plum and Van Uitert, 1978).

Levels of urinary MHPG (3-methoxy-4-hydroxyphenylglycol), considered a major product of central nervous system norepinephrine metabolism, have been found diminished in persons acutely ill with anorexia nervosa (Halmi *et al.,* 1978). Further, these levels were significantly correlated with depression on self-rating scales.

Ophthalmologic consultation is generally indicated in the evaluation of the child with anorexia nervosa and should include formal visual field testing.

Differential Diagnosis.   Anorexia nervosa must be distinguished from other causes of anorexia (see Table 10–3). These include *systemic illness* such as hepatitis, peptic ulcer, malignancy, infectious mononucleosis, cystic fibrosis, regional enteritis (Crohn disease), and ulcerative colitis among other disorders. These conditions are usually readily differentiable from classical anorexia nervosa because of symptoms such as diarrhea, constipation, blood or mucus in the stool, or vomiting (not self-induced) that suggest identifiable organic disease.

Hyperthyroidism and *diabetes mellitus* can cause marked weight loss and other constitutional symptoms without anorexia but with increased appetite.

Hypothalamic or pituitary tumor can present with many features of anorexia nervosa: weight loss, depression, and loss of appetite (Heron and Johnston, 1976; Goldney, 1978). Symptoms and signs of increased intracranial pressure, abnormalities on neurologic exam (such as papilledema, bitemporal field cut, or optic atrophy), and radiologic signs (such as suprasellar calcification or erosion of the pituitary fossa) will suggest structural disorder (see Fig. 10–2).

Drug abuse, especially with amphetamines, can cause anorexia leading to weight loss. Careful history-taking, review of past medical records, and analysis of blood and urine for toxic substances will help to clarify this possibility (see Chapter 19).

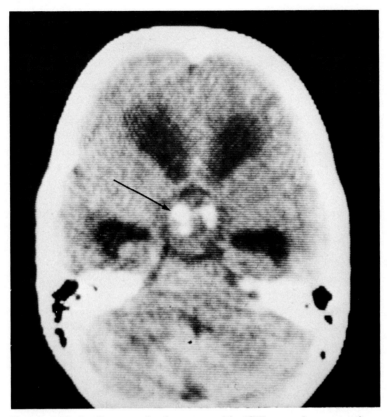

FIGURE 10–2. Computerized tomographic (CT) scan demonstrating craniopharyngioma (arrow) in a 10-year-old child.

The symptoms of *depression* variably overlap those of some syndromes of anorexia nervosa: sadness, diminished appetite, weight loss, fatigue, and reduced activity level (see Chapter 6) (see Case 10–1).

Hysterical vomiting may also suggest anorexia nervosa. With hysterical vomiting the focus is likelier to be upon swallowing difficulties rather than an obsession as to slimness. Differentiation from swallowing difficulties secondary to nasopharyngeal dysfunction (e.g., associated with tumor), pontine disease (e.g., multiple sclerosis), and botulism must be made.

Schizophrenia presenting in later childhood or adolescence may coexist with anorexia nervosa and be associated with impaired eating and weight loss.

Degenerative disorder of the nervous system may also be accompanied by profound anorexia and weight loss (see Chapter 8). Loss of intellectual function (dementia) may be demonstrable, although degenerative disorders affecting the neuromuscular system may leave the intellect intact (see Case 8–5).

Normal adolescence should not be confused with anorexia nervosa. Concerns as to a rapidly changing body (including the development of breasts) and its functions (such as menstruation) are normal. A chubby phase of ado-

CASE 10–1: DEPRESSIVE SYNDROME WITH FEATURES OF ANOREXIA NERVOSA IN A 14-YEAR-OLD BOY WITH HEADACHES AND SIXTH NERVE PALSY

R.R. was evaluated because of throbbing headaches and a sixth nerve palsy. At age 11, the boy had an exanthematous illness presumed to be viral. It was followed by a gastrointestinal syndrome manifested by diarrhea and abdominal pain. Soon thereafter, nasal stuffiness, low-grade fever, and right-sided headaches began. Headaches lasted several hours and occurred daily for nearly 2 years. They were punctuated by more intense headaches lasting several days that occurred every 2 to 3 weeks. Headaches were sometimes accompanied by nausea but not by vomiting. At 14 years, he suddenly developed double vision due to a paralysis of abduction of the right eye.

Review of systems was noteworthy for a 25-pound weight loss between the ages of 11 and 13 years. A subsequent 10-pound weight gain was followed by further weight loss. He was not known to induce vomiting. He exercised little. He was an average student but repeated sixth grade because he had been absent one-quarter of the school year.

On examination, the child was a slender, frail-appearing, and subdued boy. He acknowledged feeling depressed and having had suicidal thoughts but denied suicidal actions. Weight was 84 pounds (5th percentile) compared with height and head circumference at the 20th and 50th percentiles, respectively. General physical examination showed bilateral gynecomastia. Genitalia were normal for a male in early adolescence. On neurologic examination, optic fundi were normal. Paralysis of abduction of the right eye was evident. The face was asymmetric in smiling, the right side creasing less than the left. Deep tendon reflexes were brisk. The left plantar response was equivocal.

Investigation included measurement of serum thyroxine level and antinuclear antibody, CT scan with and without contrast, parasellar tomography, right carotid and vertebral angiography, and neuroendocrine studies. All were normal.

lescence typically precedes (though it may follow) a growth spurt and may sensitize a child as to fatness. During this stage of development, the child may embark upon a diet in order to lose weight. With anorexia nervosa, dieting persists despite loss of a reasonable amount of weight, menstrual periods cease, and emaciation results.

Etiology. The major causes of anorexia nervosa are psychologic, social-environmental, and developmental. Medical, neurologic, and toxic factors may contribute secondarily in the form of malnutrition, metabolic disturbance, and self-medication.

Medical Causes. Systemic illness associated with anorexia (as distinguished from anorexia nervosa) was discussed above in the section on DIFFERENTIAL DIAGNOSIS.

During a 2-week hospital stay, weight dropped to 75 pounds. On the ward he complained frequently of headaches and was withdrawn despite efforts to involve him in structured activities. Psychiatric evaluation further elucidated the child's depressive picture and clarified the family's pattern of interaction. Imipramine, 50 mg at bedtime, was begun. Outpatient psychotherapy was arranged.

Over the next 8 months, the child did relatively well. Regular psychotherapy continued with individual sessions every other week. Antidepressant medication was maintained. Weight increased to 120 pounds, so that he became mildly chubby. Headaches persisted but were less distressing. He attended school regularly. The neurologic examination was unchanged, including the sixth nerve palsy.

Comment. This adolescent's syndrome of depression with features of anorexia nervosa combined with headaches and paralysis of out-turning of the right eye strongly suggested intracranial pathology. The gynecomastia further indicated a lesion of the hypothalamic-pituitary axis. The sixth nerve palsy, which might have been a "false" localizing sign due to increased intracranial pressure, might also have reflected involvement of the right abducens nerve traveling adjacent to the hypothalamus and pituitary.

As his extensive evaluation demonstrated, however, his sixth nerve paralysis appeared to be an isolated finding of undetermined cause. Gynecomastia proved to be typical benign gynecomastia of adolescence. His depressive syndrome appeared to stem from developmental and familial issues accentuated by medical illness. Though problems clearly remained, he obviously benefited from psychiatric treatment that involved individual therapy, a family-based approach to his behavior, and continued use of antidepressant medication. His overall management has also included periodic neurologic reexamination.

Neurologic Causes. Hypothalamic or pituitary tumor (such as craniopharyngioma) was mentioned earlier (see DIFFERENTIAL DIAGNOSIS) as a cause of atypical syndromes of anorexia nervosa.

Psychologic Causes. Bruch (1977) views the basic psychologic issue in the young person with anorexia nervosa as that of control: being in charge of one's own body and leading one's own life. These issues are, of course, appropriate in adolescence. Rather than the development of independence, however, negativism and food refusal supervene, typically in one who previously was an excessively compliant, "model" child.

Misperception, misinterpretation, and misapplication of internal signals such as hunger or fullness are typical of persons with anorexia nervosa. Hunger may be converted into a pleasurable sensation. Hunger signals may be mistaken as satiety. Fantasies involving the gastrointestinal tract may involve the fear of oral impregnation (Bruch, 1977). In other persons guilt may render eating too pleasurable an activity to be indulged in.

Social-Environmental Causes. Social-environmental factors appear to play a significant role in causing anorexia nervosa. Affected children, typically from middle-class families, are generally described as being very good and compliant. This impression may stem from an environment in which needs have been anticipated to an exaggerated degree, and independence and assertiveness not allowed to develop. Rather than becoming a healthy adolescent with strivings toward independence, the child develops instead into an emotionally immature, negativistic teenager.

Minuchin and his colleagues (1975) have proposed that specific family patterns of interaction contribute importantly to the development of anorexia nervosa and other psychophysiologic disorders. These characteristics are enmeshment, overprotectiveness, rigidity, and lack of conflict resolution. Within this context the child's illness plays the role of maintaining the status quo of conflict avoidance.

Developmental Causes. The characteristic presentation in adolescence suggests that developmental factors, possibly mediated through or acting in conjunction with hormonal influences, play an etiologic role in anorexia nervosa.

Bruch (1977) has proposed that feeding experiences in earliest life (infancy and early childhood) lay the groundwork for later eating disturbances. For example, overanticipation of the child's needs, it is hypothesized, may lead to administration of food when the child is not hungry and thus interfere with the child's acquisition of a personal sense of hunger (and the expression of that bodily state).

TREATMENT AND OUTCOME

Management of the child with anorexia nervosa is necessarily multifaceted, involving medical, psychotherapeutic, and environmental modes of treatment (see Table 10–4). Although families may argue to the contrary, the problem has generally been a long-standing one, and therapy should be anticipated to be a relatively long-term undertaking.

The outcome varies. Apparently complete recovery from a single episode

TABLE 10–4. **Treatment of Anorexia Nervosa**

Medical	Nutritional support (by mouth, nasogastric tube, or vein)
	Treatment of intercurrent medical problems
Psychologic	Individual and family therapy
Social-Environmental	Behavior modification
Educational	Essentials of nutrition and gastrointestinal function
	Tutoring

of illness may give way to relapse when the child returns to his or her previous environment such as family and school (Bruch, 1979). Overall mortality ranges from 5 to 20 per cent (Martin *et al.*, 1977). Mortality is attributable to infection, hypocalcemia, acid-base imbalance, hypothermia, and/or suicide (Maloney and Farrell, 1980). On the other hand, Silverman (1974) reported no fatalities among twenty-nine persons followed for an average of 2 years. Three-quarters of the children, discharged from continuous treatment or maintained in regular outpatient therapy, were felt to be functioning adequately. Four children were diagnosed as schizophrenic and their prognosis considered guarded. The outlook for younger female adolescents with anorexia nervosa (ages 12–15 years) appears to be more favorable than for older girls (ages 16–19 years) (Casper *et al.*, 1981).

Early diagnosis and intervention when weight loss has not been profound and behavior patterns not yet firmly established appears to lead to a more favorable outcome and may obviate the need for hospitalization, which is necessary in more severely affected children.

Medical Management. Nutritional support is fundamental, though acceptable weight gain does not by itself constitute adequate therapy. The essential elements are calories (2,000 to 2,400 per day for the usual adolescent girl), protein (50 to 55 grams per day), vitamins, and minerals (Greene and Schubert, 1979). An oral, nasogastric, or intravenous route may be employed, depending upon the gravity of the situation and the ability of the child to participate.

Hyperalimentation can be lifesaving in cases where other nutritional approaches have failed and physical and mental deterioration associated with starvation continue. Maloney and Farrell (1980) described the use of a total parenteral alimentation regimen in which dextrose, amino acids, vitamins, electrolytes, trace metals, and fat were given intravenously to four girls with anorexia nervosa. Their mean weight loss had averaged 35 per cent of body weight. Severely marasmic upon admission to hospital, they received 12 to 44 days of hyperalimentation. During that time their mood improved and they became much better able to participate in psychotherapy. Continued weight gain was recorded in all children after a mean follow-up period of 10 months.

When the medical condition of the child permits, a baseline period of data-gathering may be valuable. A regular diet is offered to the child and the calories, protein content, food choices, and other aspects of eating behavior monitored (Greene and Schubert, 1979). Nutritional management of course should never exist in a vacuum. Close coordination with psychotherapy (individual and family-based) and with a program of behavior modification is essential.

Intercurrent medical problems such as asthma or urinary tract infection should be treated as specifically as possible.

Psychotherapy. Both individual and family psychotherapy are of demonstrated value in the treatment of anorexia nervosa. Individual therapy will include attention to the child's physical condition, fantasies and fears regarding orality and sexuality, and issues within the family. Bruch (1979) has emphasized the child's taking on an active and independent role in maintaining a healthy and appropriate body image. Minuchin and colleagues (1975), in a study including long-term follow-up, have shown the importance and effectiveness of a family approach in assessment and treatment of children with anorexia nervosa. Twenty of their twenty-five patients were considered to have recovered from their illness not only in terms of weight gain but also in adjustment in school, social, and family spheres of activity.

Social-Environmental Management.   Behavior modification can play a valuable role in the management of the child with anorexia nervosa, particularly one who has been hospitalized (Stunkard, 1972; Liebman *et al.*, 1974; Bruch, 1979; Woolston and Schowalter, 1980). A fundamental principle is that the child's access to physical activity (in some instances participation in social events as well) is made contingent upon weight gain.

Silverman (1974) has described an inpatient management protocol for children with anorexia nervosa. The child is admitted to a large ward of a general pediatric or medical service rather than to a psychiatric unit. The family is permitted to visit the child briefly once a week. The child is informed that the hospital requires each patient to consume a minimum of 1 liter per day of calorie-containing fluids. The penalty for failure to comply with this rule is intravenous fluid therapy. It is made clear to the child and family upon admission that the illness is a serious one, potentially fatal. Intensive psychiatric treatment is begun on the day of admission. The child is seen four times per week, the parents once weekly during the period of hospitalization, which averages 3 months.

Educational Management.   Therapy should include teaching of the essentials of nutrition, human energy requirements (including the meaning of calories), and the structure of the gastrointestinal system (Silverman, 1974).

When hospitalization is prolonged, it is important whenever possible to maintain educational continuity through inpatient tutoring.

SUMMARY

Anorexia nervosa is a syndrome characterized by the relentless pursuit of thinness leading to profound weight loss. It typically occurs in adolescent girls and is fatal in 5–20 per cent of cases. Diagnosis is based upon a minimum weight loss of 25 pounds (or 25 per cent of body weight), severely disturbed body image, and amenorrhea (in girls). These features are typically associated with self-induced vomiting, laxative use, and overactivity directed toward further weight loss. With atypical syndromes, true anorexia and fatigue may be present, neither of which tend to occur in classical anorexia nervosa until later stages.

Anorexia nervosa appears to result from a combination of psychologic, social, and developmental factors. It must be differentiated from other causes of profound weight loss such as brain tumor (particularly involving the hypothalamus or pituitary), gastrointestinal disorder, or malignancy. Examination is directed toward assessing the state of nutrition and hydration as well as identifying pathologic processes that might be mistaken for anorexia nervosa. Investigation should include electrolytes, complete blood count, urinalysis, and skull x-rays. Further investigation such as computerized tomographic scan of the head may be warranted. Treatment is necessarily multifaceted, involving nutritional support, psychotherapy (individual and family), and social-environmental measures. Outcome is variable. It ranges from normalcy to persisting psychopathology and, in some instances, death. Early intervention appears to contribute to a favorable prognosis.

OBESITY

Obesity in adulthood is a major problem associated with high blood pressure, diabetes mellitus, and other disease states. The difficulties of weight loss and maintenance of weight reduction are widely recognized and contribute to the morbidity of obesity. Prevention would obviously be preferable to treatment that is often unpleasant and ineffective. Although its medical morbidity is less than that in adulthood, obesity in childhood is a chronic social stress and appears to lead the way to obesity of adulthood.

Several questions pertaining to obesity will be considered in this section:

What is the definition of obesity?
What are its causes?
Do hormonal factors play a significant etiologic role?
What features of history or examination suggest underlying organic disease?
What investigations, if any, should be carried out in the obese child?
How should obesity in childhood and adolescence be treated?
Do obese children become obese adults?

DEFINITION

Obesity can be defined as excessive deposition and storage of body fat. Direct measurement of body fat can be accomplished by buoyancy testing and by measurement of skin-fold thickness. For practical purposes, obesity in childhood and adolescence is defined as weight in excess of the 97th percentile (i.e., greater than two standard deviations above the mean). This criterion cannot, however, be considered absolute. Because of changing fat composition of the body, weight alone may underestimate obesity in the younger child and overestimate it in the adolescent (Weil, 1977).

DIAGNOSIS

Clinical Process. *History.* The obese child may comment, "I'm too fat." "I'm hungry all the time." "I go on eating binges." The child, on the other hand, may have been brought for evaluation because of other problems such as depression, excessive sleepiness, or headaches. The history of the presenting problem should indicate when obesity was recognized, how it has been treated, and what the result of treatment has been. A careful history of dietary habits and eating behavior should be taken.

Jordan and colleagues (1977) have articulated eight areas for exploration:

1. Early feeding history: How did the child eat as an infant? Was he or she breast-fed or bottle-fed? When did it become possible to differentiate cries of hunger from other states of discomfort such as coldness or loneliness?

2. Parents' attitudes toward food and weight: What is the role of food in

the family? How do the parents attempt to control eating and weight? Is food used for reward or punishment?

3. Food habits and attitudes: What is the child's level of nutritional knowledge? What are preferred foods? How does the child feel before, during, and after eating—hungry, bored, angry, or depressed? Does he or she feel guilty about eating high-calorie foods? To what extent is food involved in the child's social activities?

4. Food supplies and storage: Who in the family is responsible for shopping and food preparation? What kinds of food and what quantities are generally kept at home?

5. Level of physical activity: What routine physical exercise does the child engage in? Are there additional opportunities for physical activity? Does the child walk or ride a bike to and from school? If so, does he or she stop on the way for a snack?

6. Current psychologic functioning: Have significant life changes or crises occurred recently or in the past? What have been the effects on eating behavior or weight? Are any major stresses anticipated in the near future? Have changes in mood (acute or chronic) occurred? Has schoolwork deteriorated?

7. Social relationships: What kind of support or sabotage can be anticipated from the family during a period of attempted weight loss? What interests does the patient have in addition to those of home and school? Does he or she have one, several, or no close friends?

8. Family history: Are other family members obese? Is there a history of psychiatric disturbance?

Review of systems should include inquiry as to hypersomnia or other sleep disorder, excessive urination, irregularities of body temperature, aggressive outbursts, seizures, galactorrhea, menstrual pattern, headaches, visual disturbance, preference of ambient temperature, current medications, and chronic illnesses.

Examination. The *general description* of the child should note the degree of obesity: mild, moderate, or extreme. Other striking features of the general physical examination or mental status examination that might be included here are somnolence, depression, or immaturity.

The *general physical examination* should contain careful measurement of weight, height, and head circumference. These figures should be plotted on standard growth curves along with previous growth measurements to identify the pattern and progression of excessive weight gain. The waist should be measured around the umbilicus or at the level of the iliac crest. Measurement of skinfold thickness can be accomplished with special calipers.

The distribution of fat should be noted, whether primarily truncal or more generally distributed to involve the limbs as well. Purple abdominal stretch marks (striae), reddened cheeks, a moonlike facial appearance, and a "buffalo hump" upon the shoulders are typical of Cushing syndrome. Small genitalia are characteristically seen with the Prader-Willi syndrome. Polydactyly occurs with the Laurence-Moon-Biedl syndrome, a short fourth metacarpal in pseudohypoparathyroidism. Skin texture, pulse rate, and thyroid gland size all should specifically be noted. When obesity is extreme, signs of heart failure and pulmonary hypertension may be seen (Spier and Karelitz, 1960).

The *neurologic examination* should include careful funduscopic inspection to exclude papilledema, optic atrophy, and pigmentary degeneration of the retina (retinitis pigmentosa). Visual field deficit (particularly a bitemporal quadrantic or hemianopic defect) should be sought by confrontation and with use of a tangent screen whenever possible.

The *mental status examination* should explore the child's perception of and feelings about himself or herself. Having the child draw a picture of himself alone and with his family or friends is a useful projective technique. The meaning of food to the child should also be explored. Depression or anxiety should be noted. An estimate of academic performance and overall level of intelligence should be made.

Investigation. Most children with obesity need undergo no investigation beyond that which is part of regular health care. When evidence indicates involvement of specific organs or organ systems, relevant investigation should be pursued (see Table 10–5). Obesity with excessive urination and hypogonadism, for example, will suggest hypothalamic disturbance that might appropriately be evaluated by measurement of urine specific gravity (on a random sample or following water deprivation), plain skull x-rays to assess the pituitary fossa and adjacent structures, and CT scan of the head with special attention to the suprasellar area. When thyroid dysfunction is considered, measurement of serum thyroxine (T_4), triiodothyronine (T_3), thyroid index, and thyroid stimulating hormone (TSH) are indicated. A morning cortisol level can be obtained to exclude Cushing syndrome, although additional studies of the hypothalamic-pituitary-adrenal axis may be required to characterize the problem fully. Chromosome studies are indicated when the Prader-Willi syndrome is suspected because of an associated chromosome anomaly recently described (Wisniewski *et al.,* 1980). When seizures are suggested or the person eats compulsively in binges, an electro-encephalogram should be carried out (Rau and Green, 1978).

Differential Diagnosis. Obesity must be distinguished from *excessive eating* (also called hyperphagia, megaphagia, or polyphagia) and from *bulimia,* excessive appetite. Indeed, obesity frequently results from either but need not when excessive eating occurs only in binges of several days to weeks or

TABLE 10–5. **Investigations to Be Considered in the Obese Child**

Thyroid function tests
Serum cortisol and other studies of hypothalamic-
   pituitary-adrenal function
Skull x-rays
Cranial CT scan
EEG (in awake and sleep states)
Urinalysis, including specific gravity
Water deprivation test
Chromosome analysis

when eating bouts are followed by self-induced vomiting (which may occur in anorexia nervosa). Polyphagia characteristically occurs without consequent weight gain in untreated (or undertreated) diabetes mellitus and hyperthyroidism.

Developmental "chubbiness" should also be distinguished from obesity. Infants and toddlers are normally relatively rotund. Prior to their growth spurt, adolescents also typically manifest a chubby phase.

Etiology (see Table 10–6).   Obesity ultimately results from excessive storage of fat when caloric intake is greater than expenditure. All things being equal, ingestion of 3,500 calories will result in a 1-pound weight gain whereas activity utilizing 3,500 calories will result in a 1-pound weight loss. One must therefore first determine caloric intake (the amount and kinds of food) and the level of physical activity (including intensity and duration) (Passmore and Durnin, 1955).

The situation is, however, a good deal more complicated than a simple in-and-out nutritional balance sheet. Eating is a behavior common to all but not fully understood. It involves a complex interplay of internal and external factors: hunger, satiety, mood, food availability, and social circumstances, to name a few. Furthermore, at least half of daily caloric needs are deter-

TABLE 10–6. **Causes of Obesity in Childhood**

Medical	Hypothyroidism
	Cushing syndrome
	Excessive insulin usage
Neurologic	Hypothalamic disturbance (tumor, leukemia, sarcoid, tuberculosis, trauma, postsurgical)
	Kleine-Levin syndrome
	Prader-Willi syndrome
	Laurence-Moon-Biedl syndrome
	Paroxysmal disturbance of electrical activity of brain
Toxic	Experimental toxins
	Exogenous steroids
Psychologic	Depression
	Anxiety
	Personality disturbance
Social-Environmental	Excessive response to external food cues
	Poor role models (including lack of physical exercise)
	Establishment of inappropriate eating behavior
	Boredom
Genetic-Constitutional	Hereditary factors
Developmental	Early (including prenatal) nutritional factors
	Increased number of fat cells

mined by an individual's basal metabolic rate, which may vary greatly from one person to another.

The role of activity among obese children is unclear. Waxman and Stunkard (1980), in a detailed study of four obese boys, found them to be much less active than controls at home, slightly less active outside the home, and equally active at school. Energy expenditure of the obese boys equaled or exceeded that of normal controls, while caloric intake was much increased. Food intake, then, rather than activity level appeared to maintain obesity in these children.

Medical Causes. Juvenile hypothyroidism can be associated with obesity (see Case 16–1). An overall slowing of mental and neurologic functions is characteristically seen with the appearance and often the emotional content of depression.

Cushing syndrome is the result of hypercorticism, which can occur secondary to pituitary, adrenal, or iatrogenic causes. Characteristic features on physical examination are noted above, and investigation of the hypothalamic-pituitary-adrenal axis should clarify the level of the pathologic process. Slowing of the growth rate occurs both with hypothyroidism and Cushing syndrome in contrast to an accelerated growth rate typical of exogenous obesity.

When *excessive insulin dosage* is used in the treatment of diabetes mellitus, increased appetite and weight gain can occur. The role of insulin in normal eating behavior may be significant and remains to be clarified further.

Neurologic Causes. The *hypothalamus* has been implicated (though not in all instances proved to be involved) in a number of syndromes involving obesity. In the *Kleine-Levin syndrome,* episodes of hypersomnia and megaphagia last several days to weeks (see Chapter 9). The *Prader-Willi syndrome* is characterized by hypomentia (mental retardation), hypogonadism, hypotonia, and obesity. It has, accordingly, been called the "H_3O syndrome." The obesity in the Prader-Willi syndrome is not seen in infancy. In fact, feeding difficulties and poor weight gain typify the first year of life. Obesity, hypogonadism, retinitis pigmentosa, polydactyly, and mental retardation constitute the *Laurence-Moon-Biedl syndrome.* This disorder, inherited in an autosomal recessive manner, may be associated with diabetes insipidus.

Obesity occurring with hypogonadism and diabetes insipidus suggests hypothalamic involvement, especially when associated with rage and amenorrhea (Bray and Gallagher, 1975). Several pathologic processes may cause such *hypothalamic disorder.* These include tumor (craniopharyngioma being the most common), leukemia, inflammatory disease (primarily associated with sarcoidosis or tuberculosis), head trauma, and surgery (see Case 10–2).

Rau and Green (1978) have suggested that compulsive ("binge") eating behavior (whether or not associated with obesity) can occur on a neurologic basis. They cited as evidence a high incidence of *electroencephalographic irregularities* (particularly 14-and-6-cycle-per-second sharp waves, not accepted generally as abnormal) and beneficial response to phenytoin (Dilantin) therapy among their adult patients.

Toxic Causes. Toxic agents used in experimental animals have been

CASE 10–2: OBESITY AND HYPERSOMNIA ON A HYPOTHALAMIC BASIS IN A 17-YEAR-OLD ADOLESCENT WITH A BRAIN TUMOR

A.D. was diagnosed 4 years previously as having a glioma of the right optic nerve following evaluation for progressive loss of visual acuity. Initial treatment consisted of subtotal removal of the tumor and irradiation. Hypothyroidism, hypogonadism, and diabetes insipidus occurred secondary to presumed hypothalamic involvement. They were treated with thyroxine, testosterone, and DDAVP, respectively. He also received 15 mg daily of prednisone. Over the past year he had gained 60 pounds. Within the previous 6 weeks he had several episodes per day of falling asleep during meals or at other unexpected times. Sleep paralysis, cataplexy, and hypnagogic hallucinations were not associated. He had not complained of headaches. He was not unusually depressed, but mother noted he had been irritable for several weeks.

On examination, the young man was an obese adolescent (weighing 230 pounds) who fell asleep three times within a half hour. He did not appear depressed. His face was red-cheeked and moon-shaped. Obesity was generalized. Respiratory rate, depth, and pattern were unremarkable. Neurologic examination was notable for pale optic disks and diminished visual acuity in the right eye. Investigation included a CT scan that showed no change in ventricular size but a suggestion of increase in size of the right optic glioma. Treatment was begun with dextroamphetamine sulfate, and daytime sleep episodes diminished markedly within 48 hours.

Comment. This young man's obesity was probably on a hypothalamic basis, although he did show some evidence of medication-induced Cushing syndrome. Particularly striking was his hypersomnolence. His marked obesity was a possible cause of an obesity-hypoventilation (Pickwickian) syndrome. His recent mood change suggested that depression might be playing a role. The conjunction of the large weight gain within a year, the suggestion of increased tumor size on CT scan, and the striking response to dextroamphetamine suggested, however, that direct involvement of the hypothalamus (affecting centers for satiety and alertness) was most importantly responsible for his symptoms (see Chapter 9).

demonstrated to cause both hyperphagia and excessive weight gain. Stereotaxic injection of 5, 7-dihydroxytryptamine in rats specifically destroys central serotonergic fibers (Stricker, 1978); and gold thioglucose injection in mice causes lesions in the ventromedial hypothalamus (Mayer, 1966). No such agents have been recognized in man, although exogenous steroids (such as prednisone or androgenic agents) are typically associated with weight gain.

Marijuana, reputed to be an appetite stimulant in man, has not been recognized as a cause of obesity.

Psychologic Causes. Obesity may result from overeating used to ward off anxiety or depression. Bruch (1979) has termed this pattern "reactive obesity," noting its apparent link with emotionally traumatic events.

In some children obesity is part of a pervasive disturbance in personality and behavior presumably stemming from early and sustained psychosocial influences (see SOCIAL-ENVIRONMENTAL CAUSES below).

Social-Environmental Causes. Obese persons have been considered more responsive to external food cues than persons of normal weight (Schachter, 1971). External factors include the appearance, availability, and palatability of food. The most important internal factor is hunger. Recent observations of obese adults and those of normal weight, however, have demonstrated equal responsiveness to food cues upon experimental manipulation (Meyers *et al.,* 1980). Applicability of these data to children and adolescents remains to be demonstrated.

Social and environmental influences do, it appears, shape eating behavior in childhood in several ways. Mealtime is a scheduled event in most households; and cues to stop eating often come from the parents, not the child. Further, attention and affection may be dependent upon eating behavior such as "cleaning one's plate" or asking for second helpings. Parents may further influence children's eating behavior by providing a poor role model: overeating at meals, consuming carbohydrate- and fat-laden snacks, and pursuing a sedentary life style (see Case 10–3).

Obesity may arise from establishment of inappropriate eating behaviors, for example, the use of food as an antidote to a wide variety of stresses. If an infant's cries are consistently met with food regardless of the reason for crying, it is hypothesized that in later life the child may react to stress in a similar manner: by eating. Since eating does not fully satisfy all kinds of discomfort (many of them misinterpreted as hunger), repetition of eating behavior occurs again and again with equally unsatisfying results.

Boredom appears to contribute to obesity in some instances.

Genetic-Constitutional Causes. Although it is difficult to separate familial influences from social-environmental factors, hereditary factors do appear to play a role in obesity. Twin studies, for example, show a much greater similarity in weight between identical twins than between fraternal twins (Mayer, 1966). Overall, if one parent is obese, the chance of the child's becoming obese is 40 to 50 per cent. With two obese parents the liklihood increases to 70 to 80 per cent (Knittle, 1972).

Developmental Causes. The role of early (including prenatal) nutritional influences in causing later obesity remains unsettled. Studies of young men whose mothers were pregnant during the Dutch famine of 1944–45 have shown that nutritional deprivation during the latter half of pregnancy and first few months after delivery was associated with a reduction in later obesity in their offspring. Exposure to nutritional deprivation during the first half of the pregnancy, on the other hand, was linked with an increase in obesity in their children (Ravelli *et al.,* 1976). It has been inferred from these and other findings that nutritional deprivation at a critical period may have acted to minimize numbers of fat cells.

Knittle (1972) found an increase in the number of adipose cells in subcuta-

CASE 10–3: EXOGENOUS OBESITY IN A 13-YEAR-OLD BOY

S.E. was evaluated because of obesity and behavior problems. He was the 9 pound, 5 ounce product of a pregnancy complicated by maternal obesity, diabetes mellitus, hypertension, and hyperthyroidism. He was described as "large" at 1 year of age and was placed on low-fat milk at that time. Family stresses over the years included the parents' divorce and father's incarceration. Behavior disturbances included chronic interactional difficulties between mother and son. The child's behavior tended to be immature. For example, while watching televison he sometimes sucked his thumb and played with the edge of a blanket. School performance was unremarkable.

On examination, the boy was markedly obese, mildly anxious, and immature. He weighed 90 kg, which was much greater than the 98th percentile for age. Adipose tissue was distributed most prominently over the abdomen and hips. Moon face, striae, and a buffalo hump were absent. The penis was normal in size. Neurologic examination, including funduscopic inspection and visual field testing, was normal. Investigation included normal urinalysis, fasting blood sugar, and thyroxine level. Bone age and CT scan were normal. On psychologic evaluation, the boy was felt to be neurotically conflicted and to manifest marked emotional immaturity.

Family and individual counseling in conjunction with dietary therapy was recommended. These were not pursued, however, and the child remained markedly obese 1 year following initial evaluation.

Comment. Mother's obesity and the child's history of being overweight since infancy pointed strongly toward the diagnosis of exogenous obesity. He had no evidence on examination or investigation for thyroid underactivity, congenital or acquired. Nor did he have stigmata of Cushing syndrome. He also lacked features of the Laurence-Moon-Biedl syndrome (with polydactyly and retinitis pigmentosa) and of the Prader-Willi (H_3O) syndrome.

The outcome after 1 year is familiar and somewhat discouraging. It is hoped that continued educational efforts by pediatrician and nutritionist directed toward both the behavioral and the caloric aspects of eating will break through the long-ingrained patterns that have fostered obesity in this case.

neous tissue samples from obese children. Biopsies of obese adults have also shown an increase in the number of fat cells. The implication is that during a sensitive period of development in early childhood the number of fat cells is determined. They are never lost but may be modified in terms of their fat content (Charney *et al.*, 1976).

TREATMENT AND OUTCOME

The goal of treatment in the usual case of childhood obesity should be to restore weight to normal, that is, to within two standard deviations of the mean (see Table 10–7). This goal should be approached gradually over

TABLE 10–7. **Selected Aspects of Treatment of Obesity**

Medical	Dietary management
	Appetite suppressant drugs
	Withdrawal of steroids
Neurologic	Treatment of underlying inflammatory or neoplastic disease
	Phenytoin (Dilantin)
Surgical	Stapling of stomach
	Jaw-wiring
	Intestinal bypass
	Resection of brain tumor
Psychologic	Individual therapy
	Family therapy
	Group therapy
Social-Environmental	Behavior modification
Educational	Counseling as to nutrition and eating behavior
Physical	Regular exercise

weeks and months since weight has been acquired gradually in most instances. The overall treatment plan should include dietary education, correction of abnormal eating behavior, a regular program of physical activity, and supportive counseling.

Obese children are likely to become obese adults (Charney *et al.*, 1976). Knittle (1972) has placed the likelihood at 80 per cent. Although birth weight itself does not appear to have an influence on later obesity, Charney and colleagues (1976) found that excessive weight within the first 6 months of life did predict later obesity. Whether this finding can be linked with excessive numbers of fat cells has not been determined.

It is not sufficient that the child lose weight. Altered patterns of eating must be continued if weight loss is to be maintained—a difficult process. If the family and child understand the caloric contributions of different foods, appreciate the importance of eating behavior *per se,* engage regularly in exercise, and sustain a high degree of motivation, then obesity can be dealt with successfully on a long-term basis.

Medical Management. When corticosteroids have contributed to obesity, withdrawal of medication (as indicated) will generally result in return of appetite to normal and weight loss.

Amphetamines and other appetite-suppressants typically exert a transient anorectic effect and are usually not indicated in the treatment of childhood obesity. Careful dietary management with gradual weight reduction (1 to 2 pounds per week) as a goal is the key to optimal medical treatment of obesity.

Under circumstances of extreme obesity, hospitalization and use of a protein-sparing modified fast have been effective in children and adolescents (Merritt *et al.,* 1980).

Neurologic Management.   When a hypothalamic disorder has been identified, specific therapy will depend upon the etiologic process. Tuberculosis, for example, might be treated by medical means alone, neoplasm by surgery with or without radiotherapy, and posttraumatic injury by watchful waiting unless hormone replacement therapy is indicated.

Among adults (not necessarily obese) who eat compulsively, Rau and Green (1978) identified eleven features useful in predicting beneficial response to phenytoin (Dilantin). These are rage attacks, frequent headaches, dizziness, stomach aches, nausea, perceptual disturbances, paresthesias, seizures, compulsive behaviors other than eating, family history of epilepsy, and abnormal EEG.

Surgical Management.   Surgery will rarely play a role in the management of obesity in childhood. In adults, stapling of the stomach, jaw-wiring, and intestinal bypass surgery have been employed successfully in some cases, though drawbacks to these forms of therapy are considerable (Malt and Guggenheim, 1976; Rodgers *et al.,* 1977).

When a hypothalamic or pituitary mass causes a syndrome of obesity, operative removal (with or without ventriculo-peritoneal shunting to relieve associated hydrocephalus) may be undertaken. Some diencephalic tumors can be effectively treated by radiation therapy alone. On the other hand, surgical or tumor-related injury to the hypothalamus may itself cause obesity.

Psychotherapy.   Supportive psychotherapy is always of value for the obese child and his or her family. Obese children often suffer social isolation because of their physical appearance. They are called names and excluded further from activities that they can ill afford to pass up. Mutual support groups can be of assistance, particularly with overweight adolescents. As with anorexia nervosa, a family-based approach may be beneficial since social and environmental influences are usually important (Bruch, 1979).

Persons who are losing weight should be forewarned that weight loss will not solve all their problems. Some persons experience depression during weight loss as a result of hunger or perhaps in reaction to losing a part of themselves.

Social-Environmental Management.   Behavior modification in the treatment of obesity has been written about in detail in the medical and lay press (Stuart, 1967; Stunkard, 1972). Among the elements of this approach are monitoring of eating behavior through use of a food diary, eating in the same place, keeping low-calorie foods available, and not socializing to an exaggerated degree during meals.

Educational Management.   Teaching of parents and child constitutes an important part of overall management. It must be made clear that 3,500 calories ingested equals 1 pound of weight gained (largely fat) and an equal number of calories must be "burned off" for one pound to be lost. With these figures in mind and awareness of the child's normal daily caloric needs for maintenance, a realistic program of gradual weight loss can be developed.

Physical Therapy.   Regular physical activity is an important adjunct to dietary management and behavior modification. Jogging, for example, utilizes around 100 calories per mile. Not only does running use up calories, but it further influences eating behavior because it generally precludes eating immediately before, during, and just after a run.

Physical activity should be an integral part not only of the weight-loss phase of therapy but also of the maintenance phase as well.

SUMMARY

Obesity is, by definition, an excess of body fat. In children it is usually defined by reference to standard weight curves for age. History-taking should include detailed dietary information with attention to emotional and familial factors. Examination should include plotting of current and past growth measurements. Specific abnormalities such as polydactyly, hypogonadism, mental retardation, retinitis pigmentosa, visual field deficit, or stigmata of Cushing syndrome should be sought. Investigation may range from none to extensive neuroendocrinologic studies depending upon clinical circumstances. Obesity should be distinguished from eating disturbances such as megaphagia and polyphagia, which may not be associated with obesity, and from developmental chubbiness.

Possible etiologies include endocrinologic causes such as hypothyroidism, iatrogenic causes such as steroid therapy, and neurologic causes such as craniopharyngioma. Psychologic causes include depression and personality disturbance. Social-environmental and developmental causes are probably most important in childhood and adolescence. Increase in number of fat cells due to overnutrition early in life may contribute to later obesity. Faulty eating habits and poor role models clearly are important in many instances.

Treatment is directed toward reduction in caloric intake, development of more adaptive eating behaviors, and increase in energy expenditure through regular physical activity. Supportive psychotherapy is generally indicated. More formal individual or family involvement may also be beneficial. Once weight loss has been accomplished, the maintenance phase—challenging for family, child, and professional—must be pursued with equal vigor.

ENURESIS

Enuresis has been termed the most common chronic condition seen in general pediatric practice (Starfield, 1978). In all, 15 per cent of 5-year-old children are enuretic, and 7 per cent of 7-year-old boys wet one or more times per week (Shaffer, 1977). Enuresis is defined most generally as the involuntary passage of urine at any time of day. More commonly it is used to refer to urinary incontinence during sleep. Unless otherwise specified, enuresis will be used in this chapter (and elsewhere in this book) to indicate nighttime wetting.

This section will address several questions regarding enuresis:

What are the most pertinent aspects of the history and examination to be sought in the enuretic child?

What investigations should be carried out?
What is the role of drugs in the treatment of enuresis?
Do conditioning devices work?
What is the outcome of enuresis in childhood and adolescence?

DEFINITION

As indicated above, enuresis is used here to signify the involuntary passage of urine during sleep. Since bladder control is usually established by about 5 years of age, bedwetting after this age can be considered abnormal. Distinction can be made between primary and secondary enuresis. With the former, nighttime dryness has never been established. The latter is preceded by a period of complete bladder control.

DIAGNOSIS

Clinical Process. *History.* The child being evaluated for enuresis is usually aware of the difficulty and may be reluctant to express a chief complaint. He or she should nonetheless be encouraged to articulate the problem, for it will often indicate personal repercussions of the problem. "I can't go away to camp because I still wet my bed." "I'm too embarrassed to have my friends sleep over."

The problem should be further characterized by noting its onset and pattern. Has the child ever been dry at nighttime? How often does enuresis occur per week or per month? When does wetting occur—early in the night (before 1:00 A.M.) or later? What measures (such as fluid restriction or double-voiding) have been tried? Does wetting occur during the day as well? Are episodes associated with symptoms of urinary tract infection (e.g., burning, urgency, or frequency)? Does the child sense bladder fullness? Have siblings, parents, or other family members had enuresis? Until what age? Has the child had headaches or gait difficulty? Has incontinence of stool occurred as well? Does the child have a known seizure disorder? If not, has a bitten tongue, unexplained muscle soreness, or excessive sleepiness in the morning suggested nocturnal seizure? Does the child take chronic or intermittent medication such as theophylline? Has excessive drinking or eating accompanied the urinary incontinence?

Examination. The *general physical examination* should include recording of pulse and blood pressure. Height and weight should be measured and plotted. The skin should be examined for café-au-lait spots or hypopigmented macules. The spine should be examined carefully by inspection and palpation for bony defects such as bifid spine, hairy tuft, or lipomatous mass (see Fig. 10–3).

Neurologic examination should note particularly deep tendon reflexes (often exaggerated with increased intracranial pressure), gait (frequently abnormal in multiple sclerosis), and sensation of pinprick (which may be diminished in a perineal or perianal distribution with spinal cord lesions). Funduscopic examination should be done to exclude papilledema.

Mental status examination should include attention to overall level of intelligence, affect (anxiety or depression), behavior, and degree of concern about the problem.

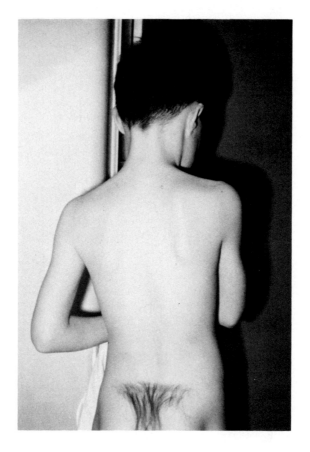

FIGURE 10–3. Hairy tuft at base of spine suggesting underlying spinal dysraphism.

Investigation. In most instances of childhood enuresis, little investigation is required (see Table 10–8). A standard urinalysis (including qualitative analysis for glucose, measurement of specific gravity, and microscopic examination of the urinary sediment) and culture of a clean-voided specimen of urine should be carried out. When indicated, an overnight fast to determine urinary concentrating ability can be performed.

When urinary tract dysfunction is suggested, radiologic investigation might include plain x-rays of the abdomen, intravenous pyelogram (IVP), voiding cystourethrogram (VCUG), abdominal CT scan, or cystoscopy. Renal function studies in blood should also be considered.

When spine or spinal cord disorder is suggested by the history or examination, plain spine x-rays, CT scan of the spine with metrizimide, pantopaque myelography, and spinal fluid examination should be considered. With signs of increased intracranial pressure, plain skull x-rays including views of the sella, cranial CT scan, and sometimes pneumoencephalography will be indicated. Visual evoked responses will often be useful in establishing the diagnosis of multiple sclerosis. When seizures are suspected, an electroencephalogram (EEG) should be carried out in the awake and sleep states. An all-night polygraphic recording will be valuable in some instances.

TABLE 10–8. **Investigations to Be Considered in the Enuretic Child**

Urinalysis
Urine culture
Renal function studies in blood (BUN, creatinine)
Testing of urinary concentrating ability
Other neuroendocrinologic studies
Plain x-rays of abdomen
Intravenous pyelogram (IVP), voiding cystourethrogram (VCUG)
Abdominal CT scan
Cystoscopy
Plain spine x-rays
CT scan of spine
Pantopaque myelography
EEG (in awake and sleep states)
All-night EEG
Visual evoked responses
CSF examination
Skull x-rays, sellar tomography
Cranial CT scan
Pneumoencephalography (PEG)

Differential Diagnosis. As mentioned earlier, enuresis is used here, unless otherwise specified, to indicate involuntary passage of urine at night. As such, it should be differentiated from daytime wetting, which more often suggests structural or other organic cause rather than developmental origin.

Etiology. Most enuresis in childhood and adolescence is developmental in nature, often with a familial contribution. It is manifested as persistence of a pattern of behavior that would be considered normal at an earlier age. Causes other than developmental should be considered as well since therapy will vary markedly depending upon the cause of the problem (see Table 10–9) (see Case 10–4).

Medical Causes. *Urinary tract infection* is the most important medical cause of enuresis. It is typically associated with incontinence of urine by day as well. Other symptoms include urgency, frequency, burning upon urination (dysuria), and hematuria. Back pain, abdominal pain, and fever may also occur.

Diabetes mellitus should also be considered. It is usually associated with increase in food and fluid intake (polyphagia and polydipsia, respectively). Abdominal pain and weight loss are frequently present at the onset of the disorder.

Genitourinary diseases of various kinds can also be associated with enuresis. Urinary concentrating ability may be defective with sickle cell disease (due to renal ischemia) or with nephrogenic diabetes insipidus (unresponsiveness to antidiuretic hormone). Structural disorder of the kidney, ureters, bladder, or urethra—particularly when associated with urinary reflux—may interfere with excretion of urine and lead to urinary tract infection.

TABLE 10–9. **Causes of Enuresis**

Medical	Urinary tract infection
	Diabetes mellitus
	Genitourinary tract disease (sickle cell disease; nephrogenic diabetes insipidus; structural abnormalities of kidney, ureter, bladder, urethra)
Neurologic	Spinal cord disease (cyst, neoplasm, spina bifida, diastematomyelia, multiple sclerosis)
	Hydrocephalus
	Nocturnal seizures
	Diabetes insipidus
	Degenerative neurologic disorder
	Disorder of arousal
Toxic	Methylxanthines: aminophylline, theophylline, caffeine
	Antipsychotic agents: thioridazine (Mellaril), haloperidol (Haldol)
Psychologic	Reactive behavioral regression
	Depression, anxiety
Social-Environmental	Substandard living conditions
Genetic-Constitutional	Familial pattern
Developmental	Central nervous system immaturity (males predominating)
	Failure to establish normal diurnal variation in urine output

Neurologic Causes. Disorders affecting the *spinal cord* must be considered in the child with enuresis. Gait disturbance, abnormal deep tendon reflexes, extensor plantar response(s), or sensory deficit should suggest spinal cord problem. Spinal disorders include cysts and tumors of the cord or meninges, spinal dysraphism (such as spina bifida or diastematomyelia), and demyelinating diseases, especially multiple sclerosis (see Figs. 10–4 and 10–5).

Hydrocephalus, which can result from many causes, may be associated with incontinence of urine by day or by night. Urinary dysfunction stems from the location of cortical neurons and associated fiber tracts concerned with bladder control. These neurons lie within the interhemispheric fissure, and their fibers course around the outer walls of the lateral ventricles on their way to the internal capsule. With hydrocephalus, these fibers are compressed by the expanding ventricles, and urinary incontinence (with gait disturbance) may result. Among possible causes of hydrocephalus are brain tumor (particularly when located in the posterior fossa) and congenital aqueductal stenosis, which may be delayed in onset of symptoms until late childhood, adolescence, or even adulthood.

CASE 10–4: ENURESIS IN A 15-YEAR-OLD BOY

C.O. was evaluated because of continued enuresis. He was fully toilet-trained by age 3 years. At 9 years, school stresses were associated with a return of nighttime wetting several times per week without other symptoms of behavioral regression. Attempted treatment by limiting fluid intake after supper, bringing him to the toilet at night, and using a buzzer-and-pad device were unsuccessful.

Past history was unremarkable. No one in the family had experienced nocturnal enuresis beyond 4 years of age. Review of systems was negative for seizure, headaches, or coordination problems.

On examination, the child was a pleasant, normally intelligent adolescent who readily expressed concerns about his wetting problem. The general physical and neurologic examinations were normal. Several urine specimens collected for culture and analysis were normal. A trial of imipramine (Tofranil) (25 mg at bedtime) stopped bedwetting within a week of use.

Comment. Although imipramine is not generally the initial treatment of choice for nocturnal enuresis, it was used here for two reasons. First, non-pharmacologic measures that are often (if not usually) effective in treating bedwetting had not helped. Second, this adolescent's self-esteem was being significantly impaired by continuation of the problem.

The side effects and toxic effects of imipramine must always be considered prior to use of this drug. It should be dispensed in childproof containers or individually wrapped sheets. It should be kept away from other children in the family. For a younger sibling (for whom wetting is age-appropriate) might ingest the medication in an attempt to emulate an older sibling and stop wetting (see Case 10–6).

Nocturnal seizures may be evidenced by little or nothing else than nighttime wetting. If the child has a known seizure disorder, then unexplained wetting should suggest nighttime seizures, particularly if associated with bitten tongue, unexplained muscle soreness ("charley horse"), or excessive morning lethargy or confusion (see Chapter 12).

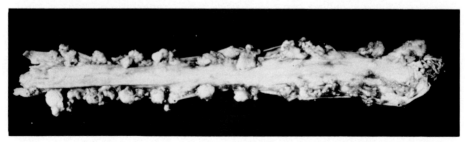

FIGURE 10–4. Specimen of spinal cord in neurofibromatosis showing multiple tumors on spinal nerve roots.

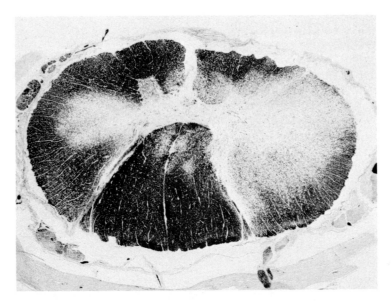

FIGURE 10–5. Myelin stain (black) of spinal cord in multiple sclerosis showing widespread demyelination.

Diabetes insipidus on a central basis is often associated with enuresis. It may be accompanied by hypothalamic signs and symptoms such as hypersomnia, rage episodes, bulimia, and amenorrhea. Optic atrophy, deafness, and diabetes mellitus also may be associated (Lessell and Rosman, 1977). Tests of urinary concentrating ability will determine the presence and degree of diabetes insipidus. Neuroradiologic investigations such as plain skull x-ray, tomography of the sella, cranial CT scan, and pneumoencephalogram, in conjunction with neuroendocrine studies, can further define the problem (see Case 10–5).

Degenerative neurologic disorders are frequently associated with loss of developmental milestones, including loss of bladder or bowel control (see Chapter 8).

Enuresis, like night terrors and sleepwalking, has been considered by some to be a *disorder of arousal* from slow wave sleep (stage 3 or 4 of non-REM sleep) (Broughton, 1968). This association, however, has not been consistently demonstrated (Shaffer, 1977; Kales *et al.*, 1977). For example, Mikkelsen and colleagues (1980), in a recent controlled study of forty severely enuretic boys, found that no particular sleep stage was associated with enuretic episodes.

Toxic Causes. Medications may cause or contribute to nighttime wetting. These include aminophylline and theophylline, methylxanthines used in the treatment of asthma, and the antipsychotic drugs thioridazine and haloperidol (Winsberg and Yepes, 1978). Caffeine, another methylxanthine (contained in cola drinks, coffee, and some teas), also can promote urine flow and cause enuresis.

Psychologic Causes. Bedwetting in a previously dry child commonly

CASE 10–5: ENURESIS SECONDARY TO DIABETES INSIPIDUS IN A 6-YEAR-OLD GIRL

J.E. wet her bed up to four times per night for several weeks prior to evaluation. She also experienced polydipsia, vomiting, anorexia, irritability, and a 10-pound weight loss over a 1-month period. Past history and family history were unremarkable. She had been fully toilet-trained for more than 3 years when nocturnal enuresis began to occur. She had been tried recently on imipramine (Tofranil), which did not diminish the enuresis.

On examination she was an alert, cooperative, well-hydrated, healthy-appearing youngster of normal intelligence. Growth parameters and vital signs were normal. Funduscopic visualization disclosed well-formed optic disks without evidence of papilledema, atrophy, or hypoplasia. Visual fields, acuity, deep tendon reflexes, and plantar responses all were normal.

Investigation included normal serum electrolytes, blood urea nitrogen, and creatinine. The specific gravity of a random sample of urine was 1.001. Urine output for 24 hours was 3 liters, which was markedly increased. Skull x-rays and hand films for bone age were normal. CT scan and pneumoencephalogram were normal. A 4-hour water deprivation test led to a 1.1 kg weight loss without appropriate urinary concentration. The child responded dramatically to intramuscular vasopressin and has been maintained on DDAVP (a synthetic analogue of vasopressin) administered intranasally. The cause for the diabetes insipidus remains obscure.

Comment. "Diabetes" refers to two conditions characterized by increased urination: diabetes mellitus and diabetes insipidus. Used alone, diabetes generally applies to diabetes mellitus, in which the urine is honeyed, or sweet. With diabetes mellitus, polyphagia is often a prominent symptom. With diabetes insipidus, however, the urine is tasteless or—as determined by more modern analytic instruments than the tongue—lacking in sugar. Excessive drinking (rather than excessive urination) may dominate the clinical picture of diabetes insipidus. This child's symptoms of vomiting, anorexia, and irritability suggested that she had become dehydrated.

The central form of diabetes insipidus, as seen in this child, is characterized by lack of antidiuretic hormone. The use of DDAVP intranasally has been a major advance in therapy since it obviates the need to use vasopressin (antidiuretic hormone) by injection. Renal resistance to antidiuretic hormone at the level of the collecting tubules causes nephrogenic diabetes insipidus, which does not respond to hormone replacement therapy.

Assessment of the child with diabetes insipidus will necessarily include attention to pituitary and hypothalamic functions. The optic disks must be visualized carefully to exclude papilledema and optic atrophy. It is also important to assess visual fields, because hypothalamic or pituitary tumors (such as craniopharyngioma) that can cause diabetes insipidus characteristically produce a bitemporal field defect due to pressure on the optic chiasm.

occurs on a reactive basis that, because of its self-limited nature, need not be considered pathologic. The majority of enuretic children appear to be psychologically normal (Werry and Cohrssen, 1965). Incontinence of urine may also represent a form of negativistic behavior or a means of asserting independence in a younger child.

Anxiety and depression have been linked with enuresis, but the nature of the association is unclear (Weinberg *et al.*, 1973; Shaffer, 1977).

Social-Environmental Causes. Social and environmental factors may concretely influence enuresis. The bathroom may be cold, poorly lighted, and located at a distance, for example.

Genetic-Constitutional Causes. The importance of genetic influences is suggested by the fact that 70 per cent of enuretic children will have an enuretic mother or father (Bakwin, 1961). Further, a high concordance for enuresis has been noted among identical twins (Shaffer, 1977). In some families cessation of wetting occurs about the same age from one generation to another.

Developmental Causes. As is true among other developmental syndromes such as hyperactivity, enuresis is more commonly encountered among males than females, though the difference is not great (Werry and Cohrssen, 1965; Forsythe and Redmond, 1974). This difference is presumed to reflect differences in central nervous system maturation.

Enuresis may be associated with diminished functional bladder capacity (the volume of urine a child can retain prior to the urgent need to void), in essence, a "small bladder" (Starfield, 1967; Troup and Hodgson, 1971).

Failure to establish normal diurnal variation in urinary output has been hypothesized as playing a role in some cases of nighttime wetting (Lewis *et al.*, 1970; Birkásová *et al.*, 1978). Normally urine output during the night is diminished. In some enuretic children, however, urine output does not fluctuate, or the day-night pattern is reversed. The basis for this diurnal variation and the significance of alterations in it are unknown. Circadian rhythms in output of antidiuretic hormone may play a role.

TREATMENT AND OUTCOME

The treatment of enuresis ranges from support, reassurance, and waiting for the bedwetting to remit spontaneously to behavioral, pharmacologic, and sometimes surgical measures (see Table 10–10). All therapies must be measured against the rate of spontaneous "cure," that is, resolution of the problem. Between 5 and 9 years, the spontaneous cure rate is 14 per cent per year, between 10 and 19 years 16 per cent per year (Forsythe and Redmond, 1974). In order to be judged efficacious, therefore, a therapy must demonstrate a success rate superior to these already impressive rates of spontaneous resolution. In addition, the benefits of therapy (e.g., drugs or surgery) must be weighed against the risks.

A difficulty in interpreting studies reporting the treatment of enuresis is that they select for the more difficult cases. Children refractory to commonly employed home management techniques such as fluid restriction after dinner, double-voiding at bedtime, and awakening the child to void are likeliest to be referred for further evaluation. Recommendations as to treatment for

TABLE 10–10. **Selected Aspects of Treatment of Enuresis**

Medical	Treatment of urinary tract infection
	Symptomatic pharmacotherapy: imipramine (Tofranil), desmopressin (DDAVP)
Neurologic	Anticonvulsant medication
Surgical	Urologic procedures for obstruction at various levels
	Neurosurgery for hydrocephalus, spinal cord cyst, diastematomyelia
Psychologic	Supportive therapy
	Therapy of depression, anxiety
Social-Environmental	Fluid restriction after supper
	Double voiding
	Nighttime awakening to void
Mechanical	Bell-and-pad conditioning

this more difficult group thus may not (indeed, *should* not) have wide applicability to enuretic children as a group.

As an overall principle the approach of Marshall and colleagues (1973) seems most reasonable and effective in the long run. They have suggested that the child take an active role in treatment of his or her enuresis rather than participating passively as with therapy involving conditioning devices, medication, or surgery alone.

Medical Management.   When urinary tract infection has been diagnosed, standard antimicrobial agents such as sulfasoxasole (Gantrisin) or ampicillin are given for 14 days. Repeat urine culture for bacterial growth is customarily obtained 2 to 3 days after antibiotic therapy is begun and 1 to 2 weeks after the course of therapy has been completed.

Imipramine (Tofranil) is the standard medication used for enuresis when drug treatment is considered advisable. Clear indications for its usage have not been defined. Most would agree, however, that an appropriate candidate is the older school-age child who feels unable to sleep at a friend's home or attend camp because of anticipated embarrassment associated with bedwetting. Before such medication is used, predisposing disorders, both renal and nonrenal, must be sought and treated as specifically as possible.

The usual therapeutic dosage range for imipramine is from 0.5 to 2.5 mg per kilogram (Rapoport and Mikkelsen, 1978). The dose may be given in mid- to late afternoon (3:00 to 4:00 P.M.) if wetting tends to occur in the early evening (before 1:00 A.M.), otherwise at around 8:00 P.M. (Alderton, 1970). A usual starting dose is from 10 to 25 mg. Dosage can be increased as needed every 2 days unless side effects such as blurred vision, dry mouth, constipation, or daytime urinary retention occur, or until a maximum of 5 mg/kg/dose is achieved (Rapoport and Mikkelsen, 1978). The dosage is maintained once a level of efficacy (say, being dry for 7 of 10 nights) has been demonstrated.

The effectiveness of imipramine may be transient, lasting 2 to 6 weeks (Rapoport *et al.*, 1980). In these circumstances it can be used intermittently, for example, during camp or on outings.

The child should periodically be free from medication several times per year to see whether it is still needed. Tapering of medication over a several-week period has been recommended, particularly for children who are taking larger doses.

The effectiveness of imipramine and other tricyclic compounds in the treatment of enuresis may be related to their peripheral anticholinergic effects on the bladder. A decrease in bedwetting is usually seen within a few days after treatment is begun, in contrast to the usual delay in clinical response of several weeks when tricyclics are employed for their antidepressant effects. Influences of imipramine upon the sleep cycle have been suggested, but these have not proved to be of significance in reducing enuresis (Rapoport *et al.,* 1980).

When imipramine is prescribed, the highly toxic nature of this drug when taken in overdosage (accidental or intentional) must be remembered. Child-proof containers or individually wrapped pills are advisable. Syrup of ipecac should be prescribed concomitantly with imipramine with instructions for its use in emergency circumstances (see Case 10–6).

Desmopressin (desamino-D-arginine vasopressin, or DDAVP) has shown promising results in the treatment of persistent nocturnal enuresis. Desmopressin, a synthetic analogue of antidiuretic hormone (ADH), is administered intranasally. In a study of twenty-two enuretic children between 4 and 12 years of age, Birkásová and colleagues (1978) found that desmopressin, taken as nosedrops in the evening, reduced bedwetting from eleven to four nights per fortnight. These results were considered to support the hypothesis that failure to establish normal diurnal variation of urine volume underlies some cases of childhood enuresis.

Neurologic Management. Seizures should be treated with standard anticonvulsant medications depending upon the seizure type and frequency (see Chapter 12).

Surgical Management. Urologic surgery has a small role to play in managing enuresis. Urethral valves, meatal stenosis, and bladder neck abnormalities all have been cited as causing significant obstruction, but the efficacy of surgical intervention (urethral dilatation or bladder neck repair, for example) has not been clearly demonstrated (Shaffer, 1977).

With neurologic problems such as hydrocephalus, spinal cord cyst, or diastematomyelia, neurosurgery is indicated.

Psychotherapy. Support is always indicated in the management of the enuretic child and his or her family. All of them may find the problem frustrating, and their patience may wear thin as they wait for the problem to resolve spontaneously.

When anxiety or depression appear to contribute to enuresis, more formal psychiatric or psychologic involvement is indicated (Weinberg *et al.,* 1973).

Social-Environmental Management. Simple measures may provide considerable relief to the child and family. Fluid restriction after supper, double-voiding (that is, having the child try to empty the bladder twice within 10 to

CASE 10–6: IMIPRAMINE INGESTION IN A 4-YEAR-OLD GIRL

E.A. was found stuporous by her mother, having ingested up to 30 imipramine (Tofranil) tablets containing 25 mg apiece. On examination in the emergency room, she was alternately obtunded and agitated. Pulse rate was 108 per minute. Cardiac rhythm was normal. Blood pressure was 125/80. Pupils were dilated and reactive to light. Deep tendon reflexes were exaggerated. Plantar responses were extensor. She was given activated charcoal by nasogastric tube to adsorb any imipramine remaining in the stomach and was brought to the intensive care unit. Cardiac status remained normal and neurologic status improved within 48 hours so she could be transferred to a general pediatrics ward by the third hospital day.

Past history was notable for hospitalization 8 months previously for propoxyphene (Darvon) ingestion. Family history was noteworthy for recent marital separation. Two older sisters were being treated with imipramine for enuresis. Discussions with the child revealed that she felt she would not wet her bed any more if she took "a whole bunch of pills."

Comment. This case illustrates a major danger of imipramine therapy, ingestion by someone other than the person for whom the medicine had been intended. In this instance the child had sought to stop her own enuresis and was fortunate that the solution was not permanent. She was apparently spared the potentially lethal cardiac arrhythmic effects of imipramine in overdosage, though she did manifest neurologic signs of central nervous system depression and adrenergic effect (pupillary dilation and hyperreflexia).

The repetition of drug ingestion is an all too common occurrence in pediatrics and merits detailed psychosocial evaluation. Assessment here clarified the roles of marital disruption and sibling rivalry in producing chronic stress that appeared to contribute to two episodes of ingestion. Following the second episode, all medicines and cleaning agents were locked up. No further ingestions occurred for at least the next 8 years.

Imipramine is, of course, not the only medication that a sibling might ingest. Anticonvulsant drugs, "cold medicines," and diet pills are among the toxic agents that may become available to children in cabinets or unattended purses. Particularly with adolescents, multiple drugs may be taken in a suicidal action.

Although not available at the time of this child's acute hospitalization, measurement of the imipramine level in blood might have been useful in her management, although there was no question that she had ingested a significant amount of the drug.

15 minutes prior to going to bed), and bringing the child to the bathroom during the night can be valuable, sheet-saving measures.

Marshall and colleagues (1973) have found active involvement of the child in his own therapy to be more effective than a passive role, such as when therapy involves medication, a conditioning device, or surgery used by itself. For example, the child monitors his or her own progress by marking on a calendar dry versus wet days and applies a star to the calendar on dry days. Reward also can be provided for withholding urination for increasingly long periods at nighttime before an alarm goes off.

When unpleasant environmental circumstances render going to the bathroom at night difficult, a bedside urinal may solve the wetting problem.

Educational Management. In order to understand and choose among the various therapies for enuresis, the family (and child, too, in some circumstances) should first learn about the likelihood of spontaneous cure. Side effects of medication such as imipramine should be discussed and precautions taken as mentioned above. Common side effects with imipramine are dizziness, headache, constipation, and dry mouth. Symptoms of overdosage include cardiac irregularities, ataxia, urinary retention, seizures, and hallucinations. Particularly when radiologic investigation and surgical treatment are being considered, a review of essential aspects of anatomy and physiology should be undertaken with the child and parents.

Mechanical Therapy. Conditioning devices can be effective in improving childhood enuresis, sometimes eradicating it (Meadow, 1974). Relapses, however, do occur in some children (Marshall *et al.*, 1973). The conventional bell-and-pad device involves a special sheet containing an electrical apparatus in which a circuit is completed by a few drops of urine. As a result, a bell or a buzzer is set off. The child is awakened and can then voluntarily empty the bladder. It appears that under this regimen children eventually become aware of bladder distension prior to passing the first drops of urine and can awaken to void.

SUMMARY

Enuresis is defined as the involuntary passage of urine during sleep. It is usually a relatively benign, self-limited condition occurring in otherwise normal children. In approaching the child with enuresis, causes of both daytime and nighttime urinary incontinence should be considered. These include urinary tract infection, diabetes mellitus, drug effect (as with aminophylline), hydrocephalus, spinal cord disorder (such as multiple sclerosis or tumor), and diabetes insipidus. Investigation should consist minimally of urinalysis (including testing for glucose, measurement of specific gravity, and microscopic inspection of urinary sediment) and bacterial culture of urine. Additional investigation may be warranted on the basis of the history and examination.

The outcome is generally favorable. A high rate of spontaneous resolution of the problem occurs. Supportive psychotherapy is always indicated; and social-environmental treatment in the form of fluid restriction after supper, double-voiding at bedtime, and nighttime awakening to urinate are also generally useful. Additional measures such as the use of conditioning devices or medication (usually the tricyclic agent imipramine) may be effective, though relapses do occur. When a specific underlying problem has been identified such as urinary tract infection, diabetes mellitus, posterior urethral valves, or diastematomyelia, these should be treated medically or surgically as indicated.

ENCOPRESIS

Encopresis is a problem that is not uncommon among school-age children. It characteristically occurs in a normally intelligent child, usually chronically constipated, who is generally able to function otherwise relatively well. The following questions concerning encopresis will be addressed in this section:

What is the definition of encopresis?
What causes it?
What conditions should be differentiated from encopresis?
What investigations are indicated in evaluating the child with encopresis?
How should it be treated?
Is psychotherapy worthwhile?
What is the outcome of encopresis in childhood?

DEFINITION

The term *encopresis* is used synonymously with incontinence of feces, or fecal soiling. Distinction is generally made between the child who has never been bowel-trained (who is said to have primary encopresis) and one who soils despite previously having been bowel-trained (who is said to have secondary encopresis). The encopresis most commonly encountered is secondary fecal soiling that occurs in an obstipated (severely constipated) child 5 years of age or older. Chronic constipation is often associated with abdominal distension due to a markedly dilated large bowel, or megacolon.

DIAGNOSIS

Clinical Process.   *History.*   The chief complaint should consist of the child's own words, although many children will be reluctant to speak about their fecal soiling. The onset of the problem should be noted, and particularly whether incontinence of feces has always been present or if it has occurred following a period of normal bowel control. Details of bowel training should be recorded. When was it begun? How was it accomplished? Was it difficult? What evaluation of the fecal soiling has been carried out? What treatment? How effective has it been?

It is important to keep in mind when obtaining a history of bowel training the difference between reflex compliance and voluntary compliance (Brazelton, 1962). The former is a manifestation of the gastrocolic reflex. It occurs within a few minutes of a meal and can be seen in an infant or toddler. Voluntary compliance implies true bowel control and is generally possible only later, beginning between ages 2 and 3 years.

It should be determined if the child feels abdominal fullness or the urge to defecate. Are stools formed or loose? Does soiling occur continuously, or is it episodic? Does the child clean, hide, or ignore soiled undergarments? How has the school handled the problem? How have friends reacted?

Associated problems such as enuresis, gait disturbance, seizures, or symptoms of behavioral regression should be sought. Recent psychosocial stresses such as deaths in the family, moves, or the birth of a sibling should be noted.

Examination. The *general description* should note the odor of feces if present and the degree of the child's concern as to the soiling problem.

The *general physical examination* should include careful abdominal and rectal examination. Examination of the abdomen comprises inspection (Is the abdomen distended? What is its girth?), auscultation (Are bowel sounds normal?), percussion (Is the abdomen tympanitic?), and palpation (Are masses felt? Are they soft, firm, or rocky? In which quadrant are they located?). The back should be examined for spinal defect, hairy tuft, or lipomatous mass.

Rectal examination should be carried out after a brief explanation of its purpose, duration, and anticipated degree of discomfort (which can be likened to feeling the urge to defecate). The anus should be inspected for fissures. Upon digital examination, tenderness should be noted and sphincter tone (patulous, spastic, or normal) described. The presence and character of stool in the rectal ampulla should be recorded. Bimanual examination, involving one hand gently pressing upon the abdomen, will allow for further characterization of an abdominal mass. The color and consistency of any stool obtained should be noted and the fecal material tested for occult blood.

At the time of rectal examination, several parts of the neurologic examination—anal wink, perianal and perineal sensation—should be assessed as well.

Neurologic examination should specifically note gait, strength of the lower extremities, deep tendon reflexes, and plantar responses. The *mental status examination* should note the child's affect (anxious, depressed, or unconcerned) and overall level of intelligence.

Investigation. Little investigation need routinely be carried out in the initial assessment of most children with encopresis (see Table 10–11). If a mass is not clearly due to fecal material, a plain radiograph of the abdomen should be obtained. When gait disturbance or other neurologic abnormality affecting the lower extremities suggesting spinal cord dysfunction is associated, x-ray of the lumbosacral spine should be carried out. When enco-

TABLE 10–11. **Investigations to Be Considered in the Encopretic Child**

Urinalysis, including specific gravity
Serum electrolytes
Thyroid function tests
Blood lead level, free erythrocyte protoporphyrin (FEP)
Plain abdominal x-rays
Lumbosacral spine x-rays
Barium enema
Sigmoidoscopy
Intestinal motility studies
Rectal pressure measurements
Gastrointestinal mucosal biopsy
EEG (in awake and sleep states)
Tests for associated enuresis, if present

presis is associated with enuresis, appropriate investigation of urinary incontinence should be pursued (see section on ENURESIS in this chapter). In the child with secondary encopresis, serum electrolytes, thyroxine, lead level, and urinalysis (including specific gravity) should be obtained. If the pattern of fecal incontinence suggests a seizure disorder, electroencephalography should be carried out.

When encopresis has not responded to an initial regimen of enemas, mineral oil, and bowel training, further evaluation of the gastrointestinal tract may be warranted. Additional investigation might include sigmoidoscopy, barium enema, intestinal motility studies, rectal pressure measurements, and mucosal biopsy.

Differential Diagnosis.   As isolated "accident" due to excitement, worry, or unavailability of a bathroom does not constitute encopresis, nor does fecal staining of underpants due to diarrhea or excessive mineral oil ingestion.

Etiology.   Encopresis, usually secondary, most commonly results from leakage of feces around an obstipated fecal mass. The mass results from chronic constipation that generally stems from a combination of medical and psychologic causes (see Table 10–12).

Medical Causes.   Among the medical causes of *constipation* in childhood are improper diet (low in bulk, high in refined sugar), hypothyroidism, lead poisoning, dehydration, and anal fissure. Anal fissure may itself result from attempts to pass rocky stools. Withholding of bowel movements avoids pain but leads to additional obstipation as more water is removed from the fecal mass.

Constipation with fecal soiling may occur secondary to *Hirschsprung disease* (aganglionic megacolon), although encopresis is rarely associated (Gar-

TABLE 10–12. **Causes of Encopresis**

Medical	Constipation due to
	    improper diet (low in bulk, high in refined sugar)
	    hypothyroidism
	    dehydration
	    plumbism
	    anal fissure
	    Hirschsprung disease

Neurologic	Mental subnormalcy Spinal cord disorder (spina bifida, tumor) Seizure disorder Degenerative disorder of central nervous system
Psychologic	Reactive behavioral regression Failure of instruction
Social-Environmental	Abuse or neglect Attention seeking

rard and Richmond, 1952). The diagnosis of Hirschsprung disease is suggested by a history of constipation since earliest childhood, even infancy. The lack of ''call to stool'' (urge to defecate) and absence of feces in the rectal ampulla further suggest aganglionic megacolon (Davidson *et al.,* 1963). Diagnosis is established definitively by barium x-ray, intestinal motility studies, and biopsy.

Neurologic Causes. Disorders affecting the *spinal cord* such as spina bifida or tumor may be associated with fecal incontinence. These disorders can be differentiated from functional encopresis by associated signs and symptoms such as gait disturbance, hyperreflexia of the legs, diminished or absent perianal sensation, or defect of the bony spine (see Case 10–7).

Mental retardation is frequently associated with delay in bowel training. Constipation and encopresis may also occur.

A generalized *seizure* may involve fecal incontinence. The temporal pattern of incontinence and associated symptomatology should, however, readily differentiate the problem from other causes of encopresis.

Degenerative disorder of the nervous system may be manifested by loss of bowel control as part of a syndrome of behavioral regression (see Chapter 8).

Psychologic Causes. Fecal incontinence or other loss of milestones can occur in a transient, self-limited manner in reaction to the birth of a sibling or other stressful event. The reappearance of wetting and other forms of regressive behavior may also be seen in imitation of the younger child.

Failure of instruction in bowel training can lead to primary encopresis, that is, in which the child has never gained control of defecation. The diagnosis of primary encopresis implies that the child is otherwise normal, specifically, without spina bifida, mental retardation, or other organic problems (see Case 10–8).

Secondary encopresis has been attributed in some instances to early and coercive bowel training (Garrard and Richmond, 1952; Hersov, 1977). A ''battle of the bowel'' is waged, which the child deals with by chronically withholding bowel movements. The result is constipation and leakage.

Social-Environmental Causes. An abused or neglected child may be soiled with feces if not given the opportunity to use a bathroom.

Fecal soiling, like other psychosomatic symptoms, may persist because of its function within the family context. For example, Sluckin (1975) described a boy whose encopresis made it necessary for his father to pay attention to him, which otherwise occurred only rarely.

Genetic-Constitutional Causes. Encopretic boys outnumber girls by nearly a four-to-one ratio. A familial incidence of encopresis has not been observed.

Developmental Causes. Bowel training is usually accomplished by 2 to 3 years of age. Failure of bowel training by 4 years is uncommon, and by 5 years abnormal. Thus, referral of an encopretic child for evaluation and treatment is often made upon entry into school, either kindergarten or first grade, when social pressures increase significantly.

Developmental issues of independence play a role in the bowel training of all children. As discussed above (PSYCHOLOGIC CAUSES), parent-child con-

CASE 10–7: INCONTINENCE OF URINE AND FECES IN A 14-YEAR-OLD GIRL

L.B. was evaluated because of bowel and bladder incontinence. She weighed 6 pounds, 4 ounces at birth following an uncomplicated pregnancy and delivery. Toilet training was achieved by 2 years by day and by 3 years by night although urinary incontinence during the day or at night occurred intermittently thereafter. At 6 years of age, urologic evaluation was carried out. It included urinalysis, urine culture, cystogram, cystourethrogram, intravenous pyelogram, and voiding cystourethrogram. All were normal.

At 12 years, nocturnal enuresis ceased, an apparent result of voluntary fluid restriction combined with high motivation to stop wetting. Incontinence of urine by day continued, however, She indicated that she did not always sense the urge to void, or she could not get to the bathroom quickly enough. She had a long-standing history of constipation and fecal soiling.

On examination, the child was an intelligent and healthy-appearing girl. Mild kyphoscoliosis was evident on inspection. Palpation of the spine disclosed no abnormalities, tenderness, or midline defects. Examination of the skin showed no neurocutaneous markings. The abdomen was not distended. No masses were palpable. Rectal examination showed no fissures. Sphincter tone was diminished. Feces were not palpable in the rectal ampulla. On neurologic examination, perianal sensation was normal. Deep tendon reflexes were normal in the upper extremities, exaggerated in the lower extremities (left greater than right). Plantar responses were normal.

Because of urinary and fecal incontinence combined with asymmetric hyperreflexia in the legs, a spinal cord lesion was suspected. Accordingly, a myelogram was carried out. It was normal.

Comment. The combination in this child of bowel and bladder symptoms, scoliosis, and hyperreflexia in the lower extremities led to the suspicion of a disease affecting the spinal cord. Intrinsic lesions would include glioma or vascular malformation. Extrinsic lesions would include neurofibroma, meningioma, arachnoid cyst, or intraspinal hemorrhage. Myelogram was essential in ruling out either kind of spinal lesion. The CT scan is becoming increasingly useful in assessing spinal problems, especially when plain films are abnormal or a level of deficit is determined on examination.

This group of findings could also be due to a cerebral rather than a spinal disorder. For example, with hydrocephalus cortical fibers subserving the legs, bladder, and bowel can be compromised as they travel around dilated lateral ventricles.

Were this teenager's problems to have pursued an intermittent course (particularly if associated with visual or other sensory disturbances), active consideration would have been given to the presence of multiple sclerosis.

flict over control of the child's sphincters may lead to a situation in which neither party wins.

CASE 10–8: ENCOPRESIS AND HYPERACTIVITY IN A 9-YEAR-OLD BOY

I.C. was referred for neurologic evaluation because of encopresis. Bladder training had been attained in part by 3 years of age, although daytime wetting occurred most days and nocturnal enuresis some three times weekly. Complete bowel training had never been accomplished. Training had been begun at 2½ years of age but was interrupted by the birth of a younger sibling. Incontinence of semiformed stool occurred almost daily. Between 5 and 7 years of age, he was provided a regimen of mineral oil and enemas that was effective for several months. The current approach was for him to sit on the toilet for 10 minutes after meals, before bedtime, and before school. He was unable to say whether he experienced bowel fullness or not.

History of pregnancy and birth was unremarkable. From early childhood, he had been considered hyperactive, impulsive, and distractible. Motor activity had declined somewhat since then, but distractibility and impulsivity had persisted. Family history was negative for spina bifida, enuresis, or hyperactivity.

On examination, the child was a pleasant, immature youngster who was self-conscious and embarrassed by his problem. His behavior was rigid and withholding at first, but soon he relaxed and became appropriately interactive. On general examination his abdomen was not distended and no fecal or other masses were palpable. Perianal sensation and sphincter tone were normal. Firm (not hard or rocky) stool filled the rectal ampulla. The back had no hairy tufts, lipomatous masses, or palpable spinal defects. Neurologic examination was normal.

Comment. Most encopretic children have secondary encopresis. They have been bowel-trained and soil around obstipated feces. This child's fecal soiling, on the other hand, can be considered primary since he never was fully bowel-trained. One gets the impression that bowel-training, interrupted by the birth of a sibling, never got back on track.

The current approach to treatment involved scheduled toileting after meals to take advantage of the gastrocolic reflex. This measure was intended to give the child an opportunity to experience gastrointestinal sensations of the urge to defecate in association with the behavior of sitting on the toilet. Such scheduled toileting thereby provides the child with some successes in a difficult and chronically failure-ridden area. Ongoing psychotherapy was recommended; and in view of the child's history of attention deficit disorder, a trial of dextroamphetamine (Dexedrine) or methylphenidate (Ritalin) was also suggested.

TREATMENT AND OUTCOME

The child with secondary encopresis will usually outgrow the problem by 16 years of age (Hersov, 1977). Few children, parents, or professionals are, however, willing to wait that long for resolution of the problem.

TABLE 10–13. **Overview of Medical Management of Encopresis**

First phase	Mineral oil by mouth Phosphate enemas (if needed)
Second phase	Bowel training (based upon gastrocolic reflex) Use of proper toilet Mineral oil, stool softeners, suppositories (if needed)
Third phase	Regular follow-up examination Telephone contact in between visits

An effective approach to managing encopresis first involves ridding the child of obstipated feces in as noninvasive a manner as possible and allowing for normalization of bowel movements through pharmacologic measures and educational-behavioral means (see Tables 10–13 and 10–14) (Halpern, 1977). A highly favorable outcome (some 90 per cent or greater cured or substantially improved) has been reported in the series of Davidson and colleagues (1963) and Levine and Bakow (1976).

Concerns as to symptom substitution (replacement of encopresis by aggressive behavior, for example) have not been supported by the recent studies of Levine and colleagues (1980).

Medical Management. If an underlying or contributing cause for constipation such as lead poisoning, hypothyroidism, or dehydration is identified, specific treatment should be undertaken.

The treatment of secondary encopresis will depend upon the duration, severity, and causes of the problem. Treatment can be divided into several phases.

TABLE 10–14. **Other Measures in the Treatment of Fecal Soiling**

Medical	Treatment of plumbism Treatment of hypothyroidism Treatment of dehydration
Neurologic	Anticonvulsant medication
Surgical	Operation for Hirschsprung disease (removal of aganglionic colon)
Psychologic	Support Treatment of any associated emotional disorder
Social-Environmental	Behavior modification (reward system)
Educational	"Demystification"
Mechanical	Child-sized diapers Instrumental learning (biofeedback)

The first phase consists of mineral oil taken by mouth to facilitate the ready passage of stools. In some circumstances phosphate enemas can be used to remove obstipated feces (Davidson *et al.,* 1963). Rectal examination may have accomplished this task already and rendered enemas unnecessary. Mineral oil is given in increasing dosages until four or five loose bowel movements occur. Because of the hyperosmolar effect of mineral oil, the child should increase fluid intake to avoid dehydration that might worsen constipation.

The next phase of treatment is bowel training. The child sits on the toilet after meals to take advantage of the gastrocolic reflex. This schedule allows the child to become more aware of the urge to defecate, which may have been blunted or absent previously when the rectum was distended with feces. The child's legs should reach the ground or some other suitable support so that the necessary increase in abdominal pressure can occur. Mineral oil, stool softeners, and rapidly acting suppositories may be of benefit during this phase of treatment.

The third phase consists of follow-up visits every few weeks or months. Telephone contact between scheduled visits may also assist the child and family (Levine and Bakow, 1976).

If the first phase of therapy is not successful, investigation including barium enema, rectal pressure measurements, and/or biopsy should be considered to diagnose Hirschsprung disease or other organic problem (Davidson *et al.,* 1963).

Neurologic Management. In persons with spina bifida or other spinal cord disorder, operant conditioning techniques appear promising (Schuster, 1974). They are designed to bring under voluntary control functions involved in bowel activity that normally are automatic and unconscious. A bowel training regimen for children with spina bifida has been described in detail by Forsythe and Kinley (1970).

Seizures should be treated with standard anticonvulsant drugs (see Chapter 12).

Surgical Management. The treatment of Hirschsprung disease consists of resection of aganglionic bowel and rejoining of the normal proximal and distal portions.

Psychotherapy. Supportive psychotherapy involving the affected child and family is always indicated. This therapeutic process usually involves several months to years.

Behavioral techniques (not far removed from those employed ordinarily in toilet training) are valuable. Initially, the child is rewarded for sitting upon the toilet, then for trying to defecate, and thereafter for productive efforts. Later rewards are contingent on greater degrees of control and independence. The reward can be in the form of stars or tokens to be "cashed in" for toys or other prizes at the end of a week.

When the child is emotionally disturbed (excessively anxious, withdrawn, or depressed) or when parent-child interaction is impaired (as with excessively demanding or highly anxious parents), formal psychotherapy is indicated (Pinkerton, 1958).

Social-Environmental Management. Behavioral techniques can be applied in a social context. By gaining control over bowel function, the enco-pretic child can, for example, "earn" time with his parents in more pleasant and socially acceptable activities than arguing over soiled underwear.

Educational Management. Levine and Bakow (1976) have emphasized the importance of "demystification" in their approach. For example, draw-ings and discussions are used to elucidate for the child (and family) relevant aspects of the structure and function of the gastrointestinal system, includ-ing both digestion and elimination. The child's fantasies about reproductive function and its connections with the gastrointestinal system may merit fur-ther exploration and explanation (MacCarthy, 1976).

Dietary counseling should also be included. The importance of eating foods containing roughage (such as celery, lettuce, and whole grains) and the advisability of avoiding highly refined, low-bulk items should be empha-sized.

Mechanical Therapy. Disposable undergarments may be useful in the management of the child with encopresis.

Biofeedback has been effectively employed in some persons with fecal in-continence (Engel *et al.*, 1974; Orne, 1979). Its applicability to the treatment of encopresis in childhood has not yet been determined.

SUMMARY

Encopresis refers to fecal soiling, usually occurring due to leakage around obstipated feces. Diarrhea, excessive mineral oil ingestion, and faulty hy-giene as causes of fecal staining should be distinguished from encopresis. Encopresis usually occurs secondary to chronic constipation with psycho-logic causes often playing an important role. Hirschsprung's disease (agan-glionic megacolon) is an unlikely cause but should be considered.

Evaluation should include abdominal and rectal examinations. Medical assessment should exclude hypothyroidism, lead poisoning, and anal fis-sure. Neurologic examination should specifically exclude a disorder af-fecting the spinal cord. Investigation will depend upon the history, examina-tion, and response to previous treatment. Therapy consists of removal of obstipated feces, use of stool-softening agents, and educational-behavioral techniques utilizing the gastrocolic reflex and reward systems. Supportive psychotherapy is always indicated. Regular follow-up appears important in ensuring a favorable outcome.

CORRELATION

Anatomic Aspects. The hypothalmus lies deep within the brain, bounded superiorly by the thalamus and inferiorly by the pituitary. Its two halves lie astride the inferior portion of the third ventricle. Anteriorly, the hypothala-mus extends above and beyond the optic tracts and chiasm. Posteriorly, the hypothalamus continues into the rostral portion of the midbrain reticular for-mation.

The descending columns of the fornix, part of the limbic system, divide each half of the hypothalamus both functionally and anatomically into me-dial and lateral parts (Martin *et al.*, 1977). The medial portion is involved in pituitary regulation and maintenance of visceral function. The lateral part is more closely connected with limbic behavioral-emotional systems.

The ventromedial nucleus of the hypothalamus (VMN) has been implicated as playing an important role in eating behavior (see Fig. 6–5) (Reeves and Plum, 1969; Plum and Van Uitert, 1978). Destructive lesions of the VMN cause increased eating, whereas electrical stimulation produces cessation of eating (aphagia). By contrast, lateral hypothalamic lesions produce aphagia and stimulation polyphagia. The lateral hypothalamic region has thus been termed a "feeding center," the ventromedial nucleus a "satiety center." Neurons producing luteinizing hormone releasing hormone, involved in regulation of menstruation, lie anteriorly and medially close to the VMN.

Although experimental studies in animals and investigations in man have supported such localization, these areas are unlikely to act in isolation. Loss or other alteration of function resulting from hypothalamic disturbance by no means implies that the function is confined to the hypothalamus. The hypothalamus is, for example, intimately connected with limbic structures that are themselves involved in complex behaviors. Martin and colleagues (1977) have suggested that the hypothalamus can act in some instances as "an amplifier of certain behavioral responses organized elsewhere in the brain, rather than as the 'center' for these responses."

Biochemical Aspects. The search for biochemical mediators of eating behavior has been wide-ranging. The central nervous system—particularly the hypothalamus—has been a major focus.

Regulation of food intake has been viewed as involving short- and long-term mechanisms. Short-term regulation of food intake has been linked with hypothalamic perception of glucose metabolism. Mayer (1966) has proposed that cells of the ventromedial nucleus of the hypothalamus act as a "glucostat," sensitive to the level of blood glucose, rate of change of blood glucose concentration, and rate of glucose utilization.

More recently, experimental evidence has suggested that peripheral glucoreceptors mediate the drive toward eating. Novin and colleagues (1973) found that infusion of 2-deoxyglucose (which blocks glucose metabolism) into the hepatic portal system initiated feeding in experimental animals. Based on these and other data, Cahill and colleagues (1979) have hypothesized that hepatic glycogen content rather than blood glucose level is the key element in short-term regulation of fuel (food) intake.

Long-term regulation of caloric homeostasis may involve a "lipostatic" mechanism (Martin et al., 1977). It has been observed that animals rendered obese through forced feeding subsequently voluntarily diminished their food intake, suggesting a homeostatic mechanism based upon body fat or a metabolite thereof (such as triglyceride).

More recent evidence suggests that central receptors for cholecystokinin, a gastrointestinal hormone, are involved in satiety (Cooper and Martin, 1980; Della-Fera et al., 1981). Diminished levels of cholecystokinin have been found in the brains of obese hyperphagic mice. Furthermore, intravenous infusion of cholecystokinin in sheep appears to curtail feeding behavior.

Physiologic Aspects. Urination results from the interaction of involuntary and voluntary muscles: detrusor and external urethral sphincter muscles, respectively. They are acted upon by both autonomic and voluntary neural input at several levels (Wright, 1975).

The process of urination is highly complex and not fully understood. Stretch receptors in the bladder wall are connected to a sacral parasympathetic center for urination at spinal cord segmental levels S_2 through S_4 (see Fig. 2–10). When bladder volume reaches 300–400 ml in the adult, sensation of the need to pass urine reaches consciousness through connections with the sensory cortex of the parietal lobes. This cortex lies within the interhemispheric fissure, deep to fibers subserving the legs. If it is inconvenient to pass urine, voluntary motor fibers of cortical origin act through the pudendal nerves to cause contraction of the external urethral sphincter. Thus, reflex emptying of the bladder is inhibited. When circumstances permit, the cortical inhibitory input is discontinued and the detrusor can act relatively unopposed. The role of sympathetic motor fibers from spinal cord segments T_{11} to L_2 and axons derived from brainstem, basal ganglia, and hypothalamus is not clear.

Similarly, the voluntary act of defecation, emptying of the large bowel, also results from interplay between autonomic and voluntary neural systems (Wright, 1975). Rectal filling is accomplished through sympathetic stimulation, which causes relaxation of the sigmoid colon and contraction of the internal anal sphincter. Parasympathetic sensory fibers derived from segmental levels S_2 through S_4 transmit the degree of rectal filling to the spinal cord. Parasympathetic motor stimulation causes contraction of smooth muscle of the rectum and relaxation of the internal anal sphinter. Once the urge to defecate has been sensed, the external anal sphincter (a voluntary muscle under cerebral cortical control) is relaxed and intra-abdominal pressure increased through muscular effort mediated via somatic motor nerves of segmental origin T_6 through T_{12}. The final step is passage of feces through another ring of voluntary muscles, the levator ani group, which make up the pelvic floor.

Intestinal pressure measurements and electromyographic recordings at various levels of the gastrointestinal tract have greatly clarified the physiology of defecation and its disorders and have led the way toward newer therapeutic techniques such as biofeedback.

CITED REFERENCES

ANOREXIA NERVOSA

Boyar, R. M. Endocrine changes in anorexia nervosa. *Med. Clin. North Am.,* **62:** 297–303, 1978.

Bruch, H. Anorexia nervosa. Pp. 101–15 in *Nutrition and the Brain,* Vol. 3. Wurtman, R. J., and Wurtman, J. J., eds. Raven Press, New York, 1979.

Bruch, H. Anorexia nervosa. Pp. 229–37 in *Psychosomatic Medicine: Its Clinical Applications.* Wittkower, E. D., and Warrens, H., eds. Harper and Row, Publishers, Hagerstown, Md., 1977.

Casper, R. C.; Offer, D.; and Ostrov, E. The self-image of adolescents with acute anorexia nervosa. *J. Pediatr.,* **98:** 656–61, 1981.

Crisp, A. H.; Palmer, R. L.; and Kalucy, R. S. How common is anorexia nervosa? a prevalence study. *Br. J. Psychiatry,* **128:** 549–54, 1976.

Diagnostic and Statistical Manual of Mental Disorders, 3d ed. American Psychiatric Association, Washington, D.C., 1980.

Goldney, R. D. Craniopharyngioma simulating anorexia nervosa. *J. Nerv. Ment. Dis.,* **166:** 135–38, 1978.

Greene, H., and Schubert, W. K. Anorexia nervosa. Pp. 350–51, in *Pediatric Nutrition Handbook.* Committee on Nutrition, American Academy of Pediatrics, Barness, L. A., chairman. American Academy of Pediatrics, Evanston, Ill., 1979.

Halmi, K. A. Anorexia nervosa: recent investigations. *Annu. Rev. Med.,* **29:** 137–48, 1978.

Halmi, K. A.: Dekirmenjian, H.; Davis, J. M.; Casper, R.; and Goldberg, S. Catecholamine metabolism in anorexia nervosa. *Arch. Gen. Psychiatry,* **35:** 458–60, 1978.

Heron, G. B., and Johnston, D. A. Hypothalamic tumor presenting as anorexia nervosa. *Am. J. Psychiatry,* **133:** 580–82, 1976.

Liebman, R.; Minuchin, S.; and Baker, L. An integrated treatment program for anorexia nervosa. *Am. J. Psychiatry,* **131:** 432–36, 1974.

Maloney, M. J., and Farrell, M. K. Treatment of severe weight loss in anorexia nervosa with hyperalimentation and psychotherapy. *Am. J. Psychiatry,* **137:** 310–14, 1980.

Martin, J. B.; Reichlin, S.; and Brown, G. M. *Clinical Neuroendocrinology.* F. A. Davis Co., Philadelphia, 1977, pp. 112–14.

Minuchin, S.; Baker, L.; Rosman, B. L.; Liebman, R.; Milman, L.; and Todd, T. C. A conceptual model of psychosomatic illness in children: family organization and family therapy. *Arch. Gen. Psychiatry,* **32:** 1031–38, 1975.

Nussbaum, M.; Shenker, I. R.; Marc, J.; and Klein, M. Cerebral atrophy in anorexia nervosa. *J. Pediatr.,* **96:** 867–69, 1980.

Plum, F., and Van Uitert, R. Non-endocrine diseases and disorders of the hypothalamus. Pp. 415–73 in *The Hypothalamus.* Reichlin, S.; Baldessarini, R. J.; and Martin, J. B.; eds. Raven Press, New York, 1978.

Rollins, N., and Piazza, E. Diagnosis of anorexia nervosa: a critical reappraisal. *J. Am. Acad. Child Psychiatry,* **17:** 126–37, 1978.

Silverman, J. A. Anorexia nervosa: clinical observations in a successful treatment plan. *J. Pediatr.,* **84:** 68–73, 1974.

Smith, N. J. Excessive weight loss and food aversion in athletes simulating anorexia nervosa. *Pediatrics,* **66:** 139–42, 1980.

Woolston, J. L., and Schowalter, J. E. Behavior modification protocols on a pediatric adolescent unit. *Pediatrics,* **66:** 355–58, 1980.

OBESITY

Bray, G. A., and Gallagher, T. F., Jr. Manifestations of hypothalamic obesity in man: a comprehensive investigation of eight patients and a review of the literature. *Medicine,* **54:** 301–30, 1975.

Bruch, H. Obesity: clinical and psychiatric aspects. Pp. 71–100 in *Nutrition and the Brain,* Vol. 3. Wurtman, R. J., and Wurtman, J. J., eds. Raven Press, New York, 1979.

Charney, E.; Goodman, H. C.; McBride, M.; Lyon, B.; and Pratt, R. Childhood antecedents of adult obesity: do chubby infants become obese adults? *N. Engl. J. Med.,* **295:** 6–9, 1976.

Jordan, H. A.; Levitz, L. S.; and Kimbrell, G. M. Psychobiological factors in obesity. Pp. 239–48 in *Psychosomatic Medicine: Its Clinical Applications.* Wittkower, E. D., and Warrens, H., eds. Harper and Row, Publishers, Hagerstown, Md., 1977.

Knittle, J. L. Obesity in childhood: a problem in adipose tissue cellular development. *J. Pediatr.,* **81:** 1048–59, 1972.

Malt, R. A., and Guggenheim, F. G. Surgery for obesity. *N. Engl. J. Med.,* **295:** 43–44, 1976.

Martin, J. B.; Reichlin, S.; and Brown, G. M. Neurologic manifestations of hypothalamic disease. Pp. 247–73, in *Clinical Neuroendocrinology.* By Martin, J. B.; Reichlin, S.; and Brown, G. M. F. A. Davis, Co., Philadelphia, 1977.

Mayer, J. Some aspects of the problem of regulation of food intake and obesity. *N. Engl. J. Med.,* **274:** 610–16, 662–73, 1966.

Merritt, R. J.; Bistrian, B. R.; Blackburn, G. L.; and Suskind, R. M. Consequences of modified fasting in obese pediatric and adolescent patients: I. protein-sparing modified fast. *J. Pediatr.,* **96:** 13–19, 1980.

Meyers, A. W.; Stunkard, A. J.; and Coll, M. Food accessibility and food choice: a test of Schachter's externality hypothesis. *Arch. Gen. Psychiatry,* **37:** 1133–35, 1980.

Passmore, R., and Durnin, J. V. G. A. Human energy expenditure. *Physiol. Rev.* **35:** 801–40, 1955.

Rau, J. H., and Green, R. S. Soft neurological correlates of compulsive eaters. *J. Nerv. Ment. Dis.,* **166:** 435–37, 1978.

Ravelli, G.-P.; Stein, Z. A.; and Susser, M. W. Obesity in young men after famine exposure in utero and early infancy. *N. Engl. J. Med.,* **295:** 349–53, 1976.

Rodgers, S.; Goss, A.; Goldney, R.; Thomas, D.; Burnet, R.; Phillips, P.; Kimber, C.; Harding, P.; and Wise, P. Jaw wiring in treatment of obesity. *Lancet,* **1:** 1221–23, 1977.

Schachter, S. Some extraordinary facts about obese humans and rats. *Am. Psychol.* **26:** 129–44, 1971.

Spier, N., and Karelitz, S. The Pickwickian syndrome: case in a child. *Am. J. Dis. Child.,* **99:** 822–27, 1960.

Stricker, E. M. Hyperphagia. *N. Engl. J. Med.,* **298:** 1010–13, 1978.

Stuart, R. B. Behavioral control of overeating. *Behav. Res. Ther.,* **5:** 357–65, 1967.

Stunkard, A. New therapies for the eating disorders: behavior modification of obesity and anorexia nervosa. *Arch. Gen. Psychiatry,* **26:** 391–98, 1972.

Waxman, M., and Stunkard, A. J. Caloric intake and expenditure of obese boys. *J. Pediatr.,* **96:** 187–93, 1980.

Weil, W. B., Jr. Current controversies in childhood obesity. *J. Pediatr.,* **91:** 175–87, 1977.

Wisniewski, L. P.; Witt, M. E.; Ginsberg-Fellner, F.; Wilner, J.; and Desnick, R. J. Prader-Willi syndrome and a bisatellited derivative of chromosome 15. *Clin. Genet.,* **18:** 42–47, 1980.

ENURESIS

Alderton, H. R. Imipramine in childhood enuresis: further studies on the relationship of time of administration to effect. *Can. Med. Assoc. J.,* **102:** 1179–80, 1970.

Bakwin, H. Enuresis in children. *J. Pediatr.,* **58:** 806–19, 1961.

Birkásová, M.; Birkás, O.; Flynn, M. J.; and Cort, J. H. Desmopressin in the management of nocturnal enuresis in children: a double-blind study. *Pediatrics,* **62:** 970–74, 1978.

Broughton, R. J. Sleep disorders: disorders of arousal? *Science,* **159:** 1070–78, 1968.

Forsythe, W. I., and Redmond, A. Enuresis and spontaneous cure rate: study of 1129 enuretics. *Arch. Dis. Child.,* **49:** 259–63, 1974.

Kales, A.; Kales, J. D.; Jacobson, A.; Humphrey, F. J., II; and Soldatos, C. R. Effects of imipramine on enuretic frequency and sleep stages. *Pediatrics,* **60:** 431–36, 1977.

Lessell, S., and Rosman, N. P. Juvenile diabetes mellitus and optic atrophy. *Arch. Neurol.,* **34:** 759–65, 1977.

Lewis, H. E.; Lobban, M. C.; and Tredre, B. E. Daily rhythms of renal excretion in a child with nocturnal enuresis. *Proc. Physiol. Soc.,* pp. 42P–43P, 1970.

Marshall, S.; Marshall, H. H.; and Lyon, R. P. Enuresis: an analysis of various therapeutic approaches. *Pediatrics,* **52:** 813–22, 1973.

Meadow, R. Drugs for bed-wetting. *Arch. Dis. Child.,* **49:** 257–58, 1974.

Mikkelsen, E. J.; Rapoport, J. L.; Nee, L.; Gruenau, C.; Mendelson, W.; and Gillin, J. C. Childhood enuresis: I. sleep patterns and psychopathology. *Arch. Gen. Psychiatry,* **37:** 1139–44, 1980.

Rapoport, J. L., and Mikkelsen, E. J. Antidepressants. Pp. 208–33, in *Pediatric Psychopharmacology: The Use of Behavior Modifying Drugs in Children.* Werry, J. S., ed. Brunner/Mazel, Inc., New York, 1978.

Rapoport, J. L.; Mikkelsen, E. J.; Zavadil, A.; Nee, L.; Gruenau, C.; Mendelson, W.; and Gillin, J. C. Childhood enuresis: II. psychopathology, tricyclic concentration in plasma, and antienuretic effect. *Arch. Gen. Psychiatry,* **37:** 1146–52, 1980.

Shaffer, D. Enuresis. Pp. 581–612 in *Child Psychiatry: Modern Approaches.* Rutter, M., and Hersov, L., eds. Blackwell Scientific Publications, Oxford, 1977.

Starfield, B. Functional bladder capacity in enuretic and nonenuretic children. *J. Pediatr.,* **70:** 777–81, 1967.

Starfield, B. Enuresis: focus on a challenging problem in primary care. *Pediatrics,* **62:** 1036–37, 1978.

Troup, C. W., and Hodgson, N. B. Nocturnal functional bladder capacity in enuretic children. *J. Urol.,* **105:** 129–32, 1971.

Weinberg, W. A.; Rutman, J.; Sullivan, L.; Penick, E. C.; and Dietz, S. G. Depression in children referred to an educational diagnostic center: diagnosis and treatment. *J. Pediatr.,* **83:** 1065–72, 1973.

Werry, J. S., and Cohrssen, J. Enuresis—an etiologic and therapeutic study. *J. Pediatr.,* **67:** 423–31, 1965.

Winsberg, B. G., and Yepes, L. E. Antipsychotics (major tranquilizers, neuroleptics). Pp. 234–73, in *Pediatric Psychopharmacology: The Use of Behavior Modifying Drugs in Children.* Werry, J. S., ed. Brunner/Mazel, Inc., New York, 1978.

ENCOPRESIS

Brazelton, T. B. A child-oriented approach to toilet-training. *Pediatrics,* **29:** 121–28, 1962.

Davidson, M.; Kugler, M. M.; and Bauer, C. H. Diagnosis and management in children with severe and protracted constipation and obstipation. *J. Pediatr.,* **62:** 261–75, 1963.

Engel, B. T.; Nikoomanesh, P.; and Schuster, M. N. Operant conditioning of recto-sphincteric responses in the treatment of fecal incontinence. *N. Engl. J. Med.,* **290:** 646–49, 1974.

Forsythe, W. I., and Kinley, J. G. Bowel control of children with spina bifida. *Dev. Med. Child. Neurol.,* **12:** 27–31, 1970.

Garrard, S. D., and Richmond, J. B. Psychogenic megacolon manifested by fecal soiling. *Pediatrics,* **10:** 474–83, 1952.

Halpern, W. I. The treatment of encopretic children. *J. Am. Acad. Child Psychiatry,* **16:** 478–99, 1977.

Hersov, L. Faecal soiling. Pp. 613–27, in *Child Psychiatry: Modern Approaches*. Rutter, M., and Hersov, L., eds. Blackwell Scientific Publications, Oxford, 1977.

Levine, M. D., and Bakow, H. Children with encopresis: a study of treatment outcome. *Pediatrics*, **58:** 845–52, 1976.

Levine, M. D.; Mazonson, P.; and Bakow, H. Behavioral symptom substitution in children cured of encopresis. *Am. J. Dis. Child.*, **134:** 663–67, 1980.

MacCarthy, D. Encopresis. *Proc. Roy. Soc. Med.*, **69:** 19–20, 1976.

Orne, M. T. The efficacy of biofeedback therapy. *Annu. Rev. Med.*, **30:** 489–503, 1979.

Pinkerton, P. Psychogenic megacolon in children: the implications of bowel negativism. *Arch. Dis. Child.*, **33:** 371–80, 1958.

Schuster, M. M. Operant conditioning in gastrointestinal dysfunctions. *Hosp. Pract.*, pp. 135–43, September 1974.

Sluckin, A. Encopresis: a behavioural approach described. *Social Work Today*, **5:** 643–46, 1975.

CORRELATION

Cahill, G. F., Jr.; Aoki, T. T.; and Rossini, A. A. Metabolism in obesity and anorexia nervosa. Pp. 1–70 in *Nutrition and the Brain*, Vol. 3. Wurtman, R. J., and Wurtman, J. J., eds. Raven Press, New York, 1979.

Cooper, P. E., and Martin, J. B. Neuroendocrinology and brain peptides. *Ann. Neurol.*, **8:** 551–57, 1980.

Della-Fera, M. A.; Baile, C. A.; Schneider, B. S.; and Grinker, J. A. Cholecystokinin antibody injected in cerebral ventricles stimulates feeding in sheep. *Science*, **212:** 687–89, 1981.

Martin, J. B.; Reichlin, S.; and Brown, G. M. *Clinical Neuroendocrinology*. F. A. Davis Co., Philadelphia, 1977.

Mayer, J. Some aspects of the problem of regulation of food intake and obesity. *N. Engl. J. Med.*, **274:** 610–16, 662–73, 1966.

Novin, D.; VanderWeele, D. A.; and Rezek, M. Infusion of 2-deoxy-D-glucose into the hepatic-portal system causes eating: evidence for peripheral glucoreceptors. *Science*, **181:** 858–60, 1973.

Plum, F., and Van Uitert, R. Non-endocrine diseases and disorders of the hypothalamus. Pp. 415–73, in *The Hypothalamus*. Reichlin, S.; Baldessarini, R. J.; and Martin, J. B., eds. Raven Press, New York, 1978.

Reeves, A. G., and Plum, F. Hyperphagia, rage, and dementia accompanying a ventromedial hypothalamic neoplasm. *Arch. Neurol.*, **20:** 616–24, 1969.

Wright, F. S. Disorders of micturition and defecation. Pp. 251–56, in *The Practice of Pediatric Neurology*. Swaiman, K. F., and Wright, F. S., eds. C. V. Mosby Co., Saint Louis, 1975.

ADDITIONAL READINGS

Allen, D. W., and Quigley, B. M. The role of physical activity in the control of obesity. *Med. J. Aust.*, **2:** 434–38, 1977.

Antelman, S. M., and Rowland, N. Endogenous opiates and stress-induced eating. *Science*, **214:** 1149–50, 1981.

Anthony, E. J. An experimental approach to the psychopathology of childhood: encopresis. *Br. J. Med. Psychol.*, **30:** 146–75, 1957.

Bruch, H. *The Golden Cage: The Enigma of Anorexia Nervosa*. Harvard University Press, Cambridge, 1978.

Bruch, H. *Eating Disorders: Obesity, Anorexia Nervosa, and the Person Within.* Basic Books, New York, 1973.

Burke, E. C., and Stickler, G. B. Enuresis—is it being overtreated? *Mayo Clin. Proc.,* **55:** 118–19, 1980.

Colvin, I.; MacKeith, R. C.; and Meadow, S. R. *Bladder Control and Enuresis.* Clinics in Developmental Medicine, 48/49. Heinemann, London, 1973.

Craighead, L. W.; Stunkard, A. J.; O'Brien, R. M. Behavior therapy and pharmacotherapy for obesity. *Arch. Gen. Psychiatry,* **38:** 763–68, 1981.

Crisp, A. H. *Anorexia Nervosa: Let Me Be.* Grune and Stratton, New York, 1980.

De Luise, M.; Blackburn, G. L.; and Flier, J. S. Reduced activity of the red-cell sodium-potassium pump in human obesity. *N. Engl. J. Med.,* **303:** 1017–22, 1980.

Glicklich, L. B. An historical account of enuresis. *Pediatrics,* **8:** 859–76, 1951.

Grossman, S. P. The neuroanatomy of eating and drinking behavior. Pp. 131–40, in *Neuroendocrinology.* Krieger, D. T., and Hughes, J. C., eds. Sinauer Associates, Inc., Sunderland, Mass., 1980.

Huschka, M. The child's response to coercive bowel training. *Psychosom. Med.,* **4:** 301–8, 1942.

Jordan, H. A.; Levitz, L. S.; and Kimbrell, G. M. *Eating Is Okay! The Behavioral Control Diet.* Rawson Associates, Publishers, New York, 1976.

Kramer, M. S. Do breast-feeding and delayed introduction of solid foods protect against subsequent obesity? *J. Pediatr.,* **98:** 883–87, 1981.

Lucas, A. R. Toward the understanding of anorexia nervosa as a disease entity. *Mayo Clin. Proc.,* **56:** 254–64, 1981.

Mason, E. E. *Surgical Treatment of Obesity,* W. B. Saunders Company, Philadelphia, 1981.

Stuart, R. B., and Davis, B. *Slim Chance in a Fat World: Behavioral Control of Obesity.* Research Press, Champaign, Ill., 1972.

Stunkard, A. J. (ed.) *Obesity.* W. B. Saunders, Philadelphia, 1980.

11 Headaches

Headache is a common and often complicated problem in childhood. Some headaches are clearly linked with medical illness such as a "flu" syndrome or sinusitis. Other headaches have a clearly emotional basis, as with a depressive syndrome stemming from the death of a family member. Other headache syndromes, however, do not fit neatly into a single category—for example, a child with a 3-month history of intermittent throbbing headaches, withdrawn behavior, and worsened school performance. With such a clinical situation, the task is to determine both the organic and the functional contributions to the problem. Indeed, it is often the case in childhood and adolescence that both elements pertain; so an either-or approach to etiology is inadequate.

The primary objective of this chapter is to provide a useful framework within which to approach the child with headaches. This approach will define several headache syndromes and describe the structural, metabolic, and emotional components to the problem. Several questions will be addressed:

What information obtained by history suggests organic disease? What aspects of the examination?
What is migraine? What forms does it take in childhood?
When is investigation indicated in evaluating the child with headache? What should it consist of?
How should headaches be treated?

HEADACHES

DEFINITION

Headache refers to pain or other significant discomfort affecting the scalp, skull, or intracranial contents. As with "depression," headache is most usefully considered part of a syndrome, not an isolated symptom. For example, a pounding bifrontal headache preceded by scintillating scotomata

TABLE 11–1. **Extracranial and Intracranial Structures Sensitive to Pain**

Extracranial	Eyes and orbits
	Ears and mastoid sinuses
	Nose and paranasal sinuses
	Teeth and oropharynx
	Scalp and skull
	Neck and cervical spine
Intracranial	Large arteries and veins
	Dura at base of skull
	Cranial nerves V, VII, X
	Upper cervical nerves

affecting one visual field and associated with nausea, irritability, and lethargy would constitute a syndrome of classical migraine.

In approaching the child or adolescent with headache, it is useful to keep in mind pain-sensitive structures and basic pain mechanisms that might be involved (see Table 11–1). Extracranially, the principal pain-sensitive structures are the eyes and orbits, ears and mastoid sinuses, nose and paranasal sinuses, oropharynx and teeth, scalp and skull, neck and cervical spine. Intracranially, major pain-sensitive structures are several of the larger blood vessels (proximal dural arteries, proximal arteries making up the circle of Willis, venous sinuses, large veins), dura at the base of the skull, certain cranial nerves (V, VII, and X), and upper cervical nerves. The brain itself is insensitive to pain.

Pain of intracranial origin is not felt at the site of origin. Rather, it is referred to other parts of the head and neck (see Table 11–2). Pain originating in the anterior two-thirds of the cranium in the anterior and middle cranial fossas, lying above the tentorium cerebelli, is felt in the frontal, parietal, and temporal regions. It is mediated through the first division of the trigeminal (fifth cranial) nerve. Pain derived from structures lying below the tentorium cerebelli in the posterior fossa (such as the cerebellum) generally projects to behind the ear, to just above the cervical-occipital junction, or to the upper neck. The ninth and tenth cranial nerves (glossopharyngeal and vagus) and

TABLE 11–2. **Pain of Intracranial Origin: Sites of Origin and Referral**

Site of Origin	Site of Referral	Nerves Involved
Anterior and middle cranial fossas (above tentorium cerebelli)	Frontal, parietal, and temporal regions	Cranial nerve V (trigeminal), first division
Posterior fossa (below tentorium cerebelli)	Behind the ear, just above cervical-occipital junction, upper neck	Cranial nerves IX and X (glossopharyngeal, vagus), C_1–C_3

the upper cervical nerves C_1, C_2, and C_3) subserve the infratentorial compartment.

These pain-sensitive structures can be involved in several ways: by inflammation, traction or displacement, muscle contraction, and/or vasodilation.

DIAGNOSIS

Clinical Process. The cause or causes of a child's headache syndrome should be identifiable by history in most instances. Examination and investigation (if any) will often confirm the diagnosis or add further data, but they will rarely provide a diagnosis not already established or strongly suspected on the basis of a careful history.

In obtaining information as to the presenting problem and past history, one is at the same time acquiring objective information as to the child's mental status (including affect, concentration, intelligence, and interactive behavior).

It is usually valuable to explore psychologic factors, whether they appear to be of primary or secondary importance, as an integral part of the interview and examination, for a return to look for emotional influences following an inconclusive examination can be felt by the child and family as "fishing" for emotional problems. Thus, referral for psychiatric evaluation, if advised, may be undermined.

History. The child should be questioned directly insofar as possible, then the parents. The chief complaint may range from the general ("I get bad headaches") to the specific ("I've got migraines"). The history of the presenting problem should characterize the headache syndrome further (see Table 11–3).

Specific features of the pain itself should be noted: its quality (aching, pounding, stabbing, pressing), location, radiation (change in location), duration, and intensity (including its interference with school or play activity). The younger child, often less verbal and more shy than an older one, nonetheless will usually be able to demonstrate by touching where the pain hurts and indicate the kind of pain by nodding "yes" or "no" to the examiner's gestures of pounding, squeezing, or stabbing.

Temporal aspects of the headache syndrome should be determined. When did your headaches begin? How frequent are they? Do you wake up with a

TABLE 11–3. **Characterization of Headaches**

Quality
Location
Radiation
Onset
Duration
Frequency
Aura
Other associated symptoms
Alteration by movement or Valsalva maneuver

headache? Do they occur on weekends as well as weekdays? Are they continuous? Does the discomfort vary, or is it always intense? Does the headache worsen with change in position or upon straining to have a bowel movement? When were you last free of headache? When was your last headache? What have you found to bring on a headache: chocolate, soft drinks, hotdogs, Chinese food, hot weather, worrying?

Associated symptoms should be identified. Do you get sick to your stomach? Have you thrown up with your headaches? Do you get any clues or warning signals before a headache comes on such as sparkling lights, loss of vision, numbness or tingling of your body or face, difficulty speaking, weakness of one side of your body, or "dizziness"? Does the headache begin suddenly or build up gradually? Does the child get pale before the headache begins?

Previous evaluation, treatment, and its efficacy should be recorded. What do you do when you get a headache? Do you lie down, take aspirin, or just keep on studying (or playing)? Does aspirin help? How much do you take? Do you feel entirely well after a nap? Are you able to resume your activities as before?

Persistent headache should direct questioning to several specific areas (see Table 11–4). Truly persistent headache pain suggests increased intracranial pressure among several other possibilities (most importantly affective disturbance, sinusitis, elevated blood pressure, nerve entrapment, or a combination of these). The pain need not be severe and may at times escape the child's awareness but still be present when he thinks about it, shakes his head, or coughs. A highly significant symptom associated with increased intracranial pressure is transient visual obscuration, which is rarely mentioned spontaneously by the child. These are brief periods of visual loss lasting only seconds. They are difficult to characterize but may be described as "graying out" or "blacking out" of vision.

Sinusitis is suggested by a frontal or infraorbital location of pain, association with allergies or "colds," chronic sore throat, or "bad breath." Emotional causes of headache are suggested by unvarying headache pain, characteristic distribution (involving the entire head or just the vertex), bizarre radiation (traveling from one temple through to the other like an arrow), unusual quality (like the pricking of a pin), and associated symptoms of depression or anxiety. Entrapment of a cervical nerve is suggested by pain localized to the cranial-cervical junction, with sensory loss in a peripheral nerve distribution, and with symptoms reproduced or worsened by local pressure. Posterior fossa tumors, too, are often associated with pain at the

TABLE 11–4. **Causes of Persistent Headache**

Increased intracranial pressure
Affective disturbance
Sinusitis
High blood pressure
Nerve entrapment
A combination of the above

back of the head and neck, but they are generally accompanied by other symptoms and signs of increased intracranial pressure. Persistent headaches may result from a combination of these factors. By no means does depression exclude the possibility of brain tumor.

Past history should include previous hospitalizations and episodes of significant head trauma. Recent medications, including vitamins A and D, tetracyclines, birth control pills, and prednisone, should be inquired about. Allergies to foods or environmental agents should be sought. Family history of headaches, especially migraine (''sick'') headaches, should be determined. Recent and chronic psychosocial stresses should be identified. These might include a family move, death of a relative or pet, impending separation or divorce of parents. The impact of the child's headache upon the family should be assessed. The personal profile of the child should include school performance (particularly any recent deterioration), temperament, and personality style (e.g., meticulous, perfectionistic, immature, or lackadaisical). Review of systems should include symptoms of systemic illness, personality change, coordinational problems, incontinence of urine, or recent weight change.

Examination.   The *general physical examination* should include full vital signs: pulse, blood pressure, temperature, and respirations. Elevated blood pressure can itself be a cause of headache. It is also an important clinical sign (in conjunction with diminished pulse and slowed respirations) of acutely raised intracranial pressure. The head circumference should be measured and plotted. In the younger child, hydrocephalus is usually associated with excessive head size or rate of growth. The head and neck should be palpated for swelling, tenderness, or other evidence of inflammation. The neck should be examined further for tenderness at the cranial-occipital junction and for stiffness or resistance to passive flexion. Meningismus may occur with meningitis, subarachnoid bleeding, or cerebellar tonsillar herniation. Evidence for upper respiratory infection (including rhinitis or pharyngitis) should be noted. Frontal and maxillary sinuses should be palpated and percussed to determine if tenderness is present. Evidence for systemic illness such as asthma, sickle cell disease, cardiac disease, or connective tissue disease (such as juvenile rheumatoid arthritis or systemic lupus erythematosus) should be noted.

Neurologic examination must include careful visualization of the optic fundi. Pupillary dilation should be carried out as indicated. It may be particularly helpful (in fact, necessary) in an uncooperative younger child in order to see the optic disks. Early signs of papilledema can be loss of venous pulsations (which are normally absent in some 20 per cent of persons) and engorgement of retinal blood vessels (especially veins). Blurring of optic disk margins and elevation of optic nerve heads are later and more reliable signs of elevated intracranial pressure (see Fig. 11–1). Retinal hemorrhages may be evident when the increase in intracranial pressure is more severe or sustained. Visual acuity, which can be diminished when intracranial pressure has been raised chronically, should be determined. Visual field testing with a small object may disclose an enlarged blind spot, an accompaniment of papilledema.

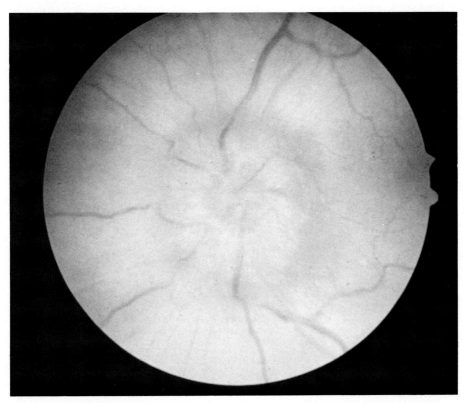

FIGURE 11–1. Optic fundus showing papilledema with blurred disk margins and elevated nerve head.

Motor and coordinational testing may show a wide-based, unsteady gait or difficulty in tandem walking with a posterior fossa tumor. With hydrocephalus of any cause, deep tendon reflexes are often abnormally brisk in the legs when compared to those in the arms; plantar responses are frequently extensor (see Table 11–5).

The *mental status examination* should note features of depression, anxiety, characterologic disturbance, or delusional thinking ("my head hurts where it's dented in like a crushed ping-pong ball").

Investigation. The extent of investigation, if any, will be determined by the history and examination (see Table 11–6). If increased intracranial pressure is suggested or evident, plain skull x-rays and computerized tomographic scan of the head should be obtained. Splitting of cranial sutures and demineralization of the sella turcica are signs of intracranial hypertension on plain radiography of the skull. CT scan will readily demonstrate hydrocephalus and may disclose a tumor causing the hydrocephalus. Infusion of contrast material may be necessary in order that a mass be visualized. With pseudotumor cerebri, ventricles will ususally be smaller than normal, often slitlike or inapparent. Cerebral arteriography may be valuable, particularly if CT scanning is unavailable.

TABLE 11–5. **Clinical Features Associated with Headache Caused by Increased Intracranial Pressure**

Symptoms	No previous headaches
	Persistent headache
	Headache present upon awakening
	Worsening of symptoms with positional and mechanical influences
	Vomiting
	Sleepiness
	Change in coordination
	Irritability or other personality change
	Transient visual obscurations
Signs	Altered mental state (lethargy, irritability)
	Change in vital signs (elevated blood pressure, slowed pulse, ataxic and/or slowed respirations)
	Papilledema
	Focal neurologic deficit(s)
	Ataxia
	Hyperreflexia
	Extensor plantar response(s)
	Stiff neck
	Diminished visual acuity

If migraine is diagnosed on the basis of history and examination, investigation is not usually necessary. If it is thought that the migraine syndrome may be due to seizure or vascular malformation, however, electroencephalography and CT scan should be carried out. With clearly defined sinus headaches, confirmatory x-rays of the paranasal sinuses need not be obtained. When meningeal infection is an important diagnostic consideration, examination of cerebrospinal fluid must be carried out. When clinical evidence of increased intracranial pressure exists, however, CT scan should be carried out first to exclude brain abscess, subdural fluid collection, or hydrocephalus (see Fig. 11–2). If, despite signs of increased intracranial pressure, it is

TABLE 11–6. **Investigations to Be Considered in the Child with Headaches**

Skull x-rays
EEG (in awake and sleep states)
Blood studies which might include CBC, blood sugar, ESR, ASO titer, antinuclear antibody (ANA), renal function tests, levels of vitamins A and D
Formal visual field examination
Cranial CT scan with contrast
Radioisotope brain scan
Lumbar puncture with measurement of CSF pressure, culture and analysis of CSF
Sinus x-rays
Arteriogram

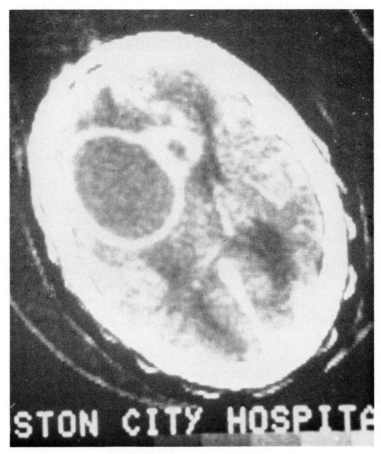

FIGURE 11–2. Computerized tomographic (CT) scan demonstrating adjacent (large and small) cerebral abscesses.

necessary to perform a lumbar puncture, a small amount of CSF can be removed through a narrow-gauge needle. An intravenous line should be in place for administration of mannitol, and equipment for hyperventilation should be immediately available should it be needed. If a lumbar puncture is done, CSF pressure should be measured.

Blood tests might include blood sugar with suspected hypoglycemia, erythrocyte sedimentation rate, and connective tissue studies in evaluation for systemic lupus erythematosus or other connective tissue disorder, kidney function tests, and antistreptococcal antibody titers for suspected glomerulonephritis. With syndromes of pseudotumor cerebri, a vitamin A level should be obtained. Electroencephalography should be carried out in cases of suspected seizure headaches, although an abnormal EEG does not exclude migraine or define a seizure disorder.

Differential Diagnosis. Several conditions must be differentiated from headache syndromes. These include pain arising from the face (including trigeminal neuralgia), eyes, ears, teeth, temporo-mandibular joints, or spine.

Papilledema may be confused with pseudopapilledema and with the normal finding of the nasal disk margin being less distinct than the temporal one.

Etiology.   Causes of headache are summarized in Tables 11–7 and 11–8.

Medical Causes.   Sinusitis is an important cause of headaches in childhood and adolescence. Because symptoms are often continuous and prolonged with sinusitis, increased intracranial pressure is frequently suggested. The diagnosis is established by periorbital headaches, usually aching in quality, associated with tenderness to pressure or percussion over the involved sinuses (see CLINICAL PROCESS: HISTORY). Sinus congestion rather than infection *per se* often contributes to migraine syndromes (see Case 11–1).

Fever itself may produce a throbbing headache.

High blood pressure is by no means limited to adults. Children, too, may suffer hypertension as defined by age-appropriate norms. For example, the normal reading of 120/80 in an adult would represent significant hypertension in a 3-year-old child in whom the measurement was taken with an appropriate-size cuff. Causes of high blood pressure in childhood include acute poststreptococcal glomerulonephritis, vascular anomalies (such as coarctation of the aorta, which can occur with Turner syndrome), pheochromocytoma, and Cushing syndrome.

TABLE 11–7. **Specific Causes of Childhood Headache**

Medical	Sinusitis
	Fever
	High blood pressure
Neurologic	Vascular headache (migraine)
	Tumor
	Hydrocephalus
	Muscle contraction (''tension'')
	Head trauma
	Meningitis
	Lumbar puncture
	Seizures
Toxic	Pseudotumor cerebri
	Foods and food additives
	Lead
	Hypoxia
	Carbon monoxide
	Caffeine withdrawal
Psychologic	Depression
	Anxiety
	Psychophysiologic reaction
Social-Environmental	Noise
	Overstimulation

TABLE 11–8. **Causes of Childhood Headache Based on Mechanism of Pain**

Disease of contiguous structures

Eyes and orbits
Ears and mastoid sinuses
Nose and paranasal sinuses
Oropharynx and teeth
Scalp and skull
Neck and cervical spine

Intracranial inflammation

Meningitis
   infectious: as with bacterial
   chemical: as with blood (subarachnoid hemorrhage)
Vasculitis
   arteritis: as with systemic lupus erythematosus
   phlebitis: as with chronic otitis media
Cranial neuritis

Traction/displacement

Following lumbar puncture
Mass with increased intracranial pressure
   tumor
   hematoma
   abscess
Increased intracranial pressure unassociated with mass
   hydrocephalus
   pseudotumor cerebri
   cerebral edema

Muscle contraction

Scalp muscles
Neck muscles
Facial muscles

Psychologic

Anxiety (hypochondriasis, conversion)
Depression
Malingering

Vascular, nonmigrainous

Febrile illness
Hypertension
Vascular malformation
Foods, especially those with nitrates, nitrites, MSG, phenylethylamine

Vascular, migrainous
Classic migraine
Common migraine

TABLE 11–8. (*Continued*)

Complicated migraine
  ophthalmoplegic
  hemiplegic
  confusional
  basilar artery
Migraine equivalent
  cyclic vomiting
  paroxysmal vertigo
  abdominal migraine
  convulsive migraine
Cluster headache

CASE 11–1: SINUS HEADACHES IN A 12-YEAR-OLD GIRL

S.T. was evaluated for periorbital headaches occurring three or four times weekly for the previous six months. Headaches were aching or stabbing in quality and were not associated with nausea, vomiting, or aura. Aspirin and rest were of symptomatic benefit. Past medical history was unremarkable. Social history indicated that her father had divorced her mother 3 years previously, had remarried, and was expecting another child soon.

On examination, the girl was an intelligent child in middle stages of adolescence who appeared neither anxious nor depressed. She had violaceous discolorations ("allergic shiners") below her eyes. Infraorbital sinuses were tender to palpation and percussion bilaterally. Examination of the nose disclosed rhinitis and erythematous nasal mucosa. The pharynx was injected without exudate. Optic disks showed sharp margins; venous pulsations were evident. Neurologic examination was normal.

She was diagnosed as having maxillary sinusitis on an allergic and infectious basis with worsening of symptoms due to situational and developmental stresses. Pharmacologic treatment was with erythromycin (250 mg four times daily for 10 days), a decongestant for 3 weeks, and continued aspirin. Mother and daughter continued in psychotherapy. Headaches improved significantly over the following weeks with a mild, brief exacerbation of symptoms around the time her half-sister was born.

Comment. This adolescent's headaches illustrate how several etiologic factors can act together to produce a prolonged headache syndrome. Sinusitis, or at least sinus congestion, was a major element. It was evident through general aspects of the examination ("allergic black eyes") and specific features (sinus tenderness). Psychosocial stresses were clearly important in augmenting the symptoms. Accordingly, management consisted of pharmacotherapy (antibiotic, decongestant, and analgesic) and psychotherapy.

Although this girl's headaches were not part of a migraine syndrome, migraines too may result from a combination of factors (e.g., upper respiratory infection, fatigue, and emotional stress).

Neurologic Causes. The neurologic categories of headache discussed in this section are migraine, increased intracranial pressure (with or without a mass lesion), muscle contraction, head trauma, meningitis, post-lumbar puncture, and seizure.

Migraine headaches are part of a larger group of *vascular headaches* that share the common quality of pounding or throbbing. The pain results from distention of pain-sensitive blood vessels in the scalp and possibly in the meninges as well (see CORRELATION: PHYSIOLOGIC ASPECTS).

Migraine is further defined as a recurrent headache with symptom-free intervals and with a variable set of associated clinical features, which would include several of the following: (1) throbbing pain, (2) neurovegetative disturbance (nausea, vomiting, abdominal pain, pallor), (3) aura, (4) relief by vomiting and/or sleep, (5) unilateral headache pain (hemicrania), (6) transient neurologic deficit, and (7) positive family history (in parents or siblings) (see Table 11–9). Migraine in childhood and adolescence is often, if not usually, bilateral and typically affects the frontal and parietal portions of the head. It may, however, be unilateral as with migraines characteristic of adulthood. Indeed, the English word *migraine* is derived from its Greek equivalent, *hemikrania*. When pain is one-sided, it tends to switch from one side to the other with different episodes of headache. A preference is often established.

Specific migraine syndromes are classic migraine, common migraine, cluster headache, complicated migraine, and migraine equivalents (see Table 11–8). Classic migraine is characterized by an aura, which usually precedes the headache by a few minutes (see Table 11–10). The aura generally lasts from several minutes to a hour. It is often visual and may take the form of sparkling lights (scintillating scotomata), geometric patterns (fortification spectra), perceptual illusions (distortions of objects so that they appear too large or too small, too near or too far away), or blind spots (gray or white areas of "nothingness," or scotomata). Because of difficulty the child may have in describing the aura, he or she should be asked to draw a picture of the visual disturbance (Hachinski *et al.,* 1973). Alternatively, if a scotomatous aura is suggested, the examiner can draw a picture in pencil and the child can erase it accordingly. Paresthesias—numbness or tingling of the nose, lips, tongue, or an entire side of the body—may also precede the headache.

TABLE 11–9. **Clinical Features of Migraine**

Recurrent headaches with at least three of the following:
    aura
    transient neurologic deficit(s)
    unilateral head pain
    throbbing headache
    nausea, vomiting, abdominal pain, pallor
    relief with vomiting and/or sleep
    family history of migraine (parents, siblings)

TABLE 11–10. **Auras of Classic Migraine**

Visual	Scintillating scotomata
	Fortification spectra
	Perceptual distortions
	Blind spots
Other sensory	Paresthesias
Behavior	Hyperactivity
	Withdrawal
Mood	Depression
	Elation
Language	Aphasia (expressive or receptive)
Memory	Forced reminiscence
	Déjà vu

Other auras can involve behavior (hyperactivity), mood (depression, elation), language (aphasia), or memory (forced reminiscence) (see Case 16–2). Particularly in childhood, an aura can occur as an isolated symptom, that is, unassociated with headache.

Common migraine by definition is not preceded by a well-defined aura, although an identifiable prodromal phase may occur first. The headache characteristically begins with mild throbbing that increases in intensity. It is less often unilateral than are the headaches of classical migraine (see Case 11–2).

Cluster headaches are severe vascular headaches occurring in rapid succession over several days to weeks. They are generally associated with conjunctival injection and increased lacrimation on the side of the headache, lasting several hours to days at a time. Cluster headaches occur only rarely in childhood and adolescence.

Complicated migraine includes syndromes of ophthalmoplegic, hemiplegic, confusional, and basilar migraine (Friedman *et al.*, 1962; Gascon and Barlow, 1970; Verret and Steele, 1971; Emery, 1977; Camfield *et al.*, 1978; Ehyai and Fenichel, 1978). With ophthalmoplegic migraine, ptosis suggests myasthenia gravis. If pupillary change occurs as well (the pupil being larger on the affected side), differentiation between ophthalmoplegic migraine and myasthenia gravis is less difficult. In hemiplegic migraine, weakness of one side of the body—which side may alternate from one episode to another—is an accompaniment of the migraine attack. Acute confusional migraine is characterized by episodes of agitation and disorientation lasting several minutes to hours. As headache may not be a prominent feature of the syndrome, the diagnosis is often delayed or missed. Basilar artery migraine can cause vertigo, ataxia, and recurrent loss of consciousness so that differentiation from seizure may be difficult.

CASE 11–2: COMMON MIGRAINE IN A 4-YEAR-OLD BOY

Between 3 and 4 years of age, this otherwise healthy child suffered six severe throbbing headaches. They affected the right forehead, were associated with vomiting and photophobia, and were not relieved by aspirin. After a brief nap, he would awaken headache-free, vigorous, and refreshed. His mother suffered from classic migraines with an aura of left-sided numbness and visual loss. The child's past medical history and development were normal. Examination was entirely unremarkable.

Comment. This boy was felt to have migraine based on the pounding nature of his headache, its association with vomiting, relief following a nap, and positive family history. Specific triggering influences (such as food, allergies, excitement, or intercurrent illness) were not identified. His parents were assigned the task of searching for provocative influences. Symptomatic treatment consisted of age-appropriate doses of aspirin or acetaminophen (4–5 grains every 4 to 6 hours by mouth or, if necessary, by rectum). Chloral hydrate, 250–500 mg orally, was also prescribed to be used as needed for sedation since the child tended to become agitated during his headache, which prevented him from getting to sleep.

The parents had suspected the diagnosis of migraine and were reassured to learn that it was not uncommon in school-age children or unheard-of in younger children. They were further reassured to learn that despite the early onset of migraines, their son was by no means destined to have severe headaches for the rest of his life.

It is of interest that the child experienced unilateral headaches. This feature is relatively uncommon in children, though typical in adults. Of further interest was the child's unusual sensitivity to spinning, which readily made him nauseated. This sensitivity, reflecting the child's autonomic reactivity, may also be manifested as car sickness, found in some 20 per cent of children with migraine. He did not have a history of cyclic vomiting.

Migraine equivalents may take several forms: cyclic vomiting, recurrent vertigo, recurrent abdominal pain (without headache), or seizures ("convulsive migraine").

Increased intracranial pressure is an important cause of headaches in childhood and adolescence. Its causes include hydrocephalus, brain tumor, and pseudotumor cerebri (see Table 11–11). Intracranial pressure is normally determined by the contents of the skull: the brain itself, the cerebrospinal fluid, and the vascular system. Problems involving one or more of these constituents can lead to elevated intracranial pressure associated with headache due to traction on or displacement of pain-sensitive structures.

Headaches associated with increased intracranial pressure have characteristic clinical features (see Tables 11–5 and 11–12). They are usually per-

CASE 11–3: MIGRAINE-LIKE SYNDROME IN AN 11-YEAR-OLD BOY WITH A BRAIN TUMOR

L.Z. was hospitalized because of 2 weeks of severe pounding right-sided supraorbital headaches associated with nausea and vomiting. Previously, headaches had been infrequent and mild. The family history was positive for migraine. He had experienced no recent intercurrent illness. School had been unusually stressful that year. Personality change had not occurred. Upon direct questioning, he acknowledged several episodes of visual loss (a "browning out" of vision) lasting less than 5 seconds.

On examination, the boy was uncomfortable and photophobic. Blood pressure was 104/70, pulse 88. The neck could not be flexed fully to the chest. Submandibular nodes were enlarged and tender. Optic disk margins were sharp temporally, mildly indistinct nasally. Venous pulsations were not evident. The optic papillae were unusually reddened throughout. Deep tendon reflexes were normally active and symmetric. Plantar responses were flexor.

Plain CT scan demonstrated mild ventricular enlargment. After infusion of contrast solution, a spherical mass estimated to be 4 cm in diameter was seen in the posterior fossa (see Figs. 11–3 and 11–4). Nearly total surgical removal of the tumor (a medulloblastoma) was accomplished. Ventriculoperitoneal shunting was not necessary because of the limited degree of hydrocephalus. He received prophylactic radiation to the craniospinal axis and did well for at least the next 10 months.

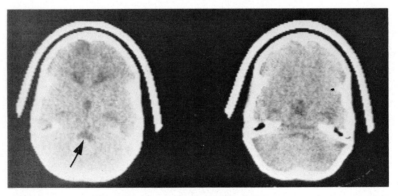

FIGURE 11–3. Plain computerized tomographic (CT) scan showing deformation of fourth ventricle (arrow) from cerebellar tumor (medulloblastoma) (Case 11–3).

Comment. This case illustrates that a clinical picture highly suggestive of migraine does not exclude the possiblity of increased intracranial pressure and brain tumor. The character of the headaches, their unilaterality, their association with nausea and vomiting, their brief course, and a positive family history all supported the diagnosis of migraine.

Clues to the presence of increased intracranial pressure were the history of transient visual obscurations and the mildly abnormal optic disks. With transient visual obscuration, visual loss lasts a few seconds only in contrast to scotomatous auras associated with migraine, which usually last 30 seconds to several minutes.

The optic disk margins themselves were actually within normal limits, for it is normal for the nasal margins to be relatively less distinct than the temporal margins. What was unusual (though not definitely abnormal) was the absence of venous pulsations, which may be absent in some 20 per cent of normal persons and which thus are not a reliable indicator of intracranial hypertension. The color of the optic disks was, however, abnormal. Instead of the characteristic light pink usually seen, the disks were decidedly redder than normal, suggesting vascular engorgement.

This case demonstrates that migraine (like hysteria) does not "immunize" a person from having a brain tumor. Although not everyone with a migraine syndrome should have a CT scan, a careful history and examination (including visualization of the optic disks) is essential. Early diagnosis benefited this child by sparing the need for shunt surgery (see Case 6–4). Furthermore, the tumor was relatively small at the time of operation and thus had less opportunity to invade local structures and to metastasize.

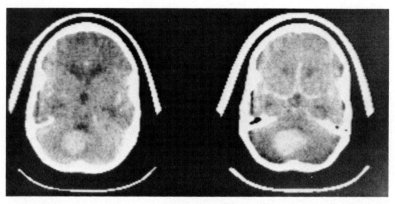

FIGURE 11–4. CT scan after contrast infusion clearly demonstrating the medulloblastoma (Case 11–3).

TABLE 11–11. **Causes of Increased Intracranial Pressure in Relation to Age***

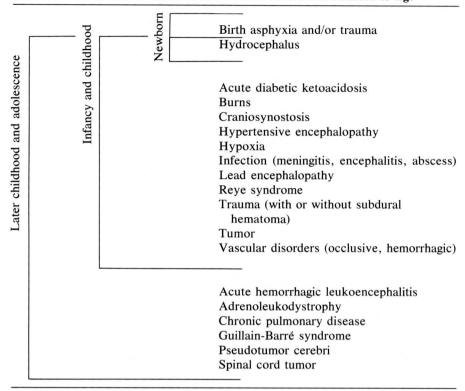

Later childhood and adolescence

Infancy and childhood

Newborn

Birth asphyxia and/or trauma
Hydrocephalus

Acute diabetic ketoacidosis
Burns
Craniosynostosis
Hypertensive encephalopathy
Hypoxia
Infection (meningitis, encephalitis, abscess)
Lead encephalopathy
Reye syndrome
Trauma (with or without subdural
    hematoma)
Tumor
Vascular disorders (occlusive, hemorrhagic)

Acute hemorrhagic leukoencephalitis
Adrenoleukodystrophy
Chronic pulmonary disease
Guillain-Barré syndrome
Pseudotumor cerebri
Spinal cord tumor

* Adapted from Rosman, N. P. Elevated intracranial pressure. In *The Practice of Pediatric Neurology*. Swaiman, K. F., and Wright, F. S., eds. C. V. Mosby Company, Saint Louis, 1975.

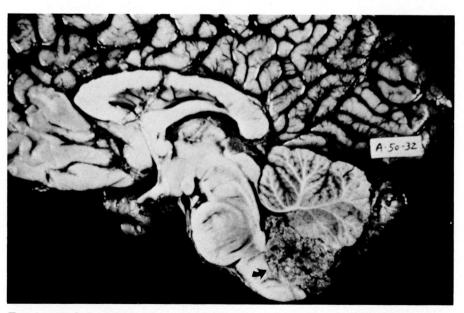

FIGURE 11–5. Lateral section of brain showing medulloblastoma of posterior inferior cerebellum (arrow).

294

TABLE 11–12. **Clinical Features of Increased Intracranial Pressure**

Acutely Elevated

altered mental state
vomiting
strabismus (CN VI, III palsies); "setting sun" sign
altered vital signs ($\uparrow$ BP, $\downarrow$ P, $\downarrow$ R)
(signs of herniation)

full fontanelle	headache
separated sutures	papilledema
(macrocrania)	
(papilledema)	
Infants	*Children*

Both

Chronically Elevated

altered mental state
vomiting
strabismus (CN VI, III palsies); "setting sun" sign

macrocrania	headache
delayed fontanelle closure	papilledema
separated sutures	macrocrania
(failure to thrive)	unfused sutures
(increased transillumination)	[open fontanelle(s)]
Infants	*Children*

Both

sistent (though not invariably so) and tend to be worsened by mechanical stimulation (such as shaking the head, coughing, or straining upon defecation). They are often present upon awakening and may be associated with forceful vomiting that occurs without antecedent nausea. Such headaches, however, may not be especially severe. Transient visual obscurations are a valuable indicator of increased intracranial pressure (see Case 11–3).

Brain tumor refers to an abnormal and excessive growth of brain tissue. It usually is circumscribed and consists of neural, vascular, and/or glial elements. The location of the tumor and its size, rather than its invasiveness or potential for metastatic spread, generally will determine its symptomatology (see Fig. 11–5). Obstruction of cerebrospinal fluid (CSF) pathways causing hydrocephalus is common in childhood, as some two-thirds of brain tumors in the pediatric age range lie in the posterior fossa in or adjacent to the midline (see Fig. 11–6). Since this area of brain is relatively "silent," symptoms

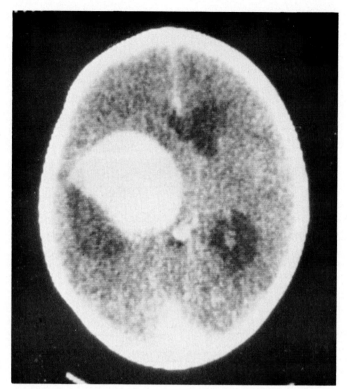

FIGURE 11–6. Computerized tomographic (CT) scan with contrast showing left cerebral mass with hydrocephalus.

typically develop slowly, insidiously, and often nonspecifically. They may be manifested solely by clumsiness of gait, irritability, poor concentration, diminished school achievement, and headaches. Specific areas of dysfunction (such as loss of vision), hypothalamic disturbances (disordered appetite, impaired temperature control, diabetes insipidus, or amenorrhea), or seizures (focal or generalized) also can result.

Hydrocephalus can occur from other causes as well. These include aqueductal stenosis, intracranial hemorrhage due to trauma or vascular malformation, and purulent meningitis. With aqueductal stenosis, the cerebral aqueduct, which connects the third and fourth ventricles, is smaller than usual. Symptoms of obstruction can occur at any time from infancy to adulthood to produce a syndrome of increased intracranial pressure. The cause of decompensation within the CSF system in a person with congenital aqueductal stenosis may not be specifically identifiable.

Head trauma or bleeding from a vascular malformation may lead to hydrocephalus. Blood within the subarachnoid space can become organized to impede flow and absorption of CSF. Purulent meningitis due to such organisms as *S. pneumoniae*, *H. influenzae*, or *M. tuberculosis* can cause hydrocephalus because of inflammatory exudate at the base of the brain that blocks the passage of CSF from the ventricular system to the surrounding subarachnoid space, thereby impeding its resorption (see CORRELATION: PHYSIOLOGIC ASPECTS).

Pseudotumor cerebri is discussed in the section on TOXIC CAUSES.

Muscle contraction headaches, so-called tension headaches, are probably less common in children than in adults. They nonetheless should be considered as a cause of headaches in childhood and adolescence. The pain is characteristically aching or pressing and affects the head in a viselike or bandlike manner. When the discomfort is pounding, a coexisting migraine syndrome should be suspected.

Such headaches result from sustained contraction of neck and scalp muscles affecting pain-sensitive nerve fibers, blood vessels, and muscle itself. They may be the result of intense concentration (as at school) or stress due to a variety of causes. Headaches attributed to "eye strain" are more likely to be due to muscle contraction than to eye problems *per se*, for squinting because of refractive error or strabismus may produce a muscle contraction headache.

Headache often occurs as a consequence of *head trauma*. Pain may be localized to the site of injury or may be generalized. Relatively insignificant head trauma may precipitate an episode of migraine. If this migraine is the child's first, then the head trauma may be blamed unjustifiably for causing the child's migraine condition.

Headache may be part of more serious syndromes of head injury as well, such as *acute epidural hematoma* or *acute subdural hematoma.* These forms of acute intracranial hemorrhage are marked by diminished level of consciousness and other signs of increased intracranial pressure. Loss of consciousness need not have occurred at the time of head injury, and focal neurologic findings may be absent. Diagnosis is established by the clinical course and confirmed, whenever possible, by radiologic studies. With acute epidural hematoma, plain skull x-rays may demonstrate fracture of the temporal bone associated with laceration of the middle meningeal artery. CT scan typically shows a lens-shaped area of blood density within the cranium with acute epidural hematoma, a crescentic outline with acute subdural hematoma. These patterns are not, however, definitively diagnostic of one form of acute intracranial hemorrhage versus the other (see Cases 11–4 and 11–5).

Later complications of head trauma include hydrocephalus (see p. 296), *chronic subdural hematoma,* and *postconcussion syndrome.* Chronic subdural hematoma is manifested by signs and symptoms of chronically raised intracranial pressure. These include irritability, abnormally rapid head growth, and delayed closure of the anterior fontanelle. Plain CT scan may fail to show a subdural mass, particularly if the hematoma is bilateral, because breakdown of extravasated intracranial blood leads to decrease in radiographic density. CT scan with contrast, radioisotope brain scan, electroencephalogram, and arteriogram may be of further diagnostic assistance.

Following cerebral concussion, several days to months of a postconcussion syndrome may ensue. Symptoms may include headache, difficulty in concentrating, postural vertigo ("dizziness"), anxiety, insomnia, and other features of depression. Chronic changes in brain, emotional upset, and litiga-

CASE 11–4: INTRACRANIAL HEMORRHAGE FOLLOWING HEAD TRAUMA IN A 14-YEAR-OLD BOY

J.M. was struck on the right occiput with a board without loss of consciousness in the early evening. After a scalp laceration was sutured in the hospital emergency room, he was sent home. He slept less well than usual that night because of pain associated with the laceration but was otherwise well until early next afternoon, when he developed a bifrontal pounding headache. Over the next several hours he vomited three times and became drowsy before his usual bedtime, which prompted his mother to bring him back to the hospital.

On examination, the boy was lethargic though easily arousable. He tended to return to sleep when not stimulated. Pulse was 100 per minute, blood pressure 128/64, and respirations 16 per minute and regular. Funduscopic examination disclosed early papilledema. Pupils were equal and reactive to light. Tone and deep tendon reflexes were increased on the left side, and a left Babinski sign was present.

Because of the left-sided pyramidal signs, early papilledema, and altered mental state, a right-sided intracranial hemorrhage was suspected. An emergency CT scan of the head was obtained while a neurosurgeon was contacted. The scan showed a lens-shaped mass consistent with a right-sided epidural hematoma. A hemorrhagic clot was surgically removed from the epidural space that evening. Recovery from surgery was uneventful. He was fully alert within 2 days. Papilledema and hyperreflexia resolved completely within several weeks.

Comment. This case illustrates several important points about epidural hematoma in particular and childhood head trauma in general. Though epidural hematoma generally poses a more acute threat to life than subdural hematoma (because blood is usually arterial in origin and accumulates more rapidly), the patient who is promptly diagnosed and treated will generally do well as did this boy, who suffered no permanent neurologic sequelae. Subdural hematoma, by contrast, usually involves less risk to life than epidural hematoma but an increased chance of permanent impairment. This morbidity is usually due to brain contusion underlying the subdural hematoma.

Although epidural and subdural hemorrhages are often acute complications of head trauma (occurring within minutes to a few hours afterward), this case demonstrates that 12 to 24 hours may elapse before symptoms of increased intracranial pressure occur. Routine "overnight" observation following head injury therefore may not be adequate, and a full day's observation in hospital may be justified if not unequivocally indicated.

tion related to the head injury have each been linked etiologically to the postconcussion syndrome.

Other neurologic causes for headache are *meningitis, lumbar puncture,* and *seizures.* Meningitis refers to inflammation of the meninges, most com-

CASE 11–5: INTRACRANIAL HEMORRHAGE IN A 7-YEAR-OLD GIRL

F.S., a previously healthy child, suddenly screamed while playing and complained of headache. Her mother had difficulty in keeping her awake. There was no history of head trauma, seizure disorder, or blood disease. On examination, the child was drowsy but arousable. Blood pressure was normal. Pulse rate was 56. Her head showed no evidence for trauma. Neck was rigid upon attempted passive flexion. Pupils were normal in size and reaction to light. Optic disks were flat. Preretinal hemorrhages were seen in the right eye. Lumbar puncture yielded frankly bloody cerebrospinal fluid. She was treated supportively over the next several hours when she had a generalized convulsion and suffered cardiac arrest, which did not respond to resuscitative measures. At postmortem examination, a vascular malformation that had bled into the brain and subarachnoid space was identified within the right temporal lobe.

Comment. This case illustrates, among other things, that "strokes" (cerebrovascular accidents) can and do occur in childhood, though usually not with this outcome (see Case 21–4). Other vascular accidents are ischemic, associated with death of cerebral tissue due to diminished blood flow, rather than hemorrhagic, as occurred here.

In this instance the patient had an unsuspected vascular malformation that bled into the brain and subarachnoid space. The subarachnoid bleeding resulted in intense headache and neck stiffness (meningismus). The hemorrhage into brain was of sufficient magnitude that it acted as a mass lesion, producing signs of increased intracranial pressure (bradycardia and retinal hemorrhages), irreversible brain damage, and ultimately death (see CORRELATION: PHYSIOLOGIC ASPECTS).

Vascular malformations are often asymptomatic. They are present since before birth in most instances and usually cause no problems whatsoever. On the other hand, they may serve as a seizure focus or may bleed into the subarachnoid space or brain to cause a stiff neck, severe headache, or signs of intracranial hypertension. CT scan (with contrast enhancement) or radioisotope brain scan will usually disclose the presence of a significant vascular malformation. Occasionally an arteriovenous malformation may be associated with such increased cerebral blood flow that the physician (with a stethoscope) or even the patient himself may hear a hum, bruit, or machinery-like sound within the cranium, especially over the eyes. Hydrocephalus may be a late complication of associated hemorrhage.

monly due to infectious agents (viruses or bacteria) (see Fig. 11–7). The clinical course is variable but consists generally of headache, photophobia, vomiting, and stiff neck. Diagnosis is made definitively by examination and culture of cerebrospinal fluid.

Headaches lasting several days may result from lumbar puncture itself

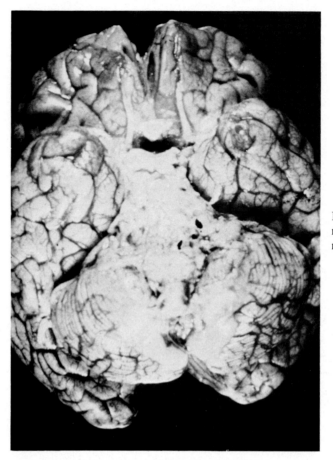

FIGURE 11–7. Basal meningitis due to pneumococcus.

(though with certain forms of increased intracranial pressure, lumbar puncture may be of symptomatic benefit). Leakage from the site of lumbar puncture following the procedure is thought to be the cause of such headaches rather than the relatively small amount of fluid removed for investigation. This loss of fluid apparently results in diminished support for the brain, causing traction on pain-sensitive brain coverings as the brain is displaced downward.

The mechanism for headaches following some seizures is unclear. It may be linked with a generalized hyperdynamic state such as occurs in some systemic illnesses and with fever. Headache as an ictal (rather than postictal) manifestation is characterized by the sudden onset of throbbing head pain. Differentiation from migraine may be difficult, although the diagnosis of seizure headache can generally be reached on the basis of clinical features such as precipitating factors (or their absence), family history, and electroencephalographic findings. It has been suggested that discharge of a temporal lobe seizure focus to vasoregulatory centers of the nearby hypothalamus accounts for the migraine-like symptomatology (Swaiman and Frank, 1978) (see CORRELATION: PHYSIOLOGIC ASPECTS) (see Case 11–6).

CASE 11–6: MIGRAINE AND CONVULSIVE ELECTROENCEPHALOGRAM IN A 9-YEAR-OLD BOY

J.L. suffered from "pounding headaches" affecting his left temple. Headaches began suddenly and were preceded by an increase in his baseline level of hyperactivity. They were accompanied by nausea without vomiting. Headaches occurred nearly daily for 2 months and were benefited by aspirin and rest. Mother and an uncle suffered from migraine. Past history included oculogyric crises of unknown cause, which the child had experienced since the age of 18 months. Social history was notable for parents' divorce, mother's remarriage, and a recent move within the preceding 2 years.

On examination, the child was hyperactive and inattentive. He was able to repeat five digits forward. Academic skills were 1 to 2 years below age level. General physical and neurologic examinations were unremarkable. EEG was markedly abnormal with 1–2 second bursts of generalized high-amplitude polyspike and slow wave discharges unassociated with clinical seizures. He was placed on phenytoin (50 mg three times daily) with complete resolution of headaches. Hyperactivity has remained the same.

Comment. Although phenytoin is not a first-line drug in treatment of migraine, it was used here because of the abnormal EEG. An EEG was obtained primarily because of the frequency of headaches and the history of episodic neurologic disorder (oculogyric crises). In general, an electroencephalogram is not needed in the evaluation of childhood migraine unless features suggest a seizure disorder or prophylactic anticonvulsant therapy is being considered.

Toxic Causes. Pseudotumor cerebri (benign intracranial hypertension) is an important cause of headache in childhood and adolescence (see Table 11–13). The CT scan is invaluable in distinguishing it among the causes of increased intracranial pressure as it characteristically shows ventricles that are diminished in size if they are evident at all. Clinically, pseudotumor cerebri is typified by the usual signs of chronically raised intracranial pressure except that the affected child is alert (see Case 11–7).

The pathophysiologic basis for pseudotumor has not been fully elucidated. It appears to involve brain swelling, interference with circulation and absorption of cerebrospinal fluid, and an increase in the size of the intracranial vascular compartment.

Many agents can cause pseudotumor cerebri. Excessive amounts of vitamin A can mimic closely the clinical features of brain tumor. Birth control pills and tetracyclines (especially those that are out of date) also can cause pseudotumor cerebri. Refeeding a malnourished child can raise intracranial pressure to the extent of splitting cranial sutures (which can be seen on skull x-rays). This result has been attributed to excessively rapid brain growth outstripping skull growth, associated with increased protein synthesis. Corticosteroid therapy (or its withdrawal) has also been associated with benign

CASE 11–7: PSEUDOTUMOR CEREBRI OF UNKNOWN CAUSE IN A 7-YEAR-OLD BOY

K.T. was evaluated because of recurrent headaches and vomiting for 1 month. He had a past history of ear infections but had recently been in excellent health. Vomiting preceded or accompanied the headaches. Otherwise no warning symptoms occurred. Headaches affected the left temporal region or the entire forehead and were described as "knifelike." They occurred once or twice daily and generally lasted an hour. Pain was alleviated somewhat by lying down in a quiet room and taking acetaminophen. For the week prior to the current evaluation, headache was continuous. He denied visual obscurations. Family history was noteworthy for migraine headaches in a maternal uncle and grandmother.

On examination, the boy was an alert, cooperative child who appeared healthy. Vital signs and head circumference were normal. Funduscopic examination disclosed tortuosity of the veins in the right eye and vascular engorgement in the left. There was blurring of the medial margins of both optic disks, particularly the left, which also was elevated. Venous pulsations were evident on the right, though were equivocal on the left. On motor examination, diminished swinging movements of the left arm occurred with walking. No drift, change in tone, or weakness was detected. Deep tendon reflexes were normal. The right plantar response was normal, the left equivocal.

A CT scan with and without infusion of contrast solution was normal. A lumbar puncture was performed. Opening pressure was 370 mm H_2O. Sufficient fluid was removed to lower the pressure to one-half that level. Complete blood count, serum electrolytes, liver function tests, and lead level all

intracranial hypertension. Obesity alone, especially in (pre)adolescent girls, may be the only apparent cause.

In susceptible individuals, reactions to foods or food additives may be manifested as severe, throbbing headaches. Among offending agents are cheese, chocolate, wine or other alcoholic beverages, monosodium glutamate (as in Chinese food), and foods containing nitrites or nitrates such as bologna, sausage, or hot dogs (see CORRELATION: PHYSIOLOGIC ASPECTS).

Other toxic causes of headache include lead encephalopathy (manifested by headache, drowsiness, and seizures), hypoxia (as in altitude sickness, manifested by a severe, pounding headache), and carbon monoxide poisoning. Withdrawal from caffeine-containing beverages (particularly coffee) can itself produce several days of a vascular headache.

Psychologic Causes.   Headache may be part of an affective syndrome involving depression or anxiety (Ling *et al.*, 1970) (see Chapter 6). Anxiety may be associated with muscle-contraction headaches or with amplification of normal sensations occurring about the head and neck (see Case 11–8).

Headaches may also occur on a psychophysiologic basis, providing the

were normal. The day after lumbar puncture, headaches were gone; but they recurred soon thereafter. He was treated initially with acetazolamide (Diamox) and furosemide (Lasix), but repeat lumbar punctures disclosed return of cerebrospinal fluid (CSF) pressure to previous elevated levels. Therefore, lumbar puncture was carried out one or twice weekly with withdrawal of sufficient fluid to lower the CSF pressure to normal. Because CSF pressures remained elevated, corticosteroids were begun. Follow-up ophthalmologic examinations disclosed no abnormalities of blind spots, peripheral visual fields or visual acuity. He continued to experience headaches intermittently, although they became less frequent and less severe.

Comment. The persistence of headaches in this boy, their association with vomiting, and the abnormalities on funduscopic examination suggested increased intracranial pressure. The left-sided arm drift and equivocal plantar response on that side hinted at a lesion of the right hemisphere. The presence of an intracranial mass, a definite consideration in this child, was excluded by the CT scan (carried out with contrast enhancement). The ventricles were not enlarged, which served to exclude the presence of hydrocephalus and confirm the diagnosis of pseudotumor cerebri.

As indicated above, management consisted of pharmacotherapy, periodic monitoring of CSF pressure, and regular neuro-ophthalmologic follow-up to prevent perhaps the most serious complication of pseudotumor: loss of visual acuity associated with optic atrophy that can result from chronically raised intracranial pressure. In cases refractory to the measures detailed above, additional medical treatment (such as glycerol) or surgical therapy (such as lumboperitoneal shunting) may become necessary before satisfactory reduction in intracranial pressure can be achieved.

child and family with a somatic focus that allows for (continued) conflict avoidance.

Social-Environmental Causes. Noise and overstimulation can also cause or contribute to headaches in childhood, particularly when a child has a coexisting attention deficit disorder.

TREATMENT AND OUTCOME

The treatment of headache will vary occording to the identified cause or causes (see Table 11–14). The therapy for migraine exemplifies the multifaceted approach to treatment that usually is most beneficial for the child. For example, management will often involve prevention of migraine by identification and avoidance of offending foods and other triggering environmental agents; use of techniques of rest, relaxation, and meditation; employment of mechanical measures such as massage to the affected portions of the head; administration of age-appropriate doses of analgesics; and consideration of prophylactic medication in an attempt to prevent future attacks.

TABLE 11–13. Causes of **Pseudotumor Cerebri***

Drug	Elevated Cerebrospinal Fluid Protein	Extracerebral Infection	Metabolic-Endocrine
Antibiotics (tetracycline, nalidixic acid, sulfonamides, penicillin, nitrofurantoin, gentamicin)	Guillain-Barré syndrome	Bronchitis	Adrenal insufficiency
Contraceptives (oral)	Poliomyelitis	Exanthems (measles, roseola, varicella)	"Catch-up" growth following malnutrition
Pesticide (chlordecone)	Spinal cord tumor	Gastroenteritis	Galactokinase deficiency
Phenothiazines		Influenza	Galactosemia
Steroids and steroid withdrawal		Mastoiditis	Hyperadrenalism
Vitamin A		Otitis media	Hyperthyroidism
		Pharyngitis	Hypoparathyroidism
		Sinusitis	Hypophosphatasia
		Tonsillitis	Obesity
		Urinary tract infection	Vitamin A excess or deficiency

Physiologic	Systemic	Trauma	Venous Abnormality
Galactorrhea	"Allergic"	Head injury with(out) skull fracture and/or intracranial venous thrombosis	Intracranial venous hypertension
Menarche	Behçet disease		Thrombosis of intracranial sinuses
Menstrual dysfunction	Histiocytosis X		
Pregnancy	Infectious mononucleosis		
	Iron deficiency anemia		
	Leukemia		
	Polycythemia vera		
	Sydenham chorea		
	Systemic lupus erythematosus		
	Wiskott-Aldrich syndrome		

* Adapted from Rosman, N. P. Elevated intracranial pressure. In *The Practice of Pediatric Neurology*. Swaiman, K. F., and Wright, F. S., eds. C. V. Mosby Company, Saint Louis, 1975.

CASE 11–8: ANXIETY DISORDER WITH HEADACHES IN A 10-YEAR-OLD BOY

C.L. was referred for evaluation because of "continuous headaches for 2 weeks." Headaches affected the right or left temple and were aching in quality. The pain was not preceded by an aura. It built up gradually in intensity, remained at a plateau for an hour, then tapered off. Aspirin and rest were of symptomatic benefit. Headaches occurred on weekdays as well as weekends an average of two or three times daily. They did not interfere with school attendance or performance. They had increased in frequency and intensity during a recent school vacation.

Mother described her son as a "worrier," particularly when he was alone and not distracted by his friends. He recently had questioned her about brain tumors, heart attacks, and going blind. Despite her explanations and attempted reassurance, he had not been reassured and continued to ask the same or related questions. For 2 weeks, he had been weepy and less involved than usual in his favorite activities. He had not experienced weight change or sleep disturbance. Past history and family history were unremarkable. No psychosocial stresses were identified.

On examination, the boy was a pleasant, alert, and anxious youngster who readily acknowledged his worries. Pulse rate was 72. The thyroid gland was not enlarged. Neurologic examination showed brisk knee and ankle jerks. Plantar responses were flexor.

Comment. This child's headaches appeared to be part of an affective disorder in which the most prominent symptom was pervasive anxiety, which interfered significantly with his activity and well-being. He manifested some depressive symptoms as well. The causes of his affective disorder were not clear, and psychiatric diagnostic evaluation was recommended. Symptomatic treatment of headaches and investigation were kept to a minimum. In fact, no investigations were pursued since the child had no evidence for hyperthyroidism, hypocalcemia, hypoglycemia, pheochromocytoma, or other organic disorder.

With other headache syndromes as with migraine, drugs should not be the sole means of therapy, particularly when emotional factors (primary or secondary) play a significant role.

Medical Management. The medical treatment of sinusitis will usually include antibiotic therapy (erythromycin or one of the penicillins), an antihistamine or decongestant, and an analgesic agent such as aspirin or acetaminophen. Antibiotics are usually taken for 10 to 14 days, antihistamines or decongestants for 2 to 3 weeks. Preventive measures might include identification of offending substances (such as feather pillows or dust) and steps to rid the environment of these agents.

When fever causes or contributes to a headache (often of the pounding, vascular type), use of standard antipyretic medications such as aspirin or ac-

TABLE 11–14. **Treatment of Headaches**

Medical	For sinusitis: antibiotics, antihistamines, decongestants, analgesics, removal of environmental allergens For fever: antipyretics, tepid bathing For high blood pressure: antihypertensive medication, salt restriction For systemic illness: treatment of pneumonia, asthma, urinary tract infection General measures: rest, relaxation, massage, local warmth or cool compress
Neurologic	Analgesia: aspirin, acetaminophen (Tylenol), codeine Antiemetic: phenothiazine Sedative: chloral hydrate Ergot alkaloid: for classic migraine Prophylaxis of migraine: phenobarbital, phenytoin (Dilantin), propranolol (Inderal), amitriptyline (Elavil), methysergide (Sansert) Avoidance of provocative food substances (such as nitrates) and environmental agents (such as feather pillows) Pseudotumor cerebri: acetazolamide (Diamox), furosemide (Lasix), ethacrynic acid; steroids; weight reduction
Surgical	Ventriculoperitoneal shunting for hydrocephalus Removal of mass lesion (may be combined with radiotherapy, chemotherapy) Removal of intracranial hemorrhage (epidural, subdural) Lumboperitoneal shunt, decompressive craniectomy for pseudotumor cerebri
Psychologic	Individual and/or family therapy
Social-Environmental	"Allergy-proofing" home (especially bedroom)
Mechanical	Massage Repeated lumbar puncture Biofeedback

etaminophen will usually be helpful, particularly when combined with rest, relaxation, and gentle massage to the scalp. The dosage is 5 grains (equivalent to one adult aspirin) for the younger school-age child, $7\frac{1}{2}$ to 10 grains ($1\frac{1}{2}$ to 2 adult aspirins) for the older child, and 10 grains (2 adult aspirins, a full adult dose) for the adolescent. Medication can be taken as needed every 4 to 6 hours.

High blood pressure, even if asymptomatic, should be treated regardless of whether a specific cause has been identified. Standard agents include methyldopa (Aldomet), propranolol (Inderal), and hydralazine (Apresoline).

Systemic illness such as pneumonia, asthma, or urinary tract infection should be treated specifically as well as symptomatically.

Neurologic Management. Treatment of migraine will depend upon its etiology and severity. Migraine occurs in susceptible persons due to one or more of the following: intercurrent illness (particularly upper respiratory infection), emotional stress (situational or developmental), allergy (such as to pollen or to food), constitutional stress (such as hunger, fatigue, or intense exercise). A wide variety of preventive and therapeutic measures thus are possible (see Table 11–15). (It is accordingly inappropriate to place a child on an ergot-containing preparation just because the diagnosis of migraine has been made. Used indiscriminately, ergot preparations probably contribute more to symptomatology than to relief.)

Mild analgesics such as aspirin or acetaminophen in age-appropriate doses are the drugs of choice for most migraine syndromes in childhood. If further analgesia is required, small amounts of codeine (15 to 30 mg by mouth) may be helpful. Prevention of vomiting is not necessarily desirable, since after one or two brief episodes the child almost always feels better. With protracted vomiting (which may extend to the point of dehydration), however, a phenothiazine antiemetic (such as chlorpromazine, 25 mg) can be given per rectum. Mild sedation with chloral hydrate may help an agitated child in obtaining a restorative nap. In cases with a well-defined aura, an ergot-containing compound such as ergotamine taken orally or sublingually can abort the headache phase of the episode. (A trial of biofeedback or, more simply, relaxation at the time of the aura might be employed before

TABLE 11–15. **Treatment of Childhood Migraine**

Categories	Examples
Acute	
analgesics	aspirin
antiemetics	chlorpromazine (Thorazine)
ergot alkaloids	ergotamine tartrate
sedative	chloral hydrate
Prophylactic	
remove "triggering event"	external, physiologic, psychologic
dietary restriction	nitrates
sedatives	phenobarbital
anticonvulsants	phenytoin (Dilantin)
beta-adrenergic blockers	propranolol (Inderal)
antidepressants	amitryptyline (Elavil), phenelzine (Nardil)
platelet antagonists	aspirin
antihistamines	cyproheptadine (Periactin)
prostaglandin antagonists	flufenamic acid
alpha-adrenergic blockers	clonidine (Catapres)
serotonin antagonists	methysergide (Sansert)
biofeedback	temperature control

ergot alkaloids are begun.) Ergot preparations are contraindicated in complicated migraine because their vasoconstrictive effect may convert a transient neurologic deficit into a permanent one.

When migraines are so frequent and intense that they interfere significantly with the child's performance at school or at home, chronic prophylactic medication should be considered. Phenobarbital in anticonvulsant dosage (4–6 mg/kg/day orally), phenytoin (Dilantin), propranolol (Inderal), or amitriptyline (Elavil) may be therapeutic. Only rarely should methysergide (Sansert), a serotonin antagonist, be used chronically in treatment of childhood migraine because of associated complications of its use that include retroperitoneal fibrosis. A listing of these and other prophylactic treatments of childhood migraine is presented in Table 11–15.

These pharmacologic measures should be employed in conjunction with modes of therapy that do not involve drugs. Indeed, relaxation and massage of affected portions of the scalp (with or without the use of a cold compress) may render little or no drug therapy necessary. Preventive measures such as avoiding provocative foods (including chocolate, nuts, or nitrite-containing items) or environmental irritants (e.g., feather pillows or dust) may prevent migraines altogether.

Because many parents know migraine only in its severe, relatively disabling form in adulthood, they may be surprised and concerned that their child has been diagnosed as having a migraine syndrome. The outlook for the child with migraine is, however, generally favorable. At least 10 per cent of all children will experience a migraine episode in childhood, not necessarily severe or recurrent, and parents can be reassured that most children will outgrow the problem.

With pseudotumor cerebri, specific therapy is indicated when a specific cause such as extreme obesity or vitamin A poisoning has been identified. Acetazolamide, furosemide, and ethacrynic acid have been used to treat pseudotumor cerebri since they can reduce cerebrospinal fluid production. Corticosteroids have also been employed, and periodic lumbar punctures are often of symptomatic benefit as well as diagnostic usefulness.

Although pseudotumor cerebri has been termed "benign intracranial hypertension," its outcome is not always favorable; prolonged elevation of intracranial pressure can lead to permanent visual loss. Regular follow-up including funduscopic examination, formal charting of visual fields and blind spots (whenever possible), sequential CT scans, and repeated lumbar punctures are indicated.

Post–lumbar puncture headaches ("spinal headaches") will be minimized by having the child maintain the horizontal position as much as possible for 12 to 24 hours following lumbar puncture and by ensuring excellent hydration (which should be achievable by mouth). Headaches may last from several hours to weeks. They should be treated with standard analgesic agents, copious fluids, and reassurance.

Muscle contraction headaches, like migraines, will generally respond to mild analgesia combined with relaxation and mechanical measures described above. An understanding of factors producing "tension" is, of course, important, and psychiatric or psychologic diagnostic evaluation may be helpful. Biofeedback directed toward relaxation of scalp and neck muscles has been effective in some adults (Orne, 1979).

Surgical Management. Hydrocephalus will generally require ventriculoperitoneal shunting to bypass the obstruction, for example, due to aqueductal stenosis. When an intracranial mass has been identified, complete surgical removal is desirable when it can be accomplished without significant damage to nearby brain and vascular tissue. Otherwise, subtotal resection with histologic evaluation of tissue removed at operation will usually be indicated.

Surgical therapy alone appears sufficient for an excellent outcome in children with cerebellar astrocytomas. Medulloblastomas, however, have a poorer (though not uniformly gloomy) outlook. Removal of the tumor is usually subtotal. Additional treatment is given in the form of radiotherapy to the craniospinal axis because of the potential for metastasis. In some centers chemotherapy, otherwise reserved for treatment of remissions or spread, is given initially along with radiation therapy.

Neurosurgery can be lifesaving in the treatment of acute intracranial hemorrhage. With acute epidural hematoma, the outlook for full recovery is excellent if the problem is recognized promptly and the hemorrhage removed without delay. With subdural hematoma death is less likely, but residual damage is more often seen, probably because of associated brain contusion underlying the subdural hematoma.

In cases of pseudotumor not responding to medical treatment, lumboperitoneal shunt, decompression of the optic nerves (to prevent progressive visual loss), and, rarely, decompressive craniectomy may be required.

Psychotherapy. Individual therapy may benefit the school-age child or adolescent with muscle contraction headaches or migraine. Emotional factors such as depression or anxiety can cause or contribute to either headache syndrome. With migraine, anxiety may be lessened by explanation of an associated aura, which can involve upsetting perceptual distortions that may occur independent of headache (see Case 11–9).

Parental or family therapy is indicated when marital stresses contribute significantly to the child's headache syndrome or when the headache syndrome functions like anorexia nervosa or asthma as a psychophysiologic (or psychosomatic) disorder (see Chapter 10).

Social-Environmental Management. The child with migraines needs a quiet, dimly lighted place to retire to as soon as possible during a severe episode. At home such a place should allow for isolation from radio, television, or other commotion. If at school the child should be permitted to go to the nurse's office, where rest should be possible and medication dispensed as indicated.

When a child suffers from recurrent sinus inflammation, allergic factors should be explored and appropriate environmental precautions taken. Such measures might include replacing feather or foam pillows with nonallergenic pillows, wiping dust-catching surfaces daily with a damp cloth, and prohibiting pets (especially cats) from entering the child's bedroom. Such measures may be highly effective even without accompanying pharmacologic treatment.

CASE 11–9: ISOLATED MIGRAINE AURA IN AN 11-YEAR-OLD BOY

L.J., a previously healthy fifth-grader, experienced a peculiar visual distur-bance while suffering from a week-long flu syndrome. Objects that he knew to be distant appeared near, as if he could touch them. "It felt like my bed was on stilts and I could just reach up and touch the ceiling," he said. This illusion lasted 15 to 20 minutes, then went away gradually over a similar pe-riod of time without subsequent headache or abdominal pain. During the next month he had six additional episodes.

Past history was unremarkable. Several family members had migraines. The child had no history of cyclic vomiting or motion sickness. Examination was normal. No investigations were carried out.

These episodes were considered to be of a migrainous nature. Precipi-tated initially by a flulike illness, they persisted despite complete recovery from that illness. Investigation was not pursued because of the benign nature of the episodes and their spontaneous decrease in frequency. Treatment consisted of explanation, reassurance, and mention that the episodes were expected to diminish further in number.

Comment. In this case, the family history of migraine, lack of evidence for seizure disorder, and normalcy of the examination led to the diagnosis of recurrent isolated migraine aura. This child's aura was a visual illusion in-volving a distortion of sensory perception suggesting *Alice in Wonderland.* The associated lack of control and peculiar symptomatology are often upset-ting to an affected child, who may nonetheless wait to tell his parents about the disturbance until long after its onset. Indeed, a child may feel he is losing his mind or "going crazy." For that reason, labeling the process as migraine often has a significant therapeutic effect in itself (see Case 16–2).

It may additionally be reassuring for a worried adolescent (without signs of increased intracranial pressure) to be told specifically that he or she does not have evidence of a brain tumor.

Educational Management.   When learning problems cause chronic stress associated with migraine syndrome or muscle contraction headaches, educa-tional assessment and remediation as indicated should be pursued (see Case 11–10).

Physical Therapy.   Although acute physical activity may cause a mi-graine, 30 to 60 seconds of intense exercise (such as push-ups or sprinting in place) may abort the headache phase of an episode (presumably by stimulat-ing release of the body's own vasoconstrictor substances, including epineph-rine).

When headache is part of a depressive syndrome, regular physical activ-ity may be of symptomatic benefit to mood as well as to headache.

Mechanical Therapy.   Gentle massage of the temples, over the eyes, or at the cervical-occipital junction may be of symptomatic benefit with migraine or muscle-contraction headaches. A cold compress, by causing constriction of scalp blood vessels, may provide additional relief, although with migraine the scalp itself may be tender and the additional pressure may cause increased discomfort.

With pseudotumor cerebri, repeated lumbar puncture (carried out as often as several times weekly) can be considered a form of mechanical therapy.

Biofeedback involving instruments such as electroencephalograph, electromyograph, and plethysmograph is another form of mechanical therapy that appears promising in the treatment of migraine and muscle contraction syndromes (Blanchard *et al.*, 1978; Dikel and Olness, 1980). Changing skin temperature in the fingers by altering blood vessel tone (that is, causing vasoconstriction) has been shown to have the opposite effect in some scalp vessels (vasodilation). This reciprocal relationship has been exploited in treating migraines.

CORRELATION

Anatomic Aspects. Hydrocephalus is a state of excessive cerebrospinal fluid (CSF) intracranially. Colloquially referred to as "water on the brain," it would in most instances be described more accurately as water *in* the brain, for hydrocephalus usually takes the form of enlarged ventricles within the brain substance (see Figs. 2–6 and 2–7).

Hydrocephalus can result in several ways: by blockage of cerebrospinal fluid flow at various places between the sites where it is formed (mostly, the choroid plexuses) up to and including the sites of resorption (mainly, the superior sagittal sinus); by overproduction of CSF; or by loss of brain tissue, permitting the secondary enlargement of CSF-containing compartments (ventricles and subarachnoid space). The last of these three is termed hydrocephalus *ex vacuo*. In contrast to the other two, it is not surgically treatable.

Obstruction to CSF flow can occur at any step along its path. For example, blockage of a single foramen of Monro (such as can occur in tuberous sclerosis) can result in dilatation of a single frontal horn of a lateral ventricle. Both frontal horns may be enlarged with a colloid cyst of the third ventricle that obstructs the foramina of Monro. The third and lateral ventricles may become dilated due to aqueductal stenosis, congenital or acquired. The entire ventricular system—both lateral ventricles, the third ventricle, and the fourth ventricle—may be enlarged secondary to blockage of openings normally permitting outflow of CSF from the fourth ventricle into the subarachnoid cisterns at the base of the brain. These openings are the two foramina of Luschka (lying at the lateral borders of the posterior fourth ventricle) and the unpaired foramen of Magendie (lying in the midline).

When the ventricular system does not communicate freely with the subarachnoid space at the base of the brain, this form of hydrocephalus is designated as "noncommunicating."

Obstruction of CSF flow may occur at more distal levels as well. Having left the fourth ventricle through the foramina of Luschka and Magendie, cerebrospinal fluid travels down into the spinal subarachnoid space, then up again into the subarachnoid cisterns at the base of the brain. From there it

CASE 11–10: MIGRAINE WITH SCHOOL PROBLEMS IN A 6-YEAR-OLD GIRL

C.R., a first-grade student, complained of "headaches and belly aches all the time." Her headaches were squeezing and pounding, lasted 4 to 6 hours, and usually were associated with nausea; less often they were accompanied by vomiting. Headaches affected her above both eyes and were not preceded by a definite aura, though her fingers tingled slightly prior to onset of headache. They occurred once weekly at the beginning of the school year and increased in frequency to three times weekly by midyear. School performance continued to be average or better. She had not missed school because of headaches. They tended to be most severe in the afternoon, when she often needed to lie down rather than play with friends after school. She awakened refreshed from these naps. Other than school, no significant stresses were identified. She had been in excellent health and had undergone no personality change other than "crabbiness" during the headaches.

Past history was essentially normal. Her mother had suffered from throbbing headaches since elementary school that were associated with nausea and vomiting and were preceded by perception of sparkling lights. Family history was negative for seizure disorder. The child had a history of car sickness.

On examination, she was an articulate, energetic youngster who was able to attend well to given tasks. She did not appear anxious or depressed. Conversational skills indicated that she was an unusually intelligent child. Her reading, however, was barely at grade level. It was accomplished with great effort as she pointed to each word individually. She reversed the number 3, recognized her error spontaneously, and corrected it. She spelled "dog" and "boy" correctly, but in so doing commented that she had trouble telling a "b" from a "d."

General physical examination was normal, including measurement of

goes over the convexities of the brain to be absorbed mainly into the superior sagittal sinus through the arachnoid granulations. Scarring from previous subarachnoid infection or hemorrhage, pressure from an overlying chronic subdural fluid collection, or underlying swollen brain can interfere with flow of CSF over the cerebral convexities and its resorption at the level of the arachnoid granulations. Since cerebrospinal fluid has entered the subarachnoid space at the base of the brain from the ventricular system unimpeded, hydrocephalus in these instances is said to be "communicating."

Communicating hydrocephalus can complicate purulent meningitis at any age. It can also result from bleeding into the subarachnoid space. Such hemorrhage typically is seen as a complication of prematurity and as a consequence of head trauma or vascular malformation in later childhood.

In contrast to these obstructive forms of hydrocephalus, it occasionally

blood pressure, palpation of paranasal sinuses, and flexion of the neck. Elemental neurologic examination was normal, including visualization of the optic disks and elicitation of deep tendon reflexes.

Comment. The quality of the headaches, the associated nausea, and the positive family history led to the diagnosis of childhood migraine. The question of what was causing them remained. In this case there was no evidence of allergy, intercurrent illness, or family stresses. She did, however, appear to have an unrecognized learning difficulty that made school a chronically stressful experience for her and contributed importantly to her headache syndrome (see Chapter 17). Although clearly above average in intelligence, she had to work unusually hard to master standard first-grade material. This difficulty led to frustration, exhaustion, and headaches that interfered with her activities and sense of well-being. Her high level of intelligence and motivation had enabled her to carry out her schoolwork satisfactorily despite her learning difficulty. As a result the classroom teacher was not aware of a problem and therefore had not transmitted any concerns to the child's parents.

Treatment was not focused exclusively, or even primarily, on the headaches themselves. The nature of the headaches was explained to the parents as was the probable role of their daughter's learning problems in causing them. The school was requested to carry out speech and language assessment as well as perceptual-motor testing to define further the child's areas of difficulty so that she might receive specific remediation. It was recommended also that she be allowed to complete her assignments at home or that her in-school workload be reduced. Continued symptomatic treatment of headaches with aspirin and rest was advised. Primary follow-up and management were through her pediatrician with neurologic follow-up on a 6-monthly basis so long as it appeared necessary.

can also result from overproduction of cerebrospinal fluid, as with a choroid plexus papilloma.

Biochemical Aspects. Biochemical factors are of unquestioned importance in the pathophysiology of migraine and other vascular headaches. A variety of foods and other dietary substances have been implicated. Some wines, cheeses (especially cheddar), and beers; marinated herring; and chicken liver contain relatively high levels of tyramine, a monoamine that causes release of norepinephrine at nerve terminals. For that reason, tyramine-containing foods are prohibited in persons (usually adults) taking monoamine oxidase-inhibiting drugs, since hypertensive crises can result as a consequence of tyramine-induced norepinephrine excess. Individual differences in tyramine metabolism have been suggested to underlie food susceptibility in some persons with migraine (Bruyn, 1980).

Chocolate can cause or contribute to headaches because it contains large amounts of phenylethylamine. It, too, is a monoamine closely related to tyramine and, therefore, to norepinephrine, epinephrine, and dopamine (see Fig. 14–2). Hot dogs and other reddened meats (such as bologna and most hams) contain nitrites and nitrates that act as vasodilators (like nitroglycerin, which promotes coronary artery vasodilation). Chinese food has been implicated in causing vascular headaches because of large amounts of monosodium glutamate, which is used as a flavor enhancer. Spoiled fish (particularly mackerel and others of the scombroid family) can cause a clinical picture of histamine toxicity (scombroid poisoning) that includes a throbbing headache and facial flushing due to elevated levels of histamine in the fish.

Serotonin, which produces constriction of extracranial and some intracranial arteries (and dilation of skin capillaries), appears to play an important though confusing role in the causation of migraine (Diamond and Medina, 1980). As evidence of this role, it has been found at the onset of a migraine attack that the serotonin level in blood (some 98 per cent of it contained in platelets) drops markedly, while urinary 5-HIAA (5-hydroxyindole acetic acid, the major metabolic product of serotonin) is increased (Bruyn, 1980). Amitriptyline, which blocks the reuptake of serotonin (hence, elevates its blood level) has been of preventive value in adults with migraine (Couch and Hassanein, 1979).

Other biochemical agents suggested as having a significant role in migraine include the prostaglandins and plasma kinins. Originally identified in human seminal fluid, prostaglandins are a group of 20-carbon fatty acids synthesized widely and found throughout the body. They have an extraordinary diversity of actions in man. Experimentally, it has been demonstrated that injection of prostaglandin PGE_1 can produce a migraine syndrome (Bruyn, 1980). Plasma kinins are a family of vasodilator peptides (including bradykinin and substance P). Some of them appear to mediate pain and other elements of an inflammatory response (Bruyn, 1980; Cooper and Martin, 1980).

Physiologic Aspects. Migraine is a disorder of the autonomic nervous system. Indeed, it appears to represent an autonomic storm, complete in many instances with premonitory lightning (visual disturbance) and thunder (pounding headache). Not surprisingly, the hypothalamus has been implicated as playing a major role. Bruyn (1980) has likened the hypothalamus to the eye of a hurricane, lying as it does at the crossroad of vegetative, affective, and behavioral functions.

Vascular events, presumably under hypothalamic influence, are of major importance in the genesis and symptomatology of migraine. With classical migraine, it has been proposed that a vasoconstrictive phase affecting both intracranial and extracranial blood vessels causes the aura (Diamond and Medina, 1980). An observant parent will often be able to recognize this stage and predict the onset of a migraine headache because of the child's appearance (very pale) or feel (hands cool to the touch). Vasoconstriction is followed by a phase of vasodilation (perhaps a secondary or rebound phenomenon) accounting for the characteristic pounding headache usually attributed to painful pulsation of extracranial (scalp) vessels.

Alternatively, vasomotor instability of the meningeal circulation has been proposed as the pathophysiologic basis for migraine (Blau, 1978). Blau has suggested that the aura results from vasoconstriction of meningeal vessels penetrating through to the cerebral cortex and that the ensuing headache results from stimulation of pain-sensitive nerve endings in the walls of meningeal vessels that are presumed to be secondarily dilated. Among the evidence cited for this hypothesis is the overlap in clinical features between the headaches of migraine and meningitis and the increase in headache severity that occurs with mechanical jolts.

Blau and others have raised the possibility that some persons with migraine are primarily vasoconstrictors, whereas others are primarily vasodilators. Perhaps this explanation can account for differences between classical and common migraine and the prophylactic efficacy of methysergide and amitriptyline despite their opposite effects on scalp blood vessels.

SUMMARY

Headaches in childhood must always be taken seriously whether the cause is medical, neurologic, psychologic, or a combination of these. Major causes of headache in childhood and adolescence are systemic illness, sinusitis, migraine, affective disturbance, and increased intracranial pressure (including hydrocephalus, intracranial mass, and pseudotumor cerebri). Diagnosis can usually be established by careful history-taking to define the character, location, intensity, time course, precipitants, and associated features of the headache. Examination should specifically seek evidence for medical illness, including sinus infection or high blood pressure. Neurologic examination must include careful funduscopic visualization to exclude papilledema. Mental status examination should note depression or anxiety. Investigation will depend upon the clinical circumstances. Testing may include skull x-rays, CT scan, EEG, or lumbar puncture. Psychiatric or psychologic consultation may be valuable. Treatment will depend upon the cause(s) of the headache syndrome. It will usually be multimodal, taking into account all contributing factors, and should not be restricted to treatment with drugs alone.

CITED REFERENCES

Blanchard, E. B.; Theobald, D. E.; Williamson, D. A.; Silver, B. V.; and Brown, D. A. Temperature biofeedback in the treatment of migraine headaches: a controlled evaluation. *Arch. Gen. Psychiatry,* **35:** 581–88, 1978.

Blau, J. N. Migraine: a vasomotor instability of the meningeal circulation. *Lancet,* **2:** 1136–39, 1978.

Bruyn, G. W. The bichemistry of migraine. *Headache,* **20:** 235–46, 1980.

Camfield, P. R.; Metrakos, K.; and Andermann, F. Basilar migraine, seizures, and severe epileptiform EEG abnormalities: a relatively benign syndrome in adolescents. *Neurology,* **28:** 584–88, 1978.

Cooper, P. E., and Martin, J. B. Neuroendocrinology and brain peptides. *Ann. Neurol.,* **8:** 551–57, 1980.

Couch, J. R., and Hassanein, R. S. Amitriptyline in migraine prophylaxis. *Arch. Neurol.,* **36:** 695–99, 1979.

Diamond, S., and Medina, J. L. Review articles: current thoughts on migraine. *Headache*, **20**: 208–12, 1980.

Dikel, W., and Olness, K. Self-hypnosis, biofeedback, and voluntary peripheral temperature control in children. *Pediatrics*, **66**: 335–40, 1980.

Ehyai, A., and Fenichel, G. M. The natural history of acute confusional migraine. *Arch. Neurol.*, **35**: 368–69, 1978.

Emery, E. S., III. Acute confusional state in children with migraine. *Pediatrics*, **60**: 110–14, 1977.

Friedman, A. P.; Harter, D. H.; and Merritt, H. H. Ophthalmoplegic migraine. *Arch. Neurol.*, **7**: 320–27, 1962.

Gascon, G., and Barlow, C. Juvenile migraine, presenting as an acute confusional state. *Pediatrics*, **45**: 628–35, 1970.

Hachinski, V. C.; Porchawka, J.; and Steele, J. C. Visual symptoms in the migraine syndrome. *Neurology* (Minneapolis), **23**: 570–79, 1973.

Ling, W.; Oftedal, G.; and Weinberg, W. Depressive illness in childhood presenting as severe headache. *Am. J. Dis. Child.*, **120**: 122–24, 1970.

Orne, M. T. The efficacy of biofeedback therapy. *Annu. Rev. Med.*, **30**: 489–503, 1979.

Swaiman, K. F., and Frank, Y. Seizure headaches in children. *Dev. Med. Child Neurol.*, **20**: 580–85, 1978.

Verret, S., and Steele, J. C. Alternating hemiplegia in childhood: a report of eight patients with complicated migraine beginning in infancy. *Pediatrics*, **47**: 675–80, 1971.

ADDITIONAL READINGS

Burnstock, G. Pathophysiology of migraine: a new hypothesis. *Lancet*, **1**: 1397–99, 1981.

Dalessio, D. J., ed. *Wolff's Headache and Other Head Pain*, 4th ed. Oxford University Press, New York, 1980.

Lance, J. W. Headache. *Ann. Neurol.*, **10**: 1–10, 1981.

Raskin, N. H. Chemical headaches. *Annu. Rev. Med.*, **32**: 63–71, 1981.

Sacks, O. W. *Migraine: The Evolution of a Common Disorder*. University of California Press, Berkeley, 1970.

12 Seizures and Other Paroxysmal Disorders of Consciousness

The dichotomy of seizure types into "grand mal" and "petit mal" has given way to recognition of varied clinical manifestations of seizures. These may take the form not only of generalized rhythmic movements associated with loss of consciousness but also more subtle kinds of dysfunction in which mental state is less profoundly affected and involuntary movements are absent. Indeed, the child with altered mental state presents a relatively common and often perplexing problem in which the question of seizure justifiably arises. For example, a child with psychomotor seizures manifested as staring spells might be considered mistakenly to be daydreaming or to be depressed.

Not every abnormal behavior of childhood should be viewed as a possible seizure, of course, although essentially *any* behavior (motor, sensory, affective, or perceptual) can itself be a manifestation of seizure. In this chapter these issues will be explored further and several questions addressed specifically:

What is the definition of seizure?
How does *seizure disorder* differ from *epilepsy?*
What are the clinical manifestations of seizures in childhood and adolescence?
What features of the history suggest or define seizure?
What aspects of the examination should specifically be sought?
When should an electroencephalogram be done? Computerized tomography of the head? Other studies?
What conditions should be differentiated from seizures?
What are the causes of seizures?
How should they be treated? Are drugs the only treatment?
What is the outcome of seizures in childhood?

SEIZURES

DEFINITION

Seizure can be defined as an episode of involuntary behavior, often recurrent, that results from abnormal electrical activity of brain. This definition embodies several important concepts. A seizure is a discrete episode of behavioral disturbance usually characterized by a well-defined period of time during which behavior is not under the control of the affected person. As behavior is not limited to visible motor activity, other spheres of activity (such as emotion, thought, and perception) can be involved as well (see Table 12–1). Ultimately, a seizure is the result of sudden and excessive electrical activity of brain and is influenced by anatomic, biochemical, and physiologic factors.

Seizure disorder is defined as more than one seizure within a given time period: infancy, childhood, or adolescence. A girl who has had three seizures between ages 14 and 16 years would thus be said to have a seizure disorder of adolescence. *Epilepsy* is used to denote recurrent seizures. Some would include as part of the definition that seizures must have recurred beyond the age of 7 years. *Convulsion* is used synonymously with motor seizure.

Seizures can be categorized in several different ways. An older classification, alluded to at the beginning of this chapter, begins with grand mal and petit mal seizures. Grand mal seizures are generalized motor convulsions involving a tonic phase (stiffening) followed by a clonic phase (rhythmic jerking). Episodes may be preceded by a warning sensation, or aura. Grand mal seizures are always associated with loss of consciousness and are followed by lethargy. Tongue-biting (not swallowing) and incontinence of urine or feces are often associated. Petit mal seizures are brief (usually 5 to 30 second) episodes of staring and rhythmic blinking that occur without warning. The child has no recall of events during the episode and is able to resume activity promptly when it has ended. Other categories of seizures included in this classification are psychomotor, focal motor, myoclonic, and akinetic.

It must be emphasized that a seizure that is not grand mal is not necessarily petit mal. The latter is a specific syndrome, distinct from other seizure types in etiology, clinical manifestations, EEG pattern, and treatment. Misuse of the term petit mal can often be avoided by employing the descriptive expression *staring spell*. Staring spell can refer to petit mal or psychomotor

---

TABLE 12–1. **Clinical Hallmarks of Seizures**

Loss or alteration of consciousness
Interruption of speech
Involuntary motor activity
Automatisms or other semipurposeful movements
Rhythmic eye-blinking
Incontinence
Tongue-biting
Postictal confusion, somnolence, headache, behavior change

seizures (as well as to episodes of simple daydreaming). These two seizure types can be differentiated in several respects (see Table 12–2). Psychomotor seizures (also called partial complex seizures) may be preceded by an aura (often abdominal discomfort) (see CORRELATION: ANATOMIC ASPECTS). Consciousness is generally altered but not fully lost during a psychomotor seizure. Automatic behaviors are often prominent during the spell; confusion, headache, and sleep usually follow. A difficult birth or significant postnatal head trauma may have occurred previously. Petit mal seizures or absence spells are generally briefer but more frequent than psychomotor seizures. They are associated with only limited automatic behaviors and complete amnesia for events during the seizure. They are not preceded by an aura, nor are they followed by postictal confusional state, headache, or sleepiness.

Seizures can alternatively be divided into two different sorts of categories: partial and generalized. Partial (or focal) seizures involve only a part of the body or a single feature of behavior as a result of a localized cerebral

TABLE 12–2. **Distinctions Between Partial Complex and Absence Seizures**

	Partial Complex (Psychomotor)	Absence (Petit Mal)
Age of onset	Any age	Usually after 3 years
Cause	Often preceded by or associated with perinatal difficulties, febrile seizures, head trauma, vascular malformation, tumor, cerebral dysgenesis	Usually none apparent (idiopathic)
Aura	Often sensory or affective: abdominal discomfort, déjà vu, dreamy feeling	None (may be vague, brief "dizziness")
Duration	Several minutes	Seconds (usually 5–30)
Automatisms	Usually prominent	Few if any
Alteration of consciousness during seizure	Partial	Complete (no awareness)
Postictal confusion, fatigue, headache	Often	Not usually
Frequency	Usually single (several per week or month)	Usually multiple (many per hour or day)
Associated other seizure types	Sometimes	Sometimes
Characteristic EEG pattern	Temporal lobe spikes, slowing; normal	3/sec. spike-and-slow-wave complexes especially with hyperventilation
Provoked by hyperventilation	Occasionally	Typically but not invariably

TABLE 12–3. **International Classification of Epileptic Seizures***

Partial seizures (seizures beginning locally)
    Partial seizures with elementary symptoms generally without impairment of consciousness, for example, focal motor seizures
    Partial seizures with complex symptoms generally with impairment of consciousness, such as temporal lobe or psychomotor seizures
    Partial seizures secondarily generalized
Generalized seizures (bilaterally symmetric and without local onset)
    Absences (petit mal)
    Bilateral massive epileptic myoclonus
    Infantile spasms
    Clonic seizures
    Tonic seizures
    Tonic-clonic seizures (grand mal)
    Atonic seizures
    Akinetic seizures
Unilateral seizures
Unclassified epileptic seizures (because of incomplete data)

---

* Adapted from Gastaut, H. Clinical and electroencephalographical classification of epileptic seizures. *Epilepsia,* **11:** 102–13, 1970.

electrical disturbance. Generalized seizures, by contrast, characteristically involve the entire body and stem from abnormal electrical activity of brain that is widespread. A partial seizure may become secondarily generalized, both electrically and clinically, but it is categorized, nonetheless, as a partial seizure.

Each of these categories, partial and generalized, is further divided into several clinical types. Partial seizures are broken down into those with elementary symptomatology (motor, sensory) and those with complex symptomatology (affect, memory, consciousness, behavior). Episodes of diminished alertness, mumbling speech, and semipurposeful movements would represent a partial seizure with complex symptomatology (a psychomotor seizure according to the older classification). Generalized seizures include tonic-clonic seizures (grand mal, as described above), absence spell (including classic petit mal and its variants), and akinetic and myoclonic seizures.

A more complete classification of seizures, adapted from the International Classification of Epileptic Seizures, is presented in Table 12–3.

DIAGNOSIS

The diagnosis of seizure is ultimately a clinical diagnosis. Examination and investigation (including EEG) often contribute to the diagnosis or, less commonly, establish it. Usually, however, the diagnosis of seizure rests upon the history: direct questioning of the affected child and parents or other person who has witnessed the behavior in question. In evaluating a child suspected of having had a seizure, there is no substitute for careful history-taking.

Clinical Process. *History.*   After a brief period of introductory conversation, the child should be asked why he or she has come for evaluation. For a generalized seizure the child may say, "I fainted in school." The child may complain of "dizzy spells" or "blurriness" in denoting partial seizures, particularly when they involve complex symptomatology such as alteration in perception or consciousness.

The child should be questioned directly as to his or her perception of the event(s) in question. What do you remember? What have others told you about the episode? Where were you when it happened? What were you doing when it began? Did you get any clue or warning that things were not quite right? What do you remember next? Have similar episodes taken place that you haven't told anybody about?

If parents have observed the episodes themselves, they should describe them in detail and not quote teachers or other sources. Focal onset, spread of involuntary behavior, and duration of the seizure should be noted. For example, they might describe a "Jacksonian march" in which rhythmic movements of the fingers of one hand progress to affect the whole extremity, then the entire body (see CORRELATION: ANATOMIC ASPECTS). If the parents can imitate the seizure episode, it will often help in characterizing it. Postictal drowsiness or the ability to resume activity immediately should be noted.

The child's general state of health and well-being should be noted. Has the child been ill recently? With fever? Has the child been unusually fatigued or sleep-deprived recently? Have episodes of head trauma occurred in which the child was knocked out or dazed?

The following symptoms are hallmarks of seizure: loss or alteration of consciousness; involuntary motor activity; incontinence of urine or feces; bodily injury, especially a bitten tongue; speech arrest; automatisms or other semi-purposeful behavior; postictal somnolence, headache, confusion, or other behavior change; rhythmic eye-blinking or staring. With speech arrest, a common feature of partial seizures, the child has a clear or mildy impaired sensorium but is unable to speak despite attempting to do so. The affected child is usually aware of this difficulty and may become anxious because of the sudden loss of language function. Automatisms of behavior can include semipurposeful actions such as buttoning and unbuttoning a shirt, walking in circles, patting the legs, or smacking the lips. Staring, with or without eye-blinking, is not normally interrupted by the examiner's hand waving or other threatening gestures if it occurs on the basis of seizure.

An aura should be sought and characterized. The aura is in fact a focal manifestation of seizure that may become secondarily generalized. It may be sensory (numbness in a hand), olfactory (burning rubber), mnestic (a frightening memory), or affective (gloom, feeling "on top of the world," or indescribable ecstasy). The diagnostic importance of the aura is its value in localizing the origin of the seizure (see CORRELATION: ANATOMIC ASPECTS). A sensory aura suggests a parietal lesion. An olfactory one suggests localization deep within the temporal lobe.

The past history should seek causes of seizures or contributing influences. Birth injury might have resulted from a prolonged labor or difficult delivery. Damage to the temporal lobes has been attributed to direct injury to their deep midline portions or, as seems more likely, compromise of the posterior cerebral arteries that subserve these parts of the brain. High fevers and prolonged seizures of early childhood have also been implicated in causing later seizures by destroying vulnerable brain cells. Again, portions of the temporal lobes appear to be particularly susceptible to such insults. Head injuries, especially when associated with contusion or laceration of brain, may cause a focal lesion that serves as a seizure focus. For example, the anterior portions of the temporal lobes, relatively silent areas of brain, may sustain contusions as they strike anteriorly and inferiorly against the sharp edges of the sphenoid wings and the roughened, irregular surface of the floor of the middle cranial fossae at the base of the skull.

Family history should include specific questions as to tuberous sclerosis and neurofibromatosis. Recent drug history should be obtained in the adolescent, since withdrawal from alcohol and barbiturates may be associated with seizures.

Examination. The *general description* should include the most marked features of the examination upon observation and interaction. Adenoma sebaceum may be obvious. Gingival changes due to chronic phenytoin (Dilantin) administration may be readily evident. Conversation may be interrupted by brief pauses, eyelid flickering, retractions of the corners of the mouth, momentary slackening of the jaw, bobbing of the head, or staring—any of which would suggest if not definitely indicate the occurrence of seizure.

The *general physical examination* should include measurement of temperature and weight. Fever may precipitate or cause seizures, and weight determination will provide a point of reference if medication (or adjustment thereof) is required. Evidence for intercurrent illness such as pharyngitis should be sought, particularly if the seizure occurred recently. The head circumference should be measured and plotted, as abnormal size (either excessively small or large) suggests abnormal brain growth. The skull and optic globes should be auscultated for bruits that would suggest vascular malformation. The tongue should be inspected for evidence of bite injury.

The entire skin should be examined carefully in evaluating the child suspected of having seizures. With tuberous sclerosis, characteristic markings are white spots ("ash leaf" macules), adenoma sebaceum, shagreen patches, and sub- or periungual fibromas (see Fig. 12–1). White spots, or hypopigmented macules, are most frequent on the trunk but may occur on any part of the body. In persons of light complexion, an ultraviolet light (Wood's lamp) may enhance the contrast between normal and affected skin, rendering a hypopigmented macule more readily visible. Adenoma sebaceum has an acneiform appearance. It typically affects the cheeks, nasal bridge, and chin. A shagreen patch is a tawny-colored, slightly elevated, and roughened area of skin, most frequently at the base of the spine. It has the appearance of untanned leather. Ungual fibromas are located under or alongside the nails. Café-au-lait macules may be seen with tuberous sclerosis or, more characteristically, with neurofibromatosis. A hemangioma of the upper face largely limited to one side is seen with the Sturge-Weber syndrome. A butterfly-shaped erythematous eruption of the upper cheeks is characteristic of systemic lupus erythematosus.

On *neurologic examination,* evidence for increased intracranial pressure and lateralizing signs should be sought. The funduscopic appearance of pa-

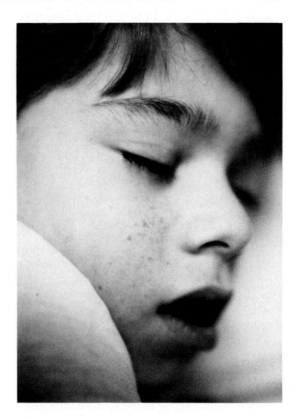

Figure 12–1. Adenoma sebaceum of cheeks in a child with tuberous sclerosis (Case 8–3).

pilledema is discussed in Chapter 11. The retinal background may show choreoretinitis resulting from intrauterine infection such as toxoplasmosis. Lateralizing findings such as reflex asymmetry, visual field deficit, or sensory abnormality would implicate focal cerebral dysfunction that might act as seizure focus.

A valuable technique for provoking petit mal or other absence seizures is hyperventilation. The child is asked to breathe in and out deeply for at least 3 minutes and is observed for staring, blinking, nodding, lip-smacking, or other form of involuntary behavior (see Table 12–2).

On *mental status examination* of the child with a seizure disorder, a variety of mental states may be seen before, during, and after seizures. These mental states can be determined through interviewing and observing the child.

Alteration in mental state before a seizure is oftentimes of an affective nature. The child may describe a feeling of being "happy," "unreal," "sad," "floating," "dreamy," or "awful." Such feelings may disappear (only to recur), or they may progress to a generalized seizure.

During a seizure mental state may be altered not at all (as with a partial seizure with elementary symptomatology), somewhat (as with a partial complex, or psychomotor, seizure), or profoundly (as with a generalized tonic-clonic convulsion). In psychomotor or petit mal status epilepticus, the child will appear alert, though perhaps not fully so, and be in an acute confusional state.

Following episodes of petit mal seizure, a child is generally able to resume his previous activity immediately or within several seconds thereafter although he will have no memory for the duration of the episode. After psychomotor or grand mal seizures, confusion or lethargy lasting several minutes to hours usually occurs.

Investigation (see Table 12–4).Routine studies in the child who has had a seizure should include a complete blood count and differential (for baseline purposes), blood sugar, and electrolytes, including calcium and magnesium. If the child is already receiving anticonvulsant medication, blood level(s) should be determined. If the head is abnormal in size or shape, skull x-rays should be obtained to look for intracranial calcification or signs of increased intracranial pressure such as splitting of cranial sutures or demineralization of the sella turcica. With focal neurologic signs or evidence of increased intracranial pressure, a CT scan of the head should be carried out with and without contrast enhancement. CT scan should disclose cerebral dysgenesis, hydrocephalus, many kinds of tumors, and vascular malformations.

Electroencephalography should be carried out both in the awake and sleep states following sleep deprivation, a nonspecific stress that facilitates the child's falling asleep without the use of sedative medication (usually chloral hydrate). It also helps to bring out EEG abnormalities that may not be apparent in the awake tracing. A particularly valuable portion of the EEG is arousal from sleep, for this is a common time of occurrence for seizures. Diagnostically useful activation procedures include hyperventilation (with suspected petit mal) and stroboscopic stimulation (with suspected photosensitive epilepsy). Use of nasopharyngeal electrodes should be considered when seizures of temporal lobe origin are suspected. Special EEG studies include 24-hour ambulatory recording, simultaneous recording of EEG activity and videotaping of behavior, and all-night polygraphic monitoring.

A word of caution with regard to the use of the electroencephalogram should be offered. The EEG may be diagnostic, may support the diagnosis of seizure disorder, may be noncontributory, or may actually interfere with the

TABLE 12–4. **Investigations to Be Considered in the Child Who Has Had Seizures**

CBC
Blood sugar
Serum electrolytes, including calcium and magnesium
Anticonvulsant blood levels
EEG (including awake and sleep tracings, hyperventilation, photic stimulation)
EEG, special studies (nasopharyngeal recording, 24-hour ambulatory recording, simultaneous video and EEG recording, all-night recording)
Skull x-rays
Cranial CT scan with and without contrast enhancement
Blood and urine amino acids, urine organic acids
Lumbar puncture
Electrocardiogram (EKG), standard and 24-hour recordings

child's well-being. With petit mal epilepsy, the tracing can be definitively diagnostic. The typical pattern is a three-per-second spike-and-wave complex that is frequently brought out by hyperventilation. In some children intermittent photic stimulation will demonstrate photosensitivity that can be of clinical significance. The EEG is less helpful within the first several days after a seizure, when it usually shows nonspecific slowing. In such cases it should generally be repeated 1 to 2 weeks later. Since EEG abnormalities are found in 10 to 15 per cent of clinically normal children, obtaining an abnormal study carries with it the risk of mislabeling a normal child as "epileptic." The reasons for obtaining an EEG and its implications for treatment must therefore be considered in advance of obtaining the test.

Further study should be undertaken based upon the specifics of the history and examination. In the child with developmental delay, for example, blood and urine should be analyzed for amino acids and urine for organic acids (see Chapters 8 and 18). When infection is suspected, cerebrospinal fluid should be examined and sent for analysis and culture unless a suspected intracranial mass lesion, thrombocytopenia, or infection of skin overlying the back preclude lumbar puncture. When cardiac disorder is being considered, a standard electrocardiogram should be obtained with a 24-hour recording arranged if indicated.

Differential Diagnosis. Because of the many different clinical manifestations of seizures, many conditions can mimic seizures and thus need to be distinguished from them (see Table 12–5).

Syncope is a fainting spell. It is the leading consideration other than generalized seizure in the school-age child who has lost consciousness for unexplained reasons. Syncope can usually be distinguished from seizure by identifying precipitating factors such as a strong emotional stimulus (e.g., seeing blood over a classmate's hand following a playground accident), systemic illness (e.g., having the "flu" for several days), or mechanical influence

---

TABLE 12–5. **Conditions to Be Differentiated from Seizures**

Syncope
Breath-holding spells
Cardiac arrhythmia
Narcolepsy, including cataplexy
Night terrors
Nightmares
Gastroesophageal reflux
Jitteriness
Spasmus nutans
Confusional migraine; other forms of migraine
Vertigo
Daydreaming
Shivering
Tics
Paroxysmal choreoathetosis
Pseudoseizures

(e.g., standing up for several hours in a stuffy gymnasium). Fainting upon assuming the upright position (sitting or standing), orthostatic syncope, is particularly common among adolescents undergoing rapid change in growth. It is usually associated with vertigo ("dizziness") that involves a sensation of motion (spinning or turning of the world or the child) (see Table 12–6) (see Case 12–1).

With syncope, loss of consciousness tends to be gradual. Vision may truly "black out" (characteristically from the periphery to the center), and the person becomes limp. Toppling over backward is unusual with syncope. Rigidity and clonic movements are seen uncommonly. Incontinence of urine or feces occurs rarely and should strongly suggest seizure, as would biting of the tongue.

Differentiation between seizure and syncope is not always easy. Indeed, the two may coexist or occur consecutively: a faint followed by a seizure. These and other points that assist in differentiating seizure from syncope are outlined in Table 12–6.

Breath-holding spells are related to syncope, though characteristically they occur in a younger child, usually between 1 and 5 years of age (Lombroso and Lerman, 1967; Stephenson, 1978). They are dramatic episodes involving brief loss of consciousness. They generally assume one of two clinical patterns: pallid or cyanotic. Pallid breath-holding spells closely resemble uncomplicated syncopal episodes of later life. A spell typically occurs following an unexpected painful stimulus. For example, a child may inadvertently strike his head against the corner of a table (without concussive loss of consciousness) or catch his finger in a door. Surprised and seemingly of-

TABLE 12–6. **Differentiation Between Seizure and Syncope***

Symptom	Seizure	Syncope
Precipitating event	Usually absent	Usually present
Loss of consciousness	Frequently >2 min	Almost always < 2 min
Premonition	Aura	Light-headed, queasy, "graying out" of vision
Incontinence	Common	Unusual
Posture at onset	Any	Usually upright
Appearance	Rubor, cyanosis, sweating	Pale, clammy, cold
Injury	May be associated	Rarely associated
Motor activity	Often prominent	Usually minimal
Pulse	Increased	Decreased and/or irregular
Resulting headache, lethargy, confusion	Frequent	Infrequent
EEG (between episodes)	Usually abnormal	Usually normal
Family history	May be positive for seizures	Often positive for syncope

* Adapted from Oppenheimer, E. Y., and Rosman, N. P. Seizures in childhood: an approach to emergency management. *Pediatr. Clin. North Am.*, **26**: 837–55, 1979.

CASE 12–1: ORTHOSTATIC HYPOTENSION WITH SYNCOPE IN A 14-YEAR-OLD BOY

L.C. experienced several episodes of near-syncope at the time of a viral respiratory infection. One week later, when seemingly healthy, he had a similar episode associated with loss of consciousness for less than 1 minute. The episode occurred some 15 seconds after he had arisen from lying. He first noted visual loss in both eyes, as darkness progressed from outside in. Voices became distant, and he became "dizzy"—both vertiginous and lightheaded. Incontinence, tongue-biting, headache, and abnormal movements were not associated.

On examination he was a tall, slender adolescent who appeared entirely healthy. Blood pressure showed a significant drop in systolic blood pressure (30 mm Hg) immediately upon arising. This drop was associated with characteristic "dizziness" but not loss of consciousness. Neurologic examination was normal; EEG, EKG, and fasting blood sugar all were normal.

Syncope was felt to be secondary to orthostatic hypotension. He was treated with leg wraps and advised to rise carefully from the lying or sitting position after "pumping" the muscles in his legs. After several weeks during which he had several more syncopal episodes, he was able to resume normal activities.

Comment. This young man's loss of conciousness was due to syncope occurring secondary to postural changes in blood pressure. Orthostatic hypotension, initially part of a viral syndrome, persisted for several weeks after he had apparently recovered. Seizure disorder and basilar artery migraine were the major alternatives considered diagnostically. The pattern of visual loss (from outside in) is characteristic of orthostatic syncope and, among other features, helped to establish the diagnosis.

The persistence of symptoms over several weeks was unusual and highly frustrating for the boy and his mother. They were reassured by the normalcy of the examination and investigations, and by the knowledge that the disorder appeared to be essentially benign. Ephedrine may be effective in some cases of recurrent postural syncope.

fended more than hurt by the incident, the child may begin to cry, then stops breathing, and falls pale and limp onto the floor. The episode usually lasts for a minute or less, and the child is soon able to resume normal activity.

The cyanotic variety of breath-holding spell usually complicates marked frustration experienced by the child, who cries intensely then stops breathing until unconsciousness supervenes. Cyanosis is characteristically associated. Muscle tone is often increased, sometimes with opisthotonic arching of the back. A few seizure-like clonic jerks may be associated with either variety of breath-holding spell (see Case 12–2).

Cardiac arrhythmia should be considered in children with unexplained

CASE 12–2: BREATH-HOLDING SPELLS AND POSSIBLE SEIZURES IN A 3-YEAR-OLD GIRL

B.B. had classical breath-holding spells of cyanotic type between 11 months and 2 years of age. After she had been free of breath-holding spells for 1 year, her mother found her one day to be blue and limp after which she had several clonic jerks followed by drowsiness. The beginning of the episode was unobserved. Subsequently, similar episodes occurred after a "clash of wills" with her mother, while others occurred without apparent provocation. Past history was negative. Examination was normal except for unusually high intelligence and heightened activity level. EEG was normal.

This child was felt definitely to have breath-holding spells of the cyanotic type and possibly to have generalized seizures as well. Because the episodes were brief, EEG was normal, and mother-child interactions were already strained, it was decided to withhold anticonvulsant medication because it was feared the side effects (or just the physical act of getting medicine into her) could make the situation even worse. Therapy thus centered on an explanation of breath-holding spells, a review of first aid for generalized seizures, and a discussion of ways to minimize confrontation with the child. A nursery school program was strongly encouraged, and within several weeks of enrollment she was free of all episodes.

Comment. As this case illustrates, the line between breath-holding spell and seizure may be very fine. A few clonic jerks at the end of a breath-holding spell are not uncommon and do not mean that a seizure disorder coexists. On the other hand, a generalized or partial seizure may be brought on by a breath-holding spell. In these circumstances anticonvulsant medication would be justified, although it would not be expected to control the breath-holding spells.

Breath-holding spells often begin in infancy and usually abate spontaneously by 3 to 5 years of age. The electroencephalogram in children with the pallid type of breath-holding spell characteristically, but not uniformly, shows marked slowing of cardiac rhythm and cerebral background activity when ocular compression, an intense vagal stimulus, is performed carefully. Anticonvulsant therapy does not benefit children with breath-holding spells unless breath-holding and seizures coexist. Because of the etiologic role of vagal stimulation in some cases, treatment with atropine has been suggested for use in some children (Stephenson, 1978).

loss of consciousness, particularly if the episodes do not appear to be due to seizure, syncope, or migraine (Schott *et al.*, 1977; Lown *et al.*, 1980). Several syndromes sharing the common feature of a long QT interval have been described (Mathews *et al.*, 1972; Frank and Friedberg, 1976; Abildskov, 1979). Family history may be positive for hearing deficit and for sudden death in young adulthood. Since the prolonged QT interval may not be evident on routine electrocardiogram, stress testing and 12–24-hour electrocardiographic monitoring may be needed to establish the diagnosis (see Case 7–3).

Other cardiac arrhythmias may be audiogenically induced. Wellens and colleagues (1972) described a 14-year-old girl with episodes of loss of consciousness associated with urinary incontinence that were triggered by loud noises (such as thunder or the ringing of an alarm clock). These produced ventricular fibrillation, which resulted in cerebral hypoxia and generalized convulsions.

Narcolepsy, characterized by sleep attacks and cataplexy, often suggests seizure disorder. Cataplexy, unlike epilepsy, is unassociated with impairment of consciousness. Associated features of the narcoleptic syndrome such as hypnagogic hallucinations and sleep paralysis should distinguish narcolepsy from seizure disorder. In addition, the EEG in narcolepsy is normal except for its direct entry into rapid eye movement (REM) sleep (see Chapter 9).

Jitteriness, particularly in the newborn, and *spasmus nutans* (head-nodding with asymmetric nystagmus) in the young infant may mimic seizure activity.

Confusional migraine may be accompanied by behavioral alterations similar to those seen in complex partial seizures (see Chapter 11).

Vertigo, the causes of which are multiple and diverse, also may mimic complex partial seizures.

Daydreaming may closely resemble petit mal seizures (see HISTORY).

Shivering associated with fever may easily be mistaken for seizure. Limbs and body are stiff. Fine, trembling movements occur. The child is less responsive (or at least less communicative) than usual and may stare straight ahead. Such an episode must be differentiated from a seizure manifested by trembling of the chin and speech arrest. Shivering, or shuddering, has also been reported with intolerance to monosodium glutamate (Reif-Lehrer and Stemmermann, 1975).

Tics, recurrent, involuntary movements characteristically seen in school-age children, may closely mimic seizures (see Chapter 13). The EEG will generally be useful in differentiating tic from seizure.

Paroxysmal choreoathetosis is a disorder characterized by recurrent tonic, dystonic, and choreoathetoid movements (see Chapter 13).

Night terrors are dramatic eruptions from sleep characterized by a state of panic, diminished responsiveness to external stimuli, incomplete arousal, automatic behavior, and amnesia for the episode. In *nightmares,* the child seems less frightened than with night terrors, is quite easily aroused, and usually recalls the event the following morning. An electroencephalogram (or all-night sleep recording) may be useful in excluding nocturnal seizures or night terrors that are triggered by abnormal electrical activity of brain (see Chapter 9).

Gastrointestinal disorder involving recurrent symptoms may imitate seizure disorder, particularly in the younger child. Gastroesophageal reflux and gastric duplication have been cited as underlying syndromes involving cyclic abdominal pain, irritability, dysphagia, or dystonia (Bray *et al.,* 1977; Rosenlund and Schnaufer, 1978).

CASE 12–3: PSEUDOSEIZURES IN A 20-YEAR-OLD WOMAN WITH DOWN SYNDROME

L.L. was evaluated because of a "seizure," she said. Earlier that day she had experienced abdominal discomfort, fell to the floor, and appeared to lose consciousness for several minutes. No abnormal movement, incontinence, or tongue-biting was observed. She resumed her normal activities within 15 minutes.

On examination, she was an alert, talkative, and cooperative young woman with obvious features of Down syndrome. She functioned at around a 6-year-old level overall. General medical examination was normal. Neurocutaneous signs were absent. Neurologic examination, including funduscopic visualization, was normal. EEG and "seizure chemistries" in blood were normal. CT scan with contrast was normal.

Comment. In a follow-up visit, this young woman spoke freely about the many seizures she had witnessed at the state school where she had resided before coming to her present community residence. Although the nature of the initial episode remained obscure, her awareness of seizures, her negative evaluation, and the lack of recurrence made pseudoseizure a likely possibility. Further questioning as to the circumstances of the episode described above revealed that the young woman had been upset by the departure of a staff person she had been close to. The staff was made aware that the pseudoseizure appeared to be part of her adjustment reaction, and this matter received further attention during group meetings at the residence. No further episodes occurred over the next several years.

Pseudoseizures can be categorized as hysterical seizures (occurring on an involuntary basis) and feigned seizures (willfully produced) (see Chapter 7). Either kind of pseudoseizure can occur in a child with a true seizure disorder (Williams *et al.*, 1978; Finlayson and Lucas, 1979; Schneider and Rice, 1979). Feigned seizures may appear as episodes of forceful eye blinking, opisthotonic writhing, or apparent loss of consciousness. Pseudoseizures may be derived from true seizures witnessed by the child (see Cases 12–3 and 12–4).

Telemetered electroencephalographic monitoring with videotaped recording of behavior can usually distinguish between true seizures and pseudoseizures (see Chapter 7).

Etiology. In considering the cause of seizures, it is essential to keep in mind that a seizure is a symptom, not a specific etiologic diagnosis. A seizure is the clinical result of invisible biochemical and electrical events occurring at the cellular level. Consideration of etiology can be reduced to two questions:

What causes the sudden discharge of excessive electrical activity?
What determines the propagation of abnormal electrical impulses?

CASE 12–4: TEMPER TANTRUMS MISPERCEIVED AS SEIZURES IN A 9-YEAR-OLD BOY

I.F. was begun on anticonvulsant medication at 4 years of age when he was observed to have an absence-like episode in his pediatrician's office. EEG at that time was normal. Episodes continued despite a variety of medications used singly and in combination. At 6 years he developed episodes of violently aggressive behavior lasting up to a half hour, for which he had no recall. Attacks were said to be unprovoked and were not associated with incontinence, tongue-biting, or somnolence. EEG was again normal. CT scan showed no abnormalities.

Past history included normal pregnancy and delivery. He had experienced no febrile convulsions, high fevers or episodes of significant head trauma. Family history was negative for seizure disorder. Mother had a history of multiple operations of the abdomen and leg. She was currently being treated for intractable pain of unknown cause.

On examination, the child was an immature youngster whose interactions with his mother were characterized by mutual provocation and manipulation. Mother reported that her son was "having a seizure" at the time the nursing staff observed a temper tantrum of gradual onset that had apparently arisen during an argument between the two. General physical and neurologic examinations were normal, as was yet another EEG.

Comment. This mother seemed to need the child's problems to be attributable to epilepsy. The reason was unclear but was probably related to her own pattern of somatization that suggested Briquet hysteria.

The normal electroencephalograms and the observed nonseizure did not, however, exclude coexisting seizure disorder in this child. Conventional recording of the electroencephalogram from scalp electrodes may not pick up deep temporal lobe discharges accessible only with nasopharyngeal or other special recording techniques if at all. The overwhelming weight of the evidence here, though, was that episodes reported by mother were temper tantrums misperceived by her as seizures.

Whether neurogenic or psychogenic in origin, the behavior was pathologic and reflected seriously disturbed mother-child interactions. Persons with such problems often produce anger in medical staff caring for them (who may feel as if the patient or the parents are trying to "fool" them). As a result, investigation may be carried out in an angry manner and referral for psychiatric evaluation or treatment may be made in an unsupportive and rejecting way. Thus, the establishment of a psychotherapeutic relationship may be impaired before it has even begun, and the maladaptive behavior becomes perpetuated.

The answers to these questions are not always, or even often, forthcoming. In childhood and adolescence the cause of seizures is usually idiopathic (unknown). Intrinsic properties of neural and glial cell membranes of the cerebral cortex and developmental-maturational influences appear to play significant roles. Factors that determine the pathway pursued by the abnormal electrical activity are unclear.

Some factors, however, can be identified that pertain directly to these two questions. Chemical influences such as hypocalcemia and hypoglycemia upset the intracellular versus extracellular ionic balance, destabilize the cell membrane, and cause an increased likelihood that a portion of brain will discharge electrically as a seizure focus (see CORRELATION: BIOCHEMICAL ASPECTS). Temperature elevation, too, can lower the membrane's potential for depolarization and thereby enhance the likelihood of seizure. Malformations of brain, gross or microscopic (such as misplaced, or heterotopic, areas of gray matter), and areas of injury (destruction of cortex secondary to trauma or metabolic insult such as hypoxia) do play a role both in creation of seizure foci and propagation of seizure discharges.

Etiology, then, must be considered on several levels—gross and microscopic; anatomic, biochemical, and physiologic—as part of the clinical diagnostic process directed toward establishing the most specific and effective therapy (see Table 12–7).

Medical Causes. Hypoglycemia, defined in childhood by a blood sugar below 40 mg/dl, can cause generalized seizures by itself or in combination with other factors such as fatigue, systemic illness, or drug use. It can result also from excessive insulin: self-administered insulin overdosage (as with diabetes mellitus), leucine-sensitive hyperinsulinemia (an excessive outpouring of insulin secondary to dietary leucine), or insulin-producing tumor of pancreatic beta cells (insulinoma). Hypoglycemia can also result from self-administration of oral hypoglycemic agents.

Adrenal insufficiency on an adrenal, pituitary, or hypothalamic basis also can be associated with hypoglycemia. Some children with ketotic hypoglycemia tolerate fasting poorly. Hypoglycemia can be manifested otherwise by sweating, tremulousness, hunger, irritability, yawning, or lethargy.

Diagnosis is based ultimately upon demonstration of low blood sugar. Hypoglycemia may not be demonstrable, however, after a generalized seizure that has itself raised the blood sugar as part of a stress response. In practice hypoglycemia is an uncommon cause of seizures in childhood and adolescence.

Hypocalcemia is another cause of generalized convulsions. A diminished calcium level (the normal being 9 to 11 mg/dl) can result from inadequate intake of vitamin D (involved in absorption of calcium from the intestine) or from disorders involving parathyroid hormone. In hypoparathyroidism, normal serum calcium levels cannot be maintained and serum phosphorus levels rise. With pseudohypoparathyroidism, parathyroid hormone *is* present but it is ineffective due to end-organ unresponsiveness. Pseudohypoparathyroidism can occur as a syndrome characterized by short stature, obesity, mild mental retardation, and minor skeletal deformities that include dysplastic feet and hands (particularly a short fourth metacarpal).

Other medical conditions that can be associated with seizures are *systemic lupus erythematosus* and *homocystinuria*. With lupus, cerebral vasculitis can be associated with headaches, affective disorder, or seizures (Ha-

TABLE 12–7. **Causes of Seizures**

Medical	Hypoglycemia (insulin excess: leucine-sensitive hyper-insulinemia, beta cell tumor of pancreas, insulin overdosage, oral hypoglycemic agent overdosage, adrenal insufficiency, ketotic hypoglycemia) Hypocalcemia (due to diminished vitamin D intake, hypoparathyroidism, pseudohypoparathyroidism) Systemic lupus erythematosus Homocystinuria Fever
Neurologic	Head trauma (at birth, during childhood) Tumor Infection (due to abscess, bacterial meningitis with or without complicating vascular thrombosis, Reye syndrome, parasitic disease) Neurocutaneous disorder (tuberous sclerosis, neurofibromatosis, Sturge-Weber syndrome) Degenerative neurologic disease (subacute sclerosing panencephalitis, adrenoleukodystrophy, ceroid lipofuscinosis) Sensory-induced (audiogenic, somatosensory, photosensitive, cognitive) Recurrent seizures (diminished anticonvulsant blood level, intercurrent illness, stress)
Toxic	Lead Insecticide Carbon monoxide (or other agent causing hypoxia) Alcohol or barbiturate withdrawal Antipsychotic drug (phenothiazine, butyrophenone)
Psychologic	Refusal to take anticonvulsant medication Self-induced
Social-Environmental	Multiple contributing factors
Genetic-Constitutional	Familial idiopathic epilepsy Specific inherited disorders
Developmental	Febrile seizures of infancy and early childhood Idiopathic epilepsy with onset in adolescence

zelton *et al.*, 1980). Homocystinuria is an autosomal recessive disorder of amino acid metabolism characterized by a "Marfanoid" body habitus, dislocated lenses, and multiple strokes secondary to repeated episodes of thromboembolism associated with seizures that are often focal.

Fever itself may cause or contribute to seizures, particularly in infants and younger children. Between the ages of 6 months and 4 years, some 3 to 5 per cent of children will have one or a few brief (less than 20 minutes), generalized seizures occurring within the first 24 hours of temperature elevation unassociated with central nervous system infection.

Although phenobarbital maintenance therapy is of demonstrated efficacy in preventing further febrile seizures in this otherwise normal group, the great majority (more than 90 per cent) of such children do not go on to develop afebrile seizures. Most children with febrile seizures outgrow them by age 5 to 7 years (Nelson and Ellenberg, 1976; Oppenheimer and Rosman, 1979).

It has not been demonstrated that phenobarbital or other anticonvulsant medication can prevent development of epilepsy in those children in whom afebrile seizures are destined to occur. If this link could be determined, then phenobarbital maintenance therapy (or rectal diazepam given at the onset of febrile illness) would be more widely recommended. Phenobarbital taken by mouth at the time a febrile illness is recognized has not proved effective in preventing febrile seizures.

Neurologic Causes.   Important neurologic causes for seizures include head trauma, tumor, infection, neurocutaneous disorder, and degenerative neurologic disease.

Head trauma at any age is an important cause of epilepsy. Some 5 per cent of children hospitalized with significant head trauma (ranging from mild concussion to more complicated injuries) will have a posttraumatic seizure. If a seizure occurs within the first week after head injury (early posttraumatic epilepsy), the risk of developing later seizures within the next 4 years is 25 per cent. With a seizure occurring in the late posttraumatic period (more than one week after head trauma), the risk of developing additional seizures during the following 4 years is further increased. Head injury complicated by prolonged unconsciousness, penetrating injury to brain, or intracranial hemorrhage are among the factors that contribute importantly to risk (Rosman and Herskowitz, 1982) (see Case 12–5).

The role of birth trauma in producing later epilepsy remains controversial, although it is doubtless of etiologic importance in some cases. It has been postulated that damage to one or both temporal lobes can occur during labor or delivery (perhaps secondary to compression of one or both posterior cerebral arteries) and that brain injury with scarring occurs along the deep, medial portions of the temporal lobe(s). These scarred areas (of incisural sclerosis) have been demonstrated to serve as seizure foci in some persons (Falconer *et al.,* 1964).

Temporal lobe seizures are of concern not only because of the morbidity associated with the seizures themselves but also because of accumulated evidence that chronic temporal lobe dysfunction causes or contributes to interictal disorders of behavior that include hyperkinetic syndromes, catastrophic rage, and psychosis (Waxman and Geschwind, 1975; Bear and Fedio, 1977; Lindsay *et al.,* 1979; Pritchard *et al.,* 1980) (see Chapter 5).

Tumors are unlikely to cause seizures in childhood as contrasted with adulthood. As discussed in Chapter 11, some two-thirds of brain tumors in childhood and adolescence occur in the posterior fossa and produce symptoms primarily through elevating intracranial pressure and secondarily by interfering with balance, gait, and other coordinative functions. Focal neurolo-

CASE 12–5: POSTTRAUMATIC SEIZURES
IN A 17-YEAR-OLD ADOLESCENT

L.Q. was observed to have a generalized tonic-clonic convulsion within several minutes of an automobile collision. Fellow passengers were unable to say if he had sustained loss of consciousness. Thirty minutes after the seizure he was awake, looked about, and walked without assistance. He was mute, however, and did not appear to recognize his family members. Except for these mental status changes, neurologic examination was unremarkable. Within an hour, he spontaneously regained his normal mental state, spoke freely and fluently, and recognized his siblings without hesitation. He was placed on phenytoin therapy. A CT scan was normal.

A friend reported 2 weeks later that the young man stared for 2 minutes, did not respond to questioning, and bent forward with his hand on his abdomen. Neither incontinence nor tongue-biting was associated. Within 15 minutes, he was normally alert and requested that the evening continue as planned. He was unaware of the lapse in behavior.

Comment. This case illustrates several important points. This young man developed a typical posttraumatic temporal lobe seizure disorder. His later seizure was partial with complex symptomatology as manifested by altered mental state, semipurposeful behavior, speech arrest, and sensory disturbance (abdominal pain). Partial complex seizures imply an epileptic focus within the temporal lobe, an area of brain frequently injured in head trauma because it lies within the middle cranial fossa that forms part of the base of the skull. The temporal lobe may readily suffer contusion, or bruising, at the time of head trauma, though symptomatology may not be manifested immediately if at all.

This young man's state of altered consciousness following his first seizure created some diagnostic uncertainty. Coexisting intoxication was considered here and excluded by examination of blood and urine for toxic substances including alcohol. Another possibility was that the abnormal behavior was itself an ictal phenomenon. The preceding generalized convulsion made it quite clear, however, that the behavior represented a postictal confusional state rather than a prolonged partial seizure.

gic findings such as reflex asymmetry, sensory loss, or visual field deficit would, however, make a supratentorial mass such as meningioma, glioma, or vascular malformation more likely, particularly if associated with a focally abnormal EEG (see Case 12–6).

Infectious causes of seizure include cerebral abscess (uncommon except among children with parameningeal infections or congenital cyanotic heart disease); acute bacterial meningitis (with or without complicating vascular thrombosis); and postinfectious encephalopathy, including Reye syndrome. Parasitic diseases such as cysticercosis can also cause seizures (see Case 12–7).

CASE 12–6: VISUAL HALLUCINATIONS AND SEIZURES IN A 9-YEAR-OLD BOY

P.C. experienced a "patch of color" in front of his right eye that was followed by a generalized convulsion. Phenytoin prevented further generalized seizures, but several times daily he had a "blurry" sensation affecting both eyes in the right visual field. The sensation was like darting lights or colored banners. Episodes lasted 10 to 15 minutes, were sometimes associated with dysfluent speech, and were followed by a throbbing, left-sided headache. Neurologic examination including funduscopic visualization, visual fields, and higher cortical functions was entirely normal. Investigation included a radioisotope brain scan, which disclosed a small lesion of the left occipital lobe consistent with a vascular malformation or neoplastic lesion. Following further investigation, the child underwent surgery. A low-grade glioma was removed in its entirety. The boy had an uneventful postoperative course and has done well subsequently.

Comment. Visual hallucinations followed by throbbing headache would suggest a classical migraine syndrome. The diagnosis of seizure disorder was suggested most directly in this case by the convulsion that followed a typical visual disturbance and by the frequency of visual symptoms. Left hemisphere localization was implied by the right homonymous field cut. The unformed character of the hallucinations suggested occipital lobe involvement. In contrast to what is seen in adults, brain tumor is an uncommon cause of seizures in childhood. But, as exemplified by this case, it must be considered an etiologic possibility in some instances.

Neurocutaneous disorders associated with seizures include tuberous sclerosis, neurofibromatosis, and Sturge-Weber syndrome. All of these disorders may be associated with the triad of mental retardation, characteristic skin lesions, and seizures.

Tuberous sclerosis is an autosomal dominant disorder with several typical skin markings: hypopigmented macules, adenoma sebaceum, shagreen patches, and sub- or periungual fibromas (see Fig. 4–2). These are described above in the section on EXAMINATION. Hypopigmented macules (white spots) are usually present at birth. Adenoma sebaceum generally develops between 2 and 5 years of age, as do shagreen patches. Ungual fibromas, by contrast, usually develop about the time of adolescence. The degree of retardation is variable, ranging from nil to profound. Seizures may be controlled easily or not at all. They result from the disorganized cortical development that typifies tuberous sclerosis, which is manifested grossly by thickened, hardened gyri that give the condition its name. The diagnosis of tuberous sclerosis is usually readily apparent on examination. Plain skull x-rays and CT scan may show confirmatory intracranial calcification protruding into the lateral ventricles (see Fig. 12–3) (see Case 8–3).

CASE 12–7: PARASITIC DISEASE AS A CAUSE FOR SEIZURE DISORDER IN AN 18-YEAR-OLD WOMAN

L.A. had a brief generalized convulsion after staying awake all night, playing volleyball for several hours, and skipping breakfast. Neurologic examination was unremarkable. Electroencephalogram, radioisotope brain scan, and skull x-rays all were normal. She was placed on anticonvulsant therapy and did well until her supervisor at work noted her to be typing nonsense. On examination she was alert, cooperative, and spoke fluently. When asked what month it was, she replied: "It's between June and August, but I can't name it." Her writing was legible but contained misspelled, incomplete, and nonsense words. Elemental neurologic examination revealed no abnormalities. CT scan disclosed a 1–2 cm mass of low density in the region of the left angular gyrus surrounded by a zone of edema (see Fig. 12–2). She underwent craniotomy and excision of the lesion, which proved to be a cysticercus cyst upon pathologic microscopic examination. She had an unremarkable postoperative course and has been seizure-free on anticonvulsant therapy.

Comment. The conditions associated with the first seizure and the negative evaluation at that time did not suggest a specific cause for the seizure. Sleep deprivation and nutritional stress may provoke seizures in susceptible persons in much the same way that fever or intercurrent illness may. The aphasic language disturbance evident upon reexamination suggested a dominant-hemisphere, that is, left-sided, lesion. The posterior location of the lesion was suspected since she had no problem in production of meaningful speech. As is characteristic of aphasia, there was associated difficulty in written (or, in this instance, typed) language.

The specific etiologic diagnosis, cysticercus cyst, was a surprise since the preoperative diagnosis was neoplastic lesion (such as low-grade glioma) or infectious process (such as tuberculoma). The young woman's country of origin (Haiti) might have suggested the diagnosis preoperatively, although parasitic disease occurs worldwide and should be considered in the diagnosis of any focal brain lesion.

Cysticercosis results from ingestion of ova of the pork tapeworm, *Taenia solium*. A period of 5 years generally elapses before neurologic symptoms develop. Seizures are the commonest central nervous system manifestation of single or multiple lesions. Hydrocephalus may also result.

Trichinosis, infestation with the roundworm *Trichinella spiralis*, can also result from ingestion of inadequately prepared pork. It usually produces a meningoencephalitis rather than convulsions. Visceral larva migrans, caused by *Toxocara* organisms from dog or cat feces, may be associated with seizures as well as meningoencephalitis. Malaria, an important cause of seizures, may present with coma, psychosis, or motor dysfunction. Diagnosis is established by recognition of intracellular parasites seen within red blood cells on peripheral blood smear.

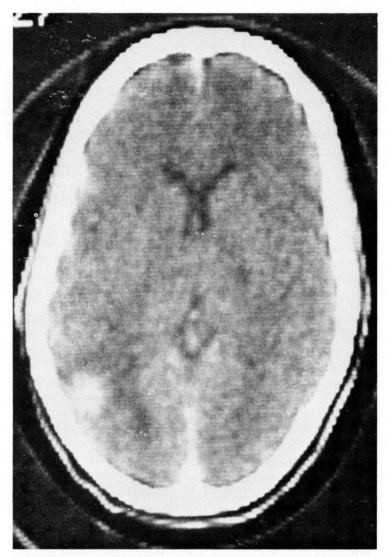

FIGURE 12–2. Computerized tomographic (CT) scan with contrast showing mass in left parieto-occipital region (Case 12–7).

Neurofibromatosis is also an autosomal dominant disorder with a variable degree of severity from one affected person to another. Mental retardation or seizure disorder occurs in about 10 per cent of cases. Characteristic skin markings are café-au-lait macules, the minimal manifestations of the disorder (see Fig. 4–1) (Whitehouse, 1966). Neurofibromatosis can be associated with spinal cord or intracranial tumors, bony abnormalities (localized overgrowth of bone, orbital dysplasia), pseudo-arthroses due to faulty healing of fractures, and plexiform neuromas. As with tuberous sclerosis, seizures and mental retardation appear to occur secondary to cerebral maldevelopment (Rosman and Pearce, 1967). Diagnosis is established by the clinical presenta-

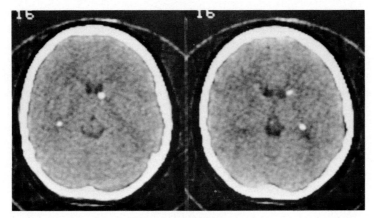

FIGURE 12–3. Intracranial calcifications on plain computerized tomographic (CT) scan of a 12-year-old boy with tuberous sclerosis.

tion, including multiple café-au-lait spots or axillary freckling, and is supported in many instances by a family history of similar skin lesions.

Sturge-Weber disease, also called encephalotrigeminal angiomatosis, involves a hemangioma of one side of the upper part of the face associated with angiomatosis of the leptomeninges overlying the same side of the brain posteriorly (see Fig. 12–4). The eyelid on the affected side is typically in-

FIGURE 12–4. Sturge-Weber syndrome (encephalotrigeminal angiomatosis) with hemangioma of left side of face.

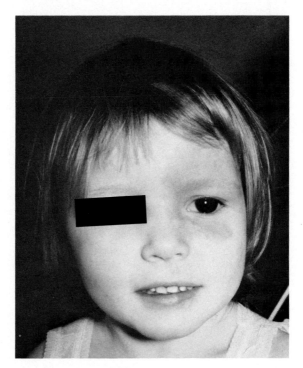

volved by the hemangioma. The eye itself may be larger than the contralateral eye and may become glaucomatous. As with tuberous sclerosis, seizures are often refractory to treatment. Mental retardation is characteristic. The diagnosis is usually readily apparent by inspection. Plain skull x-rays typically show a "railroad track" pattern in the occipital-parietal region because of calcification occurring in superficial layers of apposed gyri (see Fig. 12–5). Sturge-Weber disease occurs on a sporadic basis.

Seizures may also be part of a syndrome of *degenerative neurologic disease*. Causes include subacute sclerosing panencephalitis, adrenoleukodystrophy, and ceroid lipofuscinosis (see Chapter 8).

In some children, seizures occurring on an idiopathic basis are induced by sensory stimulation. These *sensory-evoked seizures* are among the forms of *reflex epilepsy*. Sensory-evoked seizures may be induced by stimuli of the following modalities: auditory, somatosensory, or visual. In addition, behaviors such as reading or even performing mental calculations may induce seizures in some persons (Ingvar and Nyman, 1962; Wiebers *et al.*, 1979). Within the auditory group, seizures have been induced by music, startle, and specific sounds. Seizures occurring secondary to somatosensory input can occur following painful stimulation or an unsuspected, startling

CASE 12–8: PHOTOSENSITIVE EPILEPSY IN A 9-YEAR-OLD BOY

G.J. was found in front of a television set that was flickering vertically. He was face-down on the floor with his head and arms turned to the right. His legs were stiffly extended, his arms rigidly flexed. The episode continued for some 20 seconds, after which he was mildly confused for the next hour. His parents reported that over the previous 3 to 4 years they had observed their son to have had lightning-like jerks of arm flexion and head dropping as he rode in the back seat of the car while light flashed intermittently through the rearview mirror. His 11-year-old sister was developmentally delayed and had a mixed seizure disorder, which included myoclonic seizures.

Neurologic examination showed mildly impaired fine motor coordination in both arms (left more than right) and an extensor left plantar response. With hyperventilation and photic stimulation, electroencephalogram showed generalized spike, polyspike, and slow wave activity without associated myoclonic jerks. Blue and green lenses provided partial protection from seizure discharges induced by intermittent photic stimulation (see Figs. 12–6 and 12–7).

Investigation was otherwise negative. It included CT scan, cerebrospinal fluid examination, measurement of lysosomal enzyme levels, serum calcium, and analysis of blood and urine for amino acids. He was treated with 250 mg of acetazolamide three times daily and advised to wear blue-tinted sunglasses when outdoors. Seizure control has been excellent.

Comment. One of the etiologic categories considered here was that of degenerative neurologic disease in view of the occurrence of myoclonic sei-

tap. Photosensitive epilepsy may take several forms. These include sensitivity to intermittent flashes of light, specific colors, certain patterns, and sudden exposure to bright lights (Forster, 1972). Particularly with photosensitive seizure disorders, self-induction may readily occur (Panayiotopoulos, 1979; Binnie *et al.*, 1980).

Toxic Causes. Several toxins can induce seizures in childhood. Among these is *lead,* which can also be associated with increased intracranial pressure and permanent neurologic defects including mental retardation. *Insecticide* poisoning, especially with parasympathomimetic agents, may also cause generalized convulsions. Acute *carbon monoxide* poisoning can produce generalized seizures through its hypoxic effects.

Seizures can occur as part of a *withdrawal syndrome* involving sedative drugs such as alcohol and barbiturates (see Case 19–3). Alcohol withdrawal seizures typically occur within 48 hours of cessation (or significant diminution) of alcohol intake. They are generalized, last several minutes, and usually end spontaneously. Barbiturate withdrawal seizures occur following abuse of barbiturates, not upon discontinuation of their therapeutic use (which should be carried out, nonetheless, over a period of several days to months to minimize sleep disturbances that can result).

zures in two children within the same family, one of whom was mentally retarded. Among this group of disorders is familial myoclonic epilepsy, which usually begins in early adolescence with generalized tonic-clonic convulsions. Thereafter, myoclonic seizures and mental deterioration occur. Diagnosis is made by a characteristic clinical course, positive family history, and diagnostic brain biopsy (showing so-called Lafora bodies).

This boy manifested a form of photosensitive epilepsy. By history, it was associated with flickering light from a malfunctioning television set and sudden flashes of light reflected by a mirror. The latter seizures were myoclonic. The former presumably began as myoclonic seizures, which then became generalized tonic-clonic seizures.

Photosensitive epilepsy is associated with a spectrum of clinical syndromes. At one end of the spectrum are children who show spike-and-wave bursts only in response to photic stimulation but who do not have associated clinical seizures. Other children manifest a photosensitive response on electroencephalogram and myoclonic jerks or absence spells evoked by photic stimulation, which cease when photic stimulation is discontinued. Still more severe manifestations are EEG abnormalities that persist beyond the time of photic stimulation and are associated with generalized tonic-clonic seizures.

For children who are significantly photosensitive, nonpharmacologic therapeutic measures should include explanation of the nature of photosensitivity (necessitating avoidance of flickering lights, not sitting close to the television, and minimizing sudden exposure to bright light) and the use of tinted glasses or contact lenses.

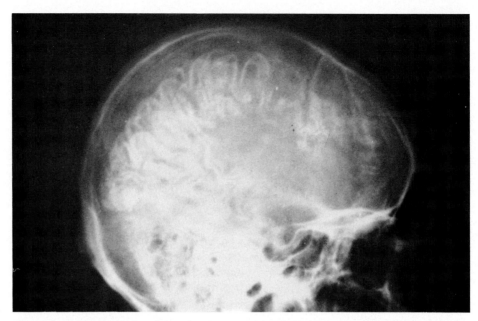

FIGURE 12–5. Skull x-ray showing intracranial calcifications ("railroad tracking") in Sturge-Weber syndrome.

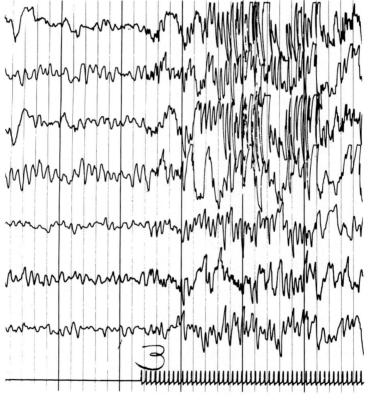

FIGURE 12–6. Electroencephalogram showing generalized poly-spike discharges occurring within 2 seconds of intermittent photic stimulation.

342

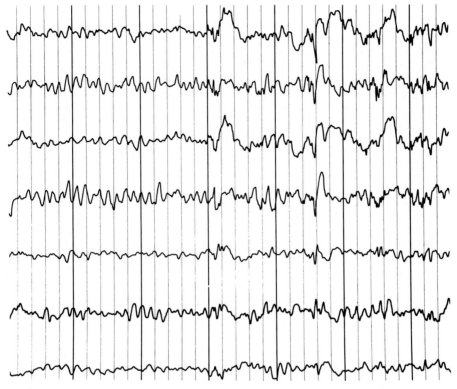

FIGURE 12–7. Electroencephalogram of same child in Figure 12–6 showing protective effect of green filter with abolition of photic-induced seizure discharges.

Antipsychotic agents of the phenothiazine and butyrophenone families appear to increase the likelihood of seizure in some persons. The mechanism has been suggested to be lowering of the seizure threshold by hypersynchronization of cerebral electrical activity (Baldessarini, 1980). Accordingly, a phenothiazine or butyrophenone should be used with caution in a person with a known seizure disorder or in one without clinical seizures whose EEG shows seizure discharges. Thioridazine (Mellaril) appears to have the least epileptogenic potential among these antipsychotic agents (see Chapter 5).

Psychologic Causes. Psychologic causes *per se* do not usually produce seizures in childhood, although refusal to take anticonvulsant medication as prescribed due to negativism, depression, or denial can lead to worsening of seizure control. Actual self-induction of seizures can also occur (see NEURO-LOGIC CAUSES). A child may hyperventilate, meditate, calculate, wave his hands in front of his face (a form of intermittent photic stimulation), or look at provocative patterns (e.g., stripes or checkerboards) to bring on seizures (see Case 12–9).

Social-Environmental Causes. Although social and environmental factors do not cause seizures, they may exacerbate a preexisting seizure problem. Family disorganization can be associated with an erratic schedule of

CASE 12–9: ANXIETY AND TEMPORAL LOBE SEIZURES IN A 19-YEAR-OLD FEMALE

R.U. began having "black-out spells" at the age of 14 years. Over the next 3 years she had episodes lasting several minutes that began with epigastric pain followed by flexion of the trunk while in the sitting position, lip-smacking, fumbling with her clothes, and angry vocalizing. One such episode occurred on the subway and resulted in her being apprehended by the police for suspected drug intoxication. The abdominal pain she experienced was a dull, burning discomfort just like what she felt when she worried about something. For that reason she feared that worrying would bring on a seizure. Past history was unremarkable except for treatment of lead poisoning at 5 years of age.

Comment. This case illustrates several points characteristic of temporal lobe epilepsy. It may present as unusual, if not bizarre, behavior not readily recognized as a seizure. A medical information bracelet or comparable form of identification can obviate this problem.

The epigastric discomfort she reported is an aura typical of temporal lobe epilepsy. It is correlated with sensory cortex mediating intra-abdominal sensation located within the insula (see Chapter 2). The suggested link between anxiety and seizures is intriguing. The psychic induction of abnormal cerebral electrical activity and clinical seizures is well recognized. The interrelations between worry, abdominal pain, and seizure in this case, however, remain speculative.

drug administration. Transportation problems and financial difficulties may lead to lapses in medication refills and failure to keep appointments for outpatient diagnostic studies (including anticonvulsant blood levels) or follow-up examinations. Chronic stresses such as poor nutrition, fatigue, and medical conditions such as asthma or diabetes mellitus can also contribute to worsened seizure control (see Case 12–10).

Undue emphasis on the seizure problem can in some instances contribute to perpetuation of the problem. Because of benefits derived from the sick role, seizures are sometimes viewed as something that must necessarily be maintained in a state of poor control. One such affected person, an adult whose life style centered on his neurologic problem, described himself as a "professional epileptic."

Genetic-Constitutional Causes. Idiopathic epilepsy is due to unidentified causes, presumably an intrinsic lowering of the seizure threshold. This tendency to have seizures may be familial or sporadic. As indicated above, seizures often occur as part of a disorder in which there is a well-recognized pattern of inheritance. These include phenylketonuria (PKU), homocystinuria, and Tay-Sachs disease, which are of autosomal recessive inheritance. Tuberous sclerosis, neurofibromatosis, and acute intermittent porphyria are autosomal dominant, whereas adrenoleukodystrophy is X-linked recessive.

CASE 12–10: PSEUDO-PSEUDOSEIZURE IN A 10-YEAR-OLD BOY

A.I., a boy with mild mental retardation, was hospitalized for management of a seizure disorder of unknown etiology. His seizures were of several kinds: generalized tonic-clonic convulsions, partial seizures with complex symptomatology (involving trancelike states with arms outstretched and speech arrest), and nocturnal awakenings with brief periods of bicycle pedaling motions of the legs.

During his hospitalization, he told the staff that he had "faked" a seizure because he did not feel he was getting enough attention. He described going toward a window, leaning against the adjacent wall, and willfully slumping to the floor to elicit help. In fact, a nurse had witnessed the episode and saw the child have a typical complex partial seizure. During the course of hospitalization, anticonvulsant medications were increased to therapeutic levels and seizures became well controlled while ongoing psychiatric care was maintained.

Comment. It is extremely difficult, if not impossible, to know precisely what happened here. Although the child claimed to have simulated a seizure, he may have been aware of the occurrence of a true seizure and said that he "faked" it in order to gain some control of an episode that was actually involuntary. Another explanation is that a pseudoseizure in some way triggered a true seizure—so that the episode involved both. Still another possibility is suggested by the child's perceptions and behavior. He approached the window with thoughts of jumping through it and might have had an hysterical seizure as a self-protective alternative.

Telemetered electroencephalography and videotaping of behavior would certainly have been helpful in unraveling these possibilities. Episodes did not recur, however, and the youngster appeared to be reassured by further explanation of the reasons for his hospitalization, the tests involved, and the anticipated duration of his stay.

Developmental Causes. As described earlier, most children with uncomplicated febrile seizures will outgrow the problem by 5 to 7 years of age. Developmental factors thus can be inferred, although the precise basis for this outcome is unknown. One has only to consider the extraordinary degree of brain growth that occurs during childhood to sense the marked maturational changes taking place in anatomic, physiologic, and biochemical parameters of development. Onset of epilepsy in adolescence also implies developmental factors.

TREATMENT AND OUTCOME

In most instances, sufficiently effective control of seizures can be achieved so that they do not interfere significantly with the child's activities at home or at school. In many cases, the child will outgrow the problem after being seizure-free on anticonvulsant medication for several years. Though pharmacologic management is the cornerstone of therapy, other modes of treatment may also play a significant role in overall management (see Table 12–8).

Medical Management. The pharmacologic treatment of seizures in childhood and adolescence will depend upon the type of seizure and the degree of urgency. Phenytoin (Dilantin), phenobarbital, and carbamazepine (Tegretol) are the standard agents for treating generalized motor and partial complex seizures. Ethosuximide (Zarontin) and valproic acid (Depakene) are drugs of choice for petit mal and other absence epilepsies. The drugs commonly used in long-term management of childhood seizures, their dosage schedules, half-lives, and therapeutic blood levels are summarized in Table 12–9. Most children can be started on oral anticonvulsant medication as outpatients. Blood tests to determine anticonvulsant levels and selected other studies (such as complete blood count, measurement of liver enzymes and serum amylase) should be carried out periodically after baseline studies have been obtained. Regular follow-up visits should be arranged with telephone contact possible in between appointed times to make adjustments in medication as necessary. Electroencephalography should be carried out at intervals of 6 months to 2 years to assess cerebral maturation and degree of seizure activity. Should the child be seizure-free for several years, the neurologic examination be normal, and the electroencephalogram show minimal or no abnormalities, consideration can be given to discontinuing anticonvulsant medication over several weeks or months (Thurston, 1973; Emerson *et al.*, 1981).

Nonpharmacologic treatment of seizure disorders in childhood can be

TABLE 12–8. **Treatment of Seizures**

Medical	Treatment of intercurrent illness
	Antipyretics for fever
	Treatment of hypoglycemia, hypocalcemia, or other electrolyte abnormality
	Treatment of lead poisoning
Neurologic	Anticonvulsant medication
	Diet (medium-chain triglyceride, ketogenic)
Surgical	Removal of tumor, cortical scar
	Section of corpus callosum
	Hemicorticectomy, hemispherectomy
Psychologic	Supportive, individual, or group therapy
Social-Environmental	Seizure precautions
	Ready access to emergency treatment
	Medical information card or bracelet
Mechanical	Tinted glasses (with photosensitivity)
	Biofeedback
	Cerebellar stimulation

TABLE 12–9. **Anticonvulsants Commonly Used in Long-Term Management of Seizures**[*]

	Daily Dose (mg per kg)	Administration (doses per day)	Half-Life (hours)	Therapeutic Blood Level (µg per ml)
Generalized motor and partial complex seizures				
Phenytoin (Dilantin)	4 to 7	1 to 2	24(±12)	10 to 20
Phenobarbital (Luminal)	2 to 5	1 to 2	60(±20)	20 to 40
Carbamazepine (Tegretol)	10 to 30	2 to 3	20(±5)	4 to 12
Primidone (Mysoline)	10 to 25	2 to 4	12	7 to 15
Valproic acid (Depakene)	15 to 60	2 to 3	6 to 12	40 to 100
Absence (petit mal) seizures				
Ethosuximide (Zarontin)	20 to 40	2 to 3	16 child 60 adult	40 to 100
Clonazepam (Clonopin)	0.1 to 0.2[†]	2 to 3	18 to 50	10 to 60 ng per ml
Valproic acid (Depakene)	15 to 60	2 to 3	6 to 12	40 to 100
Trimethadione (Tridione)	10 to 40	2 to 3	dimethadione: 72 to 144 trimethadione 10	dimethadione: 600 to 1000 trimethadione 20 to 40
Acetazolamide (Diamox)	15 to 30	2 to 3	1½ plasma 48 tissue	10 to 14
Diazepam (Valium)	0.15 to 2.0	2 to 3	24 to 42	Not established

[*] From Oppenheimer, E. Y., and Rosman, N. P. Seizures in childhood: an approach to emergency management. *Pediatr. Clin. North Am.*, **26:** 837–55, 1979.
[†] Starting dose in children: 0.01–0.03 mg per kg per day.

347

helpful in some instances. Among the most effective measures are the keto-genic and medium-chain triglyceride diets. With these diets, fats provide the majority of calories; ketosis and lowering of the blood pH (an effect opposite that produced by hyperventilation, which causes a respiratory alkalosis) result. The basis for the therapeutic efficacy of such diets in some children is not clear.

When medical illness such as diabetes mellitus, asthma, or streptococcal pharyngitis has contributed to a seizure, specific treatment will reduce the likelihood of further seizures. Fever itself, which may also precipitate seizures, should be treated with standard doses of aspirin or acetaminophen. Tepid water bathing should be employed if temperature exceeds 104 degrees rectally.

If metabolic abnormalities such as hypoglycemia or hypocalcemia have been identified, further evaluation should determine the cause of the problem and the further therapeutic course. For example, insulinoma would be treated surgically, hypoparathyroidism with oral calcium. Lead poisoning with seizures is a medical emergency since increased intracranial pressure is usually associated. Urgent treatment of intracranial hypertension is required along with anticonvulsant medication and chelating agents.

The recurrence of seizures in a child being treated with anticonvulsant medication is a common problem. The likeliest causes are inadequate blood levels of anticonvulsant medication, intercurrent illness, stress, or a combination of these factors. Worsening of the underlying disease process should be considered also, but it is usually much less likely.

A low blood level of anticonvulsant medication does not necessarily mean that the child's mother has not been giving the medicine. Other possibilities must be considered as well. Perhaps the commonest is that the child has outgrown his or her previously prescribed dosage. For example, the 20 kilogram child whose seizures were well controlled on 100 mg of phenobarbital daily (5 mg/kg/day) may have a return of seizures on the same amount of phenobarbital after a weight gain of 5 kilograms (now only 4 mg/kg/day).

A subtherapeutic blood level can also result when a child chronically pretends to take, but does not actually swallow, the anticonvulsant medication. Errors in transcription of a prescription may result in the incorrect medicine being taken or the correct medicine taken but in incorrect amounts. The preparation itself may play a role. For example, suspensions of phenytoin require vigorous shaking to achieve a homogeneous solution. Otherwise, through faulty mixing, the child may have seizures while taking the first half of the bottle and phenytoin toxicity during the second half. Out-of-date medication is another possible cause of ineffective treatment.

Intercurrent illness, often unsuspected by the parent, is a common reason for seizure recurrence in an otherwise well-controlled child. Stresses, emotional or physical, also can worsen seizure control. The increased demands of adolescence—academic, athletic, and social—render the teenager particularly vulnerable to sleep deprivation, which, when combined with poor eating habits, can significantly increase the risk of further seizures despite regular medication intake (see Case 12–11).

CASE 12–11: TEMPORAL LOBE SEIZURES PRECIPITATED BY INTERCURRENT ILLNESS IN AN 8-YEAR-OLD GIRL

K.A., treated with phenytoin for temporal lobe epilepsy of unknown cause, complained to her mother, "I can't see." In the hospital emergency room, she was awake though subdued and not normally responsive. She tended to look up and to the left, although her eyes wandered in all fields of gaze. She slapped her thighs occasionally, protruded her tongue, and made mouthing and chewing movements. When asked how many fingers the examiner held up, she guessed or said that she couldn't see. General physical examination revealed a temperature of 101.4 degrees rectally and an inflamed, bulging left tympanic membrane. She was treated with acetaminophen by mouth, and within an hour she was fully alert, normally responsive, conversing freely, and visually intact.

Comment. This child's altered mental state and behavioral automatisms constituted a partial seizure with complex symptomatology, consistent with her known temporal lobe seizure disorder (see Case 5–5). The cause for seizure recurrence appeared to be an intercurrent illness that had developed so rapidly that it was unsuspected by her mother. Inadequate level of anticonvulsant medication was another consideration but was excluded by a blood level of phenytoin within the therapeutic range.

The child's gazing up and to the left suggested the presence of a right cerebral seizure focus; and, indeed, past EEGs had shown spike-and-slow-wave complexes arising from the right temporal region (see Fig. 5–3).

Neurologic Management. Status epilepticus involving generalized motor seizures is an emergency because of the risk of brain damage due to associated cerebral hypoxia, acidosis, hypotension, hypoglycemia, hyperkalemia, hyperpyrexia, and increased intracranial pressure. Status epilepticus is defined as seizure activity persisting for more than 30 minutes or seizures occurring so often that recovery between seizures is incomplete. Drug treatment is essential but is not the first nor necessarily the most important part of therapy. Initial supportive measures involve ensuring a patent airway; providing for adequate ventilation; administering oxygen by face mask or nasal prongs; assuring that pulse rate, cardiac rhythm, and blood pressure are adequate; establishing an intravenous line for administration of medications; and rapidly assessing the nature and degree of any associated trauma that may be present.

Diagnostic studies should include blood sugar, calcium, other electrolytes, anticonvulsant levels, and complete blood count. Blood sugar determination by "Dextrostix" should be carried out at the bedside. Measurement of lead level, liver enzymes, and blood ammonia should be considered. Hypertonic glucose (25 per cent) should be given intravenously immediately after diagnostic blood samples have been obtained. Phenytoin, diazepam,

CASE 12–12: ABSENCE STATUS EPILEPTICUS PRODUCING ACUTE CONFUSIONAL STATE IN AN 11-YEAR-OLD GIRL

R.L. began having absence seizures associated with lip-smacking and provoked by hyperventilation at the age of 5 years. EEG showed spike-and-slow-wave discharges, although not the pattern of classic petit mal epilepsy. A combination of phenytoin and acetazolamide proved to be most effective in controlling her seizures.

At age 11 she was brought to the hospital because of "unusual behavior." On examination she was awake, alert, and afebrile. She was able to walk without assistance and could carry out simple commands. When asked a question, she began to answer it then drifted away without completing the sentence. She manifested an acute confusional state felt to be caused most likely by continuous absence seizure activity (status epilepticus). Accordingly, she was given 2 mg of diazepam by slow intravenous infusion, whereupon she dramatically recovered her normal state of awareness and responsivity. Over the next 2 years, this clinical picture of acute confusion returned twice. No definite cause was identified, and each episode was terminated by small amounts of intravenous diazepam.

Comment. This child met the criteria for status epilepticus, since she experienced continuous seizure activity for several hours. Status epilepticus is usually considered a medical and neurologic emergency. Indeed, it *is* an emergency when generalized motor seizures are involved since the convulsing body's consumption of oxygen and glucose can deprive the brain of necessary metabolites for its maintenance. In this case, however, with status epilepticus involving absence seizures (or with status epilepticus involving

phenobarbital, and paraldehyde are standard drugs in the treatment of status epilepticus. These drugs should be administered with continous monitoring of vital signs to detect cardiac and/or respiratory depression (Oppenheimer and Rosman, 1979) (see Case 12–12).

Surgical Management. Surgical therapy has an infrequent though important role to play in management of seizure disorders of childhood and adolescence (Falconer, 1973; Goldring, 1978; Glaser, 1980). A brain tumor producing focal seizures may be amenable to operative removal. Even when a tumor has not been identified, neurosurgical removal of a meningeal-cerebral scar or other discrete seizure focus may be beneficial when seizures are refractory to medical management. With some vascular malformations, embolization using inert materials has been employed in order to arrest enlargement of the malformation or induce it to shrink. Occasionally, as with poorly controlled seizures in children with Sturge-Weber syndrome, surgical removal of the cerebral cortex of one hemisphere can significantly improve seizure control. In other instances also involving intractible seizures, section of the corpus callosum has been carried out to prevent focal seizures from becoming secondarily generalized.

partial seizures only), the situation is far less an emergency. In fact, overly aggressive pharmacologic treatment of seizures in these instances is potentially dangerous because of the risks of overtreatment (which include respiratory arrest, particularly when diazepam and phenobarbital are used together). In this case a relatively small amount of diazepam was used, less than half the amount usually necessary to treat generalized motor status epilepticus.

The cause of the child's acute confusional state here was suggested by her known neurologic disorder. Either inadequate or excessive anticonvulsant medication may cause worsening of seizure control. Blood levels of medication can be used to confirm the clinical impression.

Acute confusional state is defined as an alteration in consciousness (in its sense of either alertness or awareness) marked by a lack of orientation and coherence in behavior, including motor activity, thought, and affect. The cause of the confusional state will usually be determined by the history and examination. Febrile delirium, insulin overdosage, drug abuse, postictal state, petit mal or complex partial status epilepticus, migraine syndrome, head trauma, central nervous system infection, and emotional stress should be considered (McBride *et al.*, 1981). Investigation might include analysis of blood, urine, and gastric contents for toxic materials; examination of cerebrospinal fluid; blood sugar determination (by laboratory as well as by "Dextrostix"); CT scan; and electroencephalogram. In some instances the etiology of an acute confusional state may be less clear or may be altogether obscure. Acute confusional state should be differentiated from such conditions as periodic paralysis or cataplexy, which are not associated with altered consciousness (see Chapters 7, 9, 11, and 19).

Psychotherapy.   Supportive therapy is always indicated in the management of the child or adolescent with a seizure disorder. Reassurance, explanation, and encouragement to participate in any and all appropriate activities will help the child and family deal with and adapt to the seizure problem with its many psychologic and social ramifications.

The child with a seizure disorder may be anxious about the problem. He may think, for example, that his seizures are contagious and not wish his friends to catch them. He may be embarrassed because of seizures that have been witnessed at school and concerned that they might occur again. Particularly with partial complex seizures involving psychic symptomatology, a child may fear he is losing his mind. The child's anxieties may be compounded by parental reluctance to let their child proceed as independently as before the onset of seizures.

It can be valuable to learn why the child feels he or she has seizures. The child may feel personally responsible for the problem and link its cause magically to simultaneous, though otherwise unrelated, events.

Group therapy may be helpful with adolescents, particularly in helping them deal with issues of chronic medication and "being different."

Social-Environmental Management. Certain precautions are advisable with the child who has had a seizure. Activities such as tree-climbing, rope-climbing, and others involving heights should be excluded. Swimming is acceptable so long as a capable person is within immediate reach of the child in the water at all times. The "buddy system" should also be practiced with bicycle riding. Bathing should take place behind an unlocked bathroom door and should be monitored. The child with a seizure disorder should not sleep on an upper bunk.

Family members, babysitters, and the school nurse should be advised as to essential first aid for a grand mal seizure: turning the child on his side to prevent aspiration of vomited material, gently extending the neck to maximize patency of the airway, and calling for help. A medical information bracelet or identification card is often indicated. It should contain, or permit immediate access to, information as to diagnosis, medications, allergies, and physicians involved in the child's care.

Mechanical Therapy. Tinted eyeglasses or contact lenses (emerald green or royal blue) may benefit some children with photosensitive epilepsy (see Figs. 12–6 and 12–7). Behavior modification techniques using the EEG for biofeedback has also been effective in some instances. Electrical stimulation of the cerebellum has been employed in some cases of seizures refractory to other modes of therapy (Grabow et al., 1974).

CORRELATION

Anatomic Aspects. Much information as to localization of function within the brain has been gained through correlation of states of abnormal function with pathologic brain anatomy. Brain injury (due to tumor, stroke, or trauma, for example) usually results in functional disturbance manifested as paralysis (partial or complete) or as seizures.

Additional knowledge of cerebral localization has been obtained through direct electrical stimulation of brain. Penfield and Rasmussen (1950) mapped the cerebral cortex of man through studies in persons with focal epilepsy. Because seizures in these persons had been unresponsive to the anticonvulsant medications available at the time, consideration was given to surgical removal of the seizure focus if it could be identified and if its removal did not present a graver risk to the patient than did the seizure disorder itself. Identification of the seizure focus was thus undertaken by craniotomy carried out under local anesthesia with exposure of the underlying brain (the overlying dura being reflected away).

Direct visualization often disclosed the area of disturbance: for example, a tumor, vascular malformation, or scar binding the meninges to a discrete portion of brain. A small amount of electric current was then applied to the brain in various locations in order to reproduce the focal seizure and determine the function of adjacent areas of brain. Since brain tissue itself is not pain-sensitive, such electrical stimulation was not painful. The comments of the fully alert patient were recorded; for the behavior generated often was not a visible movement but, rather, a sensation, emotion, or memory. Small numbered pieces of paper ("tickets") were temporarily placed upon the surface of the brain and photographed, allowing for further study and correlation.

These and other investigations have led to delineation of motor and sensory homunculi. These are maps of precentral (frontal) and postcentral (parietal) cortex correlating motor and sensory functions, respectively, with discrete areas of brain (see Figs. 2–13 and 12–8). The homunculi are cartoon-like mannikins representing the body essentially upside-down (an exception being the area representing the face) and reversed, that is, the left cortex correlated with right-sided bodily function. Relatively large cortical areas corresponding to the face and hands reflect the complexity of movement of which their component parts are capable. Also of particular note are portions of cortex lying not over the convexities but tucked into the Sylvian fissures. These infolded areas of the insula provide the anatomic basis for epigastric discomfort and other sensory auras that can occur with seizures originating from the adjacent temporal lobes (see Fig. 12–8).

The cortical representation of the upper extremities demonstrates the path of epileptic progression in a Jacksonian "march." This is a partial seizure with elementary motor symptomatology beginning with rhythmic movements of the thumb, then the fingers, hand, and entire upper limb. This

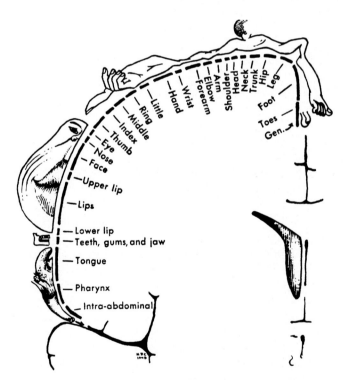

FIGURE 12–8. Sensory homunculus depicting somatotopic organization (From Penfield, W., and Rasmussen, T. *The Cerebral Cortex of Man*. Macmillan Publishing Co., Inc., New York, 1950.)

progression continues to involve one whole side of the body and may become secondarily generalized. At that point loss of consciousness occurs as the alerting mechanisms of brainstem and hypothalamus are disrupted by the abnormal electrical activity being propagated.

Biochemical Aspects.   The abnormal electrical activity involved in a seizure is determined by events at the cellular level. The cell membrane divides the electrically negative cell interior from its electrically positive surroundings. This electrical difference results from (1) movement of potassium (K^+) out of the cell and chloride (Cl^-) into the cell along an osmotic gradient and (2) pumping of sodium (Na^+) out of the cell against an osmotic gradient, a process that requires energy. Sodium is further excluded from the cell by similarly charged calcium ions (Ca^{++}) lying alongside pores or channels in the cell membrane. Glia, supporting tissue of the central nervous system, may also contribute to the ionic state by taking up potassium from the extracellular space.

Electrical discharge results from destabilization of this "ionic truce." Polarity is reversed as sodium enters the cell. The interior of the cell now becomes positive, and an electrical impulse is generated.

In normal circumstances neurotransmitters regulate ionic traffic in an orderly fashion, allowing for effective communication between different parts of the central nervous system. Acetylcholine, for example, is an excitatory neurotransmitter causing, or contributing to, depolarization. Gamma aminobutyric acid (GABA), on the other hand, is an inhibitory neurotransmitter. It renders the cell interior more negative, apparently by its effect upon chloride ion flow. GABA is made from glutamic acid, an amino acid, with pyridoxine (vitamin B_6) a cofactor in its production.

Abnormal electrical activity of brain can result when any of these mechanisms are disrupted. Hypoglycemia and hypoxia deprive the sodium pump of its fuel, permitting sodium influx and membrane depolarization. With hypocalcemia, ionic channels are unblocked and sodium ions can rush into the cell relatively unimpeded. Direct mechanical stimulation of neurons (as with head trauma) also can cause sudden membrane depolarization. The result in some instances is an immediate posttraumatic seizure.

Deficiency of vitamin B_6 (presumably leading to low levels of GABA) appears to underlie the generalized seizures of pyridoxine deficiency or dependency. These conditions are responsive to physiologic or pharmacologic doses, respectively, of this vitamin. Zinc (a trace metal) and taurine (a nonessential amino acid) have also been implicated in the pathophysiology of seizures through their effects upon cell membranes (Barbeau and Donaldson, 1974). Alterations of sodium, potassium or chloride usually do not play a major role in producing seizures, although seizures are frequent in children with water intoxication and hyponatremia.

Physiologic Aspects.   In contrast to the CT scan, the electroencephalogram provides a dynamic view of the brain, a record of its ongoing electrical activity. Pyramidal cells of the cerebral cortex appear to give rise to the slow waves characteristic of non-REM sleep (see Chapter 9). Their apical dendrites, oriented perpendicular to the cortical surface, are felt to play a particularly important role in generating this activity. The synchronization of cerebral electrical activity that normally occurs during sleep has been attributed to a "pacemaker" based in nonspecific thalamic nuclei acting in conjunction with sleep centers of the hypothalamus. Desynchronization, or activation, occurs through alerting mechanisms of the reticular activating system of the pons and midbrain.

The thalamus and other deep cerebral structures have been implicated in the production of spike-and-wave discharges such as are seen in petit mal and other so-called centrencephalic forms of epilepsy. These generalized discharges have been demonstrated to arise from direct stimulation of deep cerebral structures. Alternatively, a centrencephalic "generator" may be secondarily activated by a cortical or subcortical seizure focus. In petit mal epilepsy the first situation pertains, as structural lesions of brain are identified in this disorder exceedingly rarely. In other forms of seizure disorder involving staring spells (such as seizures of partial complex type), however, a structural lesion (for example of the medial temporal lobe) may be demonstrable and serve as a focus for the secondary spread of seizure activity to centrencephalic regions of brain.

SUMMARY

A seizure is an episode of involuntary behavior resulting from sudden, excessive electrical activity of brain. Seizures may be categorized as partial or generalized, with associated symptomatology further described as elementary or complex. The diagnosis of seizure is ultimately a clinical one, based most importantly upon a careful history elicited from the affected child, parents, and/or other observers. Examination should include a search for characteristic neurocutaneous lesions, focal neurologic signs, and abnormal response to hyperventilation. Investigation will usually include electroencephalogram, complete blood count, blood glucose, and serum calcium. Other studies such as skull x-rays or CT scan should be pursued as the clinical situation warrants.

The etiology of seizures in children is often idiopathic, influenced by developmental and maturational factors. Identifiable causes of seizure such as metabolic disturbance, tumor, vascular malformation, infection, neurocutaneous disorder, and degenerative disease should be sought. Consideration must also be given to conditions that might be mistaken for seizure. These include syncope, breath-holding spell, cardiac arrhythmia, narcolepsy, night terror, migraine, vertigo, shivering, and pseudoseizure.

Therapy will be specific when specific etiologic factors have been identified such as hypoglycemia, hypocalcemia, pyridoxine dependency, or aminoacidopathy. Otherwise, symptomatic treatment with anticonvulsant medication is pursued, the particular drug(s) depending upon the type of seizure and its frequency. The prognosis for seizure control in the majority of children is excellent. Social and psychologic factors are usually involved secondarily in seizure disorders of childhood and adolescence and must be taken into account in overall management, which should not be limited merely to drug therapy.

CITED REFERENCES

Abildskov, J. A. The prolonged QT interval. *Annu. Rev. Med., 30:* 171–79, 1979.

Baldessarini, R. J. Drugs and the treatment of psychiatric disorders. Pp. 391–447 in *The Pharmacological Basis of Therapeutics,* 6th ed. Gilman, A. G.; Goodman, L. S.; and Gilman, A., eds. Macmillan Publishing Co., Inc., New York, 1980.

Barbeau, A., and Donaldson, J. Zinc, taurine, and epilepsy. *Arch. Neurol., 30:* 52–58, 1974.

Bear, D. M., and Fedio, P. Quantitative analysis of interictal behavior in temporal lobe epilepsy. *Arch. Neurol., 34:* 454–67, 1977.

Binnie, C. D.; Darby, C. E.; De Korte, R. A.; and Wilkins, A. J. Self-induction of epileptic seizures by eyeclosure: incidence and recognition. *J. Neurol. Neurosurg. Psychiatry, 43:* 386–89, 1980.

Bray, P. F.; Herbst, J. J.; Johnson, D. G.; Book, L. S., Ziter, F. A.; and Condon, V. R. Childhood gastroesophageal reflux: neurologic and psychiatric syndromes mimicked. *JAMA, 237:* 1342–45, 1977.

Emerson, R.; D'Souza, B. J.; Vining, E. P.; Holden, K. R.; Mellits, E. D.; and Freeman, J. M. Stopping medication in children with epilepsy: predictors of outcome. *N. Engl. J. Med., 304:* 1125–29, 1981.

Falconer, M. A. Reversibility by temporal-lobe resection of the behavioral abnormalities of temporal-lobe epilepsy. *N. Engl. J. Med., 289:* 451–55, 1973.

Falconer, M. A.; Serafetinides, E.; and Corsellis, J. A. N. Etiology and pathogenesis of temporal lobe epilepsy. *Arch. Neurol., 10:* 233–48, 1964.

Finlayson, R. E., and Lucas, A. R. Pseudoepileptic seizures in children and adolescents. *Mayo Clin. Proc., 54:* 83–87, 1979.

Forster, F. M. Classification and conditioning treatment of reflex epilepsies. *Int. J. Neurol., 9:* 73–76, 1972.

Frank, J. P., and Friedberg, D. Z. Syncope with prolonged QT interval. *Am. J. Dis. Child., 130:* 320–22, 1976.

Glaser, G. H. Treatment of intractable temporal lobe-limbic epilepsy (complex partial seizures) by temporal lobectomy. *Ann. Neurol., 8:* 455–59, 1980.

Goldring, S. A method for surgical management of focal epilepsy, especially as it relates to children. *J. Neurosurg., 49:* 344–56, 1978.

Grabow, J. D.; Ebersold, M. J.; Albers, J. W.; and Schima, E. M. Cerebellar stimulation for control of seizures. *Mayo Clin. Proc., 49:* 759–74, 1974.

Hazelton, R. A.; Reid, A. C.; and Rooney, P. J. Cerebral systemic lupus erythematosus: a case report and evaluation of diagnostic tests. *J. Neurol. Neurosurg. Psychiatry, 43:* 357–59, 1980.

Ingvar, D. H., and Nyman, G. E. Epilepsia arithmetices: a new psychologic trigger mechanism in a case of epilepsy. *Neurology* (Minneapolis), *12:* 282–87, 1962.

Lindsay, J.; Ounsted, C.; and Richards, P. Long-term outcome in children with temporal lobe seizures: III. psychiatric aspects in childhood and adult life. *Dev. Med. Child Neurol., 21:* 630–36, 1979.

Lombroso, C. T., and Lerman, P. Breathholding spells (cyanotic and pallid infantile syncope). *Pediatrics, 39:* 563–81, 1967.

Lown, B.; DeSilva, R. A.; Reich, P.; and Murawski, B. J. Psychophysiologic factors in sudden cardiac death. *Am. J. Psychiatry, 137:* 1325–35, 1980.

Mathews, E. C., Jr.; Blount, A. W., Jr.; and Townsend, J. I. Q-T prolongation and ventricular arrhythmias, with and without deafness, in the same family. *Am. J. Cardiology, 29:* 702–11, 1972.

McBride, M. C.; Dooling, E. C.; and Oppenheimer, E. Y. Complex partial status epilepticus in young children. *Ann. Neurol., 9:* 526–30, 1981.

Nelson, K. B., and Ellenberg, J. H. Predictors of epilepsy in children who have experienced febrile seizures. *N. Engl. J. Med.,* **295:** 1029–33, 1976.

Oppenheimer, E. Y., and Rosman, N. P. Seizures in childhood: an approach to emergency management. *Pediatr. Clin. North Am.,* **26:** 837–55, 1979.

Panayiotopoulos, C. P. Self-induced pattern-sensitive epilepsy. *Arch. Neurol.,* **36:** 48–50, 1979.

Penfield, W., and Rasmussen, T. *The Cerebral Cortex of Man.* Macmillan Publishing Co., Inc., New York, 1950.

Pritchard, P. B., III; Lombroso, C. T.; and McIntyre, M. Psychological complications of temporal lobe epilepsy. *Neurology,* **30:** 227–32, 1980.

Reif-Lehrer, L., and Stemmermann, M. G. Monosodium glutamate intolerance in children. *N. Engl. J. Med.,* **293:** 1204–05, 1975.

Rosenlund, M. L., and Schnaufer, L. Gastric duplication presenting as cyclic abdominal pain. *Clin. Pediatr.* (Phila.), **17:** 747–48, 753, 1978.

Rosman, N. P., and Herskowitz, J. Trauma to the brain. In *The Practice of Pediatric Neurology, 2d ed.* Swaiman, K. F., and Wright, F. S., eds. C. V. Mosby Co., Saint Louis, 1982.

Rosman, N. P., and Pearce, J. The brain in multiple neurofibromatosis (von Recklinghausen's Disease): a suggested neuropathological basis for the associated mental defect. *Brain,* **90:** 829–38, 1967.

Schneider, S., and Rice, D. R. Neurologic manifestations of childhood hysteria. *J. Pediatr.,* **94:** 153–56, 1979.

Schott, G. D.; McLeod, A. A.; and Jewitt, D. E. Cardiac arrhythmias that masquerade as epilepsy. *Br. Med. J.,* **1:** 1454–57, 1977.

Stephenson, J. B. P. Reflex anoxic seizures ("white breath-holding"): nonepileptic vagal attacks. *Arch. Dis. Child.,* **53:** 193–200, 1978.

Thurston, J. H. Childhood epilepsy: the outlook for termination of therapy. *Hosp. Pract.,* October 1973, pp. 101–5.

Waxman, S. G., and Geschwind, N. The interictal behavior syndrome of temporal lobe epilepsy. *Arch. Gen. Psychiatry,* **32:** 1580–86, 1975.

Wellens, H. J. J.; Vermeulen, A.; and Durrer, D. Ventricular fibrillation occurring on arousal from sleep by auditory stimuli. *Circulation,* **46:** 661–65, 1972.

Whitehouse, D. Diagnostic value of the café-au-lait spot in children. *Arch. Dis., Child.,* **41:** 316–19, 1966.

Wiebers, D. O.; Westmoreland, B. F.; and Klass, D. W. EEG activation and mathematical calculation. *Neurology,* **29:** 1499–1503, 1979.

Williams, D. T.; Spiegel, H.; and Mostofsky, D. I. Neurogenic and hysterical seizures in children and adolescents: differential diagnostic and therapeutic considerations. *Am. J. Psychiatry,* **135:** 82–86, 1978.

ADDITIONAL READINGS

Delgado-Escueta, A. V.; Mattson, R. H.; King, L.; Goldensohn, E. S.; Spiegel, H.; Madsen, J.; Crandall, P.; Dreifuss, F.; and Porter, R. J. The nature of aggression during epileptic seizures. *N. Engl. J. Med.,* **305:** 711–16, 1981.

Freeman, J. M. Febrile seizures: a consensus of their significance, evaluation, and treatment. *Pediatrics,* **66:** 1009, 1980.

Glaser, G. H.; Penry, J. K.; and Woodbury, D. M. *Antiepileptic Drugs. Mechanisms of Action.* Raven Press, New York, 1980.

Johnston, M. V., and Freeman, J. M. Pharmacologic advances in seizure control. *Pediatr. Clin. North Am.,* **28:** 179–94, 1981.

Magnus, O., and de Haas, A. M. L. The epilepsies. In *Handbook of Clinical Neurology*. Vinken, P. J., and Bruyn, G. W., eds. North-Holland Publishing Co., Inc., Amsterdam, 1974.

Penfield, W., and Jasper, H. *Epilepsy and the Functional Anatomy of the Human Brain*. Little, Brown and Company, Boston, 1954.

Schenk, L., and Bear, D. Multiple personality and related dissociative phenomena in patients with temporal lobe epilepsy. *Am. J. Psychiatry,* **138:** 1311–15, 1981.

Scott, D. F. Psychiatric aspects of epilepsy. *Br. J. Psychiatry,* **132:** 417–30, 1978.

So, E. L., and Penry, J. K. Epilepsy in adults. *Ann. Neurol.,* **9:** 3–16, 1981.

13 Disorders of Movement: Gait Disturbance, Tic, Tremor, and Clumsiness

Movement is a pervasive and essentially continuous aspect of life, richly intertwined with thought, language, and emotion. Even during sleep, movement occurs. The thorax and abdomen are involved in breathing; the eyes make slow, rolling movements or rapid movements associated with dreaming; digestive processes continue.

In general some movements occur as part of voluntary action (getting from one place to another; carrying out specific tasks). Other movements, such as those of breathing or sleeping, are involuntary. Because of its role in behavior of all kinds, movement is altered or disturbed with many kinds of behavioral problems. Hyperkinetic behavior is an obvious example, associated with attentional problems and impulsivity (see Chapter 14). Slowed behavior and diminished movement occur with depression and hypothyroidism.

This chapter will discuss certain general aspects of movement, such as its definition, as well as specific topics. These will include the clinical approach to the child with a movement disorder, the organic basis for such disorders, and several common problems in which disorders of movement are present: gait problems, tics (which includes Tourette disease), tremor, and clumsiness. Chapters on Hysteria (7), Seizures (12), and Hyperactivity and Attentional Disorders (14) deal further with several of the problems considered here.

Several questions will be addressed in this chapter:

How is movement defined?
What is a movement disorder?
What information should be sought by history in the child with a movement problem?
What should the medical, neurologic, and mental status examinations focus upon?
What causes of movement disorder should be considered?

359

What investigation is indicated in the child with a gait disorder? With clumsiness? With tics?

What treatments are available, and what outcomes can be anticipated?

DISORDERS OF MOVEMENT

DEFINITION

Movement can be defined as the process of change in position over time. This definition encompasses many kinds of movement and provides a framework for viewing motor function and dysfunction. Position, as it applies in this definition, refers to posture, and movement can be viewed as progression from one posture to another.

A disorder of movement can involve any of these components: the process of change, the positions (or postures) involved, and the rate of change. The process of change might be jerky and discontinuous rather than smooth, interrupted by unwilled movements such as head shaking or grimacing. The position attained might not be that desired. Past-pointing or clumsiness may occur. The action might be accomplished more slowly or with more exertion than normal.

In considering movement disorders, the importance of sensory function, particularly proprioception, should not be forgotten. For example, information fed back to the central nervous system signaling the tension of muscles acting across joints is integrated into the position in space of the body part so that accurate and efficient movement can be accomplished. This process is sometimes conscious, though at most times entirely unconscious.

DIAGNOSIS

Clinical Process. The following sections on history, examination, and investigation will focus on gait problems, tics, tremor, and clumsiness.

History. The chief complaint should be recorded in the words of the child and the parent: "He's been tripping a lot lately." "I can't keep myself from barking and shaking my head." "Her left hand trembles when she reaches for an object." "He has always been clumsy, like me."

The history of the presenting problem should identify the onset of the symptom, trace its course to the present, identify associated symptoms, and record their progression. Past history of pregnancy, birth, development, and head trauma will often be relevant to the presenting problem. Family history may suggest a specific diagnosis.

Gait disturbance should be described as to its character and circumstances of occurrence. Does it involve both legs or just one? Are the legs wide apart for balance? Do the legs turn in? Does the child waddle? Is climbing stairs difficult? Which is harder, going up or down stairs? Has the child fallen? Do falls tend to occur to one side more than the other?

Additional history should include drugs, recent illnesses, and associated symptoms. Does the child take anticonvulsant medication or any other drugs regularly? Have there been any changes in medication? Is anyone else at home taking phenytoin or phenobarbital? Has the child had chickenpox or any other viral illnesses recently? Have headaches, urinary incontinence, seizures, changes in personality, memory problems, or visual loss been noted? Have family members had similar problems? Is anyone wheelchair-bound? Have any neuromuscular problems such as muscular dystrophy or myasthenia gravis occurred in the family?

Tics should be characterized as to the part or parts of the body involved, frequency of occurrence, and associated feeling state. Tics usually involve the head and neck. They may be evident as head shaking, forceful blinking, arching the eyebrows, retracting the corners of the mouth, pursing the lips, winking one eye, flaring the nostrils, sniffing, clearing the throat, or coughing. These uncomplicated, simple tics are to be contrasted with those that involve more complex actions such as jumping from one spot to another or flinging the head against a desk or table. Tics usually disappear during sleep (in contrast to seizures, which may occur only then). Reaction of family and friends to the tic(s) should be noted. Does the family call attention to the tic? Has that made it more or less frequent? How does the child feel before the tic? Is there a vague feeling of discomfort, anxious foreboding, or localizable sensory signal? Does tension build if movement is voluntarily suppressed? Does the child feel better after the tic occurs?

Tremor is defined by involuntary movement at rest, with action (e.g., with arms outstretched), or with intention (e.g., with voluntary movement). It is important to determine in what circumstances and with what activities the tremor occurs. Does it interfere significantly with activity? For example, is handwriting illegible or just sloppy? Is the child taking medication (such as aminophylline, imipramine, or lithium)? Does the child often drink caffeine-containing beverages such as coffee, tea, or soft drinks? Is the child anxious?

When the child is said to be *clumsy,* it is valuable to understand whom the symptom bothers. The child may be embarrassed by inability to ride a bicycle with friends. Parents may be concerned that the child has been bumping into things increasingly and knocking them over. The teacher may describe classmates' teasing because of awkward gait or poor athletic skills.

Clumsiness should be specified as to activities in which it is prominent. Does it occur with walking, running, skipping, balancing, throwing a ball, using a fork, or writing? The parts of the body directly involved should be noted: hands, arms, legs, or trunk. Has clumsiness always been present, or has it been noted only recently? Are other family members clumsy? How have the parents dealt with the problem? If clumsiness involves gait, further inquiry as above is suggested.

Examination. The *general description* should describe the most striking aspects of the child. Is he unusually anxious? Does he stare with eyes wide open? Are tics evident? One or many? What do they involve? If vocal tics are heard, are words recognizable?

General physical examination should include vital signs and measurement of height, weight, and head circumference. These data should be plotted and abnormalities noted in absolute size (for example, greater than two standard deviations from the mean) or rate of change (for example, weight loss or excessively rapid head growth).

The skin and conjunctivae should be examined for jaundice. Rashes, ecchymoses, and evidence for self-inflicted injuries should be noted and their distribution described. If café-au-lait spots are present, their number and size should be recorded. The back should be inspected and palpated for midline bony defect, hair tuft, or fatty mass. The thyroid gland should be assessed. Abdominal examination should include estimate of liver size and hepatic tenderness to palpation and percussion. Abdominal scars should be noted.

Although motor functions will be the primary focus of the *neurologic examination,* cranial nerves, sensation, and reflexes should not be neglected. Cranial nerve examination should include particular attention to the eyes, face, and voice.

The eyes should be examined for proptosis, ptosis (drooping of the lids), and lid-lag. Ptosis tends to become more prominent as the day progresses in myasthenia gravis. The cornea should be checked for a Kayser-Fleischer brownish-green ring at its limbus, characteristic of Wilson disease. Slit-lamp examination may be required for its detection. The bulbar conjunctivae should be inspected for prominent blood vessels as in ataxia-telangiectasia. (see Fig. 13–1). Examination of the optic fundi is essential, for it may reveal papilledema associated with hydrocephalus or other causes of increased intracranial pressure (see Chapter 11). Visual acuity and visual fields must also be assessed, as the child's clumsiness (''walking into walls'') may be secondary to amblyopia or hemianopia (see Case 17–3).

The face may show *tics* or a masklike appearance. Tics should be described as to the parts of the face involved and their frequency. It may be useful (in differentiating tic from focal seizure) to ask the child to try to suppress the tic for a brief period. A bland facial appearance lacking in ex-

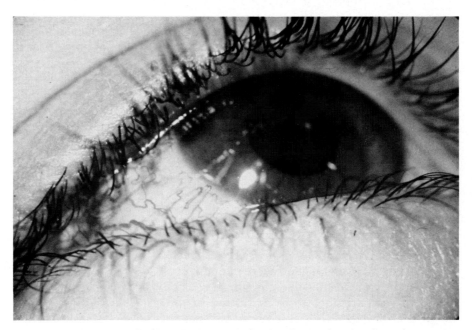

FIGURE 13–1. Conjunctival vascularization in ataxia-telangiectasia.

pression should be noted; it occurs with some muscle diseases and as a drug-related effect. Vocal tics should be described. They may be explosive, resulting from sudden diaphragmatic movements and intercostal contractions. They also may be associated with head turning, facial grimacing, or abnormal movements that literally propel the child across the room like a puppet flung by its strings.

The sensory examination is an important part of the assessment of the child with a movement disorder, especially when gait is disturbed. The position of a body part must be known to the central nervous system in order that effective movement (change in position) be carried out. Pain and temperature sensation as well as vibration, proprioception (position sense), and light touch should be examined.

Position sense can be tested in several ways. If the child can stand steadily with legs together and eyes open but falls or sways markedly when the eyes are closed, a deficit in position sense is suggested. Care must of course be taken that the child does not injure himself by falling while being tested in this way. Position sense can also be tested by the examiner grasping the child's finger or toe by its sides with thumb and forefinger and moving the digit up or down. The child is to indicate the direction of movement. Inability to detect whether movement has occurred or simply guessing supports a deficit in position sense. (With malingering, a feigned deficit in proprioception may be present, suggested by more answers being wrong than would be predicted by chance.) If a deficit at these distal-most portions of the extremities is detected, position sense should be assessed further by passive movements across the wrist and ankle joints.

Testing of deep tendon reflexes and pathologic reflexes combines aspects of the sensory and motor examinations, since reflexes by definition consist of afferent and efferent components. Reflexes may be abnormal quantitatively (that is, exaggerated or absent) or by their pattern. For example, with a hemiparesis, deep tendon reflexes will usually be brisker on the hemiparetic side of the body, often with an extensor response to plantar stimulation (Babinski sign) on that same side. Normal reflexes in the upper limbs with hyperactive reflexes in the legs (frequently associated with a bilateral Babinski sign) is often seen with spastic diplegia, hydrocephalus, and thoracic spinal cord tumor. Hypoactive reflexes, absent or elicitable only with facilitation, may be normal or associated with disease of skeletal muscle, peripheral nerves, spinal nerve roots, or spinal cord (anterior horn cells). Deep tendon reflexes are graded 0 through 4, as described in Chapter 4.

Examination of the motor system can be divided into several parts: observation, palpation, percussion, and functional testing. Striking observations such as tremor, tics, or dystonic posturing may have been included as part of the general description. Muscle bulk should be described. Are calves and deltoids enlarged? Are proximal muscles wasted? Are involuntary, worm-like muscle twitches (fasciculations) evident? Palpation can reveal a "doughy" quality to affected muscles (especially calves) in children with X-linked muscular dystrophy, because of infiltration by fat.

Palpation also includes testing of muscle tone, the resistance to passive motion across a joint. Several kinds of abnormal tone are recognized. Flac-

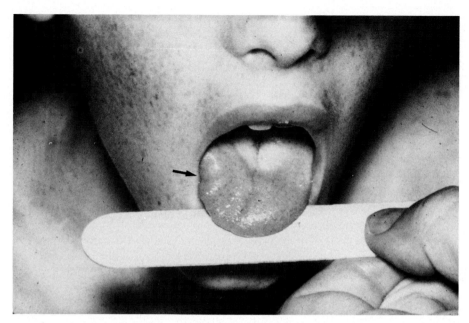

FIGURE 13–2. Percussion myotonia (persisting contraction) of the tongue (arrow).

cidity refers to looseness, floppiness, or diminution of tone. Clasp-knife rigidity refers to an initial looseness followed by increased resistance to passive movement that suddenly gives way to diminished resistance, easily permitting completion of the movement across the joint. The term clasp-knife rigidity is often used synonymously with spasticity.

Not all increase in tone, however, is spastic. Lead-pipe rigidity, or paratonia, refers to a uniformly increased resistance to passive motion. Cogwheel rigidity, seen classically with parkinsonism, is defined by a ratchety quality. Cogwheeling may be demonstrable through flexion and extension of the elbow, pronation and supination of the forearm, and flexion and extension of the wrist. Gegenhalten is said to be present when the resistance to passive movement is directly proportional to the intensity of the examiner's efforts. The harder the examiner pulls, the greater is the resistance, and vice versa.

Percussion involves striking muscle directly with a reflex hammer and observing the reaction. The deltoid, thenar, forearm, and tongue muscles are among those commonly examined in this manner. The normal response is contraction, a momentary dimpling at the site of percussion. This results from the mechanical effect of percussion. Brief flexion or extension of a joint may occur secondary to such mechanical stimulation. Sustained muscle contraction upon percussion is evidence of myotonia (see Fig. 13–2). It occurs in myotonic dystrophy, myotonia congenita, and one form of periodic paralysis. It is also manifested as an inability to relax promptly muscles voluntarily contracted, for example, with a handshake or forced eye closure.

Testing of the motor system should include assessment of individual muscle groups. Such testing should include abduction of the shoulders, flexion and extension at the elbows, wrist extension, and finger flexion (hand grip) in the upper extremities, flexion of the thigh upon the hip, flexion and extension at the knee, dorsiflexion of the ankles, and toe grip in the lower extremities.

Testing of muscle groups should identify specific areas of weakness and demonstrate whether a proximal or distal pattern of disturbance is present. Proximal weakness is characteristic of muscle diseases (such as Duchenne muscular dystrophy), metabolic myopathies (including hyperthyroidism), and inflammatory myopathies (such as polymyositis).

Functional testing of the motor system involves having the child carry out specific tasks that might be part of everyday life. The child sitting on the floor should attempt to stand up without the assistance of furniture or without climbing upon himself (Gowers sign, which is evidence of proximal muscle weakness) (see Fig. 4–5). Deep knee bends, stepping up onto a stool, climbing a flight of stairs, or reaching up to a shelf are other ways to test motor function. If a child tested by stair-walking has greater difficulty going down than up, the problem likelier involves coordination rather than strength.

When myasthenia gravis is suspected, the child should be asked to carry out repeated motor tasks in order that characteristic fatigability be elicited. For example, twenty deep knee bends, ten push-ups, or thirty forceful eye closures may be required to bring out the weakness.

Examination of *gait* is itself a form of functional testing. Before walking *per se* is observed, the distance between the feet, the base, should be noted and characterized as wide, normal, or narrow. Stability of the child's stance should be assessed and any tendency to fall one way or the other described.

Examination of gait consists of observation of the child's ordinary gait (examined without shoes or socks) and special (or stressed) gaits (walking on toes, heels, outer sides of the feet, and in tandem). Attention is directed not only to the legs but to the rhythmicity and fluidity of associated arm movements as well.

Recognizable categories of gait disorder include hemiparetic, waddling, ataxic, and hysterical. Hemiparetic gait is asymmetric. Circumduction is characteristic, with the leg swung outward about the hip rather than being brought directly forward. With more long-standing hemiparesis, toe-walking on the affected side may occur because of a tight heel cord. The arm on the affected side is held closer to the body than the contralateral limb and tends to be flexed or at least to swing less than the other. Stressed gait may bring out posturing of an affected limb that otherwise appears normal. Subtle weakness may be detected by having the child extend the arms forward with palms up, fingers outstretched, and eyes closed. Downward drift or pronation is indicative of a hemiparetic deficit on that side. The hemiparetic gait is usually accompanied by an increase in tone of spastic type. Nails, fingers, and toes on the affected side may be smaller than their counterparts.

Toe-walking affecting both legs may be seen in several conditions. These include Duchenne muscular dystrophy, associated with weakness and contracture of calf muscles; spastic diplegia, a form of cerebral palsy in which legs are more affected than arms to produce a scissoring gait; and infantile autism, in which toe-walking is a frequently seen habitual behavior. With Duchenne muscular dystrophy, weakness of proximal muscles is associated with waddling gait.

With ataxic gait, the child may assume a broad base to compensate for coordinational difficulty. Turning around may be particularly clumsy.

A characteristic feature of hysterical gait is a "stuck to the floor" quality (Dubowitz and Hersov, 1976). Astasia-abasia is described in Chapter 7.

Tremor refers to variably rhythmic, involuntary movements usually affecting the upper extremities. Tremor may also involve the head, legs, and diaphragm, the last accounting for the tremulous voice of older persons.

In examining the child with tremor, it is important to describe when it occurs (at rest, with sustained action, or with voluntary effort), its frequency, and its amplitude (coarse versus fine). The tremor in parkinsonism, although not a pediatric disorder, provides an example. It is present at rest, has a frequency of three to five oscillations per second, and disappears with intentional movement. The tremor associated with disorders of the cerebellar hemispheres is quite the opposite. It does not occur at rest but becomes evident with attempts to carry out purposeful appendicular (limb) movements. A lesion of the right cerebellar hemisphere is typically associated with an intention tremor of the right arm. Other characteristic cerebellar features are the direction of the tremor (side-to-side and perpendicular to the direction of motion) and increase in amplitude of the tremor as the goal is approached. The finger-to-nose test can illustrate these characteristics well, the tremor becoming increasingly coarse as the end point is reached. Intention tremor may be evident as the child constructs towers of blocks or copies geometric figures with pencil and paper.

The presence of tremor can be evaluated further by having the child extend the arms. This maneuver may bring out the fine action tremor of hyperthyroidism, anxiety, caffeinism, or "essential" tremor (which is often familial).

In addition to finger-to-nose maneuvers, testing of *coordinative functions* can include having the child touch the thumb to each fingertip in order; carry out rapid alternative movements (such as slapping the thighs alternately with the front and back of the hands); perform heel-to-shin maneuvers (in which the heel is brought from knee to foot in as a straight line as possible); walk in tandem, each foot touching the other in single file; and stand on one foot while the child slowly counts his age in years. Hopping, skipping, and walking down stairs can also be assessed.

Further testing of arm and hand coordination can be carried out by asking the child to imitate rhythms tapped against the thigh, draw an imaginary square in the air, pretend to screw in a light bulb, and take a small coin from the examiner by grasping it by its edges.

Since coordinative functions involve speech as well as other voluntary motor activities, the melody and the rhythm of spontaneous speech should be noted. Scanning speech is characteristic of cerebellar deficit as can occur with multiple sclerosis. It has the quality of a regular rhythm (like that of classical Latin poetry) superimposed upon that intrinsic to the words themselves. Repetition of syllables ("la-la-la . . ." or "me-me-me . . .") and phrases such as "hopping hippopotamus" also can be used to assess rhythmicity of speech.

The *mental status examination* should include special attention to affect. Affect should be noted because the child may be depressed due to his or her disability or may look depressed because of muscle weakness affecting the face causing "pseudodepression," the appearance but not the subjective feeling of depression (see Chapter 6).

Anxiety may contribute to tremor or tic and may be evidenced as fidgetiness, easy distractability, exaggerated alertness, hyperactivity, apprehension, withdrawn behavior, or expressed fear. Intelligence should be estimated, since several disorders of movement can be associated with subnormal intelligence. These include cerebral palsy and Duchenne and myotonic muscular dystrophies.

The mental status examination should include the child's perception of his or her problem, particularly with Tourette disease or with conversion reaction. With the former, the child may be able to identify sensory experiences that precede, accompany, or follow a tic (Bliss, 1980). The parents' views of the nature and seriousness of the disorder also should be explored.

Investigation. Investigation will depend upon the specific problem being considered, and especially its severity as indicated by its interference with normal activity. Since the causes of *gait disorder* range from local trauma (a stubbed toe) to distant processes (such as obstructive hydrocephalus), investigation will range from nothing at all to extensive radiologic evaluation.

When muscle disease is being considered, a complete blood count, erythrocyte sedimentation rate (ESR), thyroxine (T_4) level, and "muscle enzymes" (particularly creatine phosphokinase and aldolase) are indicated. Electromyography and nerve conduction studies can provide dynamic information about muscle and nerve. When myasthenia gravis is suspected, an edrophonium (Tensilon) test with simultaneous electromyographic monitoring will usually confirm (or exclude) the diagnosis. Muscle biopsy with routine stains, histochemical studies, and electron microscopic examination frequently provides a definitive diagnosis, particularly in disorders of muscle (dystrophies, myopathies) and spinal cord (anterior horn cell disease).

When spinal cord disorder is considered, radiologic investigation is important. Plain x-rays of the spine can demonstrate spina bifida (including diastematomyelia) or widening of interpedicular distances as with intraspinal tumor. Myelography and computerized tomography (CT) of the spine with metrizimide (water-soluble contrast) may also be carried out to determine if a pathologic process is within the spinal cord (intramedullary) or outside it (extramedullary). The assessment of multiple sclerosis, which can mimic spinal cord tumor, can include analysis of cerebrospinal fluid (with measurement of total protein and immunoglobulin G) and evaluation of visual evoked responses.

When cerebral causes for gait disorder are being considered, plain skull x-rays and cranial CT scan can determine if hydrocephalus or other cause for increased intracranial pressure is present.

Since most *tics* of childhood are so-called simple tics, investigation will usually be unnecessary. Occasionally electroencephalography should be carried out to exclude focal seizures.

For the evaluation of *tremor,* serum thyroxine (T_4) level and triiodothyronine (T_3) uptake will identify most causes of tremor due to hyperthyroidism. If the tremor appears to be on a cerebellar basis, evaluation of the posterior fossa through plain radiography and CT scan should be considered. Specialized neurophysiologic techniques may be used to characterize tremor further, monitoring and recording frequency, amplitude, and response to medication.

The mildly *clumsy* or awkward child will not usually require investigation unless a specific disorder (such as slowly progressive spinal cord tumor or muscle disease) is suggested or frequent falls have occurred (and significant associated trauma suspected).

Additional investigations are discussed with individual clinical entities in the section on ETIOLOGY.

Differential Diagnosis.   Gait disorder, tremor, and clumsiness will usually be recognized as such. With some tics, however, *focal seizures* may be difficult to distinguish from tics. Though this distinction can usually be established by careful history and examination, the electroencephalogram may be additionally helpful.

Child abuse should be considered in the clumsy child whose ecchymoses are widely distributed, not restricted to the lower extremities. Under the former circumstances, a complete blood count and platelet count should be obtained and further studies of bleeding and clotting considered (see Chapter 20).

Etiology (see Table 13–1).   *Medical Causes.   Hyperthyroidism* can cause a metabolic myopathy characterized by proximal muscle weakness (Rosman, 1976). The diagnosis of hyperthyroidism is suggested by weight loss, increased appetite, heat intolerance, and difficulty in climbing stairs. On general examination, tachycardia, exophthalmos, and goiter may be evident (see Figure 14–1). Neurologic examination will typically show a fine action tremor, proximal muscle weakness (shoulders, hips, thighs), and normally active (or heightened) patellar reflexes, which distinguish hyperthyroidism from other myopathies. Elevated blood levels of thyroid hormone definitively establish the diagnosis. Further investigation of the hypothalamic-pituitary-thyroid axis may be indicated.

Polymyositis is a connective tissue disorder in which proximal muscle weakness may be severe. It is also known as dermatomyositis when it affects the skin, characteristically over extensor surfaces of the extremities. In contrast to adult forms of the disease, polymyositis in childhood rarely is associated with malignancy.

Gait problems may be secondary to local disease or injury of the leg: skin, subcutaneous tissue, bone, or joint. Soft tissue injury and *cellulitis* will generally be readily evident. *Osteomyelitis* should be considered even if external injury is not apparent, since a puncture wound may have healed superficially days to weeks earlier. When osteomyelitis is suspected, investigation should include multiple blood cultures, erythrocyte sedimentation rate, complete blood count, plain radiographs of the affected limb, and, in se-

TABLE 13–1. **Causes of Movement Disorders**

Medical	Hyperthyroidism
	Polymyositis
	Cellulitis
	Osteomyelitis
	Joint infection
Neurologic	Muscular dystrophies (Duchenne, Becker, myotonic)
	Congenital myopathies (nemaline, central core)
	Myasthenia gravis (neonatal, congenital, juvenile)
	Neuropathy/radiculopathy (acute intermittent porphyria, diphtheria, Guillain-Barré)
	Spinal cord disorder (poliomyelitis, Werdnig-Hoffmann disease, Kugelberg-Welander disease, tumor, angioma, abscess, hematoma, cyst, motor neuron disease, vitamin B_{12} deficiency, syringomyelia, diastematomyelia, multiple sclerosis, myelomeningocele, Arnold-Chiari malformation)
	Basal gangliar disorder (Wilson disease, Sydenham chorea, dystonia musculorum deformans, Huntington chorea, Tourette disease, paroxysmal choreoathetosis)
	Cerebellar disorder (tumor: hemispheric, midline)
	Cerebral disorder (hydrocephalus, cerebral palsy: spastic, atonic, ataxic, athetoid)
	Secondary to visual deficit (optic neuritis, optic atrophy, hemianopia, tunnel vision)
	Vestibular causes
Toxic	Anticonvulsants (phenobarbital, phenytoin [Dilantin]) in excess
	Abused drugs (alcohol, barbiturates)
	Steroids
	Tremor caused by aminophylline, theophylline, caffeine, imipramine (Tofranil), lithium, valproic acid (Depakene)
	Extrapyramidal reaction caused by trifluoperazine (Stelazine), prochlorperazine (Compazine), halo-peridol (Haldol), methylphenidate (Ritalin), dextroamphetamine (Dexedrine), antihistamines
Psychologic	Hysteria
	Malingering
	Anxiety (exacerbating tics, tremor)
Genetic-Constitutional	Muscular dystrophies, myopathies, acute intermittent porphyria, Tourette syndrome, spinal muscular atrophies
Developmental	Clumsiness
	Hyperactivity

lected instances, radioisotope bone scan. Plain x-rays may be negative for 1 to 2 weeks after injury and may need to be repeated later if the diagnosis of osteomyelitis is still being considered.

Joint infection (septic arthritis) of the lower limb(s) may be gradual at onset and difficult to diagnose. A further impediment to diagnosis is that pain referred to the leg or knee may actually originate at the hip. Hip involvement may be suggested by the position of the hip joint when the child is supine. The thigh is partially flexed, abducted, and externally rotated, all of which diminish traction upon an inflamed hip joint. In addition to pain, other signs of inflammation—erythema, warmth, swelling, and diminished range of motion—may be present as well.

Neurologic Causes.   Neurologic causes of gait disorder, tic, tremor, and clumsiness will be discussed in this section. Neurologic causes of gait disturbance are considered from peripheral to central.

The most common serious muscle disorder in childhood is *Duchenne muscular dystrophy*. It is an X-linked recessive disorder, hence affects only males in its full-blown clinical picture. Duchenne muscular dystrophy usually presents insidiously in early childhood (ages 2 to 4 years) often with a delay in walking, clumsiness, inability to run, or difficulty climbing stairs.

On examination, calves are prominent ("pseudohypertrophic" due to in-filtration of fat) and feel doughy upon palpation. Deep tendon reflexes are generally diminished. Proximal muscle weakness is evident, and a Gowers sign may be seen (see Fig. 4–5). Winging of the scapulae and lumbar lordosis

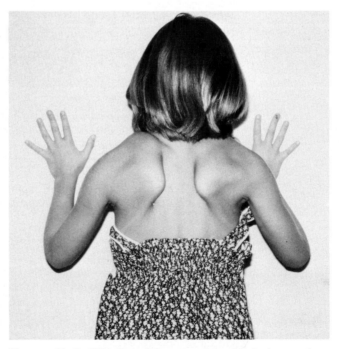

FIGURE 13–3. Winging of the scapulae with facioscapulo-humeral muscular dystrophy.

are typical (see Fig. 13–3). A waddling gait is characteristic. Toe-walking may also be seen. Mental retardation (usually mild, occasionally moderate) is often found (Rosman and Kakulas, 1966; Rosman, 1970). General examination may show tachycardia as a manifestation of cardiac involvement. Diagnosis is based upon family history, occurrence in a boy, elevated serum creatine phosphokinase (CPK) level, and characteristic muscle biopsy, showing excessive variation in fiber size and replacement of muscle with fatty and fibrous tissue (see Fig. 4–8).

A later-onset form of X-linked muscular dystrophy is the *Becker variant*. Onset is usually between 5 and 10 years of age, and the pattern of progression is less rapid than with Duchenne dystrophy. Persons affected with Becker dystrophy are unlikely to be wheelchair-bound by adolescence. In further contrast to Duchenne muscular dystrophy, the brain and heart are usually not involved.

Myotonic muscular dystrophy (Steinert disease) is an autosomal dominant disorder characterized by mental retardation, muscle weakness, myotonia, cataracts, and gonadal atrophy. Myotonic muscular dystrophy, also known as dystrophia myotonica, should not be confused with myotonia congenita. The latter, also known as Thomsen disease, is likewise a myotonic disorder of autosomal dominant inheritance. With myotonia congenita, however, mental retardation, cataracts, and gonadal atrophy are not associated.

In contrast to other muscle disorders such as Duchenne and Becker dystrophies, myotonic muscular dystrophy does not preferentially cause proximal muscle weakness. Indeed, distal weakness is often significant and more prominent than that occurring proximally. The face is usually affected as well, resulting in a characteristic transverse smile or carplike configuration of the mouth (see Figs. 13–4 and 13–5). Myotonia is of variable prominence in children. This sign can be elicited passively (by percussion of muscle) or actively (by voluntary contraction). It is manifested by sustained contraction, an inability to relax (see Fig. 13–2).

A congenital form of myotonic muscular dystrophy is characterized by poor feeding, failure to thrive, and respiratory problems. The incidence of this form of myotonic dystrophy is increased with involvement of the mother, who may be affected only minimally or not at all (see Case 18–4). Blood tests do not show specific alterations. The electromyogram can be of considerable diagnostic help, for it may show myotonic discharges on needle insertion and muscle contraction. Represented as sounds, these discharges resemble the noise of a dive bomber.

Many other muscle disorders have been identified on the basis of different clinical features, patterns of inheritance, neurophysiologic profiles, enzyme levels, and biopsy results. These include facioscapulohumeral dystrophy, limb girdle dystrophy, and *congenital myopathies* such as nemaline myopathy and central core disease.

Neuromuscular disease (that is, disorder of the neuromuscular junction) is represented by *myasthenia gravis*. The hallmark of myasthenia gravis is fatigability. With repetitive muscle contraction such as forced eye closure or deep knee bends, increasing weakness results. Frequently used muscles such as those which elevate the lids and move the eyes are generally affected

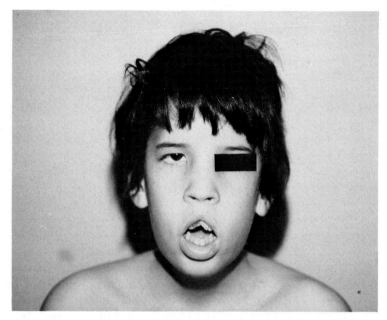

FIGURE 13–4. Expressionless face with carplike mouth in myotonic muscular dystrophy.

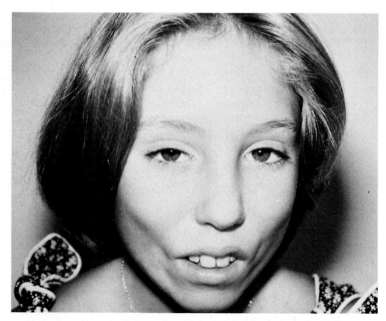

FIGURE 13–5. Transverse smile with hollowed cheeks in facio-scapulohumeral muscular dystrophy.

first, although virtually any voluntary muscle can be involved (see Fig. 13–6).

Several different forms of myasthenia gravis in childhood are recognized. A *transient neonatal* form occurs secondary to transfer of antibodies from an affected mother across the placenta. A *congenital* form is manifested within the first 1 to 2 years of life. A *juvenile* form presents characteristically in the school-age child with ptosis or other cranial nerve findings. Seizures, diabetes mellitus, asthma, and hyperthyroidism often accompany juvenile myasthenia gravis (Snead *et al.*, 1980).

The pathophysiologic basis of myasthenia gravis appears to be an autoimmune reaction involving the postsynaptic membrane, the locus of action of the neurotransmitter acetylcholine (Drachman, 1978).

Diagnosis is based upon clinical manifestations, electromyography, and a Tensilon test. This test involves observing the response to injection of edrophonium, a cholinesterase-inhibiting drug, which enhances the activity of acetylcholine at the neuromuscular junction. Assessment of the school-age child should also include determination of thyroid hormone level because of the association of hyperthyroidism with myasthenia gravis (Rosman, 1976).

Disease of *peripheral nerves* or *roots* may cause gait disturbance due to involvement of motor and/or sensory fibers. Foot drop, often unilateral, can occur secondary to trauma or can be caused by a number of toxins, including lead, that affect the anterior tibial nerves.

Acute intermittent porphyria and diphtheria are causes of demyelinative peripheral neuropathy. *Acute intermittent porphyria* is an autosomal dominant condition rare in childhood and adolescence in which a rapidly progressive peripheral neuropathy can threaten life because of respiratory

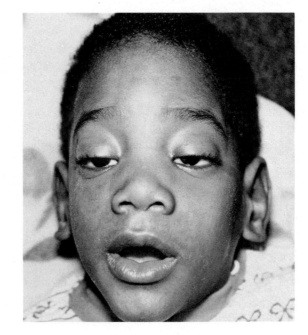

FIGURE 13–6. Bilateral ptosis and lack of facial expression in a boy with myasthenia gravis.

failure from intercostal nerve involvement. Episodes can be triggered by medical illness, barbiturates, alcohol, or other drugs. Abdominal pain may be an accompaniment and can be severe enough to mimic a surgical problem (Barclay, 1974). The urine of affected persons turns dark red upon exposure to sunlight for several hours. Analysis of urine is positive for porphyrins (including porphobilinogen), and assay of blood shows diminished urosynthetase activity.

Diphtheria, usually thought of as a severe upper respiratory illness, can also be associated with a demyelinative polyneuropathy. Clinical manifestations include loss of deep tendon reflexes and pharyngeal paralysis, characterized by hypernasal speech, impaired swallowing, and an absent gag reflex. A serious nonneurologic complication of diphtheria is myocarditis.

The *Guillain-Barré syndrome* is a disorder involving demyelination of multiple spinal nerve roots (from which peripheral nerves are derived). It classically takes the form of an ascending polyradiculopathy. The legs, subserved by the longest peripheral nerves, are involved first. The muscles of respiration and the upper extremities may be affected subsequently. Ultimately, cranial nerves may be involved in the demyelination. Diagnosis is suggested by the onset of ascending weakness with minimal sensory loss that follows an upper respiratory or gastrointestinal infection by several days to weeks. Cerebrospinal fluid examination typically shows an albumino-cytologic discrepancy, that is, elevation in protein content with little or no increase in white blood cell count.

Spinal cord disorder can interfere with gait by involving gray matter and/or white matter. *Poliomyelitis* is an enteroviral infection with a predilection for anterior horn cells, which give rise to the spinal motor nerve roots. In its bulbar form, polio affects the brainstem, thereby interfering with respiration. *Werdnig-Hoffmann disease* (infantile spinal muscular atrophy) and *Kugelberg-Welander disease* (juvenile spinal muscular atrophy) are other disorders affecting anterior horn cells. Both conditions are autosomal recessive in inheritance. They are marked by weakness, fasciculations, hypotonia, and diminished or absent tendon reflexes (see Fig. 13–7).

Multiple sclerosis, a demyelinating disease, can affect the central nervous system at any level, including the spinal cord (see Fig. 13–8). Symptoms are often sensory (hence, subjective) and are characteristically intermittent. As a result, multiple sclerosis is often mistaken for hysteria. Multiple sclerosis can cause a spastic or ataxic gait by affecting corticospinal, spinocerebellar, or proprioceptive tracts. At the level of the brainstem, the cerebellum is a favorite site of involvement (see Case 21–1).

The diagnosis of multiple sclerosis is suggested by neurologic signs and symptoms that pursue an intermittent course and indicate more than one locus of involvement within the central nervous system. Cerebrospinal fluid analysis characteristically (but not always) shows a normal (or mildly increased) protein level with elevation in immunoglobulin G content. Visual evoked responses are helpful in documenting unsuspected involvement of visual pathways.

Situated laterally in the spinal cord are the lateral corticospinal tracts, voluntary motor fibers. These may be involved by intrinsic spinal cord le-

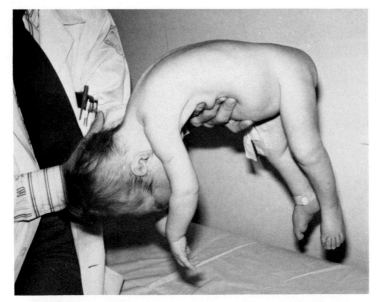

FIGURE 13–7. Marked hypotonia in an infant with Werdnig-Hoffmann disease.

FIGURE 13–8. Section of brain showing areas of acute demyelination (large one at arrow).

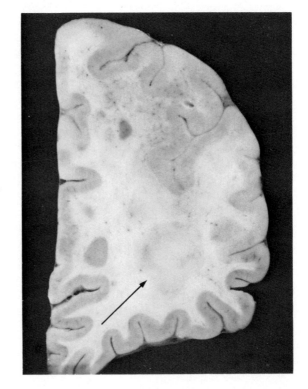

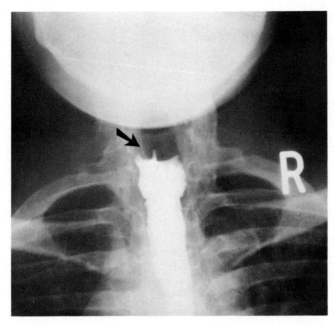

FIGURE 13–9. Myelogram demonstrating complete block due to intraspinal extramedullary mass (arrow.)

sions (glioma; demyelinative plaque) or extrinsic lesions (cyst; neurofibroma; hematoma). Deep tendon reflexes below the level of the lesion will usually be increased, and Babinski signs may be found as well.

Lateral column (corticospinal tract) disease in adulthood is classically seen in association with *motor neuron* (anterior horn cell) *disease* in *amyotrophic lateral sclerosis* (see Case 8–5). Corticospinal tract disease is also typically associated with posterior column disease in vitamin B_{12} deficiency, which may be accompanied by pernicious anemia.

An *intraspinal mass* can interfere with any aspect of spinal cord function. Clinical features combined with radiologic studies (such as plain radiography of the spine, CT scan of the spine, and myelography) will usually localize the spinal cord process (see Fig. 13–9). An intraspinal mass may be within spinal cord tissue itself (intramedullary) or within the bony spine outside of the spinal cord (extramedullary) (see Case 21–5). Glioma and vascular malformation are intramedullary lesions; neurofibroma, meningioma, and abscess are extramedullary. An arachnoid cyst, an intraspinal extramedullary lesion developing within the thoracic spine, may lead to intermittent or progressive gait disturbance easily mistaken for hysteria or multiple sclerosis.

With *syringomyelia,* a cavitation or cyst within the cervical spinal cord produces a characteristic dissociated sensory deficit and may cause a gait disturbance. Pain and temperature sensation in the upper extremities is lost. Position sense and perception of vibration are, however, preserved. This dissociation occurs because the enlarging central cyst, or syrinx, impinges upon pain and temperature fibers as they cross to the other side of the spinal cord before ascending. Fibers subserving vibration and proprioception, however, do not cross until reaching the brainstem; hence, they are affected late in syringomyelia, if at all. Because pain and temperature sensation are involved, a person with syringomyelia may traumatize his or her fingers repeatedly without promptly recognizing injury.

Diastematomyelia is a form of midline spinal defect in which a spicule of bone impales the lower spinal cord thereby dividing it. Since the bony spine grows more than the spinal cord which it houses, the spicule may interfere progressively with spinal cord function over several years (Kennedy, 1979). A typical course thus would be that of a 5-year-old child with increasing gait disturbance who has begun wetting during the day after 2 years without accidents. With forms of spina bifida such as *meningocele* and *meningomyelocele,* the neurologic problem is usually recognized at birth, and deficits tend not to occur in such an insidious manner (see Case 21–2).

Disorders of the craniocervical junction may also account for progressive gait disturbance. With the *Arnold-Chiari malformation,* for example, structures that should lie above the foramen magnum are displaced downward to lie in the cervical spinal canal. This displacement causes compression of brainstem and cerebellum, resulting in ataxia of gait and downbeating nystagmus. The latter sign is a valuable clue to the presence of craniocervical disease.

The *basal ganglia* are a collection of paired structures near the midline, lying deep to the cerebral cortex. They comprise the caudate nucleus and putamen (together known as the striatum) plus the globus pallidus. Several disorders of posture and movement are linked with the basal ganglia: Wilson disease, Sydenham chorea, dystonia musculorum deformans, Huntington disease, Tourette disease, and paroxysmal choreoathetosis.

Wilson disease, or hepatolenticular degeneration, is characterized by liver disease (hepatitis) and a wide variety of central nervous system manifestations stemming most prominently from involvement of basal ganglia (Cartwright, 1978; Dobyns *et al.,* 1979). Chorea, rigidity, or a coarse "wing-beating" tremor of the upper limbs may be seen. The Kayser-Fleischer corneal ring is a pathognomonic sign, though it often disappears with treatment. Serum ceruloplasmin is low, and copper content of liver tissue is increased.

Sydenham chorea may present as tremor or clumsiness. It is a late complication of streptococcal throat infection, perhaps the result of an autoimmune process affecting the basal ganglia. Sydenham chorea is considered a major manifestation of rheumatic fever, although active heart disease is usually not present when chorea occurs. Antecedent streptococcal infection is not always demonstrable.

Diagnosis is suspected in the school-age child with a characteristic choreiform movement disorder associated with lability of mood. An affected child may be unable to sustain contraction upon grasping the examiner's fingers ("milkmaid's grip"), maintain tongue protrusion ("darting tongue"), or hold the arms straight above the head ("pronator sign") (Aron *et al.,* 1965; Nausieda *et al.,* 1980). Restlessness, giddiness, and facial grimacing may also be seen. Elevated antistreptolysin O (ASO) titer suggests antecedent streptococcal disease. Other signs of rheumatic disease (which may or may not be

CASE 13–1: POSSIBLE SYDENHAM CHOREA IN A 5-YEAR-OLD BOY

A.D. abruptly developed involuntary facial grimacing, shoulder shrugging, posturing of his arms, and fixation of conjugate eye movements. Painful contractions of the abdominal muscles also occurred. Movements were exaggerated with anxiety and disappeared during sleep. They lasted from 5 to 30 minutes and were followed by minutes to hours of quiescence.

Past history of pregnancy, birth, and development was remarkable for choreiform movements beginning between 1 and 2 years of age. Family history was negative for movement disorder or other neurologic problems. The child had a history of sore throats but no documented streptococcal infections or evidence for rheumatic fever.

On examination, the child was an active, well-formed, and normally intelligent 5-year-old boy without pharyngitis or tonsillitis. Head circumference and optic fundi were normal. No bulbar telangiectasias or Kayser-Fleischer rings were seen. Neurologic examination showed slight hypotonia with normal strength. A mild degree of chorea was evident when arms were held outstretched. Facial grimacing and inversion of the feet occurred occasionally (see Fig. 13–10). Deep tendon reflexes were quiet and symmetric. Plantar responses were normal. Antistreptolysin O titer was 250 Todd units. Erythrocyte sedimentation rate was 12 mm per hour.

The child was placed on chlorpromazine and experienced gradual improvement over 4 months. A month later, however, while still on drug ther-

present) are carditis, migrating polyarthritis, subcutaneous nodules, a characteristic skin rash (erythema marginatum), and prolongation of the PR interval on electrocardiogram (see Case 13–1).

Dystonia musculorum deformans is a progressive disorder with onset usually in childhood. It is characterized by persistent postural abnormalities, which may result in joint deformity (see Fig. 13–11). Associated gait disturbance is often bizarre and frequently mistaken as hysterical. Two patterns of inheritance have been recognized. An autosomal recessive form occurs with increased frequency among Ashkenazi Jews and pursues a relatively rapid course of deterioration. An autosomal dominant form generally manifests a slower pattern of progression.

Huntington disease is a disorder of autosomal dominant inheritance. Loss of intellectual function (dementia), rigidity, and seizures typify the childhood form (see Fig. 13–12) (Jervis, 1963; Markham and Knox, 1965; Hansotia *et al.*, 1968) (see Chapter 8).

Tourette disease is a disorder usually beginning in childhood, manifested by multiple tics, often involving complex movements (Shapiro *et al.*, 1973). Vocal tics, particularly the explosive utterance of "dirty" words (coprolalia), are a hallmark of the syndrome. Like other tic syndromes of childhood, Tourette syndrome pursues a waxing and waning course. The anatomic and biochemical bases for Tourette syndrome are not clear. The

apy, facial grimacing, forced deviation of the eyes to the left, respiratory interruptions, and abdominal contractions recurred. Chlorpromazine was discontinued and haloperidol begun. The child did well for the next 4 years although symptoms worsened during major stresses; at such times haloperidol was increased.

Comment. Facial grimacing, choreoathetosis, and involuntary truncal movements suggested a disorder of the basal ganglia. This child did not, however, have other major stigmata of Wilson disease such as a brownish corneal ring, elevated liver enzymes, or positive family history. Huntington disease could also be excluded clinically. An autosomal dominant disorder, it characteristically assumes a rigid rather than choreoathetotic form in childhood, and is often associated with seizures. Likewise, the child lacked typical features of dystonia musculorum deformans or Hallervorden-Spatz disease. In some respects, the child's clinical picture resembled that of tardive dyskinesia, a complication of chronic antipsychotic drug use. This child did not, however, have a history of any drug use.

Perhaps the best clinical match was provided by Sydenham chorea, the poststreptococcal movement disorder, which may pursue a protracted remitting course. The child did not, however, manifest emotional lability or other typical signs of Sydenham chorea. The early history of choreoathetoid movements is intriguing and suggests that the child's neurologic substrate was not normal, perhaps unusually susceptible to streptococcal infection or other noxious agent.

basal ganglia appear to be involved, and monoamine overactivity seems to play an etiologic role (see CORRELATION: BIOCHEMICAL ASPECTS) (see Case 13–2).

Paroxysmal choreoathetosis is a rare, often familial disorder manifested by recurrent involuntary tonic, dystonic, or choreoathetotic movements. Episodes last seconds to hours and occur spontaneously or are precipitated by movement (Goodenough *et al.*, 1978; Kinast *et al.*, 1980; Tibbles and Barnes, 1980). Differentiation from seizures may be difficult.

Cerebellar disorders may be manifested as gait disturbance, tremor, or clumsiness. Lying dorsal to the brainstem, the cerebellum coordinates proprioceptive and corticospinal input so that movements are well measured and smooth. The cerebellar hemispheres primarily influence appendicular (limb) movements. The vermis, the midline portion of the cerebellum, is more involved with axial (truncal) functions, including walking. The oldest parts of the cerebellum, the flocculus and nodulus, participate in coordination of eye movements with head and body movements (see Case 13–3).

Dysfunction of different parts of the cerebellum thus will be manifested clinically by different deficits. Cerebellar tremor generally occurs as a consequence of cerebellar *hemispheric* involvement, for example, with *tumor* such as cystic astrocytoma. The tremor occurs with intention, is perpendicular to the direction of motion, and becomes greater in amplitude as the goal is

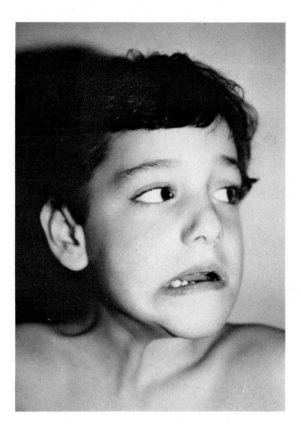

FIGURE 13–10. Facial grimacing in a 5-year-old with chorea (Case 13–1).

approached. *Midline tumors* of the cerebellum such as medulloblastoma characteristically affect axial more than appendicular structures. As a result gait may become clumsy, with walking in tandem performed very poorly (see Case 13–4).

Cerebral causes of motor disturbance include hydrocephalus and cerebral palsy. *Hydrocephalus* causes gait disturbance because dilated lateral ventricles impinge upon leg fibers that course around them from the motor cortex of the frontal lobe through the internal capsule en route to the brainstem and spinal cord. Fibers subserving the arms begin lower down along the cerebral convexities and pursue a course farther from the outer walls of the distended lateral ventricles than do the leg fibers. Thus, in hydrocephalus gait disorder usually precedes dysfunction of the upper limbs. Hydrocephalus and other causes of increased intracranial pressure are discussed in Chapter 11.

Cerebral palsy refers to a nonprogressive motor deficit stemming from prenatal or perinatal factors. These factors are at times identified; they are otherwise often presumed. Although cerebral palsy is by definition a motor deficit, other problems such as seizures and mental retardation are commonly associated.

Several forms of cerebral palsy occur. The commonest is spastic diplegia, in which the legs are affected more than the arms. A scissoring gait is typical. Deep tendon reflexes are generally brisker in the lower extremities than

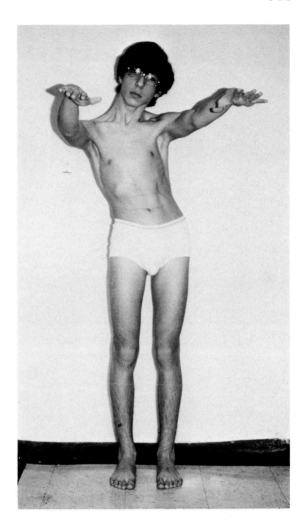

FIGURE 13–11. Dystonic posturing in an adolescent with dystonia musculorum deformans.

in the arms. This pattern of deficit has been linked with damage to periventricular white matter, presumably on an ischemic basis. As with hydrocephalus, leg fibers are preferentially affected as they pass nearest the outer walls of the lateral ventricles. Other forms of cerebral palsy are atonic, ataxic, and athetoid.

Visual disturbance—particularly loss of visual acuity or visual field defect—must always be considered in assessing the clumsy child. Severe visual loss can be associated with optic neuritis (often found in childhood multiple sclerosis) or optic atrophy (occurring secondary to optic nerve glioma or chronically raised intracranial pressure). Hemianopia can be associated with awkwardness on the side of the hemianopia. "Tunnel vision" is the characteristic visual field defect associated with pigmentary degeneration of the retina (retinitis pigmentosa). Night blindness is another typical symptom.

Vestibular causes of clumsiness include viral infection of the inner ear

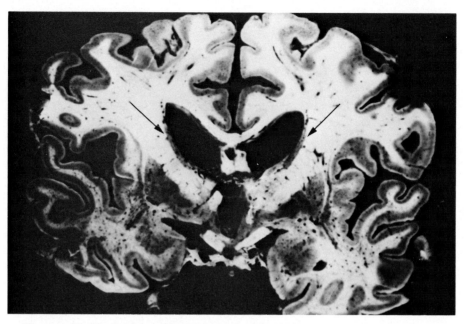

FIGURE 13–12. Section of brain demonstrating atrophy of caudate nuclei (arrows) and enlargement of frontal horns of lateral ventricles in Huntington disease.

(specifically the semicircular canals) and toxic effects, for example, due to aminoglycoside therapy (especially streptomycin).

Toxic Causes. Gait disturbance can result from use of prescribed or illicit drugs. Anticonvulsant medications are frequent offenders. Overdosage usually can be confirmed by measuring anticonvulsant blood levels. It may result from errors in writing a prescription, preparing it, or taking the medication. For example, the liquid form of phenytoin is a suspension that settles readily into a watery upper phase and a more concentrated lower phase. As a result, phenytoin toxicity (with staggering gait and slurred speech) tends to occur toward the bottom of a bottle that has not been well shaken prior to administration.

The blood level of an anticonvulsant medication can also be elevated into a toxic range by addition of a second drug that utilizes the same degradative pathway. This effect is typically encountered when sodium valproate (Depakene) is added to a regimen that consists of, or includes, phenobarbital. The phenobarbital level generally rises, often to the point of toxicity, so that it is customary to diminish its intake, at least upon initiation of sodium valproate therapy.

Drug abuse involving alcohol or barbiturates may also produce ataxia of gait. Intentional overdosage, a suicide gesture or attempt, should be considered in any child whose ataxia is due to drug overdosage (even when anticonvulsant medication has been prescribed) (see Case 6–5).

Proximal muscle weakness affecting gait can result from the use of corti-

CASE 13–2: TOURETTE DISEASE IN A 10-YEAR-OLD BOY

M.N. was considered normal until 2 years prior to hospital admission when he developed "a twitch in the shoulders" associated with shuffling of his feet. At first these involuntary movements occurred only occasionally. Later they increased in frequency and became associated with a barklike cry. Coprolalia began at 9 years of age. After blurting out obscenities, the child would often apologize. Symptoms fluctuated spontaneously. About 6 weeks before hospitalization movements became so disabling that the child was essentially bedridden.

History of pregnancy, birth, and development was unremarkable. During early elementary school years, the child was inattentive and hyperactive. He had not had recent streptococcal infection or rheumatic fever. Family history was negative for tics or other neurologic problems.

On examination, the youngster was a well-formed, mildly anxious child whose movement disorder fluctuated depending upon his state of anxiety and activity. During periods of concentration or when he was at rest, involuntary movements diminished or disappeared. When he walked, continuous truncal undulations occurred and were punctuated by lightning-like movements of the limbs and face. Movements occurred in bursts that propelled the child across the room as if he were thrown.

The general physical examination was normal. Kayser-Fleischer rings of the cornea were not evident. Neurologic examination was normal except for a fine, rapid tremor with intention and upon extension of the outstretched hands. Investigations—including erythrocyte sedimentation rate, serum electrolytes, complete blood count, liver function tests, cerebrospinal fluid examination, and EEG—were normal.

The child was placed on phenytoin with marked improvement in tics for 4 months. The tics subsequently worsened. Phenytoin was replaced with haloperidol with some improvement in symptoms.

Comment. There can be no doubt that this child suffered from Tourette disease. He manifested multiple tics—including vocal tics and coprolalia, the explosive utterance of "dirty words"—that pursued an intermittent course. Haloperidol, thought to act postsynaptically by blocking dopaminergic neurons, frequently provides a more striking benefit than was seen in this case.

costeroids. Climbing stairs or walking up hills will thus be difficult (see Case 21–1).

Several drugs may be associated with tremor. These include aminophylline, theophylline, caffeine, imipramine (Tofranil), lithium, and sodium valproate (Depakene).

Drugs can also cause movement disorders through their actions upon the basal ganglia. Phenothiazines and butyrophenones can produce dystonic posturing that often is misinterpreted as being of hysterical origin. Trifluo-

CASE 13–3: ATAXIC GAIT FOLLOWING CHICKENPOX IN A 5-YEAR-OLD GIRL

R.J. was referred for evaluation because she was "walking like a drunk." Chickenpox was recognized 2 weeks previously and lasted 10 days. It was a relatively mild case with few skin lesions and slight fever. As the rash was clearing, incoordination of legs, arms, and trunk was noted. Speech was involved also in that it was slower than usual. Neither vomiting nor headache was associated.

On examination, the child was alert and cooperative. She spoke slowly but without dysarthria. Examination of the skin revealed healing lesions of varicella. Optic disks were sharply margined and flat. She was hypotonic in all limbs. Deep tendon reflexes were quiet (1 +) and pendular at the knees. On testing of coordination, she had dysmetria of limb movements and a coarse end point tremor with intention. Rapid alternating movements were performed poorly. Gait was widely based and associated arm movements poorly coordinated. Tandem gait could be accomplished only with assistance. She was unable to balance on one leg for more than 1 second or to stand with her feet together even with her eyes open.

Comment. This child manifested a classical postvaricella cerebellar syndrome of younger childhood. The diagnosis was based upon cerebellar signs of ataxia and dysmetria following chickenpox in a child without evidence of posterior fossa mass lesion (such as signs of increased intracranial pressure or cranial nerve findings) or drug intoxication (e.g., alcohol, phenytoin, or diazepam) (see Case 20–5).

No specific therapy is available for postvaricella ataxia. The child's parents were advised as to the essentially benign nature of the pathologic process, and within 1 month the child was entirely back to normal.

perazine (Stelazine) and haloperidol (Haldol) are common offenders. The dystonic symptomatology can be quite dramatic. For example, prochlorperazine (Compazine), a phenothiazine antiemetic, can produce a syndrome involving opisthotonic posturing and "lockjaw" that suggests tetanus (Scime and Tallant, 1959) (see Case 19–2).

Methylphenidate (Ritalin), dextroamphetamine (Dexedrine), and some antihistamines have been reported to produce extrapyramidal reactions that can mimic Tourette disease (Golden, 1974; Barone and Raniolo, 1980).

Phenothiazines and butyrophenones have also been implicated in producing tardive dyskinesia, a family of disorders resulting from chronic administration of antipsychotic agents. Perhaps less likely in children and adolescents than adults, it does occur in the pediatric age group (Chiles, 1978; McLean and Casey, 1978; Gualtieri *et al.,* 1980). Tardive dyskinesia may be manifested in a buccal-lingual or facial form, in which repetitive pursing of the lips, flickering of the tongue, or grimacing occurs (see Chapter 5).

Psychologic Causes.   Hysteria is an important cause of gait disturbance in childhood. As Dubowitz and Hersov (1976) have emphasized, it frequently arises in childhood as a prolongation of an earlier organic illness. The gait characteristically has a "stuck-to-the-floor" quality. A diagnostic-therapeutic trial of suggestion is often helpful in establishing the etiology of gait disturbance as hysterical. For example, gait may improve dramatically when the child carries out the request to clap hands in time to his walking in order to "reestablish the necessary rhythm" to walk normally once again (see Case 7–4).

Astasia-abasia is a form of gait disorder associated typically with malingering, which occurs on a conscious basis in contrast to hysteria. Persons with astasia-abasia will carry out extraordinary feats of balance, skittering across the room on one leg in arduous attempts to demonstrate their disability.

Anxiety is often accompanied by tremor. It is characteristically fine, rapid (eight to ten oscillations per second), and present on action. Tremor has been attributed to catecholamines released as part of an anxiety response.

Tics of all kinds also bear a relationship to anxiety. They are typically worsened by stress, acute or chronic. With so-called simple tics of the school-age child, stresses are often age-related and developmental rather than attributable to specific environmental or social problems. Simple tics are not merely habits. They are involuntary behaviors that appear to serve as a tension-discharge device (see Case 13–5).

Genetic-Constitutional Causes.   Many conditions associated with disorders of movement have recognized patterns of inheritance. Duchenne and Becker muscular dystrophies are X-linked recessive. Myotonic dystrophy, acute intermittent porphyria, and facioscapulohumeral muscular dystrophy are autosomal dominant disorders. Tourette disease sometimes follows a parent-to-child mode of transmission and also shows an unexplained predominance of males, who are affected some three times more frequently than females (Kidd *et al.,* 1980). Werdnig-Hoffmann disease, Kugelberg-Welander disease, and limb-girdle muscular dystrophy are autosomal recessive. Tremor and clumsiness may also occur on a familial basis (see Case 13–6).

Developmental Causes.   Clumsiness in performing motor activities is generally a normal part of the process of acquiring a skill. Walking, for example, in its earlier stages of mastery is ataxic, wide-based, and dysrhythmic. Clumsiness diminishes or disappears with time and practice. As with other developmental disorders, persistence into later childhood of maladaptive behaviors characteristic of an earlier stage of development defines a developmental disorder. With developmental clumsiness, Reuben and Bakwin (1968) have noted that everyday skills such as dressing, writing, and participation in sports tend to be impaired.

Hyperactivity, often occurring on a developmental basis, may be associated with abnormal movements. These include flickering, choreiform movements of the fingers when arms are outstretched; nonspecific tremor in

CASE 13–4: CLUMSINESS DUE TO CEREBELLAR TUMOR IN A 5-YEAR-OLD GIRL

J.A. was lethargic and "sick to her stomach" after falling from a porch without losing consciousness. The following day her parents noted that her balance was "off"; and they brought her to her pediatrician. Bilateral papilledema and markedly ataxic gait were found. A CT scan demonstrated severe hydrocephalus and a posterior fossa mass. Ventriculoperitoneal shunting was carried out, and the tumor (a cerebellar astrocytoma) was excised completely. She did not receive chemotherapy or radiotherapy and has done well over the ensuing 3 years except for several shunt malfunctions (usually heralded by vomiting), which have necessitated revisions of the shunt.

Comment. Brain tumors in childhood in general do not produce acute, dramatic symptomatology. Because they typically occur in or near the midline and lie in the posterior fossa below the tentorium cerebelli, such tumors characteristically produce symptoms insidiously by obstructing cerebrospinal fluid pathways and/or by impairing coordinative functions. Accordingly, headaches (which need not be prominent in early and intermediate stages), attentional problems, and irritability result from hydrocephalus and slowly progressive clumsiness from cerebellar involvement. Seizures are a less frequent manifestation of brain tumor in children than in adults in whom tumors are more often supratentorial.

The majority (approximately two-thirds) of posterior fossa tumors of childhood are made up of astrocytomas and medulloblastomas. They each occur with about equal frequency. Medulloblastomas are usually midline in location, tend to have a shorter symptomatic course prior to presentation, and usually occur in younger children (around 2 to 5 years of age). Astrocy-

carrying out fine motor activities; and awkwardness in gross motor tasks, as impulsivity and poor motor planning stand in the way of efficient performance (see Chapter 14).

TREATMENT AND OUTCOME

The therapy and prognosis of movement disorders in childhood will vary greatly depending upon the specific disorder and its severity (see Table 13–2). Treatment will often be multifaceted, especially when chronic neurologic disorder such as Wilson disease or Duchenne muscular dystrophy is the cause. With the former, pharmacotherapy (chelation with penicillamine) and nutritional therapy (a low copper diet) are included in the treatment plan. The outlook is often favorable. For Duchenne muscular dystrophy symptomatic and supportive treatment only is available, and the prognosis is generally poor. An affected child is usually wheelchair-bound by adolescence, and death (due to respiratory or cardiac causes) typically occurs during the second or third decade of life.

Medical Management. Hyperthyroidism is treated with antithyroid drugs

tomas are less often located in the midline, typically have a more insidious onset and longer course, and are frequently found in older school-age children (10 to 12 years). These general rules, however, do not invariably apply.

The modes of therapy and the prognosis for these two different kinds of posterior fossa tumors differ greatly. The outlook is generally highly favorable with astrocytoma, which is usually treated by surgery alone. The prognosis is much less favorable for children with medulloblastoma, a malignant tumor of the brain. Subtotal resection is the rule with postoperative radiotherapy to the craniospinal axis. Chemotherapy may be employed at the time of initial diagnosis or upon relapse.

The diagnosis of posterior fossa tumor is suggested by history and by signs and symptoms of increased intracranial pressure, both chronic and acute. Funduscopic examination is essential. It must be accomplished despite difficulties engendered by the age and uncooperativeness of the younger child, whose inattentiveness and irritability may be related to tumor as well as to developmental level. Use of mydriatic eyedrops will facilitate adequate funduscopic visualization. Enlarged head circumference and delayed closure of the anterior fontanelle are signs of chronically raised intracranial pressure in the young child. On plain skull x-ray, splitting of cranial sutures and erosion of the pituitary fossa may be seen. CT scan (with and without contrast enhancement) will readily demonstrate hydrocephalus and often its cause (see Case 11–3).

Because of their position close to cerebrospinal fluid pathways, cerebellar tumors often cause symptoms of (chronically) raised intracranial pressure such as headache, irritability, or personality change long before gait disturbance, tremor, or clumsiness become major problems (see Chapter 11) (see Case 6–4).

such as propylthiouracil, surgery, or radioactive iodine (Vaidya *et al.*, 1974). Polymyositis is treated with corticosteroids or, occasionally, immunosuppressants.

Infectious processes such as septic arthritis and osteomyelitis are treated with high doses of parenteral antibiotics for several weeks, after appropriate cultures of blood, joint fluid, and/or bone aspirate have been obtained.

Tremor resulting from drugs used in the treatment of asthma, such as aminophylline and theophylline, generally does not interfere with activity. Hence specific treatment is not indicated. If tremor is associated with other symptoms such as tachycardia or headache, blood levels of medication should be determined and dosage adjusted as necessary.

When tremor results from excessive intake of caffeine, the person should be advised of the role of caffeine in producing tremor, associated features of caffeine toxicity such as irregularities of cardiac rhythm, and beverages that contain caffeine (such as coffee, tea, and cola).

Treatment of Duchenne muscular dystrophy is essentially symptomatic and supportive. Weakened respiratory effort and scoliosis frequently lead to

CASE 13–5: RECURRENT TICS IN A 9-YEAR-OLD BOY

L.G. was referred for neurologic evaluation because, he said, "I cough sometimes and laugh; but it's not real." Ticlike clearing of the throat had begun 3 years previously. Assessment then included an ear, nose, and throat evaluation, which was negative. "Phony" laughter began at 9 years. His parents also noted facial grimacing, without barking, coprolalia, or gait disturbance. Throat-clearing ceased during sleep and diminished during periods of concentration. The child denied that tension built up within him when he attempted to suppress the cough or that he experienced relief when he did cough. He continued to do well in schoolwork and athletics. Family history was negative for writer's cramp, dystonia, Wilson disease, or tics.

On examination, the child was an alert and intelligent youngster who cleared his throat nonproductively at least once every 2 minutes throughout the hour. Overall, he did not appear depressed or anxious, although he smiled continuously and grimaced when questioned directly. Coprolalia was not heard. The remainder of the examination was normal.

This boy was considered to have multiple tics, though not Tourette disease. Treatment was primarily supportive with attention directed to identifying stressful events that might be contributing to the tics and to helping the parents defuse their reaction to them. For 2 months following initial consultation he showed a dramatic reduction in throat clearing. During the next month, coincident with school-related stresses, tics again became prominent, after which they diminished once again.

Comment. The tics in this child acted as a tension discharge mechanism, increasing at times of stress. The tics themselves were a significant cause of stress. The boy's father was very strict and tolerated poorly the child's tics, which at times had a provocative edge to them. When the parents became aware of this characteristic of the tics, the overall level of tension within the family appeared to lessen. Although this child's schoolwork and social life had not suffered, evidence of chronic stress and anxiety suggested that formal psychiatric or psychologic involvement would be helpful.

---

pneumonia, which is treated with antibiotics and often with physical therapy. An associated cardiac disorder may be treated with drugs for arrhythmia or failure. Weight control is indicated so that compromise of respiratory function and mobility can be minimized.

No specific treatment exists for myotonic dystrophy. Phenytoin (Dilantin), procainamide (Pronestyl), and quinine may be of benefit in ameliorating myotonia. The disorder manifests slow progression in some of its features. Muscle wasting and contracture can develop. Cataracts may require operative treatment.

The treatment of myasthenia gravis in childhood and adolescence will depend upon the clinical syndrome manifested. The neonatal form, occurring secondary to passage of maternal antibodies, is transient and self-limited.

CASE 13–6: CONSTITUTIONAL CLUMSINESS IN A 10-YEAR-OLD GIRL

J.O. was evaluated because of gait problems and overall clumsiness. "She's always tripping," her mother said. Despite her clumsiness, she had never broken any bones or sustained significant head trauma. Her mother dated onset of clumsiness to 2 years of age, if not earlier, and felt that it was probably improving.

History of pregnancy and delivery was unremarkable. She walked at $1\frac{1}{2}$ years, pedaled a tricycle at 3 years, and rode a bicycle at 8 years. She spoke in sentences and was toilet-trained by 2 years. Family history was notable for a brother who received special assistance in school because of poor handwriting.

On examination, the child was a composed, intelligent, and mildly fidgety girl. Head circumference (53.5 cm) and funduscopic examination were normal. Gait was awkward with arm movements poorly coordinated with those of the legs. At times the left leg appeared nearly to slip away from her. She walked up or down stairs without apparent difficulty. Tandem gait was accomplished poorly. Flickering movements of the fingers occurred when the arms were outstretched. Rapid alternating movements and heel-to-shin testing were normal. She could stand on one leg for 4 seconds only. Perception of light touch, cold, and vibration was normal. Proprioception at the fingers and toes was diminished. Strength and tone were normal.

Comment. This child's clumsiness throughout her life was always exaggerated for her age and never characteristic of earlier developmental stages. Hence it is termed constitutional rather than developmental. Her clumsiness did not seem to be due to weakness, as would be the case with muscle disease. Rather, it appeared to stem most importantly from disturbances in proprioception and cerebellar function, which are closely related. Her inability to walk well in tandem implicated dysfunction of the cerebellum (particularly its midline portions), whereas problems in position sense suggested posterior column dysfunction (see Chapter 2).

Although the clumsiness was gradually getting better, it was increasingly stressful for the girl. She had been singled out for years by schoolmates because of her clumsiness. Therapy in this instance included supportive measures, emphasizing her intelligence and positive personality traits, while placing her motor problems in perspective. Formal physical therapy evaluation was also recommended with attention to be given to ways to make her gait more graceful.

Careful observation for feeding or respiratory difficulties (which may require treatment with an anticholinesterase) over the first few days to weeks of life is generally all that is required. In congenital and juvenile forms of myasthenia gravis, treatment with a cholinesterase inhibitor, pyridostigmine

TABLE 13–2. **Selected Aspects of Treatment of Movement Disorders**

Wilson disease	Chelation (with penicillamine) Avoidance of copper-containing foods
Hyperthyroidism	Propylthiouracil (PTU), thyroid surgery, radioactive iodine
Polymyositis	Steroids Immunosuppressive agents
Duchenne muscular dystrophy	Treatment of pneumonia Prevention and treatment of contractures, scoliosis, pneumonia
Myotonic muscular dystrophy	Phenytoin (Dilantin), procainamide (Pronestyl), or quinine for myotonia
Myasthenia gravis	Anticholinesterase medication Steroids Thymectomy

Neuropathies and
  polyradiculopathies
	Physical therapy
	Avoid precipitants (with acute intermittent
	  porphyria)
	Supportive measures (as with diphtheria)
	(?) Steroids (with Guillain-Barré syndrome)

Multiple sclerosis	Steroids Immunosuppressive agents Physical therapy Treatment of intercurrent illness Intrathecal interferon
Sydenham chorea	Penicillin Phenothiazine or butyrophenone
Tourette disease	Haloperidol (Haldol), clonidine (Catapres) Supportive psychotherapy
Paroxysmal choreoathetosis	Phenytoin (Dilantin), carbamazepine (Tegretol)
Hydrocephalus	Ventriculoperitoneal shunt
Dystonia musculorum deformans	Trihexyphenidyl (Artane), carbamazepine (Tegretol) Stereotaxic surgery
Cerebral palsy	Physical therapy Surgical relief of contractures (?) Cerebellar stimulation
Spinal cord tumor	Surgical removal Radiotherapy Chemotherapy

TABLE 13–2. **(Continued)**

Syringomyelia or spinal cord cyst	Aspiration of cyst Shunting of cyst
Cerebellar tumor	Surgical therapy (removal, shunt) Radiotherapy Chemotherapy
Anticonvulsant drug effects	Lower dosage Add CNS stimulant to counteract drowsiness
Acute extrapyramidal reaction	Diphenhydramine (Benadryl) or benztropine mesylate (Cogentin) IM or IV
Tardive dyskinesia	Discontinue offending drug Choline, lecithin, deanol (Deaner) Diazepam (Valium) Phenothiazine, butyrophenone (as last resort)

(Mestinon) or neostigmine (Prostigmin), usually allows for marked functional improvement.

Myasthenia gravis often takes a waxing and waning course. Its management is sometimes further complicated by difficulties in distinguishing symptoms of the disorder from drug toxicity. Hospitalization and careful withdrawal of medication are usually indicated in such circumstances.

Corticosteroids may be of benefit in treating myasthenia gravis. Surgical treatment involving removal of the thymus gland has also been of demonstrated effectiveness in some children and adolescents (Snead et al., 1980).

The polyneuropathies associated with acute intermittent porphyria and diphtheria, the polyradiculopathy of Guillain-Barré syndrome, and the motor neuron involvement of poliomyelitis may be life-threatening because of respiratory involvement. Prevention or early detection of pneumonia is essential, with antibiotics and physical therapy employed as necessary. Mechanical ventilation may be required.

Acute intermittent porphyria is best prevented by avoidance of offending agents such as barbiturates, sulfa drugs, estrogens, or alcohol. If treatment of agitation or severe abdominal pain is required, chlorpromazine (Thorazine) may be used.

Diphtheritic gait disturbance and palatal dysfunction are treated symptomatically. Tube feeding may be required to prevent aspiration. Careful attention must also be paid to myocarditis, a potentially lethal complication.

The Guillain-Barré syndrome is usually a self-limited disorder that runs its course within a few weeks. Full recovery is the rule, but a small percentage of cases will show permanent residua. Corticosteroids have been used as an adjunct to supportive therapy with favorable results in some instances (Dowling et al., 1980). Other trials have suggested that corticosteroids are of no benefit or even worsen outcome.

Treatment of Werdnig-Hoffmann disease is symptomatic. With onset of the disorder within the first few months of life, death nearly always ensues within the first 1 to 2 years due to respiratory compromise. Later-onset forms of Werdnig-Hoffmann disease and Kugelberg-Welander disease have a better outlook. Survival into adolescence and young adulthood is characteristic in the latter.

Medical treatment of multiple sclerosis may take several forms, none of which is consistently effective. Corticosteroids and ACTH may be helpful in some children, although such medication must be used with care because it may itself contribute to (or cause) a gait problem by causing a toxic myopathy (see Case 21–1). Collaborative studies have shown that steroids appear to improve neurologic function lost in acute relapses, but they may actually increase the frequency of relapses or shorten the time between relapses (Ellison and Myers, 1980). The immunosuppressive drug cyclophosphamide, an alkylating agent, has been found to diminish the number of relapses and lower cerebrospinal fluid immunoglobulin content (Ellison and Myers, 1980). Drug toxicity (including effects of infertility and malignancy) limits the use of such agents. Recent investigation has demonstrated a reduction in the number of exacerbations in some persons through the use of interferon administered intrathecally, that is, given serially by lumbar puncture (Jacobs *et al.*, 1981).

The effectiveness of any treatment of multiple sclerosis must be considered in light of the natural history of the disorder, which characteristically pursues a variable course with spontaneous remissions and exacerbations.

Wilson disease (hepatolenticular degeneration) is treated by D-penicillamine and avoidance of copper-containing foods such as chocolate, fish, and nuts. Penicillamine binds copper, thereby preventing its deposition in brain, liver, cornea, and other organs and allowing for its excretion.

The movement disorder of Sydenham chorea can be benefited in some children with chlorpromazine (Thorazine) or haloperidol (Haldol). The potential for inducing movement disorders with these drugs must be considered when they are employed (Shields and Bray, 1976). Because Sydenham chorea is part of the rheumatic fever complex, children should be placed on penicillin prophylaxis to prevent cardiac complications.

With dystonia associated with cerebral palsy or dystonia musculorum deformans, trihexyphenidyl (Artane) and carbamazepine (Tegretol) may be of symptomatic benefit.

Huntington disease is a progressively dementing disorder with a uniformly poor prognosis in affected persons. Several drugs have been employed in treating the movement disorder, but none has been consistently effective (Perry *et al.*, 1980).

A trial of L-dopa by mouth may distinguish presymptomatic persons with Huntington disease by producing transient chorea (Klawans *et al.*, 1980). Whether the medical and psychologic risks associated with this provocative test outweigh the benefits remains to be clarified.

In many children and adolescents with Tourette disease, haloperidol (Haldol) has been of benefit. Dystonic reactions and other adverse effects (such as depression and "fog states"), however, not infrequently necessitate its discontinuance (Bruun *et al.*, 1976). In their study of 78 persons with Tourette disease followed for an average of 32 months, Bruun and colleagues (1976) described complete remission in four persons. Of the 59 persons taking haloperidol at the time of follow-up, an average of 80 per cent improvement in symptoms was found.

Other agents have also appeared useful or at least promising in Tourette disease. Tetrabenazine and alpha-methyl-para-tyrosine, both dopamine and norepinephrine antagonists, have appeared to benefit some patients (Sweet et al., 1976; Bruun et al., 1976). Cholinergic agents (physostigmine and lecithin) have helped other persons with Tourette disease (Stahl and Berger, 1980; Barbeau, 1980).

Recently, Cohen and colleagues (1980) have found that clonidine (Catapres), a centrally active alpha-adrenergic agonist, benefited 23 of 25 patients (most of them children or adolescents) who had failed to respond to haloperidol or had not tolerated that medication because of its side effects.

When gait disorder or other motor disturbance occurs secondary to overmedication with anticonvulsant drugs such as phenobarbital or phenytoin, adjustment of dosage to a level that will permit improved motor function without significantly lessening seizure control should be attempted. The reason for overdosage (for example, prescription error or addition of a second anticonvulsant medication) should be identified to prevent recurrence of the problem. If ataxia or increase in seizures is caused by anticonvulsant-related drowsiness, addition of dextroamphetamine or methylphenidate to the pharmacologic regimen may be of benefit.

When a disorder of posture or movement is caused by idiosyncratic reaction to a phenothiazine or butyrophenone, administration of diphenydramine (Benadryl) 10 to 50 mg by the intravenous or intramuscular route may promptly eradicate symptoms. Alternatively, benztropine mesylate (Cogentin) can be given. The use of prophylactic "antiparkinsonian" drugs when antipsychotic medications are prescribed continues to be a matter for debate (Johnson, 1978; Chiles, 1978; Rifkin et al., 1978).

No uniformly effective treatment has been found for tardive dyskinesia. Once the problem has been recognized, medication should be discontinued as soon as possible and another antipsychotic agent employed in the lowest effective dosage should further medication appear necessary (Baldessarini et al., 1980) (see Chapter 5).

The precise pathophysiology of tardive dyskinesia has not been determined, and treatment has been largely empiric. Choline and lecithin, both acting as precursors of acetylcholine, have been effective in some adults (Growdon et al., 1977). Deanol (Deaner) and diazepam (Valium) may also be of benefit. When all else has failed and the movement disorder is severe and disabling, chlorpromazine and haloperidol themselves may help some persons.

In the treatment of paroxysmal kinesigenic choreoathetosis, phenytoin and carbamazepine have been effective (Kinast et al., 1980).

Neurologic Management. Treatment of neurologic disorders such as Wilson disease and Sydenham chorea among others is discussed above (see MEDICAL MANAGEMENT).

Surgical Management. Intraspinal lesions such as neurofibroma, arachnoid cyst, and diastematomyelia are treated surgically usually through laminectomy (Herskowitz *et al.*, 1978; Kennedy, 1979). Syringomyelia may be treated by aspiration of the cyst and by insertion of a shunt to drain fluid from the syrinx into the adjacent subarachnoid space. Gliomas and other intramedullary lesions may be inoperable, though treatable by radiation and/or chemotherapy.

Cerebellar tumors are amenable to direct surgical treatment. Cerebellar astrocytomas are frequently totally resectable. Outcome is often excellent, although some clumsiness may persist. With medulloblastomas, removal is usually incomplete. Radiation is generally delivered to the entire neuraxis (brain and spinal cord) because of the frequency of metastatic spread in the disease. Chemotherapy may also be given at the time of diagnosis (especially if metastasis has already occurred) or recurrence.

Hydrocephalus of any cause (such as cerebellar tumor or aqueductal stenosis) is usually treated surgically by ventriculoperitoneal or other shunting. Symptomatic improvement in headache and gait disturbance is often marked.

Children with dystonia musculorum deformans may be benefited by neurosurgery. Treatment consists of placement of small lesions in the ventrolateral nucleus of the thalamus. Several operations over a number of years may be necessary for continued symptomatic benefit (Cooper, 1973). Some forms of cerebral palsy have been treated by implantation of electrical stimulators into the cerebellum. Its effectiveness has not consistently been demonstrated to exceed that of placebo (Gahm *et al.*, 1981).

Surgical release of contractures (e.g., at the ankle or hip) associated with cerebral palsy and selective use of spinal fusion in persons with Duchenne dystrophy to lessen cardiorespiratory compromise are other forms of surgical therapy.

Psychotherapy. Supportive therapy involving the affected child and his or her family is always indicated in the management of movement disorders of childhood and adolescence. Treatment on an individual or family basis should include explanation, reassurance, and encouragement. Particularly with chronic progressive disorders such as Duchenne muscular dystrophy, Huntington disease, and motor neuron disease, psychotherapy is important since depression can affect any or all family members (Shoulson and Fahn, 1979) (see Chapter 21). The role of psychotherapy in the management of hysterical gait disorder is discussed in Chapter 7.

With simple tic of childhood, reassurance may itself lessen the frequency and severity of the tic, as the child may have been made increasingly anxious by parental insistence to stop the "habit" or by classmates' teasing. Parents will usually respond to requests to limit their calling attention to the tic, and peers will generally lose interest in teasing. When anxiety plays a more pervasive role in the child's life, interfering with academic or social functioning, formal child psychiatric or psychologic treatment is indicated.

Social-Environmental Management. For the wheelchair-restricted patient, a "barrier-free" environment will facilitate mobility. Access to appropriate modes of transportation will provide necessary changes of scenery, minimizing social isolation and maximizing educational opportunities.

When the child has a tic (including those of Tourette disease) or other movement disorder (such as Sydenham chorea or dystonia musculorum deformans), it will be valuable to communicate with school personnel (teacher, nurse, and principal) to coordinate medical, psychologic, and educational aspects of therapy.

Educational Management. For the child confined to a wheelchair or otherwise motorically impaired, ongoing education is an important goal, for it is a major social as well as academic activity of normal childhood. Complicating physical and emotional factors such as easy fatigability, impaired concentration, and depression need be taken into account when educational planning and performance are being considered.

Communication Therapy. In persons with cerebral palsy in whom speech and other voluntary activities are impaired, a variety of ingenious devices have been developed to facilitate oral as well as written communication. These include communication boards that enable the child to construct entire sentences by pointing (with, for example, a "head pointer") to words or pictures in sequence.

Physical Therapy. In persons with muscular dystrophy or motor neuron disease, active and passive range-of-motion exercises are valuable in preserving function and mobility. Chest physical therapy can be useful in assisting the child to clear secretions from the respiratory tract, thereby helping to prevent pneumonia.

The clumsy child will often benefit from physical therapy or adaptive physical education to improve skills and gain confidence in areas of difficulty (McKinlay, 1978).

Mechanical Therapy. With severe motor handicap, wheelchairs (which may be conventional or motorized, controlled by hand or mouth) can offer a considerable increase in freedom and allow for development of greater independence.

Splints and braces, used in conjunction with a program of physical therapy, are designed to prevent contracture and to increase or preserve function.

CORRELATION

Anatomic Aspects. Although it is somewhat artificial to tease apart the motor system, it has proved clinically useful to view motor function from the standpoint of pyramidal, extrapyramidal, and cerebellar motor systems.

The pyramidal (voluntary motor) system begins in the precentral cortex of the frontal lobe, the so-called motor strip. Giant pyramidal neurons of Betz send axons from the motor cortex through the internal capsule to the brainstem en route to the spinal cord. There lie the anterior horn cells, ultimate destination of corticospinal fibers.

Throughout its course, the voluntary motor system is organized somatotopically. The motor homunculus, a more or less upside-down caricature of a human being, was described in Chapter 12 (see CORRELATION). Leg fibers originate from the area of the interhemispheric fissure. Arm fibers are derived from the convexity of the hemisphere. Mouth, face, and tongue fibers arise close to the Sylvian fissure. After passing through the internal capsule, pyramidal fibers enter the midbrain, where they run within the cerebral peduncles. Here, face fibers are represented medially, leg fibers later-ally, and arm fibers in between. From there, they course through the basal portions of the pons to make up the pyramids of the medulla. The pyramids cross, or decussate, and continue in the spinal cord as the lateral cortico-spinal tracts, which are contralateral to the cerebral hemisphere of origin. Corticospinal fibers end upon anterior horn cells of the spinal cord. These give rise to spinal nerve roots, which become organized to form peripheral nerves.

A "leg fiber" from the motor cortex of the left hemisphere thus will origi-nate near the interhemispheric fissure, course around the lateral wall of the left lateral ventricle, make up part of the internal capsule, traverse the brain-stem, cross to the opposite side of the central nervous system in the medulla, and travel in the right lateral corticospinal tract to end upon motor neurons of anterior horn cells in the lumbosacral region of the spinal cord on the right.

The extrapyramidal motor system is rooted in the basal ganglia, a set of deep, paired structures near the midline that are involved in posture and movement. The head of the caudate nucleus lies anteriorly, indenting the medial wall of the frontal horn of the lateral ventricle. The body and tail of the caudate nucleus travel posteriorly along the wall of the lateral ventricle. The globus pallidus and putamen are basal ganglia separated from the cau-date nucleus by the anterior limb of the internal capsule. These structures are richly interconnected. They also communicate intimately with pyramidal and cerebellar motor systems, the hypothalamus, and other portions of the limbic system.

The cerebellar system begins with the cerebellum, a distinctive-appearing structure lying at the base of the brain in the posterior fossa. Its primary con-nections are not to the cerebrum or spinal cord but to the brainstem, from which it originates embryologically. Lying between cerebrum and spinal cord, the cerebellum is well situated to correlate and coordinate information from higher and lower centers of the nervous system.

Like the cerebrum, the cerebellum is divided into two hemispheres. Each is primarily involved in appendicular (limb) movements rather than axial (truncal) movements. In contrast to cerebral hemispheres, cerebellar hemi-spheres influence ipsilateral (rather than contralateral) limb movements (see Fig. 13–13). The midline portion of the cerebellum is called the vermis be-cause of its wormlike appearance. The anterior portion of the vermis influ-ences axial (truncal) motor activity such as walking. It appears to be the site of the wide-based "cerebellar gait" caused by agents such as alcohol and phenytoin in toxic amounts. Other portions of the cerebellum include the flocculus and nodulus, phylogenetically old structures that are involved in coordination of eye movements with those of the head and neck.

Biochemical Aspects.   Experimental and clinical evidence has indicated that normal movement depends upon a proper biochemical balance between dopamine and acetylcholine.

In idiopathic parkinsonism, a disorder of adulthood characterized by bra-dykinesia (diminished movement) and tremor at rest, dopamine appears to be deficient. The substantia nigra of the midbrain in affected persons is paler than normal due to dopamine depletion. L-Dopa, a dopamine precursor, is

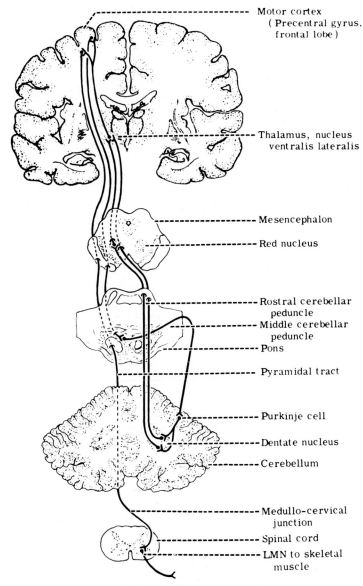

Motor cortex
(Precentral gyrus,
frontal lobe)

Thalamus, nucleus
ventralis lateralis

Mesencephalon

Red nucleus

Rostral cerebellar
peduncle
Middle cerebellar
peduncle
Pons

Pyramidal tract

Purkinje cell

Dentate nucleus

Cerebellum

Medullo-cervical
junction
Spinal cord
LMN to skeletal
muscle

FIGURE 13–13. Cerebellar pathways (From DeMyer, W.
Technique of the Neurologic Examination, 3rd ed. Copyright
© 1980, McGraw-Hill Book Company. Used with the permission
of McGraw-Hill Book Company.)

able to improve motor function significantly in many persons with parkinsonism. L-Dopa is used instead of dopamine because, given orally, it is
able to cross the blood-brain barrier. Overdosage or intolerance of L-dopa
can produce a movement disorder characterized by involuntary movements.

The role of acetylcholine has been suggested by the effectiveness of anticholinergic agents in the treatment of parkinsonism and dystonic reactions

to antipsychotic drugs. Anticholinergic drugs include trihexyphenidyl (Artane) and benztropine mesylate (Cogentin).

An important cholinergic role in movement disorders is further indicated by atrophy of the caudate nucleus (which appears to produce acetylcholine) in persons with Huntington disease (Enna *et al.*, 1976). Atrophy of the head of the caudate can be seen by CT scan, pneumoencephalography, or postmortem examination as dilatation of the frontal horn of the lateral ventricle (see Fig. 13–12). The beneficial response to cholinergic agents such as dietary choline and lecithin in some persons with tardive dyskinesia demonstrates additionally the significance of acetylcholine in motor function.

Serotonin may also play an important biochemical role in motor function. Studies of persons with Tourette disease have demonstrated a reduction in metabolites of serotonin (Cohen *et al.*, 1978). It has been suggested that diminished inhibitory serotonergic input contributes to the dopaminergic overactivity seen in affected persons.

Overall, then, too little movement is associated with dopamine depletion (as in parkinsonism), too much movement with acetylcholine deficit (as in Huntington disease) or dopamine excess (as in overdosage with L-dopa). Hypersensitivity to dopamine may underlie tardive dyskinesia.

Physiologic Aspects. The neuromuscular unit consists of an anterior horn cell (motor neuron), motor nerve roots (axons derived from a single motor neuron), neuromuscular junctions, and muscle fibers upon which the axons of a single anterior horn cell end. A motor neuron whose cell body lies in the anterior horn of the spinal cord or correspondingly within the brainstem may end upon a few or many motor fibers. With muscles supplying the eye, three muscle fibers may be subserved by one motor neuron. In limb or trunk muscles, however, an anterior horn cell may supply hundreds of muscle fibers. In general, the more discrete the motor movement, the fewer skeletal muscle fibers supplied by a single motor neuron.

Muscle contraction normally results from propagation of an electrical impulse away from the body of the motor neuron along its axon to its distal, or presynaptic, portion. When an electrical threshold has been exceeded, acetylcholine released presynaptically at the neuromuscular junction acts upon a receptor at the postsynaptic membrane, a portion of the muscle cell. This causes depolarization of the muscle cell membrane in that region, further transmission of the electrical impulse, and ultimately muscle contraction.

The molecular basis of muscle contraction rests upon the structure and interaction of the proteins actin and myosin (Fenichel, 1975). Filaments of actin and myosin overlap one another to make up myofibers. Projections from actin and myosin filaments prevent them from slipping over each other until the process of contraction is initiated.

Contraction involves the simultaneous shortening of all myofibers of a muscle cell. It results from acetylcholine-mediated depolarization of the postsynaptic membrane, the motor end plate. Consequently calcium is released, ATPase is activated, and ATP broken down into ADP and high-energy phosphate. The energy generated permits actin and myosin filaments to overlap further. As they slip over one another, the myofiber is shortened.

Relaxation occurs when calcium is re-bound, and thus made unavailable to participate further in contraction.

SUMMARY

Movement plays a key role in essentially all behavior and is affected in a wide variety of behavioral and emotional problems of childhood and adolescence. Gait disorders, tics, tremors, and clumsiness are frequently encountered problems in pediatrics. Their management is based upon characterization of the child's particular syndrome through history-taking, examination, and investigation. In general the onset and tempo of the problem should be documented with precipitating influences and associated features identified. Family history and medication history may be relevant. The examination will serve to identify the nature and degree of deficit. Investigation will depend upon relevant diagnostic possibilities suggested through interview and examination. Treatment will be determined by the cause and severity of the movement disorder. It may involve specific treatment, as with Wilson disease, or exclusively symptomatic measures, as with Duchenne muscular dystrophy. Supportive therapy is always of value. Anatomic, biochemical, and physiologic factors involved in movement provide the basis for a rational approach to management of these common and often difficult disorders.

CITED REFERENCES

Aron, A. M.; Freeman, J. M.; and Carter, S. The natural history of Sydenham's chorea: review of the literature and long-term evaluation with emphasis on cardiac sequelae. *Am. J. Med.,* **38:** 83–95, 1965.

Baldessarini, R. J.; Cole, J. O.; Davis, J. M.; Simpson, G.; Tarsy, D.; Gardos, G.; and Preskorn, S. H. Tardive dyskinesia: summary of a task force report of the American Psychiatric Association. *Am. J. Psychiatry,* **137:** 1163–72, 1980.

Barbeau, A. Cholinergic treatment in the Tourette syndrome. *N. Engl. J. Med.,* **302:** 1310–11, 1980.

Barclay, N. Acute intermittent porphyria in childhood. *Arch. Dis. Child.,* **49:** 404–6, 1974.

Barone, D. A., and Raniolo, J. Facial dyskinesia from overdose of an antihistamine. *N. Engl. J. Med.,* **303:** 107, 1980.

Bliss, J. Sensory experiences of Gilles de la Tourette syndrome. Cohen, D. J., and Freedman, D. X., eds. *Arch. Gen. Psychiatry,* **37:** 1343–47, 1980.

Bruun, R. D.; Shapiro, A. K.; Shapiro, E.; Sweet, R.; Wayne, H.; and Solomon, G. E. A follow-up of 78 patients with Gilles de la Tourette's syndrome. *Am. J. Psychiatry,* **133:** 944–47, 1976.

Cartwright, G. E. Diagnosis of treatable Wilson's disease. *N. Engl. J. Med.,* **298:** 1347–50, 1978.

Chiles, J. A. Extrapyramidal reactions in adolescents treated with high-potency antipsychotics. *Am. J. Psychiatry,* **135:** 239–40, 1978.

Cohen, D. J.; Shaywitz, B. A.; Caparulo, B.; Young, J. G.; and Bowers, M. B., Jr. Chronic, multiple tics of Gilles de la Tourette's disease. *Arch. Gen. Psychiatry,* **35:** 245–50, 1978.

Cohen, D. J.; Detlor, J.; Young, J. G.; and Shaywitz, B. A. Clonidine ameliorates Gilles de la Tourette syndrome. *Arch. Gen. Psychiatry,* **37**: 1350–57, 1980.

Cooper, I. S. *The Victim Is Always the Same.* Harper and Row, New York, 1973.

Dobyns, W. B.; Goldstein, N. P.; and Gordon, H. Clinical spectrum of Wilson's disease (hepatolenticular degeneration). *Mayo Clin. Proc.,* **54**: 35–42, 1979.

Dowling, P. C.; Bosch, V. V.; and Cook, S. D. Possible beneficial effect of high-dose intravenous steroid therapy in acute demyelinating disease and transverse myelitis. *Neurology* (Minneapolis), **30**: 33–36, 1980.

Drachman, D. B. Myasthenia gravis. *N. Engl. J. Med.,* (first of two parts), **298**: 136–42, (second of two parts), **298**: 186–93, 1978.

Dubowitz, V., and Hersov, L. Management of children with non-organic (hysterical) disorders of motor function. *Dev. Med. Child Neurol.,* **18**: 358–68, 1976.

Ellison, G. W., and Myers, L. W. Immunosuppressive drugs in multiple sclerosis: pro and con. *Neurology* (Minneapolis), **30**: 28–32, 1980.

Enna, S. J.; Bird, E. D.; Bennett, J. P., Jr.; Bylund, D. B.; Yamamura, H. I.; Iversen, L. L.; and Snyder, S. H. Huntington's chorea: changes in neurotransmitter receptors in the brain. *N. Engl. J. Med.,* **294**: 1305–09, 1976.

Fenichel, G. M. Normal muscle: structure, function, and development. Pp. 927–38 in *The Practice of Pediatric Neurology.* Swaiman, K. F., and Wright, F. S., eds. C. V. Mosby Company, Saint Louis, 1975.

Gahm, N. H.; Russman, B. S.; Cerciello, R. L.; Fiorentino, M. R.; and McGrath, D. M. Chronic cerebellar stimulation for cerebral palsy: a double-blind study. *Neurology* (New York), **31**: 87–90, 1981.

Golden, G. S. Gilles de la Tourette's syndrome following methylphenidate administration. *Dev. Med. Child Neurol.,* **16**: 76–78, 1974.

Goodenough, D. J.; Fariello, R. G.; Annis, B. L.; and Chun, R. W. M. Familial and acquired paroxysmal dyskinesias. *Arch. Neurol.,* **35**: 827–31, 1978.

Growdon, J. H.; Hirsch, M. J.; Wurtman, R. J.; and Wiener, W. Oral choline administration to patients with tardive dyskinesia. *N. Engl. J. Med.,* **297**: 524–27, 1977.

Gualtieri, C. T.; Barnhill, J.; McGimsey, J.; and Schell, D. Tardive dyskinesia and other movement disorders in children treated with psychotropic drugs. *J. Am. Acad. Child Psychiatry,* **19**: 491–510, 1980.

Hansotia, P.; Cleeland, C. S.; and Chun, R. W. M. Juvenile Huntington's chorea. *Neurology* (Minneapolis), **18**: 217–24, 1968.

Herskowitz, J.; Bielawski, M. A.; Venna, N.; and Sabin, T. D. Anterior cervical arachnoid cyst simulating syringomyelia: a case with preceding posterior arachnoid cysts. *Arch. Neurol.,* **35**: 57–58, 1978.

Jacobs, L.; O'Malley, J.; Freeman, A.; and Ekes, R. Intrathecal interferon reduces exacerbations of multiple sclerosis. *Science* **214**: 1026–28, 1981.

Jervis, G. A. Huntington's chorea in childhood. *Arch. Neurol.,* **9**: 244–57, 1963.

Johnson, D. A. W. Prevalence and treatment of drug-induced extrapyramidal symptoms. *Br. J. Psychiatry,* **132**: 27–30, 1978.

Kennedy, P. R. New data on diastematomyelia. *J. Neurosurg.,* **51**: 355–61, 1979.

Kidd, K. K.; Prusoff, B. A.,; and Cohen, D. J. Familial pattern of Gilles de la Tourette syndrome. *Arch. Gen. Psychiatry,* **37**: 1336–39, 1980.

Kinast, M.; Erenberg, G.; and Rothner, A. D. Paroxysmal choreoathetosis: report of five cases and review of the literature. *Pediatrics,* **65**: 74–77, 1980.

Klawans, H. L.; Goetz, C. G.; Paulson, G. W.; and Barbeau, A. Levodopa and presymptomatic detection of Huntington's disease: eight-year follow-up. *N. Engl. J. Med.,* **302**: 1090, 1980.

Markham, C. H., and Knox, J. W. Observations on Huntington's chorea in childhood. *J. Pediatr.,* **67**: 46–57, 1965.

McKinlay, I. Strategies for clumsy children. *Dev. Med. Child Neurol.*, **20**: 494–96, 1978.

McLean, P., and Casey, D. E. Tardive dyskinesia in an adolescent. *Am. J. Psychiatry,* **135**: 969–71, 1978.

Nausieda, P. A.; Grossman, B. J.; Koller, W. C.; Weiner, W. J.; and Klawans, H. L. Sydenham chorea: an update. *Neurology,* **30**: 331–34, 1980.

Perry, T. L.; Wright, J. M.; Hansen, S.; Allan, B. M.; Baird, P. A.; and MacLeod, P. M. Failure of aminooxyacetic acid therapy in Huntington disease. *Neurology,* **30**: 772–75, 1980.

Reuben, R. N., and Bakwin, H. Developmental clumsiness. *Pediatr. Clin. North Am.,* **15**: 601–10, 1968.

Rifkin, A.; Quitkin, F.; Kane, J.; Struve, F.; and Klein, D. F. Are prophylactic antiparkinson drugs necessary? *Arch. Gen. Psychiatry,* **35**: 483–89, 1978.

Rosman, N. P. Neurological and muscular aspects of thyroid dysfunction in childhood. *Pediatr. Clin. North Am.,* **23**: 575–94, 1976.

Rosman, N. P. The cerebral defect and myopathy in Duchenne muscular dystrophy: a comparative clinicopathological study. *Neurology* (Minneapolis), **20**: 329–35, 1970.

Rosman, N. P., and Kakulas, B. A. Mental deficiency associated with muscular dystrophy: a neuropathological study. *Brain,* **89**: 769–88, 1966.

Scime, I. A., and Tallant, E. J. Tetanus-like reactions to prochlorperazine (Compazine): report of eight cases exhibiting extrapyramidal disturbances after small doses. *J.A.M.A.,* **171**: 1813–17, 1959.

Shapiro, A. K.; Shapiro, E.; and Wayne, H. L. The symptomatology and diagnosis of Gilles de la Tourette's syndrome. *J. Am. Acad. Child Psychiatry,* **12**: 702–23, 1973.

Shields, W. D., and Bray, P. F. A danger of haloperidol therapy in children. *J. Pediatr.,* **88**: 301–3, 1976.

Shoulson, I., and Fahn, S. Huntington disease: clinical care and evaluation. *Neurology* (Minneapolis), **29**: 1–3, 1979.

Snead, O. C., III; Benton, J. W.; Dwyer, D.; Morley, B. J.; Kemp, G. E.; Bradley, R. J.; and Oh, S. J. Juvenile myasthenia gravis. *Neurology,* **30**: 732–39, 1980.

Stahl, S. M., and Berger, P. A. Physostigmine in Gilles de la Tourette syndrome. *N. Engl. J. Med.,* **302**: 298, 1980.

Sweet, R. D.; Bruun, R. D.; Shapiro, A. K.; and Shapiro, E. The pharmacology of Gilles de la Tourette's syndrome (chronic multiple tic). Pp. 81–105 in *Clinical Neuropharmacology,* Vol. 1. Klawans, H. L., ed. Raven Press, New York, 1976.

Tibbles, J. A. R., and Barnes, S. E. Paroxysmal dystonic choreoathetosis of mount and reback. *Pediatrics,* **65**: 149–51, 1980.

Vaidya, V. A.; Bongiovanni, A. M.; Parks, J. S.; Tenore, A.; and Kirkland, R. T. Twenty-two years' experience in the medical management of juvenile thyrotoxicosis. *Pediatrics,* **54**: 565–70, 1974.

ADDITIONAL READINGS

Barbeau, A.; Growdon, J. H.; and Wurtman, R. J. *Choline and Lethicin in Brain Disorders.* Raven Press, New York, 1979.

Dubowitz, V. *Muscle Disorders in Childhood.* W. B. Saunders Ltd., London, 1978.

Evarts, E. V. Brain mechanisms of movement. *Sci. Am.,* **241**: 164–79, September 1979.

Gordon, N., and McKinlay, I. (eds.). *Helping Clumsy Children.* Churchill Livingstone, Edinburgh, 1980.

Poskanzer, D. C.; Walker, A. M.; Prenney, L. B.; and Sheridan, J. L. The etiology of multiple sclerosis: temporal-spatial clustering indicating two environmental exposures before onset. *Neurology* (New York), **31:** 708–13, 1981.

Roueché, B. Live and let live. *The New Yorker,* July 16, 1979, pp. 82–87. Reprinted in *The Medical Detectives,* by Roueché, B. New York Times Book Co., New York, 1980, pp. 345–60.

Weingarten, K. Tics. Pp. 782–803 in *Handbook of Clinical Neurology,* Vol. 6. Vinken, P. J., and Bruyn, G. W., eds. North-Holland Publishing Company, Amsterdam, 1968.

Young, R. R., and Delwaide, P. J. Spasticity. *N. Engl. J. Med.,* **304:** 28–33, 1981.

14 Hyperactivity and Attentional Disorders

Hyperactivity, the symptom, is but one aspect (a highly visible one at that) of a syndrome of attentional disturbance, an attention deficit disorder. The problem is a common one and often involves parents, teacher, pediatrician, neurologist, psychologist, and psychiatrist because of its widespread behavioral repercussions and its multifactorial etiology. As with other behavioral and emotional problems of childhood, attention deficit disorder is a descriptive term, not an etiologic diagnosis. It represents a final common pathway, the outward manifestations of one or several influences upon the developing nervous system of the child.

This chapter will define hyperactivity and attention deficit disorder, examine their causes, discuss conditions that might be mistaken for them, and present a comprehensive approach to treatment. The notion of "the hyperactive child" as a single entity responsive to a single treatment (drugs) is false and stands in the way of more specific and comprehensive treatment (which may include medication) based upon individualized evaluation.

Several questions will be addressed in this chapter:

What is the difference between hyperactivity and overactivity?
What is the definition of attention deficit disorder? How does it differ from hyperactivity or the hyperkinetic syndrome?
Can a child who is quiet and cooperative in an office setting be considered hyperactive?
Is the child who is hyperactive secondary to emotional stresses truly hyperactive or, rather, emotionally disturbed?
What medical or neurologic conditions should be considered in the evaluation of a hyperactive child?
What nonpharmacologic measures can be employed in the treatment of attention deficit disorder?
When should medication be employed? What drug, in what dosage, how often, and for how long?

What is the outcome in adolescence and adulthood of persons who were
hyperactive as children?

HYPERACTIVITY AND ATTENTIONAL DISORDERS

DEFINITION

Hyperactivity is a term used to describe motor behavior that is felt to be
excessive for age. Attempts to quantitate movement (such as by recording
the number of times a child interrupts a photoelectric beam) have proved of
little diagnostic or therapeutic usefulness. In fact, some children with motor
behavior equal to or less than that of so-called normal children are functionally hyperactive because they move in ineffectual patterns. For example,
they may turn distractedly this way or that in response to noise in the classroom and not be able to carry on with school work. By contrast, a classmate
chewing gum and tapping his feet may be able to work productively despite
nearly continuous motor activity. The hyperactive child, then, often exists
in a chronic state of "spinning his wheels" with a great deal of energy ex-
pended and movement generated, but very little to show for it.

To a certain degree the use of the term "hyperactive" relates to the eye of
the beholder. Children virtually never identify themselves as such, parents
do so much more often, and teachers perhaps most of all. A hyperactive
child running in and out of the home to play will not excite much attention,
but the same degree of motor activity at school—manifested as getting out
of the seat, wandering around the classroom, and tapping a pencil on the
desk—can be highly disruptive.

Hyperactivity is commonly encountered as part of the syndrome of *attention deficit disorder* (see Table 14–1). As with any syndrome, not all features
need be present for the diagnosis to apply. Indeed, attention deficit disorder
can be diagnosed *without* hyperkinesis (used here synonymously with hyperactivity). The essential features of attention deficit disorder are: inattention, impulsivity, and hyperactivity. Overexcitability, impersistence, and
dysphoria are often associated. One or two of the three major criteria will
generally predominate in a child with attention deficit disorder. Thus, hyperactivity may be much less prominent than impulsivity or inattentiveness.

When hyperactivity is a prominent symptom, the designation *hyperkinetic syndrome* is used interchangeably with that of attention deficit disorder,
though the latter has the advantage of underscoring the important (and perhaps primary) role of attentional disturbance.

Brain damage has over the years been an area of concern in the evaluation
of hyperactive children. Inattention and hyperactivity following encephalitis
or obvious brain trauma have indeed been identified as part of a syndrome of
brain damage. Many more hyperkinetic children, however, lack convincing
evidence of significant brain damage by history or upon examination. Thus the
concept of "minimal brain damage" came into wider use, later supplanted
by "minimal brain dysfunction," which most recently has yielded to "attention deficit disorder." It is certainly possible that brain damage, minimal or
otherwise, underlies the attention deficit disorder of some such children; but
the normalcy of the neurologic examination in most instances and the fre-

TABLE 14–1. **Diagnosis of Attention Deficit Disorder**[*]

Attention Deficit Disorder with Hyperactivity
    Inattention
        doesn't finish tasks
        doesn't seem to listen
        distractible
        has difficulty concentrating on tasks
        has difficulty sticking to play
    Impulsivity
        acts before thinking
        shifts from one activity to another
        has difficulty organizing work
        needs much supervision
        often calls out in class
        has difficulty awaiting turn
    Hyperactivity
        runs or climbs excessively
        has difficulty sitting still
        has difficulty staying seated
        restless during sleep
        always "on the go"
    Onset: before 7 years (usually by 3 years)
    Duration: at least 6 months

Attention Deficit Disorder Without Hyperactivity
    As above, except for absence of hyperactivity

[*] Adapted from *Diagnostic and Statistical Manual of Mental Disorders,* 3d ed. (American Psychiatric Association, Washington, D.C., 1980).

quently familial nature of the problem render across-the-board judgments as to the presence of brain damage difficult, if not impossible, to sustain.

DIAGNOSIS

Clinical Process. *History.* A parent's chief complaint will often bring out which symptom is foremost in the child's syndrome: hyperactivity, impulsivity, inattention, or overexcitability. "He can't sit still." "The teachers say he never pays attention in class." "He doesn't take the time to think." "He gets as high as a kite when he is excited." The child may be aware of the problem, but it does not usually bother him. "They say I've got the wiggly worms," one child recounted.

The history of the presenting problem should provide the framework within which referral for evaluation has occurred. A typical situation would involve a boy in kindergarten or first grade not felt ready to advance to the next grade because of a high activity level associated with poor pencil and paper skills or inability to master rudiments of reading. Another common scenario is the 9-year-old boy whose academic achievement is two grade levels below that predicted by his intelligence and who has few friends among classmates because of his "bossiness." The history of the major presenting symptom (e.g., hyperactivity) should be traced to the present and associated features of impulsivity, inattention, and overexcitability likewise described.

School evaluation, remediation efforts, and their effectiveness should be noted. Particulars of the current classroom setting should be determined. How many students are in the classroom? How many teachers or aides? Is the classroom open or contained? How are desks arranged—in rows or in circular islands? Where does the child sit—in the back or up front, near the teacher? Such information should be sought directly from school personnel: teacher, psychologist, or principal. The Conners Abbreviated Rating Scale has proved valuable in the diagnosis of hyperactivity syndromes and in studies of medication and other therapies (Sleator and Ullman, 1981) (see section on MEDICAL MANAGEMENT).

The past history should include information as to pregnancy, labor, delivery, and the neonatal period. Prenatal infection (e.g., with rubella) can lead to a wide variety of behavioral disturbances in the child, including hyperactivity. Activity level *in utero* is often but not invariably noted to be increased in children who later prove hyperactive. Toxemia of pregnancy, protracted labor, breech delivery, fetal distress, small size for gestational age, or low Apgar scores suggest possibly harmful effects upon the developing brain.

Within the first weeks or even days of life, an infant may be recognized to have a characteristic style of temperament, the substrate of emerging personality and behavior. For example, a neonate may show an increased activity level by traveling from one end of the crib to the other when placed down for a nap or by consistently wriggling out of booties. Thomas and colleagues (1968) noted that features such as activity level, distractability, and persistence, which declared themselves early in life, carried on into later childhood and often played important roles in later behavior disorders.

Some behaviors of infancy appear to antedate later attention deficit disorder. These include jitteriness in the newborn period; irregular sleep patterns, colic, and feeding difficulties in early infancy; head banging, rocking, and teeth grinding in later infancy.

Family history should note the occurrence of hyperactivity in parents (when they were children) or in siblings. A parent's impulsive and distractable style of conversation may readily be apparent during the interview, even if increased motor activity is not.

Additional information should be sought as to nocturnal enuresis, sleep disturbance, heat intolerance, seizures, allergies, medications, recent streptococcal infections, and lead poisoning. Enuresis frequently accompanies hyperactivity, particularly when it occurs on a developmental-familial basis. Restless sleep, particularly when associated with snoring, suggests an obstructive sleep apnea syndrome. Heat intolerance, weight loss (despite increased appetite), and a racing heart should suggest hyperthyroidism in the hyperactive and easily distracted child. A history of seizures of temporal lobe origin—for example, manifested by staring spells—should be inquired about. Allergies to environmental agents and food substances should be sought. Among medications, phenobarbital and antihistamines have been associated with hyperactivity. Recent streptococcal infection or past history of rheumatic fever might suggest Sydenham chorea. Past history of lead poisoning should also be sought.

Examination. The hyperactive child may be anything but that in a stimulus-poor, highly structured setting. The *general description* should note the motoric activity of the child, whether increased or not. Some children are able to sit calmly during the interview. Others fidget and have difficulty staying in their chairs. Still others manifest continuous, driven activity. They are out of the seat, under the desk, out the door, playing with the telephone, tugging at the window shade, opening and shutting drawers—in general, acting impulsively and often provocatively.

The *general physical examination* should include pulse rate and blood pressure, inspection and palpation of the thyroid gland, and recording of height, weight, and head circumference. Examination may disclose one or more minor somatic anomalies such as abnormal palmar skin creases and irregular ear shapes found with increased frequency among hyperactive children (Waldrop *et al.,* 1978). Their significance is unclear.

The *neurologic examination* should include careful visualization of the optic fundi to exclude papilledema. Hearing impairment should be noted. Lateralizing findings suggestive of focal brain injury and coordinative difficulties should be sought (Denckla and Rudel, 1978). Evidence for seizures should be looked for: characteristic birth marks on the skin, bitten tongue, staring spells provoked by 2 to 3 minutes of hyperventilation. Minor neurologic signs may include mirror movements (synkinesis) and choreic flickering of hands and fingers when arms are held outstretched with the eyes closed. The diagnostic usefulness of such signs appears to be limited (McMahon and Greenberg, 1977; Camp *et al.,* 1978).

Mental status examination should include description of the child's affect: for example, depressed, anxious, or unconcerned. Overexcitability may be manifested by silliness, giddiness, or tantrums. Attention and distractability can be evaluated by the child's recall of digits given 1 second apart, ability to count backward or to subtract serially three's or seven's from 20 or 100, ability to complete assigned tasks such as writing the numbers 1 through 100, printing the alphabet, or drawing a picture of a person. The child's reaction to ambient noise should be noted. For example, does he look out the window every time a car passes by?

Overall intelligence should be estimated. Reading ability should be determined. Impulsiveness and inattentiveness may be evident in reading by errors of word substitution, poor sound-blending, and difficulty in sounding out words of two or more syllables. Mental arithmetic will often be carried out rapidly and inaccurately.

Investigation. Investigation should not be considered routine in the child with an attention deficit disorder but, rather, should be individualized (see Table 14–2). When hyperthyroidism is considered, thyroid function studies should be obtained. If lead poisoning has occurred or is suspected, measurement of blood lead and erythrocyte protoporphyrin levels should be carried out. Antistreptolysin O (ASO) titer and serum ceruloplasmin level should be obtained when a movement disorder such as Sydenham chorea or Wilson disease is being considered.

TABLE 14–2. **Investigations to Be Considered in the Child with Attention Deficit Disorder**

Thyroid function tests
Blood lead level, free erythrocyte protoporphyrin (FEP)
Psychologic testing
EEG (in awake and sleep states)
EEG, special studies (nasopharyngeal recording; all-night recording)
ASO titer
X-rays of nasopharynx to assess obstruction
Auditory evoked responses
Cranial CT scan
Serum ceruloplasmin
Catecholamine metabolites in urine

Electroencephalography (to include waking and sleep studies and, as indicated, recording with nasopharyngeal leads) should be carried out when seizure disorder, particularly of temporal lobe origin, is under active consideration (see Chapter 12). An EEG is not routinely indicated in the evaluation of a hyperactive child. (Nonspecific slowing and other minor irregularities often found do not justify the use of anticonvulsant medication.) An all-night sleep study with monitoring of brain wave activity, respirations, and other functions should be carried out when sleep apnea is a possibility (see Chapter 9). Lateral radiographs of the pharynx will aid in assessment for adenoidal obstruction.

Cranial CT scan should be carried out if structural abnormality of brain or increased intracranial pressure is suspected. Measurement of urinary MHPG (3-methoxy-4-hydroxyphenylglycol) levels and other catecholamine metabolites are currently under investigation. They have not yet proved consistently useful in diagnosis or management (Shekim *et al.,* 1979; Khan and Dekirmenjian, 1981). Nor has the benefit of evoked potential studies in children with attentional problems yet been demonstrated for routine purposes.

Psychologic testing is often valuable in determining overall intelligence level and detecting frequently associated cognitive difficulties such as visual-motor dysfunction.

Differential Diagnosis (see Table 14–3). *Normal behavior* is sometimes misinterpreted as hyperactivity. The motor activity of normal 1½- to 3-year-old children is generally greater than that of children 5 to 7 years old. This increased activity, combined with age-appropriate striving for independence, may surprise and frustrate parents, who label the child "hyperactive."

Within an age group activity level does vary from one child to another. Children who are relatively more active than usual for age thus might be termed "overactive." This term (of limited use) does not connote a syndrome of attention deficit disorder or other behavior disorder.

Active, outgoing, and athletic ("*boyish*") *behavior* in a school-age girl may be misinterpreted as hyperactivity because it does not conform to stereotypes of how little girls should behave.

TABLE 14–3. **Differential Diagnosis of Attention Deficit Disorder**

Normal activity and behavior for age ("terrible twos")
"Boyish" activity in a girl
Tics
Dystonia or other extrapyramidal movement disorder
Conduct disorder

Tics, simple or complex, should be readily distinguishable from hyperactivity by their pattern of occurrence. *Dystonic movements* affecting the trunk or arms that cause the child to squirm in his seat can appear to be hyperactivity though without associated features of impulsivity, distractability, or excitability (see Chapter 13).

Attention deficit disorder should be distinguished from a *conduct disorder* of undersocialized aggressive type (*DSM* III, 1980). The two disorders frequently coexist.

Etiology. Causes of attention deficit disorder are summarized in Table 14–4. Most syndromes of attention deficit disorder occur on a constitutional-developmental basis, often with familial and genetic influences. These factors make up an organic substrate for a hyperkinetic syndrome, which is expressed as a result of physical, psychologic, and social stresses. Even though a child may be "born hyperactive," it is valuable from both the diagnostic and the therapeutic standpoints to identify factors that bring out or worsen the symptoms of attention deficit disorder. Other causes of hyperactivity and attentional problems will also be discussed in this section.

Medical Causes. *Hyperthyroidism* is associated with an increased rate of essentially all functions, including motor activity. Schoolwork may suffer because of diminished attention, and papers may be produced in uncharacteristically hasty and sloppy fashion (see Case 16–1). The onset of symptoms is often insidious, with behavioral and personality features prominent. Affected children tend to be irritable and difficult to live with. Appetite increases though weight remains stable or decreases. Sweating increases, and heat is tolerated poorly. Menstrual periods, if present, may become irregular. Excessive fatigue, particularly upon climbing stairs, is common.

Examination will show a variable array of signs: tachycardia, widened pulse pressure, exophthalmos, lid lag, enlarged thyroid gland, fine tremor, proximal muscle weakness, and hyperreflexia (see Fig. 14–1) (Vaidya *et al.,* 1974; Rosman, 1976). Diagnosis is suggested by the clinical picture and established by thyroid function tests.

A *sleep apnea syndrome* may be associated with hyperactivity, inattention, irritability, chronic fatigue, and daytime napping. These behaviors appear to result from chronic sleep deprivation due to respiratory obstruction or impairment of respiratory function on a central neurologic basis. Upper respiratory obstruction (due to excessive adenoidal tissue, for example) is suggested by fitful, restless sleep and snoring or other noisy breathing during sleep in addition to respiratory pauses of 30 to 60 seconds (see Chapter 9).

TABLE 14–4. **Causes of Attention Deficit Disorder**

Medical	Hyperthyroidism
	Sleep apnea syndrome
	Pinworms
	Intercurrent illness
Neurologic	Prematurity
	Congenital infection
	Difficult delivery
	Perinatal asphyxia
	Head trauma
	Encephalitis (particularly from *Herpes simplex*)
	Sydenham chorea
	Temporal lobe epilepsy
Toxic	Phenobarbital
	Antihistamines
	Lead
	Phenothiazines
	Alcohol *in utero*
	Food substances
Psychologic	Anxiety
	Depression
	Manic syndrome
Social-Environmental	Overstimulation
	Boredom
	Failure of limit-setting
	(?) Fluorescent lighting
Genetic-Constitutional	Familial pattern
	Temperament
Developmental	Relatively slower CNS maturation in males

The diagnosis of sleep apnea syndrome is suggested by disturbed night-time sleep combined with daytime hypersomnolence alternating with hyperkinesis. ENT consultation, radiologic studies, and polygraphic sleep studies will generally confirm or establish the diagnosis.

Pinworm infestation may be associated with fidgety, hyperactive behavior.

Intercurrent medical illness, such as chronic middle ear disease, may bring out or worsen hyperkinetic behavior problems (see Case 14–1).

Neurologic Causes. *Brain injury* is occasionally identifiable in the child with a hyperkinetic syndrome. It is suggested historically by such factors as extreme *prematurity, maternal infection during pregnancy* (with rubella, toxoplasmosis, or cytomegalovirus), *difficult delivery, perinatal asphyxia,*

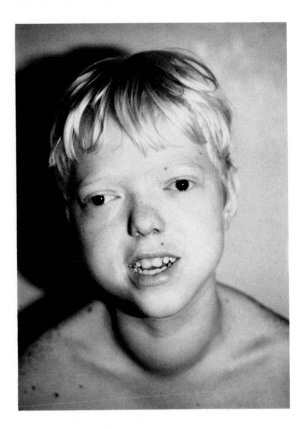

FIGURE 14–1. Hyperthyroidism with goiter in a schoolage boy.

head trauma, or *postnatal encephalitis* (e.g., with *Herpes simplex*). Microcephaly, abnormal patterns of deep tendon reflexes, and mental retardation may support the diagnosis of brain injury (see Case 14–2). Computerized tomographic scan should be considered if focal brain deficit is suggested by examination.

Sydenham chorea may present with hyperactivity (motor restlessness) and emotional lability (giddiness, silliness) of new onset in the school-age child. Antecedent streptococcal infection, rheumatic fever, or a choreic syndrome itself may have preceded the current motor disturbance. Examination characteristically will show choreiform movements, facial grimacing, "darting tongue," "milkmaid's grip," and a pronator sign (Aron *et al.,* 1965). Diagnosis is suggested by history of antecedent streptococcal infection, increase in anti-streptolysin O (ASO) antibody titer, and present or past evidence of acute rheumatic fever: migratory polyarthritis, erythema marginatum, subcutaneous nodules, or carditis.

Children with *seizure disorders* appear to have an increased incidence of hyperkinetic behavior beyond that which is caused or exacerbated by anticonvulsant medication such as phenobarbital. The association of hyperactivity particularly with seizures of complex partial type suggests that in some circumstances temporal lobe dysfunction may cause excessive electrical ac-

CASE 14–1: HYPERKINETIC SYNDROME EXACERBATED BY HEARING DEFICIT IN A 5-YEAR-OLD BOY

I.M. was evaluated because of hyperactivity and inattention. His mother remarked on the child's ability to "tune her out" and noted that he got along poorly with other children. Past history was of a 6 pound, 13 ounce product of a full-term uncomplicated pregnancy, delivered vaginally though a breech presentation. No neonatal depression occurred. As an infant he screamed a great deal and was described as colicky. Early development was normal. Neither seizures nor significant head trauma had occurred. His father, as a child, was recalled to have been similar to his son in temperament and behavior.

On recent hearing assessment, a 30–40 decibel hearing loss was found bilaterally, apparently due to middle ear effusions possibly linked with milk allergy.

On examination, the child was a well-formed youngster who appeared and acted immature. Head circumference (53 cm) was normal. Examination of the skin showed no neurocutaneous signs. Neurologic examination was normal except for mild conductive hearing deficit.

At the time of follow-up examination 2 months later, polyethylene tubes had been inserted in the middle ears. Mother reported that once the tubes were in place, the child interacted better with peers, played longer with his toys, and began a new activity: coloring. He was able to engage in conversation with his mother for the first time.

Comment. This case illustrates how a coexisting medical problem (in this case, hearing deficit secondary to middle ear effusion) can significantly worsen a hyperkinetic syndrome. It also demonstrates how attacking a primary problem directly made symptomatic treatment with psychoactive drugs unnecessary. It further illustrates that failure to pay attention may be the result of failure to hear.

tivity of brain (temporal lobe epilepsy) and increased motor activity (hyperkinesis) (Lindsay *et al.*, 1979) (see Case 14–3).

Toxic Causes. A significant proportion of children treated with phenobarbital on a long-term basis will manifest a hyperkinetic syndrome (Stores, 1975; Wolf and Forsythe, 1978). Hyperactivity *per se* only rarely necessitates discontinuation of phenobarbital; a change in medication is more often necessitated by irritability and lability of mood.

Lead poisoning (including asymptomatic plumbism) has been implicated in causing a hyperkinetic syndrome as well as lowered intelligence in some children (de la Burdé and Choate, 1972; Needleman *et al.*, 1979; Rutter, 1980).

Phenothiazines may produce a movement disorder, akathisia, in some children characterized by excessive activity ("ants in the pants"). Such movements should be distinguished from other extrapyramidal reactions as-

CASE 14–2: HYPERACTIVITY AND MENTAL RETARDATION IN AN 8-YEAR-OLD BOY

L.S. was the 6 pound, 13 ounce product of an uncomplicated full-term pregnancy. He was delivered after 22 hours of labor and had Apgar scores of 1 at one minute, 2 at two minutes, and 3 at three minutes. Head circumference at birth was 36.75 cm (75th percentile). At 1 day of age he had focal seizures and apneic spells. At 12 days his EEG was normal. Since his seizures had ceased, anticonvulsant medication (phenobarbital) was discontinued after 6 weeks. At 14 months he had several generalized convulsions with fever. He was placed on phenytoin and was seizure-free over the next 7 years, when anticonvulsant medication was discontinued. At 8 years, he was referred for pediatric neurologic consultation because of poor school performance, hyperactivity, and impulsive behavior.

On examination, the boy was an immature, talkative youngster in constant motion. He interrupted conversations and played distractedly with anything in sight or reach. Head circumference was 50.5 cm (10th percentile). He was left-handed and manifested posturing of the right arm while walking on heels or toes. Deep tendon reflexes were exaggerated in the legs, normal in the arms. He could repeat only two digits forward. Figure drawings were scored at the 5-year level. EEG showed excessive background slowing without paroxysmal activity. Psychologic testing showed an intelligence quotient of 57 on the Stanford-Binet. In addition to social and environmental measures, his treatment included dextroamphetamine, 5 mg twice daily. His behavior improved, particularly in his interactions with his mother, who previously had felt exhausted and frustrated by her child.

Comment. This case illustrates a syndrome of attention deficit disorder that does appear to be associated with brain damage. This child had several neonatal seizures following perinatal asphyxic insult, manifested a falloff in head growth (from the 75th percentile at birth to the 10th percentile at 8 years), and was left-handed in a family otherwise without left-handers. The last-mentioned suggests injury to the left cerebral hemisphere resulting in right cerebral dominance and "pathologic" left-handedness.

sociated with phenothiazine use. These include bradykinesia, dystonia, and tardive dyskinesia (see Chapter 13).

Alcohol exposure *in utero* has been implicated in determining later attention deficit syndromes in some children (Shaywitz *et al.*, 1980).

The role of food substances, artificial flavors, coloring agents, preservatives, and natural salicylates in producing hyperactivity in some children has been the subject of much concern and debate (Feingold, 1975; Wender, 1977; Bierman and Furukawa, 1978; Conners, 1980). Controlled studies have demonstrated inconsistent findings, although it appears that a small subgroup of hyperkinetic children will benefit from dietary manipulation (Con-

CASE 14–3: HYPERACTIVITY AND SEIZURE DISORDER IN A 5-YEAR-OLD BOY

I.F. was first evaluated at 3 years of age because of "mean behavior." He was considered to have a hyperkinetic syndrome and was treated with methylphenidate, 5 mg three times daily. Hyperactivity diminished, but his mood and "meanness" did not. An EEG was obtained. It was abnormal because of spike-and-slow-wave activity. Because of this result methylphenidate was discontinued and phenytoin begun, although the child had never been observed to have clinical seizures.

Confused about the switch in medication, the parents obtained a second neurologic opinion. It was felt that there was no reason for continuing anticonvulsant medication in this child without seizures, so phenytoin was discontinued over several days. A week later the child had a generalized convulsion lasting 30 seconds. He was placed on phenytoin once again, and seizures have not recurred.

Following a family move, the child was reevaluated because of continuing behavioral problems. Mother described her son's behavior as "nasty and destructive." Instead of saying "hello" to his friends, he hit or threw things at them. As a consequence he had no friends.

Past history was that the child weighed 7 pounds, 12 ounces at birth following an uncomplicated pregnancy and delivery. Mother smoked one pack of cigarettes per day. At 10 days of age, the child was hospitalized because of lethargy and was found to have otitis media and *E. coli* sepsis (without meningitis), treated with parenteral antibiotics. Subsequent development was normal, although mother felt he had been "on the go" since 18 months of age. Family history was negative for hyperactivity. A maternal aunt had epilepsy beginning in childhood.

On examination, the child was a well-formed, fidgety youngster of normal intelligence who settled down once his activity was structured. Head circumference (50 cm) was normal. A roughened patch of skin at the base of the spine suggested a shagreen patch. Adenoma sebaceum and hypopigmented macules were absent. Neurologic examination was normal.

Because of his continued hyperkinetic syndrome (attention deficit disor-

ners *et al.*, 1976; Mattes and Gittelman-Klein, 1978; Harley, Ray *et al.*, 1978; Harley, Matthews, and Eichman, 1978; Lipton *et al.*, 1979; Swanson and Kinsbourne, 1980; Weiss *et al.*, 1980; Mattes and Gittelman, 1981). The characteristics of this population remain to be defined.

Psychologic Causes. Affective disturbance can cause or contribute to hyperkinetic behavior and attentional problems. Fidgeting, restlessness, and inattention are often seen with anxiety. Difficulty in concentrating is a hallmark of depression. Dysphoric mood, a fundamental aspect of many depressive syndromes, occurs in many children with hyperkinetic syndromes. Certainly their academic problems and lack of social success contribute to

der), he was begun on dextroamphetamine; phenytoin was continued. Mother described the child as "a completely different person" on dextroamphetamine, which was maintained at $7\frac{1}{2}$ mg in the morning, 5 mg at midday, and $2\frac{1}{2}$ mg in the afternoon. He was much better able to play with siblings and friends, and he appeared happier.

Comment. This case illustrates several points regarding hyperkinetic syndromes and the confusion that may result from the use of electroencephalography.

The diagnosis of attention deficit disorder in this case was based upon the child's activity level, impulsive behavior, and dysphoria. Inattention was not a prominent symptom. The etiology of the hyperkinetic syndrome was not clear. Cigarette smoking has been implicated in causing or contributing to hyperactivity, but a major influence in this case was probably neonatal sepsis (which was not, however, associated with meningitis). The apparent shagreen patch combined with the seizure disorder raised the possibility of tuberous sclerosis (see Chapter 12). He clearly did not manifest tuberous sclerosis in its classical form, however, but may have a forme fruste of the disorder.

This case shows further how a different dosage of medication can be used depending on the time of administration. Midday and afternoon doses will often be less than the morning dose in order to minimize interference with sleep. Many children actually have less trouble getting to sleep after a small afternoon dose of medication than on no medication at all, as it seems to help prevent the extreme disorganization that some hyperkinetic children manifest around bedtime.

The decision as to whether to obtain an electroencephalogram on a hyperkinetic child is a matter of judgment. It is not valuable on a routine basis but should be obtained in the child with known or suspected seizures. In this case the electroencephalogram created more confusion than clarification at first. Eventually the seizure disorder declared itself unequivocally and the child proved to benefit from both anticonvulsant and "stimulant" medication.

secondary, or reactive, depression. It has been suggested that in addition a primary depressive component (presumably biochemically mediated) is present (Wender, 1971).

Unipolar or bipolar affective disorders with manic episodes or even recognizable manic-depressive cycles may present with hyperkinetic and aggressive behavior (see Chapter 6) (see Case 14–4).

Social-Environmental Causes. A noisy, disorganized home environment with televisions, radios, and tape recorders blaring continuously, siblings trooping in noisily with their friends, and parents unavailable for assistance or support will interfere with the quality and quantity of schoolwork accomplished at home. Likewise, a work area cluttered with model airplanes and baseball cards provides ready distraction for any child, particularly one with an attentional problem.

Within the classroom the child whose intelligence is either unusually high or low may have attentional difficulties. The dull child cannot keep up with assigned tasks and becomes inattentive. The bright child finds the work too easy and becomes bored. In either instance, daydreaming and fidgeting may ensue.

The hyperactivity of some children appears to be "needed" by certain depressed parents who derive benefit from the constant stimulation provided by the child, which serves to drive away painful thoughts. This situation is reminiscent of "superego lacunae" in some children that result from unconscious parental sanction of acting-out behavior. Problems in limit-setting and a resulant hyperkinetic syndrome may also stem from a child's recovery from an earlier life-threatening illness (Green and Solnit, 1964; Benjamin, 1978).

The role of fluorescent light in causing or contributing to hyperactive behavior is under investigation (Mayron, 1978).

Genetic-Constitutional Causes.   That boys with attention deficit disorder far outnumber similarly affected girls by a five- to tenfold ratio has been attributed to the slower rate of central nervous system maturation in boys.

Hyperkinesis appears to run in families and to follow a polygenic mode of inheritance (Morrison and Stewart, 1973). Some 10 per cent of hyperactive children will have a parent who was hyperactive in childhood.

The importance of constitutional factors in behavior disorders of childhood has been emphasized by Thomas and colleagues (1968). They found temperamental features such as activity level and reaction to environmental change to characterize a child's behavior from earliest life, to serve as the basis for personality development, and to play a role in later behavior problems.

Developmental Causes.   This category encompasses most cases of hyperactivity and attention deficit disorder. The problem is considered developmental not because the child is certain to outgrow it eventually but because the abnormal behavior is, in most respects, consistent with development that is normal at an earlier age (Werry, 1968; Routh *et al.*, 1974; Levy, 1980). A hyperactive 9-year-old boy of normal intelligence thus may act like a 4-year-old in terms of activity level and impulse control. The different rate of neurologic maturation in boys and girls was mentioned above as contributing to the greater frequency of attention deficit disorder in boys (see Case 14–5).

TREATMENT AND OUTCOME

Although drug therapy is often an essential part of the management of attention deficit disorder, it must not be the sole focus of therapeutic attention. As presented above, the usual child with an attention deficit disorder has an organically based capability of manifesting a hyperkinetic syndrome. Such behavior is potentiated by stress, which may result from a variety of factors. A plan of therapy then will be based not only upon fundamental causes of the

CASE 14–4: ATTENTION DEFICIT DISORDER WITH FEATURES OF MANIC SYNDROME IN A 12-YEAR-OLD BOY

A.L. was referred for neurologic evaluation because of "erratic and impulsive behavior," according to his father. Hyperactivity and diminished attention had been noted since 2 years of age. At 9 years, the child was placed on dextroamphetamine, $2\frac{1}{2}$ mg twice daily, for 2 weeks without beneficial effect. Recent behavior was marked by provocativeness, impulsivity, and overexcitability with rapid escalation to temper tantrums. Schoolwork continued to be satisfactory.

History of pregnancy, delivery, and early milestones was unremarkable. Family history was noteworthy for mother's "hyperactivity" in childhood and depressive illness in adulthood, treated effectively with imipramine and psychotherapy. The paternal grandmother had been treated with lithium for behavioral changes of adult onset.

On examination, the child was an intelligent, articulate boy whose only abnormal findings were symmetrically exaggerated deep tendon reflexes. Plantar responses were flexor. Optic disks showed no elevation. Investigation included normal serum calcium and thyroxine levels.

Because of the child's apparent attention deficit disorder, he was begun on methylphenidate. This medication was of no benefit despite doses that reached 20 mg twice daily. Dextroamphetamine was equally ineffective, and imipramine was employed in low dosage (25 mg at bedtime). Behavior was improved for 5 months. Then agitation, impulsivity, and hyperactivity increased to reach a new baseline level worsened by episodes of attacking and self-injurious behavior. Examination showed a resting pulse rate of 100/minute, pressured speech, and hyperreflexia. Because of the possible effect of imipramine in contributing to behavioral deterioration, it was discontinued. Therapy with lithium carbonate was begun 2 weeks later. It was discontinued several weeks later while still at a subtherapeutic level because of comprehensive reevaluation to be undertaken while the child was on no medication.

Comment. This child's attention deficit disorder was manifested by extreme impulsivity, overexcitability, and hyperactivity. Prior treatment with dextroamphetamine appeared to be without benefit, but the dosage employed was so low that the child could not be considered to have had an adequate trial. Subsequent attempts at pharmacotherapy (combined with regular individual and family psychotherapy) demonstrated that neither dextroamphetamine nor methylphenidate were helpful. Imipramine seemed beneficial for a while, until behavior worsened to reach a chronic hypomanic state. Possible causes for this deterioration included hyperthyroidism (excluded by previous blood tests, which were nonetheless repeated and again proved to be normal), tricyclic drug toxicity, and hypomanic state. Treatment with lithium was begun in view of manic symptoms (including prominent aggressive behavior) and the family history of a relative who had responded positively to lithium treatment.

CASE 14–5: ATTENTION DEFICIT DISORDER ON A DEVELOPMENTAL-MATURATIONAL BASIS IN A 6-YEAR-OLD BOY

K.A. was brought for neurologic evaluation by his mother because of "aggressive, unmanageable, wild, impulsive, and obnoxious behavior." He fought constantly with his sister, could not maintain any friendships, and could not be brought shopping with his mother. He was described otherwise as highly intelligent and capable of being "totally adorable."

Hyperactive behavior was noted at 9 months when he began walking. By 18 months, his mother recalled him to be "uncontrollable." He touched things he should not, did not listen, and did not respond to the word "no." Recognizing the potential for child abuse, mother referred herself to a protective services unit and met regularly with a unit social worker.

History of pregnancy and delivery was unremarkable. As a neonate, the child had been unusually active and startled excessively to noise. Development was normal to accelerated. Nocturnal enuresis occurred occasionally. Family history was negative for hyperactivity or attentional problems.

On examination, the child was a well-formed, intelligent youngster whose behavior was disruptive, annoying, and provocative. He spun himself in a chair, pounded his mother with a toy hammer, and interrupted conversation. When firm limits were provided, he quieted down and remained manageable for nearly 45 minutes, after which behavior deteriorated seriously. General physical and neurologic examinations were normal. Speech was immature. Digit span was three forward.

His response to medication was striking. On a dosage of 7.5 mg of methylphenidate in the morning and 5 mg at noon, he was able to accompany his mother shopping for the first time, and he experienced new and unaccustomed successes in making friends. In addition, enuresis diminished. Medication was continued on weekends in order to avoid a "yo-yo" (rebound behavioral) effect.

Comment. This child was in trouble. As recognized by his mother, he was at great risk for physical abuse because of his wild and provocative behavior. He seemed never to have left the "terrible twos." In addition, he was failing socially, making friends with great difficulty and not able to keep them.

Pharmacologic treatment was the cornerstone of therapy in this case. Child guidance counseling continued, and mother further sought out and applied information on behavior management she learned from books on hyperactivity. She was also eager to meet with other parents of hyperactive children to share their experiences in a group setting.

In this child a third daily dose of methylphenidate was considered but withheld, because his behavior was relatively acceptable later in the day and he had no significant difficulties in getting to bed.

TABLE 14–5. **Treatment of Hyperactivity and Attentional Disorders**

Medical	Symptomatic pharmacotherapy (see Table 14–6)
	Treatment of underlying or contributing medical illness: hyperthyroidism, lead poisoning, Sydenham chorea, seizure disorder
Neurologic	See MEDICAL TREATMENT
Surgical	Adenoidectomy, tracheostomy with nighttime mechanical ventilation for sleep apnea
	Stereotaxic amygdalotomy for refractory epileptic hyperactivity
Psychologic	Treatment of depression, anxiety
	Explanation to the child
	Parental counseling
	Behavior modification
Social-Environmental	Quiet environment
	Stimulus-poor area for doing homework
	Scheduled activities
	Time off for parents
Educational	Remediation for associated learning problems
	Preferential seating arrangements
	Four-walled classroom
	Small teacher-to-student ratio
Physical	Adaptive physical education
	Encouraging of athletic abilities

behavioral syndrome, but also on those activities and experiences that bring out the maladaptive behavior (see Table 14–5).

The outcome in hyperkinetic children, treated or untreated, remains somewhat unclear. As the child attains and passes through adolescence, hyperactivity *per se* tends to diminish (Menkes *et al.*, 1967). Despite this change, problems remain. Attention continues to be impaired, academic performance is poor, self-esteem remains low, and behavioral problems persist (Minde *et al.*, 1972; Hoy *et al.*, 1978; Wender *et al.*, 1981). On the other hand, one study of hyperactive adults found them to fare as well as persons without hyperactivity when evaluated by their employers (Weiss *et al.*, 1978). A hyperkinetic behavior disorder in childhood appears to be associated in later life with an increased risk of developing a sociopathic personality disorder or alcoholism (Cantwell, 1972; Kinsbourne and Caplan, 1979).

It is clear, however, that many bright, quick-witted, verbal, and successful adults, representing virtually all professions, manifested attention deficit disorders as children and compensated for these problems so that the need for evaluation never arose.

Medical Management.   Treatment with drugs such as dextroamphetamine (Dexedrine), methylphenidate (Ritalin), or pemoline (Cylert) for attention deficit disorder will depend upon the degree of impairment in academic, social, or other spheres of activity and the response to nonpharmacologic measures. Hyperactivity itself does not automatically justify the use of psychoactive drugs. They should be employed only after serious, not superficial, consideration—not in routine or "knee-jerk" fashion when the diagnosis of hyperkinetic syndrome or attention deficit disorder has been made.

Who will benefit from pharmacotherapy is a key question. Formal office examination often is not useful in that regard, since hyperactive children frequently function in a correct and composed manner in this setting. This response in itself suggests that environmental measures can have a beneficial effect. Nor have laboratory investigations been very helpful in predicting favorable response to medication. Electroencephalography, cortical evoked potentials, pupillography, and measurement of catecholamine metabolites in urine and cerebrospinal fluid have been employed with variable results in the assessment of central nervous system arousal, responsiveness, and maturity in hyperactive children. The further refinement of such investigations is expected to provide important diagnostic and therapeutic information in such cases.

Information obtained from parents and teachers is generally the cornerstone upon which is placed the decision to treat or not to treat with medication. The Conners Abbreviated Symptom Questionnaire can be valuable in assessing the child with an attention deficit disorder. Its usefulness is enhanced when responses are obtained from both parents and classroom teachers (Kinsbourne and Caplan, 1979).

The ten items on the scale are as follows:

1. Restless or overactive, excitable, impulsive
2. Disturbs other children
3. Fails to finish things started
4. Short attention span
5. Constantly fidgeting
6. Inattentive, easily distracted
7. Demands must be met immediately, easily frustrated
8. Cries often and easily
9. Mood changes quickly and drastically
10. Temper outbursts, explosive and unpredictable behavior

The items are graded on a scale of 0 through 3: "not at all," "just a little," "pretty much," or "very much," respectively.

Kinsbourne and Caplan (1979) have found that children who score 15 points or more on the scale according to both parents and teachers almost always respond favorably to pharmacotherapy with "stimulant medication." This scale (or some other relatively objective measure) can also be employed in evaluating the response of hyperactive children to treatment.

The pharmacotherapy of attention deficit disorder is summarized in Table 14–6. Dextroamphetamine (Dexedrine) and methylphenidate (Ritalin) are

TABLE 14–6. **Pharmacologic Treatment of Hyperactivity and Attentional Disorders**

Drug	Initial Dosage	Usual Therapeutic Dosage
Dextroamphetamine (Dexedrine)	2.5 mg 2–3 times daily	1 mg/kg/day
Methylphenidate (Ritalin)	5 mg 2–3 times daily	0.3–2 mg/kg/day
Pemoline (Cylert)	18.75 mg each morning	75 mg/day (in single dose)
Imipramine (Tofranil)	10 mg 2 times daily	20–100 mg/day
Chlorpromazine (Thorazine)	10 mg 2 times daily	20–120 mg/day (0.5–2.0 mg/kg/day)
Thioridazine (Mellaril)	10 mg 2 times daily	20–60 mg/day (0.5–1.0 mg/kg/day)
Lithium carbonate (Eskalith)	150 mg 3 times daily	450–1,200 mg/day
Caffeine	50 mg 2 times daily	150–200 mg/day

the medications of choice in the drug treatment of attention deficit disorder affecting children 6 years of age and older. Dextroamphetamine is available in scored tablets containing 5 or 10 mg. An elixir containing 1 mg per ml is also available as are sustained-release capsules. Methylphenidate comes in 5, 10, and 20 mg scored tablets.

Medication is begun only.after the parents and child have understood the reason for its use and its possible side effects (see Table 14–7). Anorexia or sleep disturbance is usually transient, lasting several days to a week. Weepiness, irritability, anxiety, depression, hallucination, or development of involuntary movements usually indicate overdosage or idiosyncratic effect.

The choice of dextroamphetamine versus methylphenidate is an individ-

TABLE 14–7. **Side Effects of CNS Sympathomimetic Drugs**

Anorexia Insomnia Stomach ache Headache	Relatively common, usually transient; generally does not necessitate discontinuation of drug
Irritability Excessive sensitivity Depression Tremor and tics	Relatively common, often transient; may necessitate discontinuation of drug
Tachycardia Mild hypertension	Not uncommon, often persistent; clinical significance unclear
Involuntary movements Psychosis	Infrequent; necessitates reduction in or discontinuation of drug
Suppression of growth, especially weight	Of uncertain frequency; probably only occasionally clinically significant

ual matter. Dextroamphetamine is considered likelier than methylphenidate to cause disturbances in appetite and sleep, though the difference is not felt to be great (Cantwell, 1977). A disadvantage to the use of methylphenidate is that, unlike dextroamphetamine, it is vulnerable to destruction by gastric juices. Hence it should be taken at least a half-hour before meals, not with meals or soon thereafter (Kinsbourne and Caplan, 1979).

The initial dosage should be small: 2.5 mg of dextroamphetamine or 5 mg of methylphenidate. Onset of action is $\frac{1}{2}$ to 1 hour after administration, and peak effect occurs between 2 and 3 hours following ingestion. Usually little or no effect remains by 4 hours even if a sustained-release preparation of dextroamphetamine is taken (Brown et al., 1980). Twice-daily administration of the drug is necessary for effectiveness throughout the school day, three times a day for coverage that includes the late afternoon and early evening. The last dose should be given no later than 4:00 P.M. to minimize interference with sleep. This dose may be smaller than the previous two.

If neither beneficial effect nor adverse response is evident after 3 or 4 days at a given dosage level, the amount of medication can be increased gradually: from 2.5 to 5 mg of dextroamphetamine; 5 to 7.5 or 10 mg of methylphenidate. The decision to increase medication usually can be made on the basis of telephone contact between family and physician. Subsequent adjustments can be made as indicated by 2.5 to 5 mg increments for dextroamphetamine and 5 to 10 mg for methylphenidate. Maximum individual doses are generally around 30 mg for dextroamphetamine (approximately 1 mg per kg per day) and 60 mg for methylphenidate (approximately 2 mg per kg per day).

These maximum doses should be approached with the work of Sprague and Sleator (1977) and Brown and Sleator (1979) in mind. They found that for both learning and impulsivity, a methylphenidate dosage of 0.3 mg per kg was superior to placebo or to a dosage of 1 mg per kg, even though the higher methylphenidate dose was associated with reduced activity level. On the other hand, Charles and colleagues (1981) did not find differences in optimal dosage levels of methylphenidate for behavior and cognitive performance.

Once a therapeutic dosage has been reached, it should be maintained for several days to weeks and then cautiously increased by a small amount to see if additional gains can be made.

Improvement can be seen in several ways (Lerer et al., 1977; Swanson et al., 1978; Charles et al., 1979). Classroom assignments may be completed during school hours. Accuracy and neatness may be enhanced. Fidgetiness and disruptive behavior may be diminished. Nighttime sleep may be less fitful. Concentration may be obviously improved. One mother described her 12-year-old son as being able to help her wash and dry dishes for the first time.

Whether medication should be taken two or three times daily, on weekends as well as weekdays, will depend upon the child and individual circumstances. Twice-daily administration is sufficient if the child's problems are confined to school. If, on the other hand, impulsivity and excitability are associated with constant fighting, inability to make friends, difficulty in getting along with family members, and battles in going to sleep, then a third dose of medication should be considered. As indicated above, this third dose need not be in the same amount as earlier in the day. A third dose may diminish rebound behavioral effects and enhance learning during evening study.

These same principles hold true for medication on weekends and during brief school holidays. During summer vacation the child should probably be given a 1- to 2-week "drug holiday" to test the need for continued medication. If no change in behavior is seen, then increase in dosage or discontinuation of the drug should be considered.

Height, weight, pulse rate, and blood pressure should be checked every 3 months or so while the child is on medication because of monoaminergic effects upon the cardiovascular system and because of issues raised (but not settled as yet) as to possible growth suppression. Some blunting of weight gain and height acquisition has been noted with use of these medications, but a return to previous growth curves generally occurs when medication is discontinued (Safer et al., 1972; Gross, 1976; Roche et al., 1979).

The duration of therapy is another matter of importance. As noted earlier, hyperactivity—a prominent symptom during elementary school years—normally diminishes as the child approaches and enters adolescence. Distractability and impulsiveness typically remain, however, often interfering significantly with academic and social performance. For that reason medication use should be considered in individual cases into adolescence and young adulthood, although the long-term consequences of such drug use are not known (Wender et al., 1981). It is known, however, that medication such as dextroamphetamine or methylphenidate used within a medical context are not addicting, do not produce a "high," are not associated with habituation, and do not appear to lead to later drug abuse (Beck et al., 1975).

Studies of cognitive and behavioral effects of dextroamphetamine on non-hyperactive prepubertal boys of above-average intelligence have shed further light on the role of medication in treatment and the pathophysiologic basis of attention deficit disorders. In a double-blind investigation, Rapoport and colleagues (1978) found that dextroamphetamine produced a marked decrease in motor activity and improved performance on cognitive testing. These results demonstrate that beneficial effects of "stimulant" medication do not define the child as hyperactive and that a therapeutic response should not be considered a paradoxical effect.

Other medications that have been employed in the treatment of hyperkinetic syndromes are magnesium pemoline (Cylert), phenothiazines, imipramine (Werry et al., 1980), lithium (DeLong, 1978), and caffeine (Firestone et al., 1978). Kinsbourne and Caplan (1979) found that pemoline may have a longer duration of action in some children than dextroamphetamine or methylphenidate. It is given usually as a single morning dose, initially 18.75 mg, which can be raised incrementally as needed to 75 mg. Like dextroamphetamine and methylphenidate, there is evidence to suggest that pemoline may interfere with growth (Dickinson et al., 1979).

Thioridazine (Mellaril), chlorpromazine (Thorazine), and haloperidol (Haldol) may be of value in hyperkinetic children, especially those less than 3 years of age, in whom dextroamphetamine and methylphenidate are usually ineffective. Thioridazine may also be of benefit in mentally retarded hyperactive children who have not responded well to dextroamphetamine or methylphenidate. It is generally used in a daily dosage of 20 to 60 mg (0.5–1.0 mg per kg per day). Imipramine (Tofranil) has been found effective in some children with hyperactivity (Werry *et al.*, 1980). Possible serious effects of overdosage such as cardiac arrhythmia should be kept in mind when imipramine use is being considered (see Case 10–6). Lithium has benefited some children whose syndrome of hyperkinesis and aggressive behavior suggests manic disorder (DeLong, 1978) (see Case 15–4).

The results of caffeine use in children with attention deficit disorder have been inconclusive, although it may benefit some (Firestone *et al.*, 1978; Elkins *et al.*, 1981). Harvey and Marsh (1978) found that one cup of coffee (containing 100 mg of caffeine) consumed at breakfast and another upon returning home from school helped some children with behavioral problems.

When underlying medical illness causes a hyperkinetic syndrome, specific therapy should be given. For example, with hyperthyroidism, the overactive thyroid gland can be treated with propylthiouracil, radioactive iodine, or surgery. Lead poisoning is treated with chelating agents (calcium EDTA, BAL, or penicillamine) and removal from the leaded environment. The involuntary movements of Sydenham chorea can be treated with chlorpromazine (Thorazine) or haloperidol (Haldol). If other major clinical manifestations of rheumatic fever are present, treatment may include penicillin, anti-inflammatory agents (aspirin, corticosteroids), and occasionally digitalis. Chorea may last from 1 month to several years and may recur.

Anticonvulsant medication is employed in children with absence spells or other seizures that interrupt consciousness and interfere with attention. Ethosuximide (Zarontin) or valproic acid (Depakene) can be used for such episodes. Complex partial or major motor seizures can be treated with drugs such as phenytoin (Dilantin) or carbamazepine (Tegretol). Phenobarbital should generally be avoided, because it can cause or contribute to hyperactivity (see Chapter 12).

In the hyperactive child without clinical seizure activity who nonetheless shows spike discharges or other paroxysmal activity on electroencephalogram, anticonvulsant medication may be tried. Only a minority of such cases are benefited, however. If significant improvement does not result, dextroamphetamine or methylphenidate can be added or substituted.

Neurologic Management.   The use of dextroamphetamine, methylphenidate, and other psychoactive medicines is presented in MEDICAL MANAGEMENT above.

Surgical Management.   Sleep apnea associated with adenoidal obstruction may be dramatically cured by adenoidectomy. Sleep apnea of central origin may require a tracheostomy and even nighttime mechanical ventilation (see Chapter 9).

Neurosurgery has benefited some children with intractible hyperactivity (Narabayashi, 1977). Such surgery has involved stereotaxic amygdalotomy. It should be considered only in extreme circumstances when all other more conservative approaches have failed.

Psychotherapy.   Psychotherapy is a valuable adjunct to other modes of therapy (Satterfield *et al.*, 1981). Discussion with parents should explain the nature of attention deficit disorder and the multifaceted approach to therapy that is usually most effective. The analogy of a 6-year-old hyperactive child acting like a 2-year-old provides a vivid picture of the child's behavior in a developmental context. When the child has an attention deficit disorder without hyperactivity, it will be important to indicate to the parents that attentional problems and impulsivity are the target symptoms rather than hyperkinesis.

If medication is part of the treatment plan, discussion with the child should clarify his or her understanding as to why it is being given. Responsibility for behavior cannot be disavowed because of attention deficit disorder, nor can the child look to medication as the answer to all behavior problems. Rather the child should understand that medication is given in order to assist in behavior, to give him increased control over his behavior, and to help him sort out different choices in academic and social situations so that the first possibility (right or wrong) is not always the one acted upon.

Counseling for parents is essential, as their approach to the child requires understanding, cooperation, and establishment of firm, consistent, and predictable limits. The destructive, provocative, and frustrating behavior of many hyperactive children very frequently makes anticipatory counseling about the prevention of inflicted injury worthwhile.

Behavior modification therapy will often benefit the hyperactive child (Christensen and Sprague, 1973; Wolraich *et al.*, 1978; Bidder *et al.*, 1978; O'Leary and Pelham, 1978). A desired behavior is identified (for example, eating with fork rather than fingers; not fighting with a younger sister; picking up in one's room), and successful performance is recorded daily on a calendar chart. Tokens earned in this manner are "cashed in" on a daily or weekly basis. A token system should give way to praise as reinforcement, ultimately with self-praise becoming the usual reward.

Undesired behavior (such as temper tantrum or swearing) can be dealt with by ignoring it insofar as possible or, if appropriate, placing the child in an *ad hoc* isolation (quiet or "time-out") room. This room should not be viewed as a padded cell. Rather, it is an area identified beforehand where the child knows he or she will be sent (or brought) and will remain until self-control is regained (Wender and Wender, 1978).

Social-Environmental Management. The hyperactive child should have an unstimulating space to retreat to when overstimulation is a problem or homework needs to be completed. The room should be quiet—without radio, television, or record player nearby. The desk should be well lighted and cleared of distracting debris such as half-completed models, jigsaw puzzles, or comic books. Wallpaper and wall hangings should be of simple design and subdued hue rather than of dazzling colors, engaging patterns, or flying superheroes.

A daily or weekly schedule can be used to let the hyperactive child know what is expected of him or her. Constructed with the child's participation, it should contain events and times. The schedule might also include regular household responsibilities, time set aside for homework, bedtime, and selected television programs. Such a schedule will often help the child make transitions from one activity to another without surprises or confrontations that lead to tantrums. Such a chart can also be used as a part of a behavioral program to record successful behavior.

Getting the attention of the hyperactive child (and keeping it long enough to get a message across) can be a problem. For that reason, gently holding the child by the shoulders or head in order to establish eye contact prior to speaking may prove useful.

An important adjunct to social-environmental management is "time off" for the parents, particularly the mother, who is often subjected to chronic stresses that render a sustained patient and understanding approach to the child virtually impossible (Schmitt, 1977).

Educational Management.   The many benefits of one-to-one interaction between the hyperactive child and his or her teacher are widely recognized. Though this ratio is rarely attainable for an entire school day, the child should receive as much individualized educational input as possible. Otherwise, small student-to-teacher ratios are beneficial. Sitting near the teacher to minimize distraction and increase supervision may be additionally helpful.

Seating arrangements in which children face each other in square or circular arrays are to be avoided, for they allow for more distraction than conventional rows facing forward. Likewise, the traditional four-walled, enclosed classroom provides structure and limits distraction for many inattentive children.

Since specific learning disabilities are frequently found among children with attention deficit disorders, they should be sought and included with the child's individualized educational plan (see Chapter 17).

The importance of clear and ongoing communication between the child, parent, teacher, physician, and psychiatrist or psychologist cannot be overemphasized. Though parents are the ultimate "signal-callers," major input as to treatment choices should be made available to them by the professionals working with their child.

Physical Therapy.   Clumsiness and poor motor planning may be reasons for teasing and embarrassment of some hyperactive children. For that reason adaptive physical education should be considered as part of the child's overall educational plan.

If the child is physically gifted, for example, fleet of foot (as many hyperactive children are), then such ability should be encouraged. Athletics offers a socially acceptable mode of expression for the child's high level of motor activity and an opportunity to build self-esteem and learn how to get along better with peers.

CORRELATION

Anatomic Aspects.   Attention requires alertness, which is a state of consciousness mediated through the reticular activating system. It "lights up" the cerebral cortex. The reticular activating system, involved in both sleeping and waking, originates within the core of the brainstem and extends from the medulla through the pons and midbrain to the hypothalamus (see Chapter 9).

The reticular activating system does not merely "broadcast." It receives input from above and below within the central nervous system. The cerebral cortex sends down visual, auditory, and affective information. The spinal cord sends along tactile, thermal, and proprioceptive data, so that the physical state of the body has an ongoing influence upon behavior. Arousal is thus maintained through the interaction and mutual stimulation of the reticular activating system, cerebral cortex, and spinal cord.

Norepinephrine, a neurotransmitter closely identified with the reticular activating system, is produced within the central nervous system in two major cell clusters in the pons: the locus coeruleus and the lateral tegmental neurons. The locus coeruleus consists of pigmented neurons located caudally within the pontine gray matter. Its major connections include the cerebral cortex, hypothalamus, and spinal cord. The lateral tegmental neurons, more loosely arrayed than those of the locus coeruleus, lie further from the midline. These neurons appear to send fibers to limbic structures including the amygdaloid nuclei (Cooper *et al.*, 1978).

Although importantly involved in arousal, norepinephrine pathways to the hippocampus and cerebral cortex have generally been demonstrated in experimental situations to have inhibitory effects upon spontaneous discharge of these structures (Cooper *et al.*, 1978). In this way norepinephrine is thought to play a role in attention, enabling one to focus as well as to exclude selectively.

Biochemical Aspects. A catecholamine is an organic compound that consists of a catechol and an amine group. In general use, catecholamine refers to dopamine, norepinephrine, or epinephrine. Similar in structure but not strictly catecholamines are phenylethylamine (contained in chocolate), phenylpropanolamine (included in many "cold" medicines and decongestants), tyramine (found in marinated herring, chopped liver, and other foods), ephedrine, and amphetamine (see Fig. 14–2). This last group of compounds differs from catecholamines in that they are effective by the oral route.

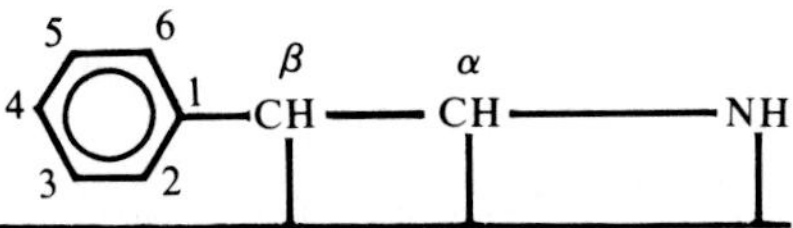

		β	α	
Phenylethylamine		H	H	H
Epinephrine	3-OH,4-OH	OH	H	CH$_3$
Norepinephrine	3-OH,4-OH	OH	H	H
Dopamine	3-OH,4-OH	H	H	H
Tyramine	4-OH	H	H	H
Amphetamine		H	CH$_3$	H
Methamphetamine		H	CH$_3$	CH$_3$
Ephedrine		OH	CH$_3$	CH$_3$
Phenylpropanolamine		OH	CH$_3$	H

FIGURE 14–2. Structural formulas of monoamines, amphetamines, and closely related drugs.

Amphetamine lacks the hydroxyl groups that would make it a catechol. Amphetamine (Benzedrine) was used by Bradley (1937) in his initial pharmacologic trials involving children with behavior disorders. It consists of a racemic mixture of dextro and levo forms of the molecule. The dextro isomer (dextroamphetamine) is three to four times as potent as the levo form (Weiner, 1980). Dextroamphetamine sulfate (Dexedrine) is the amphetamine preparation most commonly employed in the treatment of attention deficit disorder. Methylphenidate, another noncatechol, is not an amphetamine either but is structurally related to this group of compounds.

Amphetamines, methylphenidate, and imipramine appear to act primarily by blocking reuptake of norepinephrine (and dopamine) at the presynaptic membrane. Since reuptake is the major mode of inactivation of monoaminergic neurotransmitter, blockage of reuptake allows more catecholamine to be available to act postsynaptically. To a lesser degree amphetamines also act by promoting release of neurotransmitter (Cooper *et al.*, 1978).

Dopamine has also been implicated as playing a significant role in hyperkinesis in clinical and experimental studies. Levels of homovanillic acid, a principal metabolite of dopamine, were found to be diminished in the cerebrospinal fluid of a group of hyperkinetic boys as compared with a control group (Shaywitz *et al.*, 1977). Furthermore, an animal model for hyperactivity has been developed in rat pups by producing a state of dopamine depletion (Shaywitz *et al.*, 1978). Studies in progress should clarify further the role of dopamine in attention deficit disorders.

Physiologic Aspects.   Kinsbourne (1977) has proposed a model for problem-solving that incorporates many features of the abnormal behavior seen in children with attentional disorders. The major steps involved are activation, selection, and processing.

In normal circumstances recognition of a problem leads to *activation,* a generalized state of arousal mediated by the reticular activating system (see Fig. 14–3). This state is superseded by a more specific, focused state through the process of *selection.* Selection involves the channeling and fil-

PROCESSORS

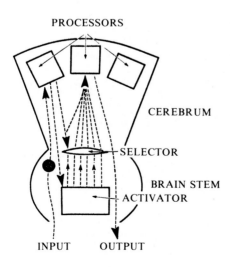

CEREBRUM

SELECTOR

BRAIN STEM

ACTIVATOR

INPUT   OUTPUT

FIGURE 14–3. Schematic representation showing relationship of activator, selector, and processors. (Reprinted by permission from Figure 2, page 301, in *Topics in Child Neurology* by Michael E. Blaw, Isabelle Rapin, and Marcel Kinsbourne [eds.] Copyright 1977, Spectrum Publications, Inc., New York.)

tering of information relevant to the task at hand to appropriate cerebral processing mechanisms. The selection process includes not only the onward routing of relevant information but the exclusion of data found not to be pertinent. *Processing* can then occur to allow for decision-making as to how the problem can best be solved. The result is a behavioral output, for example, a symbol written on a piece of paper or a change in body position.

Interference with this process of problem-solving can occur at any step along the way from activation to selection to processing. The result will usually be either too much or too little information. Too much information can result from inadequate filtering of information or from an excessive amount of time devoted to the processing of a single problem. The consequence can be confusion (the result of stimulus overload) or stereotyped behavior (which might include obsessional thinking). Too little information can result from orientation to a new problem before adequate information needed for decision-making has been channeled forward, from random or faulty choice of cerebral processor, or from lack of time spent in processing itself. The result will be faulty decision-making.

With this model in mind, one can view the child with an attention deficit disorder as maintaining a relatively steady level of ongoing stimulation by changing focus and position frequently rather than by organizing and otherwise reworking information at hand. The result is a vicious cycle in which the hyperkinetic syndrome (or other attentional disorder) becomes self-sustaining.

SUMMARY

Hyperactivity is but one symptom of a syndrome comprising hyperkinesis, impulsivity, inattention, and overexcitability. These can generally be subsumed under the diagnosis of attention deficit disorder, which may occur with or without hyperactivity. Attention deficit disorder typically occurs in a school-age boy and is often on a developmental, frequently familial, basis. Hyperactivity must be distinguished from normal activity for age and from tics. Hyperactivity can be seen with hyperthyroidism, Sydenham chorea, drug use, and seizure disorder, particularly of temporal lobe origin. Learning disability frequently accompanies attention deficit disorder, adding stress that often worsens behavioral problems.

History should include standard inquiry as to past history, development, and school performance. Examination in the office setting is often normal, without evidence of increased motor activity. Minor neurologic signs, such as awkwardness and synkinesis may be evident. Investigation will usually be nil or minimal in the assessment of most hyperactive children. Blood studies (such as thyroid hormone level), psychologic testing, and electroencephalography may, however, be indicated.

Treatment is almost always multifaceted, involving child, parent, teacher, and professional (often pediatrician, neurologist, and psychiatrist). Pharmacotherapy may be of dramatic benefit, though it should not be considered the sole mode of therapy. Regular follow-up to assess positive versus negative effects of medication and to consider the need for its further use are essential. The outlook for the child with attentional problems is for diminution of increased motor activity in adolescence and young adulthood. Impulsivity, distractability, and overexcitability often persist and, with them, social and academic difficulties. The lifelong effects of the disorder and its treatment are unknown.

CITED REFERENCES

Aron, A. M.; Freeman, J. M.; and Carter, S. The natural history of Sydenham's chorea: review of the literature and long-term evaluation with emphasis on cardiac sequelae. *Am. J. Med.,* **38:** 83–95, 1965.

Beck, L.; Langford, W. S.; MacKay, M.; and Sum, G. Childhood chemotherapy and later drug abuse and growth curve: a follow-up study of 30 adolescents. *Am. J. Psychiatry,* **132:** 436–38, 1975.

Benjamin, P. Y. Psychological problems following recovery from acute life-threatening illness. *Am. J. Orthopsychiatry,* **48:** 284–90, 1978.

Bidder, R. T.; Gray, O. P.; and Newcombe, R. Behavioural treatment of hyperactive children. *Arch. Dis. Child.,* **53:** 574–79, 1978.

Bierman, C. W., and Furukawa, C. T. Food additives and hyperkinesis: are there nuts among the berries? *Pediatrics,* **61:** 932–34, 1978.

Bradley, C. The behavior of children receiving benzedrine. *Am. J. Psychiatry,* **94:** 577–85, 1937.

Brown, G. L.; Ebert, M. H.; Mikkelsen, E. J.; and Hunt, R. D. Behavior and motor activity response in hyperactive children and plasma amphetamine levels following a sustained release preparation. *J. Am. Acad. Child Psychiatry,* **19:** 225–39, 1980.

Brown, R. T., and Sleator, E. K. Methylphenidate in hyperkinetic children: differences in dose effects on impulsive behavior. *Pediatrics,* **64:** 408–11, 1979.

Camp, J. A.; Bialer, I.; Sverd, J.; and Winsberg, B. G. Clinical usefulness of the NIMH physical and neurological examination for soft signs. *Am. J. Psychiatry,* **135:** 362–64, 1978.

Cantwell, D. P. Psychiatric illness in the families of hyperactive children. *Arch. Gen. Psychiatry,* **27:** 414–17, 1972.

Cantwell, D. Hyperkinetic syndrome. Pp. 524–55 in *Child Psychiatry: Modern Approaches.* Rutter, M., and Hersov, L., eds. Blackwell Scientific Publications, Oxford, 1977.

Charles, L.; Schain, R.; and Zelniker, T. Optimal dosages of methylphenidate for improving the learning and behavior of hyperactive children. *Dev. Behav. Pediatr.,* **2:** 78–81, 1981.

Charles, L.; Schain, R. J.; Zelniker, T.; and Guthrie, D. Effects of methylphenidate on hyperactive children's ability to sustain attention. *Pediatrics,* **64:** 412–18, 1979.

Christensen, D. E., and Sprague, R. L. Reduction of hyperactive behavior by conditioning procedures alone and combined with methylphenidate (Ritalin). *Behav. Res. Ther.,* **11:** 331–34, 1973.

Conners, C. K. *Food Additives and Hyperactive Children.* Plenum Press, New York, 1980.

Conners, C. K.; Goyette, C. H.; Southwick, D. A.; Lees, J. M.; and Andrulonis, P. A. Food additives and hyperkinesis: a controlled double-blind experiment. *Pediatrics,* **58:** 154–66, 1976.

Cooper, J. R.; Bloom, F. E.; and Roth, R. H. *The Biochemical Basis of Neuropharmacology,* 3d ed. Oxford University Press, New York, 1978.

de la Burdé, B., and Choate, McL. S., Jr. Does asymptomatic lead exposure in children have latent sequelae? *J. Pediatr.*, **81:** 1088–91, 1972.

DeLong, G. R. Lithium carbonate treatment of select behavior disorders in children suggesting manic-depressive illness. *J. Pediatr.*, **93:** 689–94, 1978.

Denckla, M. B., and Rudel, R. G. Anomalies of motor development in hyperactive boys. *Ann. Neurol.*, **3:** 231–33, 1978.

Diagnostic and Statistical Manual of Mental Disorders, 3d ed. American Psychiatric Association, Washington, D.C., 1980, pp. 41–45.

Dickinson, L. C.; Lee, J.; Ringdahl, I. C.; Schedewie, H. K.; Kilgore, B. S.; and Elders, M. J. Impaired growth in hyperkinetic children receiving pemoline. *J. Pediatr.*, **94:** 538–41, 1979.

Elkins, R. N.; Rapoport, J. L.; Zahn, T. P.; Buchsbaum, M. S.; Weingartner, H.; Kopin, I. J.; Langer, D.; and Johnson, C. Acute effects of caffeine in normal prepubertal boys. *Am. J. Psychiatry,* **138:** 178–83, 1981.

Feingold, B. F. *Why Your Child Is Hyperactive.* Random House, Inc., New York, 1975.

Firestone, P.; Davey, J.; Goodman, J. T.; and Peters, S. The effects of caffeine and methylphenidate on hyperactive children. *J. Am. Acad. Child Psychiatry,* **17:** 445–56, 1978.

Green, M., and Solnit, A. J. Reactions to the threatened loss of a child: a vulnerable child syndrome. *Pediatrics,* **34:** 58–66, 1964.

Gross, M. D. Growth of hyperkinetic children taking methylphenidate, dextroamphetamine, or imipramine/desipramine. *Pediatrics,* **58:** 423–31, 1976.

Harley, J. P.; Matthews, C. G.; and Eichman, P. Synthetic food colors and hyperactivity in children: a double-blind challenge experiment. *Pediatrics,* **62:** 975–83, 1978.

Harley, J. P.; Ray, R. S.; Tomasi, L.; Eichman, P. L.; Matthews, C. G.; Chun, R.; Cleeland, C. S.; and Traisman, E. Hyperkinesis and food additives: testing the Feingold hypothesis. *Pediatrics,* **61:** 818–28, 1978.

Harvey, D. H. P., and Marsh, R. W. The effects of de-caffeinated coffee versus whole coffee on hyperactive children. *Dev. Med. Child Neurol.,* **20:** 81–86, 1978.

Hoy, E.; Weiss, G.; Minde, K.; and Cohen, N. The hyperactive child at adolescence: cognitive, emotional, and social functioning. *J. Abnorm. Child Psychol.,* **6:** 311–24, 1978.

Khan, A. U., and Dekirmenjian, H. Urinary excretion of catecholamine metabolites in hyperkinetic child syndrome. *Am. J. Psychiatry,* **138:** 108–110, 1981.

Kinsbourne, M. The mechanism of hyperactivity. Pp. 289–306 in *Topics in Child Neurology.* Blaw, M. E.; Rapin, I.; and Kinsbourne, M., eds. Spectrum Publications, Inc., New York, 1977.

Kinsbourne, M., and Caplan, P. J. *Children's Learning and Attentional Problems.* Little, Brown and Company, Boston, 1979.

Lerer, R. J.; Lerer, M. P.; and Artner, J. The effects of methylphenidate on the handwriting of children with minimal brain dysfunction. *J. Pediatr.* **91:** 127–32, 1977.

Levy, F. The development of sustained attention (vigilance) and inhibition in children: some normative data. *J. Child Psychol. Psychiatry,* **21:** 77–84, 1980.

Lindsay, J.; Ounsted, C.; and Richards, P. Long-term outcome in children with temporal lobe seizures: III. psychiatric aspects in childhood and adult life. *Dev. Med. Child Neurol.,* **21:** 630–36, 1979.

Lipton, M. A.; Nemeroff, C. B.; and Mailman, R. B. Hyperkinesis and food additives. Pp. 1–27 in *Nutrition and the Brain,* Volume 4: *Toxic Effects of Food Constituents on the Brain.* Wurtman, R. J., and Wurtman, J. J., eds. Raven Press, New York, 1979.

Mattes, J. A., and Gittelman, R. Effects of artificial food colorings in children with hyperactive symptoms: a critical review and results of a controlled study. *Arch. Gen. Psychiatry*, **38**: 714–18, 1981.

Mattes, J., and Gittelman-Klein, R. A crossover study of artificial food colorings in a hyperkinetic child. *Am. J. Psychiatry*, **135**: 987–88, 1978.

Mayron, L. W. Hyperactivity from fluorescent lighting—fact or fancy: a commentary on the report by O'Leary, Rosenbaum, and Hughes. *J. Abnorm. Child Psychol.*, **6**: 291–94, 1978.

McMahon, S. A., and Greenberg, L. M. Serial neurologic examination of hyperactive children. *Pediatrics*, **59**: 584–87, 1977.

Menkes, M. M.; Rowe, J. S.; and Menkes, J. H. A twenty-five-year follow-up study on the hyperkinetic child with minimal brain dysfunction. *Pediatrics*, **39**: 393–99, 1967.

Minde, K.; Weiss, G.; and Mendelson, N. A 5-year follow-up study of 91 hyperactive school children. *J. Am. Acad. Child Psychiatry*, **11**: 595–610, 1972.

Morrison, J. R., and Stewart, M. A. Evidence for polygenetic inheritance in the hyperactive child syndrome. *Am. J. Psychiatry*, **130**: 791–92, 1973.

Narabayashi, H. Stereotaxic amygdalotomy for epileptic hyperactivity: long-range results in children. Pp. 319–31 in *Topics in Child Neurology*. Blaw, M. E.; Rapin, I.; and Kinsbourne, M., eds. Spectrum Publications, Inc., New York, 1977.

Needleman, H. L.; Gunnoe, C.; Leviton, A.; Reed, R.; Peresie, H.; Maher, C.; and Barrett, P. Deficits in psychologic and classroom performance of children with elevated dentine lead levels. *N. Engl. J. Med.*, **300**: 689–95, 1979.

O'Leary, S. G., and Pelham, W. E. Behavior therapy and withdrawal of stimulant medication in hyperactive children. *Pediatrics*, **61**: 211–17, 1978.

Rapoport, J. L.; Buchsbaum, M. S.; Zahn, T. P.; Weingartner, H.; Ludlow, C.; and Mikkelsen, E. J. Dextroamphetamine: cognitive and behavioral effects in normal prepubertal boys. *Science*, **199**: 560–63, 1978.

Roche, A. F.; Lipman, R. S.; Overall, J. E.; and Hung, W. The effects of stimulant medication on the growth of hyperkinetic children. *Pediatrics*, **63**: 847–50, 1979.

Rosman, N. P. Neurological and muscular aspects of thyroid dysfunction in childhood. *Pediatr. Clin. North Am.*, **23**: 575–94, 1976.

Routh, D. K.; Schroeder, C. S.; and O'Tuama, L. A. Development of activity level in children. *Dev. Psychol.*, **10**: 163–68, 1974.

Rutter, M. Raised lead levels and impaired cognitive/behavioural functioning: a review of the evidence. *Suppl. Dev. Med. Child Neurol.*, **22**: 1–26, 1980.

Safer, D.; Allen, R.; and Barr, E. Depression of growth in hyperactive children on stimulant drugs. *N. Engl. J. Med.*, **287**: 217–20, 1972.

Satterfield, J. H.; Satterfield, B. T.; and Cantwell, D. P. Three-year multimodality treatment study of 100 hyperactive boys. *J. Pediatr.*, **98**: 650–55, 1981.

Schmitt, B. Guidelines for living with a hyperactive child. *Pediatrics*, **60**: 387, 1977.

Shaywitz, B. A.; Cohen, D. J.; and Bowers, M. B., Jr. CSF monoamine metabolites in children with minimal brain dysfunction: evidence for alteration of brain dopamine. *J. Pediatr.*, **90**: 67–71, 1977.

Shaywitz, S. E.; Cohen, D. J.; and Shaywitz, B. A. Behavior and learning difficulties in children of normal intelligence born to alcoholic mothers. *J. Pediatr.*, **96**: 978–82, 1980.

Shaywitz, B. A.; Klopper, J. H.; and Gordon, J. W. Methylphenidate in 6-hydroxy-dopamine-treated developing rat pups: effects on activity and maze performance. *Arch. Neurol.*, **35**: 463–69, 1978.

Shekim, W. O.; Dekirmenjian, H.; Chapel, J. L.; Javaid, J.; and Davis, J. M. Norepinephrine metabolism and clinical response to dextroamphetamine in hyperactive boys. *J. Pediatr.*, **95**: 389–94, 1979.

Sleator, E. K., and Ullmann, R. K. Can the physician diagnose hyperactivity in the office? *Pediatrics*, **67**: 13–17, 1981.

Sprague, R. L., and Sleator, E. K. Methylphenidate in hyperkinetic children: differences in dose effects on learning and social behavior. *Science*, **198**: 1274–76, 1977.

Stores, G. Behavioural effects of anti-epileptic drugs. *Dev. Med. Child Neurol.*, **17**: 647–58, 1975.

Swanson, J. M., and Kinsbourne, M. Food dyes impair performance of hyperactive children on a laboratory learning test. *Science*, **207**: 1485–87, 1980.

Swanson, J.; Kinsbourne, M.; Roberts, W.; and Zucker, K. Time-response analysis of the effect of stimulant medication on the learning ability of children referred for hyperactivity. *Pediatrics*, **61**: 21–29, 1978.

Thomas, A.; Chess, S.; and Birch, H. G. *Temperament and Behavior Disorders in Children.* New York University Press, New York, 1968.

Vaidya, V. A.; Bongiovanni, A. M.; Parks, J. S.; Tenore, A.; and Kirkland, R. T. Twenty-two years' experience in the medical management of juvenile thyrotoxicosis. *Pediatrics*, **54**: 565–70, 1974.

Waldrop, M. F.; Bell, R. Q.; McLaughlin, B.; and Halverson, C. F., Jr. Newborn minor physical anomalies predict short attention span, peer aggression, and impulsivity at age 3. *Science*, **199**: 563–65, 1978.

Weiner, N. Norepinephrine, epinephrine, and the sympathomimetic amines. Pp. 138–75 in *The Pharmacological Basis of Therapeutics*. 6th ed. Gilman, A. G.; Goodman, L. S.; and Gilman, A., eds. Macmillan Publishing Co., Inc., New York, 1980.

Weiss, B.; Williams, J. H.; Margen, S.; Abrams, B.; Caan, B.; Citron, L. J.; Cox, C.; McKibben, J.; Ogar, D.; and Schultz, S. Behavioral responses to artificial food colors. *Science*, **207**: 1487–89, 1980.

Weiss, G.; Hechtman, L.; and Perlman, T. Hyperactives as young adults: school, employer, and self-rating scales obtained during ten-year follow-up evaluation. *Am. J. Orthopsychiatry*, **48**: 438–45, 1978.

Wender, E. H. Food additives and hyperkinesis. *Am. J. Dis. Child.*, **131**: 1204–06, 1977.

Wender, P. H. *Minimal Brain Dysfunction in Children.* John Wiley and Sons, Inc., New York, 1971.

Wender, P. H.; Reimherr, F. W.; and Wood, D. R. Attention deficit disorder ('minimal brain dysfunction') in adults. *Arch. Gen. Psychiatry*, **38**: 449–56, 1981.

Wender, P. H., and Wender, E. H. *The Hyperactive Child and the Learning Disabled Child.* Crown Publishers, Inc., New York, 1978.

Werry, J. S. Developmental hyperactivity. *Pediatr. Clin. North Am.*, **15**: 581–99, 1968.

Werry, J. S.; Aman, M. G.; and Diamond E. Imipramine and methylphenidate in hyperactive children. *J. Child Psychol. Psychiatry*, **21**: 27–35, 1980.

Wolf, S. M., and Forsythe, A. Behavior disturbance, phenobarbital, and febrile seizures. *Pediatrics*, **61**: 728–31, 1978.

Wolraich, M.; Drummond T.; Salomon, M. K.; O'Brien, M. L.; and Sivage, C. Effects of methylphenidate alone and in combination with behavior modification procedures on the behavior and academic performance of hyperactive children. *J. Abnorm. Child Psychol.*, **6**: 149–61, 1978.

ADDITIONAL READINGS

Chiel, H. J., and Wurtman, R. J. Short-term variations in diet composition change the pattern of spontaneous motor activity in rats. *Science,* **213:** 676–78, 1981.

Davis, R. E. Manic-depressive variant syndrome of childhood: a preliminary report. *Am. J. Psychiatry,* **136:** 702–6, 1979.

Deuel, R. K. Minimal brain dysfunction, hyperkinesis, learning disabilities, attention deficit disorder. *J. Pediatr.,* **98:** 912–15, 1981.

Jankovic, J. Treatment of hyperkinetic movement disorders with tetrabenazine: a double-blind crossover study. *Ann. Neurol.,* **11:** 41–47, 1982.

Mesulam, M.-M. A cortical network for directed attention and unilateral neglect. *Ann. Neurol.,* **10:** 309–25, 1981.

Rutter, M. Syndromes attributed to "minimal brain dysfunction" in childhood. *Am. J. Psychiatry,* **139:** 21–33, 1982.

Schreier, H. A. Mania responsive to lecithin in a 13-year-old girl. *Am. J. Psychiatry,* **139:** 108–10, 1982.

Swanson, J. W.; Kelly, J. J., Jr.; and McConahey, W. M. Neurologic aspects of thyroid dysfunction. *Mayo Clin. Proc.,* **56:** 504–12, 1981.

Weiss, G., and Hechtman, L. The hyperactive child syndrome. *Science,* **205:** 1348–54, 1979.

Youngerman, J., and Canino, I. A. Lithium carbonate use in children and adolescents. *Arch. Gen. Psychiatry,* **35:** 216–24, 1978.

15 Aggressive and Violent Behavior

Aggression and violence are increasingly a part of everyday life, contributing importantly to morbidity and mortality in childhood and adolescence (Holinger, 1980). One has only to listen to the radio, watch television, or read a newspaper to be impressed by the frequency of aggressive and violent acts; those reported are surely a minority. Social and environmental influences have long been recognized as contributing to aggressive and violent behavior. The organic role has been more recently explored and is the primary focus of this chapter.

Several questions will be addressed:

What is the definition of aggressive behavior? Violent behavior?
What are their causes in childhood?
What investigations, if any, should be undertaken in assessing such behavior in childhood?
How should aggressive and violent behavior in childhood or adolescence be treated?
What is the prognosis?

AGGRESSIVE AND VIOLENT BEHAVIOR

DEFINITION

Aggression refers to behavior directed against another person, an inanimate object, or at times oneself, with the goal generally to establish a position of control, dominance, or superiority. Anger, hostility, rage, and fear are commonly associated feeling states. From a developmental perspective, aggression is closely related to inquisitiveness, activity, and mastery—behaviors that are a natural and important part of the developmental process.

Violence is an extreme form of aggression. It is used to describe behavior involving, or promising to involve, bodily injury or damage to property. As with suicidal actions, a spectrum of likelihood exists. It is, therefore, best to

435

describe the behavior in question as "threatening" or "potentially violent" rather than "violent" if destructive behavior has not been attempted or consummated.

Aggression has been categorized largely based upon observations of animals: predatory, fear-induced, irritable, territorial, maternal, sex-related, intermale, and instrumental (Corning and Corning, 1975). These categories are applicable to human beings at least in part. For example, maternal aggression applies to protective actions of a mother in guarding her offspring. Fear-induced and irritable forms of aggression are self-explanatory. Instrumental aggression involves learned behavior used in a rational fashion for advantage.

Aggression and violent behavior are common in syndromes of behavioral disturbance. Among adults, explosive personality disorder and antisocial personality disorder are diagnostic categories involving varying degrees of aggressive and violent behavior (*DSM*-III, 1980). In childhood "poor impulse control" and "acting-out" may, in fact, refer to aggressive and violent actions occurring with syndromes of attention deficit disorder, affective disturbance, or conduct disorder.

Rage lies at the core of violent behavior. An enraged infant provides a ready example of the intensity and lack of control that characterize this emotional state. Everyday experience demonstrates that such behavior in pure form is relatively uncommon in later life, as it has been modulated by experience (especially within the family) against a backdrop of central nervous system growth and maturation. Feelings of anger or even rage, however, continue to occur, but they are generally handled in a more adaptive manner.

DIAGNOSIS

Clinical Process. *History.* The chief complaint should be recorded in the words of the child, parent, teacher, or other observer. "He starts attacking children for no reason at all." "He always hits. He can't seem to control himself." "I can't help it. I just feel like exploding and have to strike out." It is always valuable to obtain several viewpoints, particularly in assessing the element of provocation.

The history of the presenting problem should elaborate further the chief complaint and determine specifically why (and by whom) evaluation has been sought. The associated affect and social circumstances of alleged incidents should be noted in detail. Was the child involved in a game at the time of an outburst? Or did he "pick a fight" with a classmate in the school cafeteria? Has fighting occurred repeatedly with another child in particular? Have attacks been planned or carried out impulsively? What has provoked the episodes?

It is too simple to say that an attack was "unprovoked" as opposed to "provoked," for subjective and objective aspects of the episode must be appreciated in order that a clearer picture of the violent behavior may emerge. How did the child feel before the attack: scared, angry, anxious? How does he or she feel during it and afterwards? Does he recall the episode? Previous similar incidents should be noted and their circumstances defined.

Associated features of behavior such as headache, confusion, semipurposeful behavior, abdominal pain, and drug use should be sought.

The past history should include information as to pregnancy, birth, development, major illnesses, hospitalizations, episodes of head injury, allergies, and medications. Perinatal difficulties, significant head trauma, central nervous system infection (such as encephalitis or abscess), and prolonged febrile seizures have been associated with later development of temporal lobe epilepsy, which has been linked with aggressive and violent behavior in some children.

Family and social history should include delineation of the family picture: members of the household, recent or anticipated changes, parents' work schedules, past or impending moves, and recent deaths, for example. Information should also be obtained as to modes of discipline, circumstances under which it has been administered, the child's reaction to discipline, and the effectiveness of disciplinary measures. As with the problem of child abuse, discipline experienced by the parents when they were children may be relevant to the child's problem. When a child has attempted suicide, family history of suicide or major depressive illness should be sought (see Chapter 6).

Examination. The *general description* should note whether the child is irritable, anxious, depressed, belligerent, or threatening. These aspects of mood and behavior are part of the mental status examination as well but may be striking enough to warrant inclusion here.

The *general physical examination* should seek signs of systemic illness such as asthma or duodenal ulcer, which might contribute to irritability and predispose to aggressive or violent behavior. Examination of the skin should note evidence of injury (self-inflicted or acquired otherwise), neurocutaneous signs (as with tuberous sclerosis), and acne (as with the XYY syndrome). Evidence for, and effects of, drug use, including alcohol, should also be recorded. Height and weight should be measured and plotted.

On *neurologic examination,* pupillary abnormalities may be found with drug use: dilated pupils with cocaine, small pupils with opiates. Nystagmus, ataxia, and dysarthria can be seen with abuse of alcohol, barbiturates, diazepam, or phencyclidine ("angel dust") (see Chapter 19).

The *mental status examination* should provide objective data as to personality, behavior, and parent-child interaction. Disorientation may be seen as part of a confusional state. Activity level may be increased, attention diminished, and behavior impulsive with hyperkinetic children. If the child actively provokes a parent in the office, the parent may be unable (or unwilling) to resist hitting the child despite the examiner's presence. On the other hand, the child's behavior may be unchecked by the parent, who delivers ineffectual "lip service" to limit-setting, thereby implicitly sanctioning the child's aggressive misbehavior.

The child's affect and mood should be noted and explored as to appropriateness. Anger, for example, may be part of a depressive syndrome secondary to death, divorce, or other major loss. The content of the child's speech should be examined for depressive, psychotic, or suicidal ideation. Halluci-

TABLE 15–1. **Investigations to Be Considered in Children with Aggressive or Violent Behavior**

Blood, urine for toxic screen
EEG (in awake and sleep states)
EEG, special recording techniques (nasopharyngeal or
    sphenoidal recordings; 24-hour ambulatory
    recording; simultaneous video recording)
Psychologic testing
Visual field examination
Skull x-rays
Cranial CT scan
CSF examination
Neuroendocrinologic studies
Radioisotope brain scan
Pneumoencephalogram (PEG)
Chromosome analysis
Brain biopsy

nation should be considered. It may be valuable to ask specifically whether violent behavior (including attempted suicide) was carried out in response to perceived commands (auditory hallucinations).

Investigation.   The investigation of the child with aggressive or violent behavior will be determined by the history and examination (see Table 15–1). Use of the EEG should be guided by the clinical features of the abnormal behavior and particularly by suspicion that a seizure disorder coexists. Electroencephalography may disclose nonspecific abnormalities in persons with aggressive, violent, and criminal behaviors. Such persons may also have definite seizure discharges on EEG. Such findings do not, however, determine that seizures have necessarily occurred or that such occurrence is necessarily related to the deviant behavior. Further, temporal lobe epilepsy, the seizure type most often associated with aggressive and violent behavior, may be accompanied by an EEG that is entirely normal. In some such circumstances electroencephalographic abnormalities are not found because only conventional scalp electrodes, which record electrical activity only from the cerebral convexities, are used. Seizure discharges emanating from deep, medial portions of the temporal lobe may be accessible only by special techniques such as recording with nasopharyngeal or sphenoidal electrodes. Oftentimes, temporal lobe seizure discharges are found only on an EEG recorded during sleep. Finally, regardless of recording techniques employed, it is by no means rare that clinically evident temporal lobe seizures may be accompanied by repeatedly normal electroencephalograms.

Special electroencephalographic techniques, including ambulatory monitoring over a 24-hour period and simultaneous recording of EEG activity and behavior (by videotaping) may be useful in clarifying the possible relationship between aggressive behavior and seizures.

Formal psychologic assessment, including both intellectual (psychometric) and projective testing, is often indicated. Neuropsychologic assessment may be valuable in delineating areas of disordered hemispheric function. For example, impaired auditory verbal memory is characteristically seen with lesions of the left temporal lobe (Luria and Karasseva, 1968).

When a structural lesion affecting the hypothalamus or other part of the limbic system is suspected, radiologic studies such as plain skull x-rays, computerized tomographic (CT) scan, isotope brain scan, and pneumoencephalography should be considered. When an infectious etiology is suspected, particularly limbic encephalitis of viral origin, examination of cerebrospinal fluid for sugar, protein, cell count, viral antibody titers, and growth of viral or other pathogens is indicated. When *Herpes simplex* encephalitis is of particular concern, brain biopsy is usually required for its definitive diagnosis.

When drug use is suspected, analysis of blood and urine for toxic substances should be carried out. When suspicion of an XYY syndrome or other chromosomal disorder is high, chromosomal analysis should be considered. Formal neuro-ophthalmologic assessment (including measurement of visual fields) and neuroendocrinologic studies are indicated when a disorder of the hypothalamus or neighboring structures is suspected.

Differential Diagnosis. Aggressive and violent behaviors are symptoms, not diagnoses. As such, there is little that they can be mistaken for, if abnormal behavior has been observed and described accurately.

Etiology. As with other behavioral problems in childhood and adolescence, it is an oversimplification to view aggressive or violent behavior as stemming solely from one cause. In most instances etiology is multifactorial. An organic (often neurologic, that is, brain-based) abnormality is frequently demonstrable, and social and environmental influences (such as family upbringing, socioeconomic circumstances, or drugs) lead to expression of the aberrant behavior (see Table 15–2).

Medical Causes. Systemic illness, previously recognized or not, can contribute to or cause irritability that predisposes to aggressive behavior. Chronic renal disease, cardiac disorders, asthma, cystic fibrosis, ulcerative colitis, and regional enteritis exemplify conditions that may weaken the child, interfere with interest and initiative, and lead to a state of chronic irritability. Moreover, as with any chronic illness, a depressive syndrome may be associated.

Lability of mood associated with *hyperthyroidism* and *Sydenham chorea* may also contribute to aggressive behavior.

Neurologic Causes. Seizure disorders have been linked with violent behavior, although the nature of the association remains unclear. *Temporal lobe epilepsy* has been singled out as being associated with hyperkinetic syndromes and catastrophic rage (Lindsay *et al.,* 1979; Pritchard *et al.,* 1980). The left temporal lobe in particular appears to be related to those temporal lobe epilepsies in which violent behavior or psychosis have been associated (Krynicki, 1978; Lindsay *et al.,* 1979) (see Case 15–1).

Aggressive and violent behavior rarely (if ever) occurs as a seizure manifestation itself. Rather, rage episodes are typically interictal behavioral disturbances felt to result from an abnormal brain (and its environment), whose malfunction is also evident as epilepsy. The specific behavior problems man-

TABLE 15–2. **Causes of Aggressive or Violent Behavior**

Medical	Systemic illness
	Hyperthyroidism
	Sydenham chorea
Neurologic	Temporal lobe epilepsy (postictal state; interictal behavior)
	Limbic encephalitis (particularly from *Herpes simplex*)
	Hypothalamic disorder
	Migraine
Toxic	Barbiturates, including primidone (Mysoline)
	Diazepam (Valium)
	Alcohol
	Hallucinogens
	Cocaine
	Amphetamines
Psychologic	Depression
	Anxiety
	Anger
	Psychosis
Social-Environmental	Lack of limit-setting
	Implicit sanction
	Culturally acceptable
	(?) Television
Genetic-Constitutional	XY (normal male) karyotype
	XYY syndrome
Developmental	Sibling rivalry

ifested between seizures presumably reflect disturbances involving the temporal lobe and connected structures such as the hypothalamus (see Case 15–2).

Catastrophic rage was studied in children with temporal lobe epilepsy by Ounsted and co-workers (1966). They found 26 of 63 boys (41 per cent) and 10 of 37 girls (27 per cent) to manifest this symptom. The rage episodes sometimes took the form of murderous assault. Fewer than one-half of the children with catastrophic rage had an associated hyperkinetic syndrome.

In adults, the high frequency of EEG abnormalities (particularly involving the temporal lobe) among persons jailed for crimes of aggression and violence has frequently been cited (Williams, 1969; Pincus and Tucker, 1978). Krynicki (1978) found paroxysmal activity frontally to typify the electroencephalograms of repetitively assaultive adolescent males.

The connection between temporal lobe seizures and violence has been the subject of considerable investigation. Rodin (1973) explored the possible relationship by recording some forty psychomotor seizures and postictal states photographically and electroencephalographically. He found only one instance in which aggressive behavior was threatened. It was avoided when efforts to restrain the patient were abandoned.

The problem of epilepsy and violence not infrequently arises in court. A careful analysis of cases in which defense was attempted on the basis of associated epilepsy was presented by Gunn and Fenton (1971). They concluded that automatic behavior rarely, if ever, could explain the crimes of epileptic patients. In a follow-up study Gunn (1978) described temporal lobe seizures occurring in an adult who had apparently committed homicide during a prolonged postictal state. More recently, Delgado-Escueta and colleagues (1981) in an extensive review of the subject have concluded that epileptic seizures *per se* only rarely can be considered the cause of acts of violence. Studies carried out by Mark and Ervin (1970) have also investigated the role of seizure activity in producing violent behavior through the use of indwelling electrodes deep within the temporal lobes. These studies are presented in further detail in the section on CORRELATION: PHYSIOLOGIC ASPECTS.

One should also keep in mind the possibility of pseudoseizure—either hysterical or feigned. Telemetered electroencephalography and simultaneous videotape recording will often be able to confirm the diagnosis of pseudoseizure (see Chapter 7).

The combination of organic susceptibility and environmental influence in problems of aggression and violence has been emphasized by Mark and Ervin (1970) and Bach-y-Rita and colleagues (1971), who described an "episodic dyscontrol syndrome" in adults. This disorder is characterized by a state of heightened susceptibility to alcohol ("pathological intoxication") such that violent acts are carried out when blood levels of ethanol are in a range that would be considered only mildly intoxicating in most persons. Though the episode of dyscontrol is not itself a seizure, a therapeutic trial of phenytoin or other anticonvulsant medication may occasionally benefit a person even if the EEG is normal (Monroe, 1975). The relevance of this syndrome to childhood and adolescence has not been established.

In childhood aggressive and violent behavior may be seen with a hyperkinetic syndrome. Impulsivity, "bossiness," and dysphoria contribute to behavioral problems (see Chapter 14).

Central nervous system infection, particularly limbic *encephalitis*, can be associated with aggressive or violent behavior. *Herpes simplex* is a viral agent with a known predilection for the limbic system, particularly the temporal lobes. It may present as an organic psychosis or with other manifestations of intracranial mass. Diagnosis is established definitively by a brain biopsy (see Chapter 5). Rabies is another viral illness whose clinical and pathologic manifestations reflect preferential involvement of the temporal lobes.

Hypothalamic disorder, such as might result from neoplasm, infection, hamartoma, or trauma, can be associated with rage among other symptoms, which might include diabetes insipidus, obesity, and visual impairment (Plum and Van Uitert, 1978).

CASE 15–1: TEMPORAL LOBE SEIZURES AND RAGE EPISODES IN A 14-YEAR-OLD BOY

S.V. was evaluated because of a mixed seizure disorder and recent development of aggressive behavior. Seizures began at 8 years of age. The first kind consisted of staring episodes lasting less than 1 minute associated with turning of his head to the left. Afterward he returned promptly to a state of normal consciousness. The second seizure type was a generalized tonic-clonic convulsion. The third consisted of an aura of "dizziness" followed by abdominal pain, staring, immobility, and a bad taste in the mouth. These last episodes, 3 to 5 minutes long, were followed by fatigue and sometimes headache.

Since the age of 13 years, behavior had deteriorated. The boy had violent, angry outbursts when he felt pressured or was disciplined. At first he would be silent then would strike out suddenly at his mother, gym instructor, classroom teacher, or others. He once chased his brother with a knife. Outbursts lasted 20 minutes and were associated with facial flushing. He did not have amnesia for the episodes. Recovery took several minutes and was unaccompanied by headache, sleepiness, or confusion.

Past medical history included normal pregnancy, labor, and delivery. Early developmental milestones were normal. No head injury of significance or infections of the central nervous system had occurred. Family history was negative for seizures or emotional disturbance.

General examination was normal. It included measurement of head circumference, visualization of the optic fundi, and inspection of the skin for neurocutaneous signs. Neurologic examination, including visual field testing, was likewise unremarkable. Electroencephalography showed bitemporal and bifrontal spike-and-slow-wave discharges occurring in bursts during the awake and sleep states. Pneumoencephalography demonstrated attentuation of the left temporal horn.

Migraine headaches are commonly accompanied by irritability and may be associated with behavioral disturbances as well (see Case 15–3).

Toxic Causes. Several drugs have been implicated in producing or contributing to aggressive or violent behavior. These include barbiturates, diazepam, hallucinogenic agents, cocaine, amphetamines, and alcohol (see Chapter 19). Pathologic intolerance to alcohol was described above. Although alcohol may be used to ward off feelings of depression and anxiety, intoxication may produce further despondency and heightened anxiety. This effect may underlie the increased risk of suicide with alcoholism (Mendelson and Mello, 1979). With psychoactive drugs in general and alcohol in particular, aggressive and violent behavior may involve motor vehicles used intentionally or otherwise as agents of destruction.

Phenobarbital and other members of the barbiturate family such as primidone (Mysoline) or mephobarbital (Mebaral) may cause personality change

Treatment consisted essentially of pharmacotherapy (primidone and phenytoin) and family-centered psychotherapy.

Comment. This teenage boy suffered from a mixed seizure disorder consisting of focal motor, grand mal, and psychomotor (partial complex) seizures. The seizures associated with stomach ache, bad taste in the mouth, and staring strongly suggested temporal lobe origin. The cause for his seizure disorder was not determined by history, examination, or investigation. Head trauma can result in bruising of the temporal lobe against the sharp and firm anterior border of the middle cranial fossa, but no significant head trauma had occurred in this case. Birth trauma has also been invoked as a cause of temporal lobe injury leading to seizures. Perinatal events were, however, quite unremarkable here. Nor did he have a history of asphyxia or prolonged fevers in early childhood, which have been implicated in causing temporal lobe damage. Tuberous sclerosis would be another etiologic possibility. The skin examination and pneumoencephalogram excluded that diagnosis.

This child exemplifies the association of rage episodes with temporal lobe epilepsy in childhood. The rage episodes themselves are not ictal phenomena. Rather, they reflect disordered brain function, perhaps a disinhibition of aggressive behaviors normally held in check.

This adolescent with temporal lobe epilepsy by clinical as well as electroencephalographic criteria did not manifest the interictal personality disorder of adults with temporal lobe epilepsy. This syndrome includes such features as hyperreligiosity, hypergraphia, and "stickiness." The full-blown syndrome is felt to result only after years of having had temporal lobe seizures. The effect of treatment of temporal lobe epilepsy upon development of later personality disturbance is uncertain.

in some children manifested by irritability and unusually aggressive behavior (Stores, 1975).

Psychologic Causes. Depression, anxiety, anger, and psychosis may be associated with aggressive or violent behavior in childhood. Depression may be overt, with obvious features of sadness, low self-esteem, somatic complaints (such as headache), and psychomotor slowing; or hyperactive, criminal, or violent behavior may mask depressive symptoms at the core of a behavioral disturbance (see Chapter 6).

Aggressive behavior may occur as part of a separation reaction. Younger children especially may react with anger rather than with joy when a parent returns after a period of separation.

Psychosis also may be associated with aggressive and violent behavior. Catatonic excitement can occur in some forms of schizophrenia and rage in acute paranoid states.

CASE 15–2: VIOLENT BEHAVIOR AND SEIZURES IN A 15-YEAR-OLD GIRL

P.B. was evaluated because of generalized seizures and recurrent episodes of violent behavior. The violent behavior consisted of screaming, throwing things, and destroying objects. A typical temper outburst, lasting more than an hour, was provoked by the girl's sister taking a bath before she did. During these outbursts or shortly afterward she was noted to become ''chalky white'' and to have ''blue lips.'' The episodes were often associated with automatic behavior, unresponsiveness, urinary incontinence, or tongue-biting.

Generalized tonic-clonic convulsions began at 7 years of age. The first seizure lasted for 2 hours. Early history was of normal pregnancy, labor, and delivery. She banged her head as an infant and had been considered overactive since that time. Temperamentally, she had always been easily frustrated and had tended to be irritable. Social history was noteworthy for the child's mother being wheelchair-bound due to arthritis. Her teenage sister had a background of scholastic and interpersonal difficulties.

The general physical and neurologic examinations were normal. Electroencephalogram was mildly abnormal, with slowing of background activity and occasional sharp waves. CT scan was normal. Psychometric testing showed intelligence in the borderline range. Projective testing clarified the importance of stresses caused by her mother's chronic illness, her own neurologic problems, and her impaired ability to learn.

Comment. As is often found with seizure disorders in childhood, the etiology in this case remained obscure. This child's behavior problems were much more disabling than her seizure disorder, which was under excellent pharmacologic control. In this case situational stresses were poorly tolerated by a child whose central nervous system was not normal. For that reason, family-based therapy was an integral part of her treatment plan.

Another consideration in the behaviorally disturbed child being treated for epilepsy is medication effect. Phenobarbital and primidone (Mysoline) are common offenders. They may cause a ''Jekyll and Hyde'' personality transformation that makes it necessary to change to other anticonvulsant drugs.

Complicating effects of drugs, prescribed or taken illicitly, should be considered even when another cause for affective disturbance has been identified. For example, an adolescent may use alcohol to deal with angry feelings toward a parent (see Case 19–3). Alcohol may, however, promote acting-out against the parent or lead to aggressive and violent behavior directed toward others.

Social-Environmental Causes. Social and environmental factors are of great importance in the genesis of aggressive and violent behavior. Seen in its most primitive form in earliest childhood, the rage of the young infant is molded by maternal and other family interactions as neurologic maturation

CASE 15–3: SLEEP DISTURBANCE AND PREVIOUS AGGRESSIVE BEHAVIOR IN A 12-YEAR-OLD BOY

L.J. was referred for neurologic evaluation because of "nightmares." Sleep disturbance probably began at 1 year of age when he had episodes lasting 5 minutes during which he produced guttural sounds, flailed his arms, appeared frightened, and failed to recognize his parents. At 6 years of age, behavior at school deteriorated and led to his expulsion the next year in the second grade when he was described as "uncontrollable." Typical behaviors included spitting at teachers and fighting with classmates.

Since 11 years of age, he had experienced occasional night terrors lasting 15 to 20 minutes. They began with a cry approximately 2 hours after falling asleep. When mother entered his room, he was wide-eyed and agitated, and did not recognize her. He was unresponsive to mild stimulation and had no recollection of the episode in the morning. Review of systems was negative for seizures or headaches, although he sometimes experienced the illusion of being "small and tiny," as if he were in a huge room. Past history of pregnancy and birth was unremarkable. Mother had a history of classic migraines preceded by paresthesias and visual illusions.

On examination, the child was an intelligent, articulate youngster without evidence of anxiety or depression. Head circumference (54 cm) and neurologic examination were normal.

Comment. Establishing the basis for this child's aggressive behavior several years previously could not be accomplished with certainty. His uncontrollable behavior suggested catastrophic rage such as is characteristically seen in children with temporal lobe epilepsy. He had never been observed to have seizures, however, of generalized or partial complex type (although his sleep disturbance was consistent with either night terror or psychomotor seizure). Nor had he apparently experienced birth trauma, prolonged febrile seizures, or significant head injury that might have produced temporal lobe damage.

Another possibility for this child's behavioral disturbance during his early school years was that he suffered from a complicated migraine syndrome. One can postulate that, stressed by the transition from kindergarten to first grade, he experienced episodes of confusional migraine (see Chapter 11). Alternatively, he may have had migrainous episodes of dysphoria and irritability associated with aggressive behavior.

progresses. As a result, strategies for dealing with frustration and anger are acquired, and nonviolent ways of responding are learned to supplant instinctual rage.

The continuation of aggressive behavior into later childhood can result from faulty parenting. Persistent failure to set limits, difficulty in extinguishing previously established maladaptive behavior patterns, and implicit (often unconscious) sanctioning of aggressive behavior are among the causes

(Johnson, 1949; Johnson and Szurek, 1952). As a result the child, when thwarted, may have little to resort to other than a temper tantrum that may include attacking behavior.

Inadequate supervision of children may lead to unbridled expression of jealous feelings that may result in serious injury to an essentially defenseless younger child (Adelson, 1972). In other words, through lack of awareness or concern, parents may allow a jealous 4-year-old to remain unattended in the room of an infant sibling, against whom expressions of anger and rage may reach murderous proportions.

Previous child abuse has been found to be of increased frequency among violent adolescents (Lewis et al., 1979; Pincus, 1980). A high incidence of grand mal seizures, electroencephalographic abnormalities, and symptoms of psychomotor epilepsy also characterized the more violent offenders in a series of ninety-seven incarcerated males reported by Lewis and colleagues (1979).

Styles of aggression differ among socioeconomic groups as well as from one family to another. Thus, the tendency to fight back, to respond physically if verbally or physically attacked, will vary.

The role of television cartoons, sports telecasts, and crime programs in contributing to aggressive and violent behavior is unclear but may be significant (Report to the Surgeon General, 1972). Younger children appear to be more vulnerable than adolescents. Kniveton and Stephenson (1975) found an increase in fighting among young boys who had previously watched a film involving two children fighting over cars.

Genetic-Constitutional Cases. It is widely recognized that the XY (male) karyotype carries with it a greater likelihood of aggressive behavior. Werry and Quay (1971) assayed fifty-five behavioral symptoms in an entire kindergarten-through-grade-two population of a Midwestern university town (926 boys and 827 girls). They found acting-out or disruptive behavior to be significantly more prevalent among boys in this 5- to 8-year range.

Differences in aggressive behavior between males and females have been linked with hormonal differences. Increased levels of testosterone in males postnatally appear to be related to this behavioral difference (Rubin et al., 1981). Females given male hormone pursue more ''boyish'' activities than untreated members of their gender. In males, diminished aggressiveness has been noted among teenage boys who were exposed *in utero* to female hormones (estrogen and progesterone) taken by their mothers (Yalom et al., 1973; Ehrhardt and Meyer-Bahlburg, 1981).

Males with an XYY sex chromosome constitution have been found to be overrepresented among criminally institutionalized males as determined by karyotypic screening (Walzer et al., 1978). The incidence of this sex chromosome anomaly among males approximates 1:500 to 1:1,000 in the general population (Grumbach, 1977; Walzer et al., 1978). Tall stature and severe acne are characteristic features. Undescended testes and hypogonadism are sometimes present. Impulsivity, sociopathy, and mental subnormalcy are less clearly associated. Marfan syndrome and homocystinuria should be considered in the differential diagnosis of the XYY syndrome.

Since the XYY karyotype does not preclude normal development, the value (versus the risk) of screening and early identification is dubious.

Developmental Causes. As indicated above (SOCIAL-ENVIRONMENTAL CAUSES), development often plays a role in the expression of aggressive or violent behavior. Examples might include jealousy toward a sibling and anger expressed toward a parent following separation and return.

Hyperactivity and impulsivity, frequently seen as part of a developmental syndrome of attention deficit disorder, may also be associated with aggressive and violent behavior (see Chapter 14).

Adolescence, particularly in males, is associated with an increase in aggressive and violent behavior. Elevation in testosterone production appears to play a role in this change (Mattsson *et al.*, 1980) (see GENETIC-CONSTITUTIONAL CAUSES).

TREATMENT AND OUTCOME

The relationship between behavior disorders of childhood and those of adulthood is a matter of great interest and concern. Pincus and Tucker (1978) present a relatively gloomy outlook for the child who has been criminally aggressive. They cited evidence that fewer than 20 per cent would be "well-adjusted" as adults, and 20 per cent would be psychotic. From a more specific diagnostic standpoint, Henn and colleagues (1980) found aggressive behavior as part of an undersocialized conduct disorder likely to lead to antisocial personality disorder after the age of 18 years.

One can only hope that these statistics can be improved upon by further understanding of the organic bases of aggression and violence, of social and environmental influences, and of the effects of early identification and intervention (see Table 15–3).

Medical Management. Treatment of systemic illness can be expected to restore a greater sense of well-being and energy to the affected child, to reduce irritability, and to diminish the likelihood of aggressive behavior.

The person with catatonic excitement must be treated actively because of the danger of exhaustion in addition to the possibility of damage to self or others. Standard pharmacologic agents are chlorpromazine (Thorazine), haloperidol (Haldol), and phenobarbital given by injection during acute phases of treatment. Phenothiazines and butyrophenones are also effective in the acute treatment of violent behavior that is part of a psychotic syndrome.

When aggressive behavior occurs with a hyperkinetic syndrome, a multifaceted approach to treatment (pharmacologic, behavioral, and/or other modes) will often alleviate this symptom among others (impulsivity, distractibility, overexcitability).

When aggressive or violent behavior occurs as part of a manic syndrome (in a unipolar or bipolar affective disorder), lithium carbonate has been reported to benefit some children (DeLong, 1978; Youngerman and Canino, 1978). Periodicity of mood disturbance and history of a beneficial response to lithium in a close family member suggest a relatively favorable outcome with lithium use in a child (see Case 15–4).

Antiandrogenic agents have been used effectively in treating some men with disorders of sexual aggression (Rubin *et al.*, 1981).

TABLE 15–3. **Selected Aspects of Treatment of Aggressive or Violent Behavior**

Systemic illness	Specific and/or symptomatic treatment
Catatonic excitement	Chloropromazine (Thorazine), haloperidol (Haldol), or phenobarbital
Acute psychosis	Phenothiazine, butyrophenone
Acute mania	Phenothiazine, butyrophenone (lithium for prophylaxis)
Sexually aggressive males	Antiandrogenic agents, propranolol (Inderal)
Temporal lobe epilepsy	Phenytoin (Dilantin), carbamazepine (Tegretol), phenobarbital, primidone (Mysoline), stereotaxic lesions of amygdala and other parts of temporal lobe
Episodic dyscontrol syndrome	Phenytoin (Dilantin)
Depression	Counseling; pharmacotherapy
Homicidal, suicidal behavior	Hospitalization; continuous supervision; removal of dangerous objects; physical and/or chemical restraint as necessary

Propranolol, a beta-adrenergic blocking agent, when given in high doses, appears promising in the treatment of rage and violent behavior. Yudofsky and colleagues (1981) described a strongly positive beneficial response to propranolol in daily doses of 320–520 milligrams in persons with a variety of neurologic disorders (posttraumatic encephalopathy, temporal lobe epilepsy, Wilson disease, and mental retardation) who had not responded to other drugs.

Neurologic Management. Carbamazepine (Tegretol), phenytoin (Dilantin), phenobarbital, and primidone (Mysoline) are drugs of choice in the treatment of temporal lobe seizures in childhood and adolescence. As noted above, aggressive and violent behavior is rarely, if ever, an ictal event. Such behavior might, however, occur during a postictal confusional state, when there is an altered state of consciousness. For that reason improved seizure control might be associated with improvement in behavior.

Treatment of adults with an episodic dyscontrol syndrome with anticonvulsant medication (usually phenytoin) may occasionally be beneficial even when clinical seizures have not been observed (Monroe, 1975; Pincus and Tucker, 1978).

Surgical Management. In a small group of severely disabled persons with seizure disorders whose aggressive and violent behavior has not responded to medical therapy, neurosurgical treatment involving placement of small brain lesions merits consideration. Stereotaxic lesions in the medial amygdala have benefited some epileptic children with severe aggressive behavioral disturbances (Narabayashi, 1977). Not only behavior but also seizure control improved among Narabayashi's patients. Preoperative symptoms in-

CASE 15–4: RAGE EPISODES AND ATTENTION DEFICIT DISORDER WITH MANIC SYMPTOMS IN A 16-YEAR-OLD GIRL

I.G. was evaluated because of longstanding behavior problems. She was considered hyperactive in elementary school and was treated briefly with methylphenidate. It was discontinued because of excessive sedation. Over the next several years hyperkinesis diminished while impulsivity and distractability persisted. In addition, she periodically had episodes of rage during which she described the feeling of adrenalin going through her body. She felt "paranoid" at these times of increased vigilance and sometimes struck out at persons or destroyed property. Rage episodes typically lasted for periods of several minutes to a few days. Past history included normal to accelerated development. Family history was positive for migraine and unipolar affective disorder (depression).

On examination, the young woman was an intelligent, articulate, and fidgety youngster. She had a high pressure of speech and was unable to stay more than briefly on a topic of conversation. General physical and neurologic examinations were normal. Pulse rate was 60 per minute. Deep tendon reflexes were normally active.

She was treated with lithium carbonate, and rage episodes diminished over several months. She found it increasingly possible to control herself and to walk away from provocative situations that otherwise would have been explosive. Her parents had their most tranquil months in years. Regular individual psychotherapy continued, while lithium blood levels, serum electrolytes, and thyroid function tests were closely followed.

Comment. This adolescent's behavior disturbance appeared to be an attention deficit disorder with features of unipolar (manic) affective disorder on a constitutional-familial basis. Indeed, she did have all the essential elements of a hyperkinetic child syndrome: hyperactivity, distractability, impulsivity, overexcitability, and dysphoria (see Chapter 14). Accordingly, she had been treated with methylphenidate, with negative effects. Because symptoms were of a depressive nature, she was tried on imipramine. It was not beneficial either. The positive response to lithium was described above.

The episodes of explosive rage had a striking adrenergic flavor to them, remarked upon by the young woman herself. For that reason, urine was collected for 24 hours for vanillylmandelic acid (VMA) to exclude further the unlikely possibility of pheochromocytoma, a catecholamine-secreting tumor.

cluded uncontrollable rage, explosive behavior, hyperexcitability, lability of mood, hyperactivity, and shortened attention span. Complications of temporal lobe destruction such as memory loss, sexual dysfunction, overly placid behavior, and appetite change were not found beyond several weeks after surgery.

Mark and Ervin (1970) also carried out temporal lobe surgery among selected patients with epilepsy and behavior disorders. The special diagnostic techniques employed (utilizing electrodes implanted within the temporal lobes) and treatment (selective destruction of portions of the temporal lobe) are discussed more fully in the section on CORRELATION: PHYSIOLOGIC ASPECTS.

Psychotherapy. When aggressive behavior stems from ineffective limit-setting, counseling of parents in child management should be undertaken.

Play therapy may also be of benefit. Acting out aggressive feelings with toys in a therapeutic setting provides a more acceptable mode of expression for the child than such activity directed against people. It may further provide useful insights into why aggressive behavior has been pursued (for example, sibling jealousy or anger due to separation).

The treatment of depression, which often underlies aggressive behavior, is discussed in Chapter 6.

Social-Environmental Management. Several general measures merit consideration in the social-environmental management of the aggressive or violent child. Guns, knives, pills, and other potentially injurious agents should be removed from the home or made otherwise inaccessible to the child. Jealous older children must be supervised and not left alone with infants.

Behavior modification can play a significant role in the management of children with aggressive and violent behavior. Positive reinforcement of acceptable behavior is coupled with consistent nonresponse to disruptive conduct or other unacceptable behavior. Such a program of behavior modification should be pursued not only in the classroom but at home as well so that gains can be carried over throughout the day and from one day to the next.

When behavior is so violent that injury to self or others is likely or has already occurred, hospitalization on an emergency basis is required. Careful and continuous observation by trained personnel will be an essential part of the inpatient treatment plan. Physical and/or chemical restraint should be used as needed to prevent damage to the child, other persons, or surroundings. Management of the suicidal child is discussed in Chapter 6.

CORRELATION

Anatomic Aspects. Two C-shaped groups of structures making a limbic circuit were described in CORRELATION: ANATOMIC ASPECTS in Chapter 5. A third "limbic C" appears to play a major role in aggressive and violent behavior. This C is made up of the stria terminalis, an efferent bundle from the amygdala to the septal nuclei.

The amygdala is an almond-shaped structure lying deeply within each anterior temporal lobe close to the midline (see Fig. 15–1). Its name is taken from the Greek word for *almond*. Rather than being a homogeneous mass of cells, the amygdala includes some nine to fourteen cell groups that appear to be of different functional significance (Mark and Ervin, 1970).

The septal nuclei lie above the amygdala on each side. They are situated anteriorly within or near the walls of the septum pellucidum, which separates the right lateral ventricle from the left. Anteriorly, the diagonal band of Broca connects each amygdala with ipsilateral septal nuclei. The C of each side is thereby made into a complete loop. The loops are themselves connected by the anterior commissure, which joins right and left amygdalas.

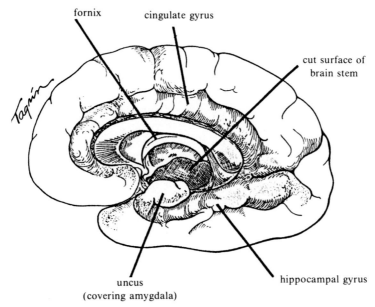

fornix   cingulate gyrus

cut surface of
brain stem

uncus   hippocampal gyrus
(covering amygdala)

FIGURE 15–1. Sagittal section of brain indicating position of
amygdala. (From Mark, V. H., and Ervin, F. R. *Violence and the
Brain*. Harper and Row, Publishers, Hagerstown, Md., 1970.)

The amygdala and the stria terminalis are areas targeted for stereotaxic
lesions in the neurosurgical treatment of violent behavior in persons with epilepsy (Mark and Ervin, 1970; Narabayashi, 1977).

The amygdala is also richly connected to the hypothalamus (Goldstein,
1974). The anatomic relationship between the amygdala and the hypothalamus (particularly the ventromedial and lateral nuclei) is reflected in emotional
and motivational aspects of eating behavior (see Chapter 10: CORRELATION).

Biochemical Aspects.   Clinical and experimental evidence has shown that
monoamines, cholinergic agents, and serotonin each play a role in aggressive and violent behavior (Goldstein, 1974). Epinephrine, a monoamine released peripherally by the adrenal medulla, causes a "fight or flight" response: tachycardia, elevated blood pressure, increased alertness, and
readiness for defense, attack, or fleeing. Centrally, norepinephrine appears
to play a major role in violent behavior. In animals operated upon to produce
rage behavior the intensity of rage display appears to be proportional to the
amount of norepinephrine released from brain. Rage behavior can be
blunted by drugs that inhibit central effects of norepinephrine.

Acetylcholine and other cholinergic drugs injected into the cerebral ventricles or directly into the hypothalamus or amygdala can produce anger and
rage. The importance of serotonin has been demonstrated in rats given septal lesions to produce spontaneous aggression; aggressive behavior is prevented by administration of parachlorophenylalanine, a drug that blocks the
first enzyme in production of serotonin from tryptophan (Cooper *et al.*,
1978).

Physiologic Aspects.   Experimental studies in animals and clinical investigations in man have elucidated the function of several portions of the brain involved in aggressive and violent behavior. Bard (1928) produced hypothalamic lesions in cats and thereby induced striking emotional reactions of rage. Further experimental work showed that lesions of the ventromedial nucleus of the hypothalamus could produce permanently ferocious animals (Pincus and Tucker, 1978). The opposite effect, rendering wild animals placid, was accomplished by resecting the anterior temporal lobes, including both amygdalas, bilaterally (Klüver and Bucy, 1939). Flynn (1969) demonstrated that electrical stimulation of the amygdala inhibited aggressive behavior associated with hypothalamic lesions.

In studies of persons with uncontrollably violent behavior and seizure disorders, Mark and Ervin (1970) implanted tiny wire electrodes into several sites within the amygdalas. Electrical activity from various portions of the amygdala could thus be recorded and correlated with observed behavior (such as aggressive activity and affective facial display) and with the patient's subjective experiences. These objective and subjective data were also elicited upon stimulation of selected portions of the amygdala directly or at a distance through radio signals. Depending upon the pathophysiologic-behavioral correlations, electrical destruction of small parts of brain could then be carried out.

One patient described by Mark and Ervin was a 34-year-old man with psychomotor seizures and episodes of violent behavior. He had apparently suffered asphyxic injury to his temporal lobes due to shock 14 years previously when a peptic ulcer had perforated. Episodes of rage typically were preceded by severe abdominal or facial pain. He would then take offense from an innocuous comment, brood over this "insult," argue, and reach a state of violent frenzy. This rage usually lasted 5 to 6 minutes and was followed by a brief nap that was fully refreshing. The man's rage episodes were unresponsive to psychoactive medications used individually or in combination. These included anticonvulsant and tranquilizing drugs. Subsequently, electrodes in the form of wire strands were implanted into the amygdalas and other portions of the temporal lobes, and they were used to localize further areas of electrical abnormality. Electrical stimulation of the amygdala in one area produced a typical complaint of pain and a feeling that he was losing control. Brief stimulation in another area terminated the pain and changed his mental state from one of brooding to relaxation. This relaxed state was maintained for 4 to 18 hours. Daily stimulation of this area kept the man free of rage attacks for nearly 2 months. After careful consideration and discussion involving the patient, it was decided to carry out neurosurgical destruction of the area of the amygdala that led to violent behavior when stimulated electrically. This procedure left the man free of rage episodes for at least the next 4 years, although occasionally he did have psychomotor seizures.

Based upon this case and others involving damaged brains, Mark and Ervin have placed emphasis upon "trigger areas" within the brain that can produce violent behavior in susceptible persons. They have drawn attention as well to brain mechanisms apparently involved in the suppression of violence, not just its production.

SUMMARY

Aggressive behavior, an intrinsic part of animal behavior, comes increasingly under voluntary control in man through maturation and socialization during childhood and adolescence. In some circumstances, however, primitive rage becomes expressed as violent behavior.

Several factors can contribute to aggressive and violent behavior in childhood. Medical conditions, by causing fatigue and irritability, can predispose to such behavior. Temporal lobe epilepsy has been associated with aggressive behavior, although the link between seizures, abnormal electrical activity of brain, and behavior disturbance awaits further delineation. Toxic influences include drugs used illicitly or by prescription. Affective disturbance (depression, anger, or anxiety) and psychosis are other causes of or contributors to aggression and violence. Family instability, poor supervision of jealous siblings, and ineffective limit-setting are social-environmental causes. Chromosomal and hormonal factors may also contribute to aggressive and violent behavior.

Treatment, often multifaceted, will depend upon the severity of the behavioral disturbance and its cause or causes. Outcome will vary accordingly.

CITED REFERENCES

Adelson, L. The battering child. *JAMA*, **222**: 159–61, 1972.

Bach-y-Rita, G.; Lion, J. R.; Climent, C. E.; and Ervin, F. R. Episodic dyscontrol: a study of 130 violent patients. *Am. J. Psychiatry*, **127**: 1473–78, 1971.

Bard, P. A diencephalic mechanism for the expression of rage with special reference to the sympathetic nervous system. *Am. J. Physiol.*, **84**: 490–513, 1928.

Cooper, J. R.; Bloom, F. E.; and Roth, R. H. *The Biochemical Basis of Neuropharmacology*, 3d ed. Oxford University Press, New York, 1978, p. 218.

Corning, C. H., and Corning, P. A. Biological aspects of aggressive behavior. Pp. 310–16 in *Comprehensive Textbook of Psychiatry*, 2d ed. Freedman, A. M.; Kaplan, H. I.; and Sadock, B. J., eds. Williams and Wilkins Co., Baltimore, 1975.

Delgado-Escueta, A. V.; Mattson, R. H.; King, L.; Goldensohn, E. S.; Spiegel, H.; Madsen, J.; Crandall, P.; Dreifuss, F.; and Porter, R. J. The nature of aggression during epileptic seizures. *N. Engl. J. Med.* **305**: 711–16, 1981.

DeLong, G. R. Lithium carbonate treatment of select behavior disorders in children suggesting manic-depressive illness. *J. Pediatr.*, **93**: 689–94, 1978.

Diagnostic and Statistical Manual of Mental Disorders, 3rd ed. American Psychiatric Association, Washington, D. C., 1980, pp. 45–50, 295–98, 317–21.

Ehrhardt, A. A., and Meyer-Bahlburg, H. F. L. Effects of prenatal sex hormones on gender-related behavior. *Science*, **211**: 1312–18, 1981.

Flynn, J. P. Neural aspects of attack behavior in cats. *Ann. N.Y. Acad. Sci.*, **159**: 1008–12, 1969.

Goldstein, M. Brain research and violent behavior: a summary and evaluation of the status of biomedical research on brain and aggressive violent behavior. *Arch. Neurol.*, **30**: 1–35, 1974.

Grumbach, M. M. Abnormalities of sex differentiation. P. 1709 in *Pediatrics*, 16th ed. Rudolph, A. M., ed. Appleton-Century-Crofts, New York, 1977.

Gunn, J. Epileptic homicide: a case report. *Br. J. Psychiatry*, **132:** 510–13, 1978.

Gunn, J., and Fenton, G. Epilepsy, automatism, and crime. *Lancet*, **1:** 1173–76, 1971.

Henn, F. A.; Bardwell, R.; and Jenkins, R. L. Juvenile delinquents revisited. *Arch. Gen. Psychiatry*, **37:** 1160–63, 1980.

Holinger, P. C. Violent deaths as a leading cause of mortality: an epidemiologic study of suicide, homicide, and accidents. *Am. J. Psychiatry*, **137:** 472–76, 1980.

Johnson, A. M. Sanctions for superego lacunae of adolescents. Pp. 225–45 in *Searchlights on Delinquency*. Eissler, K. R., ed. International Universities Press, Inc., New York, 1949.

Johnson, A. M., and Szurek, S. A. The genesis of antisocial acting out in children and adults. *Psychoanal. Q.*, **21:** 323–41, 1952.

Klüver, H., and Bucy, P. C. Preliminary analysis of functions of the temporal lobes in monkeys. *Arch. Neurol. Psychiatry*, **42:** 979–1000, 1939.

Kniveton, B. H., and Stephenson, G. M. The effects of an aggressive film model on social interaction in groups of middle-class and working-class boys. *J. Child Psychol. Psychiatry*, **16:** 301–13, 1975.

Krynicki, V. E. Cerebral dysfunction in repetitively assaultive adolescents. *J. Nerv. Ment. Dis.*, **166:** 59–67, 1978.

Lewis, D. O.; Shanok, S. S.; Pincus, J. H.; and Glaser, G. H. Violent juvenile delinquents: psychiatric, neurological, psychological, and abuse factors. *J. Am. Acad. Child Psychiatry*, **18:** 307–19, 1979.

Lindsay, J.; Ounsted, C.; and Richards, P. Long-term outcome in children with temporal lobe seizures: III. psychiatric aspects in childhood and adult life. *Dev. Med. Child Neurol.*, **21:** 630–36, 1979.

Luria, A. R., and Karasseva, T. A. Disturbances of auditory-speech memory in focal lesions of the deep regions of the left temporal lobe. *Neuropsychologia*, **6:** 97–104, 1968.

Mark, V. H., and Ervin, F. R. *Violence and the Brain*. Harper and Row, Publishers, Hagerstown, Md., 1970.

Mattsson, Å.; Schalling, D.; Olweus, D.; Löw, H.; and Svensson, J. Plasma testosterone, aggressive behavior, and personality dimensions in young male delinquents. *J. Am. Acad. Child Psychiatry*, **19:** 478–90, 1980.

Mendelson, J. H., and Mello, N. K. Biologic concomitants of alcoholism. *N. Engl. J. Med.*, **301:** 912–21, 1979.

Monroe, R. R. Anticonvulsants in the treatment of aggression. *J. Nerv. Ment. Dis.*, **160:** 119–26, 1975.

Narabayashi, H. Stereotaxic amygdalotomy for epileptic hyperactivity: long-range results in children. Pp. 319–31, in *Topics in Child Neurology*. Blaw, M. E.; Rapin, I.; and Kinsbourne, M., eds. Spectrum Publications, Inc., New York, 1977.

Ounsted, C.; Lindsay, J.; and Norman, R. M. *Biological Factors in Temporal Lobe Epilepsy*. Clinics in Developmental Medicine, No. 22, Spastics International Medical Publications, London, 1966.

Pincus, J. H. Can violence be a manifestation of epilepsy? *Neurology*, **30:** 304–7, 1980.

Pincus, J. H., and Tucker, G. J. Violence in children and adults. *J. Am. Acad. Child Psychiatry*, **17:** 277–88, 1978.

Plum, F., and Van Uitert, R. Non-endocrine diseases and disorders of the hypothalamus. Pp. 415–73, in *The Hypothalamus*. Reichlin, S.; Baldessarini, R. J.; and Martin, J. B., eds. Raven Press, New York, 1978.

Pritchard, P. B., III; Lombroso, C. T.; and McIntyre, M. Psychological complications of temporal lobe epilepsy. *Neurology* (Minneapolis), **30:** 227–32, 1980.

Report to the Surgeon General (Cisin, I. H., *et al.*). *Television and Growing Up: The Impact of Televised Violence.* U.S. Government Printing Office, Washington, D.C., 1972.

Rodin, E. A. Psychomotor epilepsy and aggressive behavior. *Arch. Gen. Psychiatry,* **28:** 210–13, 1973.

Rubin, R. T.; Reinisch, J. M.; and Haskett, R. F. Postnatal gonadal steroid effects on human behavior. *Science,* **211:** 1318–24, 1981.

Stores, G. Behavioural effects of anti-epileptic drugs. *Dev. Med. Child Neurol.,* **17:** 647–58, 1975.

Walzer, S.; Gerald, P. S.; and Shah, S. A. The XYY genotype. *Annu. Rev. Med.,* **29:** 563–70, 1978.

Werry, J. S., and Quay, H. C. The prevalence of behavior symptoms in younger elementary school children. *Amer. J. Orthopsychiatry,* **41:** 136–43, 1971.

Williams, D. Neural factors related to habitual aggression. *Brain,* **92:** 503–20, 1969.

Yalom, I. D.; Green, R.; and Fisk, N. Prenatal exposure to female hormones: effect on psychosexual development in boys. *Arch. Gen. Psychiatry,* **28:** 554–61, 1973.

Youngerman, J., and Canino, I. A. Lithium carbonate use in children and adolescents. *Arch. Gen. Psychiatry,* **35:** 216–24, 1978.

Yudofsky, S.; Williams, D.; and Gorman, J. Propranolol in the treatment of rage and violent behavior in patients with chronic brain syndromes. *Am. J. Psychiatry,* **138:** 218–20, 1981.

ADDITIONAL READINGS

Cannon, W. B. The emergency function of the adrenal medulla in pain and the major emotions. *Am. J. Physiol.,* **33:** 356–72, 1914.

Fields, W. S., and Sweet, W. H., eds. *Neural Bases of Violence and Behavior.* Warren H. Green, Inc. Saint Louis, 1975.

Green, M., and Solnit, A. J. Reactions to the threatened loss of a child: a vulnerable child syndrome. *Pediatrics,* **34:** 58–66, 1964.

MacLean, P. D. Contrasting functions of limbic and neocortical systems of the brain and their relevance to psychophysiological aspects of medicine. *Am. J. Med.,* **25:** 611–26, 1958.

Papez, J. W. A proposed mechanism of emotion. *Arch. Neurol. Psychiatry,* **38:** 725–43, 1937.

Pincus, J. H. Violence and epilepsy. *N. Engl. J. Med.,* **305:** 696–98, 1981.

Reinisch, J. M. Prenatal exposure to synthetic progestins increases potential for aggression in humans. *Science,* **211:** 1171–73, 1981.

Schachter, S., and Singer, J. E. Cognitive, social, and physiological determinants of emotional state. *Psychol. Rev.,* **69:** 379–99, 1962.

Stevens, J. R., and Hermann, B. P. Temporal lobe epilepsy, psychopathology, and violence: the state of the evidence. *Neurology* (New York), **31:** 1127–32, 1981.

16 Memory Disturbances

Memory is fundamental to learning and is involved in many other behaviors of childhood and adolescence as well. It is frequently the focus of complaints by parents and teachers and when it represents a change from previous levels of functioning, the question of degenerative disease often will be raised. Memory difficulties are commonly encountered with mental retardation, in which the acquisition of new information is chronically impaired. This chapter will look broadly at memory disturbances in childhood, considering its definition, neuroanatomic substrate, important biochemical factors, and specific syndromes in which memory is disordered. Several questions will be addressed:

Do primary memory disorders exist in childhood, or do memory problems occur only secondary to other difficulties?
What types of memory disturbance occur in children and adolescents?
What aspects of the history and examination suggest memory disturbance to be on an organic basis (for example, with petit mal seizures) as opposed to a functional basis (secondary to depression or anxiety)?
What office tests can be employed to evaluate memory?
What laboratory investigations are indicated in assessing the child with memory disturbance?
What conditions cause memory problems in childhood?
How are they treated and what is their outcome?

MEMORY DISTURBANCES

DEFINITION

Memory is essentially an informational storage mechanism of brain that allows for comparison of past data with present and future (anticipated) data. This process involves the feeding back of information from both internal and external sources to be matched with information stores already

456

within the central nervous system so that adjustment in behavior (posture, position, movement, language, or affect) can be made and the goal of behavior accomplished.

If one keeps this definition in mind, it is evident that memory plays a much more pervasive role in everyday life than one generally considers. For example, the position of a child's limbs at a given moment while climbing a tree must be recorded at least briefly so that this position may be compared with that anticipated according to visual, tactile, proprioceptive, and vestibular inputs. Storage and matching of information thus permit the successful climbing of one tree and provide for further successes when other trees are encountered because of the benefit of experiential memory.

Memory has been divided into functional categories: immediate, short-term, and long-term. Immediate memory depends largely upon attention and involves the registration of memory traces. Through the processes of repetition and rehearsal, these memory traces become consolidated to enter short-term memory. Immediate memory is familiar through everyday experience, as when one obtains a telephone number from the operator and retains that information long enough to dial it. Should dialing the number be delayed by several seconds and interfering stimuli (such as a pot boiling over) prevent repetition of the number, it usually will be lost. Once entering short-term memory (lasting hours to days), information is further consolidated and stored as long-term memory, available for use through the process of retrieval.

Amnesia refers to loss of memory. When an identifiable event such as head trauma or major illness has interfered with memory, it may be useful to categorize amnesia as anterograde (occurring after the event) or retrograde (occurring before the event). Anterograde amnesia can also be considered an inability to acquire new information, that is, to lay down new memories.

DIAGNOSIS

Clinical Process. *History.* The chief complaint should be recorded in the words of the child as well as the parent. A child might complain that "I always forget what I learn in school" or "I can't remember anything unless I write it down." The parents may remark, "She can't remember anything any more" or "His memory has always been poor and the school asked that he be evaluated."

The time course of the memory disturbance should be defined. Some children will never have been able to retain information well, and recent academic demands may have accentuated a long-standing problem. In other children, previously adequate or otherwise unremarkable memory may have given way to currently impaired recall. Precipitating incidents such as severe illness, significant head trauma, or major psychosocial stress (such as a death in the family, a move, or a divorce) should be sought.

In many children memory lapses are circumscribed and intermittent. Migraines or seizures thus are suggested. Associated or antecedent feelings such as déjà vu or of being in a dream, epigastric discomfort, a terrible smell, or "dizziness" will support either of these diagnostic possibilities. A history of loss (or alteration) of consciousness, abnormal movements (such as tonic-clonic movements, rhythmic eye-blinking, or other automatisms of behavior), and headache should be sought. It should be recalled (see Chapter 11) that in a migraine syndrome of childhood an aura can occur in the absence of headache.

Memory disturbance following head trauma can take several forms. Cerebral concussion, usually defined as posttraumatic loss of consciousness, is associated with several types of memory loss (amnesia). Some are transient, others permanent. The period of memory loss for events occurring prior to impact (retrograde amnesia) generally shrinks considerably within minutes to hours after head injury (Benson and Geschwind, 1967). The period immediately preceding impact in most instances is forever lost to recall. Hence the person is said to have a permanent retrograde amnesia. This memory loss, even though brief, can be upsetting to children, who may behave as if something has been taken away from them.

The most striking form of memory deficit following concussive head injury is anterograde amnesia. This amnesia is manifested by an inability over the minutes to hours following the injury to learn new material. For example, the head-injured child will ask the same question repeatedly even though the question has been answered repeatedly. For example, a 9-year-old boy who had lost consciousness for 3 minutes asked his mother a dozen times in 10 minutes, "Where's Dad?" Though the child had recovered consciousness promptly, his mother feared that her son had lost completely his ability to remember anything. In characteristic fashion, however, the boy regained the ability to acquire new information within 24 hours.

In assessing the child with a memory disturbance, it is important to exclude problems of hearing, attention, or comprehension. Hearing difficulty will be suggested by unresponsiveness to sounds, speaking in a loud voice, and sometimes faulty comprehension. Attentional problems can occur as part of a hyperkinetic syndrome that may include impulsivity and excitability (see Chapter 14). Understanding may be impaired with receptive language disorder or with more global cognitive impairment (see Chapters 17 and 18).

If change in personality and loss of previously acquired functions accompany memory disturbance, a syndrome of behavioral regression should be considered (see Chapter 8).

Past history should include inquiry as to seizures (generalized or partial), medications (including those used for control of seizures or taken without prescription), and major illnesses.

Psychosocial data should include the following considerations. The home environment may be so noisy that focusing upon schoolwork and mastering new material is impossible. Sleep may be disturbed so that drowsiness and inattentiveness interfere with learning. Recent stresses may have caused or contributed to depression or anxiety.

Examination. The *general description* should note the most striking aspects of the child's appearance and behavior. Is he distractable and hyperactive? Is he depressed or anxious? Do flickering facial movements, a suddenly slackened jaw, rhythmic blinking, or episodes of staring suggest absence seizures?

The *general physical examination* should seek to identify systemic illness that might cause fatigue, irritability, and inattentiveness. The pulse and weight should be recorded and the neck examined to estimate the size and consistency of the thyroid gland. The head should be examined for evidence of trauma.

The *neurologic examination* should include visualization of the optic disks to exclude papilledema. Focal neurologic signs should be sought. Hyperventilation is a useful provocative technique in children with suspected petit mal or other absence seizures. Since memory loss may be but one sign of a progressive neurologic disorder, other evidence of neurologic dysfunction—such as visual loss, weakness, and ataxia—should also be sought.

Testing of memory should include evaluation of immediate, short-term, and long-term memory functions (see Table 16–1). Immediate memory ("registration") is tested by the child's recall of digits presented at one-second intervals. Three repetitions by the examiner may be given. A 6-year-old child should be able to repeat four or five digits forward, a 9-year-old five or six digits, a 12-year-old six or seven. Attention can also be assessed by having the child count backward from 100 or name the months in reverse order. Immediate memory can be tested further by having the child repeat increasingly complex sentences or story paragraphs.

Short-term memory (the ability to learn new information) can be evaluated by asking the child what he or she ate for breakfast or lunch that day. More formal testing can involve the child's recall of three or four unrelated objects 5 to 10 minutes after presentation. The younger school-age child will generally be able to name two of three objects. The third may be recalled with assistance; that is, given a choice of items, the child is able to identify the missing one.

The ability to repeat a short story after 5 to 10 minutes can also be used to test short-term memory. A standard tale is "the fishing story," containing some twelve bits of information: "Tom and Bill went fishing. It was a beautiful Sunday. They each caught three black bass and rode home on their bicycles to have the fish for lunch."

A paired word test is another means of evaluating short-term memory (Strub and Black, 1977). Four word pairs are presented in whole or in part a

TABLE 16–1. **Memory Testing**

Immediate Memory	Digit span (1 digit per second)
	Immediate repetition of sentences or short story
Short-Term Memory	Recall of three or four objects after 5 or 10 minutes
	Repetition of short story after 5 or 10 minutes
	Paired-word test
	Hidden object test
	Drawing of geometric figures briefly presented
Long-Term Memory	Recall of past experiences and events (such as birthdays, holidays, major news stories)

total of three times. Two pairs are closely related: e.g., shoe-heel, pants-pocket. Two are not obviously related: e.g., table-automobile, sink-rug. After all four word pairs have been read, the first word only of each pair is presented in a different order and 5 seconds allowed for completion of each pair. Following this first testing, a second presentation (in yet another order) is carried out and recall tested.

An adult normally will recall accurately both closely related pairs and one of the two other pairs upon the first trial. All four pairs should be recalled upon the second trial. Although norms for children are not described, this technique may nonetheless prove useful in assessing their short-term memory function.

Short-term memory can be evaluated nonverbally by the hidden object test (Strub and Black, 1977). The examiner hides three or four small objects (such as a comb, paper clip, pencil, and watch) while the person is watching. He is then requested to locate all objects after 5 to 10 minutes. Other nonverbal techniques of assessing short-term memory include drawing geometric figures that have been briefly presented visually.

Long-term, or remote, memory can be evaluated by having children describe events from summer vacations, recall presents received on their birthdays, recall major news stories, or name their classroom teachers of previous years.

Mental status examination should include specific attention to mood and affect, particularly anxiety or depression.

Investigation.   The history and examination may suggest specific areas for investigation (see Table 16–2). The possibility of chronic illness, suggested by fatigue, weight loss, and recurrent fevers, may prompt evaluation of the genitourinary and gastrointestinal tracts. If evidence of increased intracranial pressure has been found, plain radiography of the skull and cranial CT scan should be carried out. With a possible seizure disorder, electroencephalography is essential. Recording in the awake state with 3 to 4 minutes of hyperventilation included in the tracing will usually detect petit mal epilepsy. Audiometry and tympanometry should be carried out in order to ex-

TABLE 16–2. **Investigations to Be Considered in the Child with Memory Disturbance**

Toxic screen of blood and urine
Thyroid function tests
Psychologic testing (psychometric, projective)
Specific memory testing
Audiometry and tympanometry
EEG (in sleep and awake states, including hyperventilation)
Skull x-rays
Cranial CT scan
CSF examination, including measurement of immunoglobulins and measles antibody titers
Adrenal function tests

clude hearing deficit. When attention and immediate memory are affected most prominently, thyroid function tests (T_4, T_3 uptake, thyroid index, and TSH) should be considered. If drug effects are suspected, toxicologic analysis of blood and/or urine should be carried out. If a degenerative disorder such as subacute sclerosing panencephalitis or adrenoleukodystrophy is being considered, examination of cerebrospinal fluid with measurement of measles antibody titers and immunoglobulins for the former and adrenal function tests for the latter should be pursued.

Formal psychologic testing should be carried out when memory deficit appears to be part of a syndrome of intellectual decline (dementia). Such testing will be especially valuable when it is compared with results obtained at other times. When anxiety or depression appears to contribute to memory disturbance, projective testing (in conjunction with psychometric testing) can be helpful in differentiating affective disturbance from dementia.

Memory evaluation can be pursued formally through the use of specifically designed tests. These include the Benton Visual Retention Test (Benton, 1974), Wechsler Memory Scale (Wechsler and Stone, 1973), Supraspan Digit Storage Test (Drachman and Leavitt, 1974), Free Recall Word Storage Test (Drachman and Leavitt, 1974), and the "selective reminding" and "restricted reminding" techniques of Buschke and Fuld (1974).

Differential Diagnosis. Hearing deficit and receptive language disorder must be differentiated from memory disturbance. What the child cannot hear or understand, he surely will not be able to remember.

Hearing deficit will be suggested through whisper, watch tick, and finger-rubbing tests. When hearing impairment is definite, suggested, or equivocal on office testing, formal audiologic assessment is indicated. It can characterize further the hearing impairment (if any) in terms of sound frequencies involved and degree of hearing loss. Tympanometry should be part of the audiologic evaluation to exclude middle ear disease.

With *receptive language disorder,* testing of memory and repetition will be difficult to carry out because of the child's problems in comprehension of language.

Auditory sequencing difficulties should be distinguished from memory deficit *per se,* although they may be considered a form of memory disturbance. Formal testing through the Illinois Test of Psycholinguistic Abilities (ITPA) can be useful in defining a problem in auditory sequencing.

Etiology (see Table 16–3). *Medical Causes.* Intercurrent *medical illness* may be associated with fatigue, anxiety, and depression that interfere with attention, motivation, remembering, and learning. Many disorders could cause these symptoms, and they need not be enumerated exhaustively here. A few merit specific mention, however. Gastrointestinal disorders such as ulcerative colitis or regional enteritis (Crohn disease) may be insidious in onset and progression. *Thyroid disorder* (hypo- or hyperthyroidism) can also be associated with disturbances in memory and learning. With these or other medical problems (such as asthma or anticipation of surgery), memory may be impaired because of secondary anxiety or depression (see Case 16–1).

Neurologic Causes. Head trauma is a common cause for memory disturbance in children. Memory disturbance is typically associated with loss of

TABLE 16–3. **Causes of Memory Disturbance**

Medical	Chronic systemic illness causing fatigue or apathy
	Hypo- or hyperthyroidism
Neurologic	Head trauma
	Attention deficit disorder
	Seizures (particularly petit mal seizures, complex partial seizures)
	Migraine (including confusional and basilar artery forms)
	Increased intracranial pressure (from tumor or other cause)
	Sleep disturbance (causing daytime hypersomnolence)
	Mental subnormalcy
	Autism
	Dementia (as with subacute sclerosing panencephalitis, adrenoleukodystrophy, ceroid lipofuscinosis, multiple sclerosis)
	Thiamine deficiency
	Leigh disease
	Herpes simplex encephalitis
	Temporal lobe damage (due to tumor, abscess, trauma, hemorrhage, infarction)
	Electroconvulsive therapy
Toxic	Antihistamines, anticonvulsants, or sedatives causing drowsiness
	Scopolamine
	Flashbacks following hallucinogen use or with seizure
Psychologic	Anxiety
	Depression
	Hysteria
	Conflict
Social-Environmental	Excessive noise
	Overstimulation

consciousness, but amnesia can occur when loss of consciousness has not resulted from head trauma (Fisher, 1966; Yarnell and Lynch, 1970 and 1973). These effects have been attributed to torsion of the upper brainstem, temporal lobes, and associated vascular structures as a consequence primarily of rotational accelerative influences upon the brain (Ommaya and Gennarelli, 1975).

Characteristic retrograde and anterograde amnesias were described above (see HISTORY). The reversibility of most of the retrograde amnesia implies that this memory deficit involves failure of retrieval of available information rather than disruption of registration or dissolution of previously formed memory traces (Benson and Geschwind, 1967). Anterograde amnesia, by contrast, appears to result from interference with consolidation.

CASE 16–1: MEMORY DISTURBANCE AND POOR SCHOOL PERFORMANCE IN AN 11-YEAR-OLD GIRL WITH THYROID DYSFUNCTION

K.N., a sixth-grade student, complained of "forgetting" for several months. She and her parents dated the onset of school problems to 1 month after treatment with thyroid hormone had begun. The diagnosis of hypothyroidism had been established 8 months previously based upon symptoms of obesity and apathy. Blood tests confirmed the clinical diagnosis.

Since thyroid hormone treatment was begun, her grades in school deteriorated from A's to C's. Her drawing ability, previously above average and a source of considerable pleasure for her, worsened as well. When asked to carry out a simple task such as getting something from a table, she would return empty-handed several minutes later and not recall the request. Teachers noted a decline in both the amount and the quality of her schoolwork. On a positive note, while on thyroid replacement therapy she lost 30 pounds, found it no longer necessary to watch her diet, and became much more outgoing. Past history was unremarkable.

On examination, the child was a pleasant, attentive girl without evident anxiety or depression. She was able to repeat seven digits forward and recall four of four objects after 20 minutes. Remote memory (tested by having her recall Christmas presents she received the previous year) was also normal. General physical examination showed a resting pulse of 93 per minute. Her eyes were not proptotic. The thyroid gland was neither enlarged nor tender. Neurologic examination was normal except for mild proximal weakness as evidenced by difficulty in walking up stairs two steps at a time. With her arms outstretched, no tremor was seen.

Investigations included thyroid function tests, which were mildly elevated. An electroencephalogram in the awake state was normal. The child was seen in endocrinologic consultation, and it was recommended that her dosage of thyroid medication be diminished slightly. On a reduced amount of thyroid hormone, school work and drawing ability improved; proximal muscle weakness disappeared; and dietary discretion became necessary once again.

Comment. Development of either hypothyroidism or hyperthyroidism may be associated with personality change, alteration in weight, and deterioration in school performance. In this case replacement with thyroid medication appeared to produce a mildly hyperthyroid state associated with diminished attention and haste in carrying out school assignments.

Often with the return to a euthyroid state, a previously quiet, "good" hypothyroid child is replaced by a more normal, sometimes mischievous youngster who may catch the teacher's attention because of uncharacteristically poor performance. In this case the child's personality change was decidedly for the better and was associated with weight loss that made her feel better about herself. Although pleased about the loss of pounds, she was unhappy about her loss of drawing skill. Adjustment of her dosage of thyroid medication allowed for an acceptable compromise.

463

Head trauma does not usually produce severe ongoing memory disturbance unless bilateral temporal lobe damage has occurred (see CORRELATION: ANATOMIC ASPECTS). On the other hand, damage to the dominant (usually left) temporal lobe has been implicated in significant disturbances in auditory memory (Luria and Karasseva, 1968).

Attention deficit disorder, with or without hyperkinesis, is another common and important cause of memory difficulties (see Chapter 14). With attentional problems, the first step in the memory process, registration, is interfered with; subsequent steps (consolidation, storage, and retrieval) become impaired or impossible. Associated dysphoria (primary or secondary) and learning disability frequently compound the child's school difficulties.

Seizures are an important consideration in the child with memory deficit. "Daydreaming" episodes in the classroom, during which the child has no recollection of ongoing events, should suggest petit mal or partial complex seizures. Such seizures may be so brief or subtle as to escape detection (see Chapter 12).

Petit mal seizures are defined electroencephalographically by three-per-second spike-and-wave complexes. Clinically, they are characterized by several seconds of staring with associated rhythmic eye-blinking. Partial complex seizures, or psychomotor seizures, are generally associated with somewhat longer periods of staring (15 to 30 seconds) and semipurposeful behaviors such as lip-smacking, chewing, or picking at the clothes. After typical petit mal seizures, the child is usually able to resume activities promptly. Psychomotor seizures, however, are often followed by a brief state of disorientation, and sometimes by agitation or lethargy (see Table 12–2).

With generalized seizures of the grand mal type, the child will have memory loss for the duration of the seizure and for the period of postictal confusion or lethargy as well, when new memories cannot be formed.

Migraine syndromes of childhood and adolescence can be associated with several kinds of memory disturbance: amnesia, forced reminiscence, and the illusion of memory (such as déjà vu) (see Chapter 11). Amnesia is characteristic of confusional migraine and is, of course, associated with loss of consciousness occurring as part of a basilar artery migraine syndrome. Forced reminiscence, involuntary "playback" of brief stretches of memory, can occur as a migraine aura that precedes a headache or may occur independently of headache (see Case 16–2).

Brain tumor or other cause of increased intracranial pressure may be associated with memory deficit on a specific or relatively nonspecific basis. The former can be seen with tumors that involve the limbic system. These include tumors in the area of the third ventricle and in the hippocampal portions of the temporal lobes (Adams, 1969; Muramoto *et al.,* 1979) (see CORRELATION: ANATOMIC ASPECTS). Relatively nonspecific effects of increased intracranial pressure include inattention, lethargy, and irritability. Any or all of these symptoms can interfere significantly with memory and learning.

Any form of *hypersomnia* (such as a sleep apnea syndrome) will impair memory functions since it interferes with arousal and attention (see Chapter 9).

Mental retardation implies an associated memory deficit, which reflects or underlies a global inability to learn (see Chapter 18).

Memory disturbance in *autism* is striking, as is well known to those who have endeavored to teach something new to an autistic child. These children learn in an extraordinarily concrete manner, and their learning is not readily transferrable to other situations. On the other hand, the insistence of autistic children upon sameness implies a very precise memory for certain aspects of their physical and social environments. Changes within these contexts are met with anxiety and tantrums, as if widespread and irrevocable destruction threatens to take place. These disturbances in memory and behavior are among the clinical features of autism that indicate involvement of the limbic system, particularly the temporal lobes (see Chapter 5).

Dementia, the loss of intellectual function, usually includes memory disturbance, which may be the first sign of a degenerative neurologic disorder (see Chapter 8). Typical examples in the school-age child would be subacute sclerosing panencephalitis (SSPE), adrenoleukodystrophy, and ceroid lipofuscinosis, which are associated with dementia and personality change. Multiple sclerosis, which characteristically involves multiple sites of demyelination and subsequent scarring (plaque formation) within the central nervous system, may also be associated with memory deficit. Alternatively, intercurrent illness or depressive reaction should be considered to cause or contribute to memory problems in persons with multiple sclerosis.

Thiamine deficiency is an important cause of memory deficit in adults. It is typically associated with the Wernicke-Korsakoff syndrome in alcoholics (Adams, 1969). This syndrome involves a retrograde amnesia and a striking anterograde amnesia: an inability to acquire new information. This failure to lay down new memories is permanent, in contrast to that occurring in some children who have suffered head trauma (see above). With Wernicke-Korsakoff syndrome digit span will usually be normal, but if the examiner leaves the room for a few minutes and returns, the patient will not recall having met him. The tendency of persons with Wernicke-Korsakoff syndrome to provide answers to questions despite their severely impaired memory is termed confabulation.

Thiamine deficiency in childhood and adolescence is uncommon. It has been described secondary to incomplete artificial formulas in infancy (Cochrane *et al.,* 1961). It is possible that a restricted diet taken for purposes of weight loss (with anorexia nervosa, for example) might lead to clinically significant thiamine deficiency (see Chapter 10). Such should be suspected in any malnourished child with memory deficit or confusional state.

Deficiency of thiamine has been implicated clinically, biochemically, and neuropathologically in *Leigh disease* (subacute necrotizing encephalomyelopathy) (Sipe, 1973; Plaitakis *et al.,* 1980). The disorder has been linked with a factor in body fluids (urine, blood, and cerebrospinal fluid) that blocks the formation of thiamine triphosphate (see Chapter 8). Memory functions *per se* have not been detailed in reported cases, although intellectual subnor-

CASE 16–2: MEMORY DISTURBANCE (FORCED REMINISCENCE) IN A 9-YEAR-OLD GIRL WITH MIGRAINE

K.B. experienced headaches two or three times weekly for nearly 6 months. They were preceded by "dizzy spells." The headaches were not severe: 5 to 10 minutes of bitemporal aching relieved by aspirin and rest. The dizzy spells consisted of 20–30 seconds during which she said, "I can't control my thinking." The content of thought for each of these episodes was not itself stereotyped but, rather, was a recapitulation of actual events from the day before. Preceding other headaches she experienced difficulty reading. At such times she indicated that she could see the words but "they didn't make sense to me." These episodes frightened her. On several occasions she ran to her mother fearing that she was losing her mind. Still other headaches were preceded by tingling and numbness around her nose.

Past medical history was unremarkable. Mother suffered from severe headaches as a child that were preceded by numbness of the lips and tongue. The family was in the process of moving out of the state at the time of neurologic evaluation.

On examination, the child was a serious and thoughtful girl of normal intelligence, who did not appear depressed or anxious. General physical and neurologic examinations were normal. EEG was normal.

She was diagnosed as having a classic migraine syndrome with amnestic, aphasic, and paresthetic auras. Headaches appeared to be provoked by social and familial stresses. Treatment included mild analgesia with rest at times of headaches. The nature of migraine auras and headaches was explained to the child and her parents. She was reassured that her problem had a name (migraine) and that she was not losing her mind. Further discussion

malcy is characteristic of persons with subacute and chronic forms of the disease.

Herpes simplex *encephalitis* is a well-established cause of persistent and severe memory loss (Bell and McCormick, 1975; Peters and Levin, 1977). The infecting organism, herpesvirus hominis (type I), has a predilection for the temporal lobes, whose involvement can cause acute psychosis and memory impairment. Typical presenting features include fever, vomiting, convulsions (focal or generalized), and memory disturbance. Acute disturbances in mental state also include restlessness, irritability, hyperactivity, disorientation, and hallucinations. Such symptoms frequently suggest an intracranial mass lesion. Herpetic lesions ("fever blisters") on the face or buccal mucosa may be absent.

In general *temporal lobe damage,* particularly if bilateral, will result in memory dysfunction. Tumor, abscess, hemorrhage, or infarction can cause such lesions. Hemorrhage can occur secondary to head trauma or hematologic disorder such as platelet deficiency associated with leukemia. Occlusion of the posterior cerebral arteries (as can occur with herniation of the

about the impending move was recommended and additional visits to their new home were suggested. Because unresolved issues between the parents appeared to contribute to their daughter's headaches, psychiatric consultation was recommended. Soon after neurologic assessment, the memory problem and other migrainous disturbances ceased, and the move occurred without incident.

Comment. The diagnosis of migraine was suggested by headaches (even though they were not pounding) preceded by several kinds of auras. The memory disturbance, which took the form of forced reminiscence, was especially interesting. This aura was stereotyped not in content but in form. Memories from a fixed, specific time in the past and of a specific duration were replayed as if a "memory cassette" had been plugged in to the present.

Seizure disorder (of temporal lobe origin) was another diagnostic consideration here because of the recurrent episodes of forced reminiscence. The multiplicity of sensory disturbances, the characteristic sequence of events including headache, and the normal EEG helped to exclude this possibility.

The striking improvement in symptoms emphasizes the value of explanatory counseling and supportive therapy. This case further illustrates the importance of understanding exactly what the child means by such phrases as "dizzy spells" or statements that "words didn't make sense" (see Case 16–3).

Disturbances of memory such as occurred in this case do not necessarily imply migraine. They may occur (relatively infrequently) as part of normal experience, or they may represent focal epileptic symptoms suggesting temporal lobe origin.

brain) can cause infarction of the hippocampi, resulting in profound memory deficit.

Electroconvulsive therapy (ECT) produces a characteristic memory disturbance (Cronholm, 1969). It is manifested by total amnesia for the period of unconsciousness during the time of electrical stimulation of brain and for the confusional period immediately following. In addition, a brief period of retrograde amnesia and a patchy anterograde memory loss occur. The mechanism for memory disturbance is unknown but appears to involve interference with consolidation of immediate into short-term memory.

Toxic Causes. Memory disturbance due to toxic causes is probably most often associated with the sedative effects of medication. Antihistamines, for example, frequently used in the treatment of allergies and upper respiratory symptoms, often cause drowsiness. Anticonvulsant medication, particularly phenobarbital, may cause sedation, especially during the first several days of use (MacLeod *et al.*, 1978). Later drowsiness should lead one to suspect overdosage, which can be confirmed by determining anticonvulsant blood levels.

Scopolamine, also known as hyoscine, has been found to impair short-term memory specifically (Safer and Allen, 1971; Crow, 1979). It has, in fact, been used to study memory processes in man (see CORRELATION: BIOCHEMICAL ASPECTS). Scopolamine is closely related to atropine, which competitively inhibits the widely distributed neurotransmitter acetylcholine. Scopolamine has often been used for obstetric purposes since it typically induces an amnestic state of "twilight sleep" (Weiner, 1980). In addition to amnesia it causes drowsiness, sleep, and euphoria. Restlessness, excitement, and hallucinations may also occur. Scopolamine is found in some over-the-counter drug preparations, including sedative and anti–motion sickness preparations.

Flashbacks are memories, characteristically with visual, auditory, and affective content, that can follow usually unpleasant drug-related experiences (Zeidenberg, 1973). These may occur after marijuana or other psychoactive drug use. Their pathophysiologic basis is not understood. Less commonly, a flashback may occur as a manifestation of focal seizure suggesting temporal lobe origin. For example, Penfield and Rasmussen (1950) described a girl who suffered frightening, stereotyped reminiscences of being scared by a stranger in a park, an experience that had actually happened several years earlier. The episodes of recollection sometimes preceded a motor seizure. Surgery disclosed a scar affecting the meninges and temporal lobe cortex that appeared to stem from earlier-life brain injury.

Psychologic Causes.   Anxiety and depression are important causes of memory disturbance in childhood and adolescence (see Case 16–3).

Anxiety, manifested by apprehension, fidgeting, tachycardia, and increased perspiration, among other signs, generally occurs in anticipation of loss or change. The anxious person is characteristically unfocused and inattentive. Depression, on the other hand, can be described as reaction to loss (see Chapter 6). With depression, a brooding person is overfocused and inattentive. Since depression often occurs in reaction to physical illness and disability, memory and learning can be further impaired because of fatigue and pain.

Conflict frequently underlies ordinary forgetting, as Freud (1904) described in the *Psychopathology of Everyday Life*. By encouraging the person with a memory "block" to say the first word that comes to mind, by following this word through associative techniques, and by understanding the context in which the memory lapse occurred, it is often possible to determine the apparent reason why the word was prevented from reaching consciousness more directly. Hysterical memory loss presumably involves similar psychologic mechanisms.

Social-Environmental Causes.   A noisy, stimulus-laden environment may overwhelm the child's capabilities to attend and to remember. If, for example, the child's study area overlooks a busy street or siblings pass by continually distracting the child, attention will certainly suffer and, with it, memory for tasks at hand. In these circumstances not only registration but rehearsal is interfered with so that both immediate and short-term memory are impaired.

Genetic-Constitutional Causes.   In some circumstances memory prob-

CASE 16–3: DIZZY SPELLS AND MEMORY DIFFICULTIES IN A 13-YEAR-OLD GIRL WITH DEPRESSION

L.L. was evaluated because of "dizzy spells" which had begun 2 years previously and were becoming longer. Episodes lasted up to 3 hours and were associated with derealization ("It's like I'm dreaming and I'm not really there"). She acknowledged feeling depressed and thinking about jumping from a tall building or throwing herself in front of a car, but she denied making such plans or attempts. When a dizzy spell occurred during cheerleading practice, she forgot completely where she was in the routine. Schoolwork had not deteriorated. Past medical history was unremarkable. Social and family history was negative for depressive illness or suicide. Psychosocial history disclosed no recent stresses of significance.

On examination, the girl was a pleasant, well-groomed adolescent with flattened facial expression. She maintained a somewhat unfocused expression of her eyes and spoke with diminished intensity of speech. Digit span and recall of three objects after 5 minutes were normal. General physical and neurologic examinations were normal.

Comment. This adolescent was clearly depressed, which could amply account for the memory difficulties she experienced. It was unclear what was causing the depressive syndrome, and referral for psychiatric diagnostic evaluation was made. Suicide was discussed openly with both child and parent, and precautions (such as ensuring that weapons and unnecessary medicines be removed from the home) were reviewed. As with Case 16–2, this case illustrates the importance of understanding exactly what the child means by such expressions as "dizzy spells" or "blurry vision."

lems can be attributed to intrinsic or constitutional causes that may affect other family members as well (see Case 16–4)

Developmental Causes. One can postulate a developmental form of memory dysfunction analogous to other developmental disorders of childhood. Memory, like other functions (motor, language, and cognitive), grows and becomes increasingly useful with age. Within the first 3 years of life, for example, memory develops as language and other capabilities evolve. As one result a child becomes better able to tolerate separation from parents because of knowledge gained through experience, particularly the memory that the parent has returned in similar circumstances in the past. A lag in memory functions such that memory was at an earlier developmental level while other skills were more appropriate for chronologic age would constitute a specific developmental disorder of memory. Attention deficit disorder might be included within this category of developmental memory disorder.

Treatment and Outcome

Memory disturbances in childhood and adolescence range from the benign and self-limited (as with a posttraumatic Korsakoff syndrome) to the permanent and severe (for example, following *Herpes simplex* encephalitis).

CASE 16–4: SHORT-TERM MEMORY DYSFUNCTION AND LEARNING DISABILITY IN AN 8-YEAR-OLD BOY

I.E. was evaluated because of language difficulties, memory problems, and poor school performance. Past history was unremarkable in terms of pregnancy and birth. He spoke in word combinations between 3 and 4 years of age. Family history was notable only for a maternal cousin who was mentally retarded.

On examination, the child was initially shy, withdrawn, and fidgety. He soon relaxed somewhat, although he volunteered little speech under any circumstance. He did not know the month or the year, nor could he recite the days of the week. He could not provide his telephone number or street address. He was unable to read a first-grade-level story. Digit span was only four forward. He was unable to carry out three-part commands, nor was he able to recall the month 5 minutes after it was told to him. Figure drawings were richly detailed without being bizarre. He was able to print his first name crudely.

General physical examination was unremarkable. Elemental neurologic examination was notable only for brisk, symmetric deep tendon reflexes and extensor plantar responses. He was right-handed.

Investigation included formal psychologic testing, which demonstrated intelligence in the low-normal range. CT scan suggested absence of the usual asymmetry between left and right parieto-occipital portions of the cerebrum. The left was no larger than the corresponding part on the right.

Treatment is essentially symptomatic, generally directed at associated problems such as intercurrent illness or affective disorder (see Table 16–4). With attentional disorders, pharmacotherapy can benefit memory dysfunction. With other memory disorders, clinical trials with physostigmine, vasopressin and its analogues, and other neuroactive peptides indicate exciting future directions for therapy (see CORRELATION: BIOCHEMICAL ASPECTS).

Medical Management.   Treatment of intercurrent medical illness that has interfered with memory through systemic effects can be expected to result in improvement of memory functions, reversing the process that produced the deficit.

In children with attention deficit disorders, treatment with dextroamphetamine (Dexedrine) or methylphenidate (Ritalin) has been demonstrated to improve memory and learning (see Chapter 14). In employing these medications, one must be careful not to use them in excessively high dosage, for at a dosage level of methylphenidate that diminishes motor overactivity, cognitive gains seen at lower dosage levels may be lost.

Neurologic Management.   With posttraumatic memory deficit, treatment is essentially supportive. Acute complications of head injury such as

Comment. This boy had an extraordinarily severe learning problem with difficulties in both language and memory. If his drawing skills had not been unusually good and if formal psychometric testing had not demonstrated normal ability in nonverbal tasks, he might have been misdiagnosed as globally mentally retarded.

His deficits in immediate and short-term memory were especially striking. He was unable to repeat more than four digits forward and could not remember a single item after 5 minutes. This performance was puzzling, as he did not seem unusually distractable and appeared to be trying very hard. Perhaps he had learned how to look attentive (with appropriate orientation of body, head, and eyes) despite impaired cerebral processing. Another possible explanation for his difficulty with digits and other sequences would be that he had a specific deficit in auditory sequential memory.

The primary thrust of management has been special education individually suited to the child's needs. His parents had always encouraged him in areas of relative strength, and they were supported in continuing these efforts.

The CT scan provided visual evidence for the presumed organic basis of this child's problems. In most right-handed persons, the left hemisphere is larger than the right in its parieto-occipital dimensions and is dominant for language (and memory). In this right-handed child loss of the usual asymmetry was seen, a finding reported in several conditions involving language disorder, namely autism and dyslexia.

In this case it was presumed because of an essentially negative past history that constitutional and perhaps familial factors accounted for the child's syndrome. The significance of the extensor plantar responses is unclear.

seizures or intracranial hemorrhage should be identified and treated promptly. The retrograde amnesia associated with cerebral concussion shrinks considerably, although the child is left with a small mnemonic lacune, which includes the time of impact. Anterograde amnesia, an inability to form new memories, usually clears completely within 24 hours of the trauma. Recall of events occurring within the first several hours after head injury, however, will often continue to be patchy.

The treatment of seizures will depend upon the type of seizure, its frequency, and the associated electroencephalographic findings. Ethosuximide (Zarontin) is a standard drug for absence (petit mal) seizures, carbamazepine (Tegretol) for partial complex (psychomotor) seizures, and phenytoin (Dilantin) or phenobarbital for grand mal (major motor) seizures (see Chapter 12). Treatment of increased intracranial pressure, as with brain tumor or hydrocephalus, is presented in Chapter 11. Progressive neurologic disease may not be specifically treatable (see Chapter 8). SSPE, for example, is managed symptomatically and supportively with treatment of seizures and maintenance of nutritional state.

Herpes simplex encephalitis is treated acutely with adenine arabinoside

TABLE 16–4. **Selected Aspects of Treatment of Memory Disturbance**

Chronic Systemic Illness	Symptomatic and supportive therapy
Attention Deficit Disorder	Dextroamphetamine (Dexedrine), methylphenidate (Ritalin)
Thyroid Disease	Thyroid hormone replacement for hypothyroidism PTU, radioiodine, or surgery for hyperthyroidism
Head Trauma	Supportive care; specific treatment of complications: seizures, intracranial hemorrhage
Seizures	Supportive, general measures; anticonvulsant therapy
Increased Intracranial Pressure	Medical and surgical therapies
Herpes simplex *Encephalitis*	Adenine arabinoside (Ara-A) for infection Physostigmine for memory disorder
Anxiety, Depression	Individual therapy Antidepressant medication
Idiopathic-Constitutional	Mnemonic techniques Use of note pad Repetition Regular schedule

(Ara-A) (Hirsch and Swartz, 1980). The resulting memory disturbance has been treated with physostigmine with beneficial results (Peters and Levin, 1977).

Psychotherapy. The treatment of depression is discussed in Chapter 6. Psychotherapy is often valuable in treating anxiety disorders as well.

Periods of amnesia, even when brief, may be upsetting to the child. With posttraumatic memory loss, the child and parents should be informed as to the kinds of memory disturbance that occur with head injury. Emphasis should be placed upon that which has cleared, the circumscribed nature of the persisting deficit, and the normalcy of current memory in terms of learning new material.

When memory disturbance has been of longer duration (days to weeks), as may follow a period of coma, it may be valuable to consider what the child has missed in terms of a birthday party, Christmas celebration, or family vacation. Specific "remediation" can then be undertaken.

Mnemonic techniques can improve memory function. One technique involves associating "peg" words with vivid mental images to facilitate memorizing brief lists of items. Peg words might be as follows: 1-bun, 2-shoe, 3-tree, 4-floor, 5-hive, 6-sticks, 7-heaven, 8-gate, 9-line, 10-hen. To remember the first item in a list (for example, a book to be returned to the library), one might imagine a book in the shape of a steaming bun sliced nearly in half with print covering both halves. Bizarre mental imagery appears to make elements of the list more memorable (Patten, 1972). Forgetting fortunately comes to the aid of the mnemonicist, as mental images from different days rarely intrude upon each other.

A memory device for recalling numbers utilizes a letter code in the construction of words. One is represented by T, 2 by N, 3 M, 4 R, 5 L, 6 G (or J), 7 K (or hard C), 8 F, 9 P (or B), 0 (zero) S (or Z). The number 1946, for example, would correspond to the letters T,B,R,G. A word constructed from that sequence would be Tuborg, a brand of beer.

There is no substitute for rehearsal (repetition) in improving recall. Repeating out loud or to oneself items to be remembered is valuable in converting immediate into short-term memory.

Social-Environmental Management. Diminishing distraction by establishing a quiet, stimulus-poor environment for studying is valuable not only for children with attention deficit disorders, but for others as well. A regular schedule will also usually benefit children with memory problems. For example, if homework is always to be done upon returning home from school, a minimum of reminding will be necessary.

Educational Management. When children have problems in auditory memory or sequencing, their school performance can suffer not from lack of intelligence, attention, or motivation but because of difficulties in handling instructions given orally by the teacher. Such children should be allowed to write down instructions, or they should be provided them in written form.

Mechanical Therapy. Calendars, notebooks, and appointment books can be of great value to the older school-age child or adolescent with a memory problem. Wristwatch alarms can act as a sophisticated string around the finger.

CORRELATION

Anatomic Aspects. Abnormalities of the limbic system have been implicated in numerous studies of persons with memory disorders (Luria and Karasseva, 1968; Adams, 1969; Penfield and Mathieson, 1974; Muramoto *et al.*, 1979). The failure of anatomic studies to account for much that is known about memory and its disorders, however, underscores the importance of biochemical factors. Nonetheless, several important pathologic-anatomic links have been established and merit review.

Bilateral lesions of the limbic system have been the most consistent gross anatomic findings associated with significant and persistent memory deficits (Adams, 1969). Affected regions have included medial portions of the temporal lobes (specifically the hippocampi, amygdaloid nuclei, and parahippocampal gyri), the fornix (arching around the lateral ventricles to link the hippocampus with the ipsilateral mammillary body), and the anterior commissure (which connects one temporal lobe with the other) (see Fig. 2–11).

Several pathologic processes can affect the limbic system to produce serious memory disturbance. These include infection (as with *Herpes simplex* encephalitis), infarction (secondary to occlusion of branches of the posterior cerebral arteries), or trauma (associated with cerebral contusions, for example). Unilateral injury to medial portions of the left temporal lobe has been implicated in disturbances of verbal memory (Luria and Karasseva, 1968).

Detailed neuropathologic studies of the Wernicke-Korsakoff syndrome have indicated the importance of the thalamus and brainstem in associated memory disorders. The striking short-term memory deficit that characterizes this syndrome has been linked most consistently with lesions of the medial dorsal nuclei of the thalami (Adams, 1969). The mammillary bodies are also often affected, but they may show significant abnormalities in persons without memory deficit. Other portions of the brain frequently affected in the Wernicke-Korsakoff syndrome are the walls of the third ventricle, periaqueductal regions of the midbrain, and the floor of the fourth ventricle.

As noted earlier the chronic memory disturbance seen with Wernicke-Korsakoff syndrome consists of a profound anterograde amnesia (an inability to learn new material) and a less marked retrograde amnesia often associated with confabulation. Affected persons are normally alert and attentive. Their digit span is normal. Little, if any, intellectual change can be determined upon psychometric testing. Yet such persons typically will not remember any of three objects after 5 minutes and may not even remember that they were asked to recall anything at all.

Acutely, the Wernicke-Korsakoff syndrome is manifested by the development over several days of ocular palsy, nystagmus, ataxia of gait, and mental status changes (confusion, apathy, or delirium). Following administration of thiamine (vitamin B_1), these symptoms disappear. The characteristic memory deficit emerges, however, and persists despite vitamin therapy.

Biochemical Aspects.   Biochemical aspects of memory appear to be of great importance and are the subject of extensive ongoing investigations (Drachman and Sahakian, 1979; Weingartner et al., 1981).

Scopolamine, a centrally acting anticholinergic agent related to atropine, has long been known to have effects upon memory. It has been used for years as premedication for obstetric and operative purposes because of its ability to produce a "twilight state." The clinical impression that memory is temporarily impaired by scopolamine has been borne out by several controlled studies (Safer and Allen, 1971; Crow, 1979). Short-term memory appears preferentially affected, as immediate recall is only mildly impaired by administration of scopolamine, whereas recall after 20 seconds is markedly reduced.

If scopolamine interferes with short-term memory, is memory enhanced by physostigmine, a centrally acting cholinesterase inhibitor (thus, a cholinergic agonist)? The results of trials utilizing physostigmine in man have been inconclusive but suggest a significant cholinergic role in memory function.

Peters and Levin (1977) gave intramuscular physostigmine to a young woman who had suffered *Herpes simplex* encephalitis 2 years previously. Her illness had left her with a severe anterograde amnesia, although she had retained the ability to repeat 8 digits forward. Significant improvement in short-term memory followed treatment with physostigmine.

When administered to normal volunteers, physostigmine has not consistently been found to enhance memory (Drachman and Leavitt, 1974; Davis *et al.,* 1978). On the other hand, the cholinergic agents arecholine and choline have been found to improve serial learning in normal persons (Sitaram *et al.,* 1978).

Age-related changes in cholinergic systems (most notably the limbic and reticular activating systems) have been hypothesized as underlying the dementia of Alzheimer disease (Drachman and Leavitt, 1974). Preliminary trials of physostigmine used in combination with lecithin (an acetylcholine precursor) demonstrated an improvement in memory in five persons with Alzheimer disease (Peters and Levin, 1979).

Vasopressin and the synthetic analogue DDAVP (1-desamino-8-D-arginine vasopressin) have been demonstrated to improve memory in man (Oliveros *et al.,* 1978; de Wied and Versteeg, 1979; Cooper and Martin; 1980; Weingartner *et al.,* 1981). Employing a vasopressin nasal spray several times daily, Oliveros and colleagues (1978) described improvement in memory in three adults who had sustained major head trauma. One of these was a 21-year-old man who had been comatose for 15 days following an automobile accident and who had been left with severe retrograde and anterograde amnesias. Within a week of beginning vasopressin (five puffs per day), memory was considered "completely recovered." Clinical gains (including improved memory, mood, and self-confidence) were maintained when placebo was later substituted for vasopressin.

Weingartner and colleagues (1981) found improvement in memory in three groups of volunteers who took DDAVP intranasally three times a day. The study involved six normal college students, four depressed patients, and two persons undergoing unilateral electroconvulsive therapy for treatment of mood disorder. Significant enhancement in learning was found in all groups, characterized by improved completeness, organization, and reliability of recall.

Other peptides, naturally occurring and synthetic, also have been found to have beneficial effects upon memory and learning (Sandman *et al.,* 1977; de Wied and Bohus, 1979; Cooper and Martin, 1980). Sandman and colleagues (1977) studied the effects upon attention and learning of MSH/ACTH 4-10, a polypeptide subunit of melanocyte-stimulating hormone (MSH) and adrenocorticotropic hormone (ACTH). Their investigation, involving eleven healthy adult male volunteers, supported previous studies demonstrating enhanced attention with MSH/ACTH 4-10. This neuropeptide facilitated the processes of detection and discrimination, seemingly acting as part of a "filtering mechanism" for protection from "perceptual noise."

Long-term storage of information in macromolecules has been recognized to play an important role in growth, development, and maintenance of health. DNA (deoxyribonucleic acid), for example, is a storehouse of information enclosed in nucleotide sequences. Indeed, the entire immune system of man can be considered a molecularly based long-term memory mechanism. Thus, the role of macromolecules in long-term memory and learning is strongly suggested, although it remains to be clarified (Doty, 1979).

Physiologic Aspects. Experimental work on memory and learning carried out in lower organisms suggests mechanisms that may pertain to man. The mollusc *Aplysia californica,* a relatively simple organism containing only some 15,000 neurons, has been the subject of considerable investigation. Research has been facilitated by the large size of these neurons, some of which measure one millimeter, hence are visible to the unaided eye.

Studies have looked into two important properties of the gill withdrawal reflex, habituation and sensitization (Kandel, 1979A and B). Habituation is defined as "a decrease in behavioral response that occurs when an initially novel stimulus is repeatedly presented" (Kandel, 1979A). Memory is implied in this process, as stimuli that are no longer novel elicit less of a reaction. They are, so to speak, to a greater or lesser degree ignored.

The gill withdrawal reflex involves sensory neurons, motor neurons, and connecting interneurons. Because the number of cells in the reflex is relatively small, fewer than fifty, it has been possible to isolate responses (excitatory postsynaptic potentials) in individual motor neurons following electrical stimulation of single sensory neurons. With continued stimulation, a decremental response in the excitatory postsynaptic potential occurs until nearly no response is elicitable.

The duration of habituation varies with the amount of "training" (Kandel, 1979B). A single session involving ten sensory neuron stimulations produced a habituating effect lasting minutes to hours. If training sessions were carried out daily for 4 consecutive days, however, the memory for habituation lasted for more than 3 weeks.

The basis for this effect has been determined to be diminution of neurotransmitter released presynaptically. This effect reverts to normal within 15 minutes to several hours after stimulation has ceased. Thereafter, presentation of the sensory stimulus, once again perceived as novel, triggers the motor neuron involved in the reflex.

Sensitization is essentially the opposite of habituation. It is defined as "the process whereby an animal learns to increase a given reflex response as a result of a noxious or novel stimulus" (Kandel, 1979B). Instead of a decrease in excitatory postsynaptic potential as occurs with habituation, an increase occurs with sensitization. This effect is felt to result from an increase in the level of cyclic AMP (adenosine monophosphate), which leads to an increase in calcium ion within the neuron.

As Kandel (1979B) has noted, learning at the cellular level need not involve anatomic rearrangement. Rather, the function of already existing neurons and synapses can be modified by "experience," as sensory stimulation produces alterations in calcium flow, in the amount of neurotransmitter released, and in the magnitude of excitatory postsynaptic potentials.

SUMMARY

Memory, rooted in the limbic system, plays a fundamental role in learning, among other behaviors. Hence it is often involved in emotional and behavioral disturbances of childhood and adolescence. Evaluation begins with characterization of the memory disturbance, including onset and associated features such as headache, staring spells, or personality change. Relevant past history should include inquiry about head injury, major illnesses (particularly encephalitis), and drug use (including anticonvulsant medications). Examination should assess immediate, short-term, and long-term memory. Affect and intelligence should be noted. Systemic medical illness should be identified. Neurologic examination should seek lateralizing findings or evidence of raised intracranial pressure. Investigations may include psychometric evaluation, formal memory testing, electroencephalography, radiologic investigation, or blood studies (including measurement of thyroid hormone levels). Major causes of memory deficit in childhood include intercurrent illness, anxiety, depression, attention deficit disorder (with or without hyperkinesis), mental retardation, head trauma, seizures, and sleep disturbances. Hearing impairment and receptive language disturbance should be distinguished from memory dysfunction.

Treatment will depend upon the cause(s) identified. Pharmacologic treatment may be included in the management of attentional and affective disorders. Psychologic techniques involving mental imagery may be of benefit. Social-environmental and mechanical modes of therapy are often helpful.

Recent investigations into the structural and biochemical bases for memory and its disorders indicate that further important advances in our understanding and treatment of memory problems will be made within the current decade.

CITED REFERENCES

Adams, R. D. The anatomy of memory mechanisms in the human brain. Pp. 91–106 in *The Pathology of Memory*. Talland, G. A., and Waugh, N. C., eds. Academic Press, New York, 1969.

Bell, W. E., and McCormick, W. F. Herpesvirus hominis (simplex) encephalitis. Pp. 194–203 in *Neurologic Infections in Children*. W. B. Saunders Co., Philadelphia, 1975.

Benson, D. F. and Geschwind, N. Shrinking retrograde amnesia. *J. Neurol. Neurosurg. Psychiatry,* **30:** 539–44, 1967.

Benton, A. *Benton Revised Visual Retention Test*. The Psychological Corporation, New York, 1974.

Buschke, H. and Fuld, P. A. Evaluating storage, retention, and retrieval in disordered memory and learning. *Neurology,* **24:** 1019–25, 1974.

Cochrane, W. A.; Collins-Williams, C.; and Donohue, W. L. Superior hemorrhagic polioencephalitis (Wernicke's disease) occurring in an infant—probably due to thiamine deficiency from use of a soya bean product. *Pediatrics,* **28:** 771–77, 1961.

Cooper, P. E. and Martin, J. B. Neuroendocrinology and brain peptides. *Ann. Neurol.,* **8:** 551–57, 1980.

Cronholm, B. Post-ECT amnesias. Pp. 81–89 in *The Pathology of Memory*. Talland, G. A., and Waugh, N. C., eds. Academic Press, New York, 1969.

Crow, T. J. Action of hyoscine on verbal learning in man: evidence for a cholinergic link in the transition from primary to secondary memory? Pp. 269–75 in *Brain Mechanisms in Memory and Learning: From the Single Neuron to Man*. Brazier, M. A. B., ed. Raven Press, New York, 1979.

Davis, K. L.; Mohs, R. C.; Tinklenberg, J. R.; Pfefferbaum, A.; Hollister, L. E.; and Lopell, B. S. Physostigmine: improvement of long-term memory processes in normal humans. *Science,* **201:** 272–74, 1978.

de Wied, D., and Bohus, B. Modulation of memory processes by neuropeptides of hypothalamic-neurohypophyseal origin. Pp. 139–49 in *Brain Mechanisms in Memory and Learning: From the Single Neuron to Man*. Brazier, M. A. B., ed. Raven Press, New York, 1979.

de Wied, D., and Versteeg, H. G. Neurohypophyseal principles and memory. *Federation Proc.*, **38:** 2348–54, 1979.

Doty, R. W. Neurons and memory: some clues. Pp. 53–63 in *Brain Mechanisms in Memory and Learning: From the Single Neuron to Man*. Brazier, M. A. B., ed. Raven Press, New York, 1979.

Drachman, D. A., and Leavitt, J. Human memory and the cholinergic system. *Arch. Neurol.*, **30:** 113–21, 1974.

Drachman, D. A., and Sahakian, B. J. Effects of cholinergic agents on human learning and memory. Pp. 351–66 in *Nutrition and the Brain*, Vol. 5. Barbeau, A.; Growdon, J. H.; and Wurtman, R. J., eds. Raven Press, New York, 1979.

Fisher, C. M. Concussion amnesia. *Neurology* (Minneapolis), **16:** 826–30, 1966.

Freud, S. *The Psychopathology of Everyday Life*. Brill, A. A., trans. Macmillan Publishing Co., 1904.

Hirsch, M. S., and Swartz, M. N. Antiviral agents. *N. Engl. J. Med.*, **302:** 903–7, 1980.

Kandel, E. R. Cellular aspects of learning. Pp. 3–16 in *Brain Mechanisms in Memory and Learning: From the Single Neuron to Man*. Brazier, M. A. B., ed. Raven Press, New York, 1979A.

Kandel, E. R. Psychotherapy and the single synapse. *N. Engl. J. Med.*, **301:** 1028–37, 1979B.

Luria, A. R., and Karasseva, T. A. Disturbances of auditory-speech memory in focal lesions of the deep regions of the left temporal lobe. *Neuropsychologia*, **6:** 97–104, 1968.

MacLeod, C. M.; Dekaban, A. S.; and Hunt, E. Memory impairment in epileptic patients: selective effects of phenobarbital concentration. *Science*, **202:** 1102–4, 1978.

Muramoto, O.; Kuru, Y.; Sugishita, M.; and Toyokura, Y. Pure memory loss with hippocampal lesions. *Arch. Neurol.*, **36:** 54–56, 1979.

Oliveros, J. C.; Jandali, M. K.; Timsit-Berthier, M.; Remy, R.; Benghezal, A.; Audibert, A.; and Moeglen, J. M. Vasopressin in amnesia. *Lancet*, **1:** 42, 1978.

Ommaya, A. K., and Gennarelli, T. A. Experimental head injury. Pp. 67–90 in *Handbook of Clinical Neurology*, Vol. 23. Vinken, P. J., and Bruyn, G. W., eds. North-Holland Publishing Co., Amsterdam, 1975.

Patten, B. M. The ancient art of memory. *Arch. Neurol.*, **26:** 25–31, 1972.

Penfield, W., and Mathieson, G. Memory: autopsy findings and comments on the role of hippocampus in experiential recall. *Arch. Neurol.*, **31:** 145–54, 1974.

Penfield, W., and Rasmussen, T. *The Cerebral Cortex of Man. A Clinical Study of Localization of Function*. The Macmillan Company, New York, 1950, pp. 164–67.

Peters, B. H., and Levin, H. S. Memory enhancement after physostigmine treatment in the amnesic syndrome. *Arch. Neurol.*, **34:** 215–19, 1977.

Peters, B. H., and Levin, H. S. Effects of physostigmine and lecithin on memory in Alzheimer disease. *Ann. Neurol.*, **6:** 219–21, 1979.

Plaitakis, A.; Whetsell, W. O., Jr.; Cooper, J. R.; and Yahr, M. D. Chronic Leigh disease: a genetic and biochemical study. *Ann. Neurol.*, **7:** 304–10, 1980.

Safer, D. J., and Allen, R. P. The central effects of scopolamine in man. *Biol. Psychiatry*, **3:** 347–55, 1971.

Sandman, C. A.; George, J.; McCanne, T. R.; Nolan, J. D.; Kaswan, J.; and Kastin A. J. MSH/ACTH 4-10 influences behavioral and physiological measures of attention. *J. Clin. Endocrinol. Metab.*, **44:** 884–91, 1977.

Sipe, J. C. Leigh's syndrome: the adult form of subacute necrotizing encephalomyelopathy with predilection for the brainstem. *Neurology* (Minneapolis), **23**: 1030–
38, 1973.

Sitaram, N.; Weingartner, H.; and Gillin, J. C. Human serial learning: enhancement
with arecholine and choline and impairment with scopolamine. *Science,* **201**: 274–
76, 1978.

Strub, R. L., and Black, F. W. Memory. Pp. 63–83 in *The Mental Status Examination in Neurology.* F. A. Davis Co., Philadelphia, 1977.

Wechsler, D., and Stone, C. *Wechsler Memory Scale.* The Psychological Corporation, New York, 1973.

Weiner, N. Atropine, scopolamine, and related antimuscarinic drugs. Pp. 121–28 in
The Pharmacological Basis of Therapeutics, 6th ed. Gilman, A. G.; Goodman,
L. S.; Gilman, A., eds. Macmillan Publishing Co., Inc., New York, 1980.

Weingartner H.; Gold, P.; Ballenger, J. C.; Smallberg, S. A.; Summers, R.; Rubinow,
D. R.; Post, R. M.; and Goodwin, F. K. Effects of vasopressin on human memory
functions. *Science,* **211**: 601–3, 1981.

Yarnell, P. R., and Lynch, S. Retrograde memory immediately after concussion. *Lancet,* **1**: 863–64, 1970.

Yarnell, P. R., and Lynch, S. The "ding": amnestic states in football trauma. *Neurology* (Minneapolis), **23**: 196–97, 1973.

Zeidenberg, P. Flashbacks. *Psychiatr. Ann.,* **3**: 14–19, 1973.

ADDITIONAL READINGS

Breslow, R.; Kocsis, J.; and Belkin, B. Contribution of the depressive perspective to
memory function in depression. *Am. J. Psychiatry,* **138**: 227–30, 1981.

Ericsson, K. A.; Chase, W. G.; and Faloon, S. Acquisition of a memory skill.
Science, **208**: 1181–82, 1980.

Lorayne, H., and Lucas, J. *The Memory Book.* Ballantine Books, New York, 1974.

Saltz, E., and Donnenwerth-Nolan, S. Does motoric imagery facilitate memory for
sentences? A selective interference test. *J. Verbal Learning Verbal Behav.,* **20**:
322–32, 1981.

Victor, M.; Adams, R. D.; and Collins, G. H. *The Wernicke-Korsakoff Syndrome.*
F. A. Davis Co., Philadelphia, 1971.

Whitley, R. Diagnosis and treatment of herpes simplex encephalitis. *Annu. Rev.
Med.,* **32**: 335–40, 1981.

17 Learning Disabilities and Disorders of Speech and Language

Learning problems are among the commonest, though often the most confusing, of childhood difficulties that confront professionals, parents, and children themselves. By the time a child reaches school age, mental retardation is usually evident; hence only rarely is it found to be the primary cause of unanticipated learning failure in school. Neurosensory deficit such as deafness or blindness is unlikely to have been overlooked. Severe behavioral disturbance such as extreme hyperactivity or psychosis generally will also have become readily evident early in life. With these categories excluded, one must consider learning disability as a cause for learning problems, although it is by no means a diagnosis of exclusion.

Learning disability is invoked increasingly frequently to account for school problems. The result is sometimes beneficial to the child; at other times it is not. Simply identifying the problem as a circumscribed difficulty and giving it a name may be helpful and reassuring to the family and child. Identification of the problem can also facilitate specific academic remediation. On the other hand, use of the term ''learning disability'' or ''dyslexia'' may have the unfortunate effect of crystallizing the notion of a child's defectiveness, particularly since brain damage has so often been implied by the use of these terms. In addition, programs designed to help children with learning disabilities through early intervention can have negative effects by identifying children inappropriately early or by categorizing them as ''different.'' The negative impact upon the child may be further compounded by removing him or her from activities of interest, success, and personal reward to participate in a well-intentioned program of remediation.

This chapter will focus upon learning disabilities and disorders of speech and language. Several key terms such as learning, learning problem, learning failure, learning disability, dyslexia, and aphasia will be defined. The normal processes of speech and language development will be reviewed. Pertinent aspects of history, examination, and investigation will be presented with emphasis upon remediable aspects of childhood learning problems. The bio-

480

logic basis for learning disabilities and disorders of speech and language will be discussed.

Several questions will be addressed:

How is the diagnosis of learning disability established?

What causes learning disabilities?

What is the relationship between learning disabilities and hyperactivity?

What medical, neurologic, and psychologic signs should be sought in evaluating the child with a suspected learning disability? The child with speech delay?

What is the significance of "soft" neurologic signs in the learning-disabled child?

When should the child with a learning problem be referred for neurologic or psychologic evaluation?

What is the value of therapy in the learning-disabled child?

Is a multidisciplinary approach to learning disabilities most beneficial for the child?

Are learning-disabled children brain-damaged?

LEARNING DISABILITIES

DEFINITION

Learning, the primary task of the school-age child, is defined as the acquisition of information. Learning involves the perception, organization, storage, and retrieval of information, which knowledge helps to shape a child's behavior.

A *learning problem* occurs when the child has difficulty in acquiring information. Such problems may be compensated for or not, and compensation may occur unbeknownst to teacher or parents. For example, giving a child an extra 10 minutes to complete a task at his or her own pace may allow the child to compensate for a problem with no further intervention required.

Learning failure occurs when compensatory strategies have not been developed or instituted and the child falls increasingly behind his classmates.

Learning disability is defined by a child's relatively low performance in school subjects (such as reading, writing, or arithmetic) contrasted with his or her overall level of intelligence. A significant gap between school performance and intelligence is generally taken to be two grade levels. For example, a fourth-grade child of normal intelligence who reads at a first- or second-grade level would be defined as having a learning disability. On the other hand, a normally intelligent fourth-grader reading at a third-grade level or a first-grader reading at a kindergarten level would not, according to this definition, have a learning disability.

This definition of learning disability can be applied usefully to persons who are either below or above average in intelligence. For example, a 15-year-old child who is functioning overall at a 10-year level but who is unable to read at all would qualify as having a specific learning disability in the area of reading in addition to mental retardation. The fifth-grader with an intelligence quotient of 140 who reads at a fifth-grade level might well have a learning disability, for his anticipated reading performance would be considerably higher than grade level.

In the instances described above, the child would be said to have a specific reading disability, or *dyslexia*. Comparable specific deficits in the areas of writing and arithmetic are termed *dysgraphia* and *dyscalculia*, respectively.

Developmental learning disability implies that the school problem is developmental in nature. It suggests that the learning problem represents a specific lag when the child's performance is compared with that of peers. Stated differently, the child's performance in a specific academic area is like that of a younger child in whom it would be considered normal.

The use of the word "developmental" should not be taken to mean that the problem will always be outgrown entirely, although such an outcome is possible. More likely, adaptation and compensation will occur over time, with some difficulty or deficit persisting.

Minimal brain dysfunction is a term that has been used to encompass broadly the conditions of specific learning disability (particularly when it is developmental in nature) and hyperkinetic syndrome (or attention deficit disorder with hyperkinesis). The two disorders frequently coexist. As both clinical categories have become better understood and as their therapies have diverged increasingly, the concept of minimal brain dysfunction has become of diminishing usefulness.

Language is a symbolic system learned and used for communication between persons (Swisher *et al.*, 1977). It has also been defined as a symbolic code for the generation of novel messages (Rutter, 1977). The elements of language are words, which can be spoken, printed, or formed with the hand in accordance with a set of organizing principles. The term *speech*, by contrast, is generally used in a narrower sense, restricted to the process of production of spoken language, including its articulation.

TABLE 17–1. **Normal Speech Development**

Age	Speech Development
Birth	undifferentiated cry
2–3 months	differentiated cry
3–4 months	random babbling
5 months	40+ sounds used in later speech
6–7 months	rhythmic babbling
7–8 months	self-imitation
8–10 months	echolalia
1 year	1–2 words
2 years	2-word combinations; 200–300 words
3 years	3–4-word combinations
4 years	5-word combinations; 1,000 words
5 years	6-word combinations
7 years	7-word combinations; 20,000 words (± 10,000 words)
8 years	8-word combinations

Speech delay is defined by failure of acquisition of words by 24 months or of phrases by 3 years of age. Normal speech undergoes extraordinary development, from no words during the first 6 months of life to 10,000 words or more by 7 years (Rutter, 1977; Moskowitz, 1978). During early infancy undifferentiated crying progresses to differentiated crying by 2 to 3 months, when cooing is usually first heard. Rhythmic babbling develops over the next 6 months, and one or two words are usually evident by 1 year of age. Between 18 months and 2 years, vocabulary builds to 200 or so words and, generally, word combinations are first heard. Between 2 and 5 years of age, the mean phrase length increases from two to six words and vocabulary grows to hundreds of words (see Table 17–1).

Aphasia is defined as the loss of previously acquired, linguistically correct speech. According to this definition, a child who has never developed normal speech cannot be said to be aphasic, although he clearly may be suffering from a disorder of language development.

DIAGNOSIS

Clinical Process. All portions of the clinical process—history, examination, and investigation—play an important role in the assessment of the child with a learning problem. The history includes standard medical and neurologic data-gathering as well as detailed school history. Examination consists of the fundamental general physical examination, neurologic examination, and mental status examination supplemented by office testing of intelligence and school-related skills. Investigation will often include psychologic testing and speech and language assessment.

History. A teenage boy may complain that "I have never been able to read." The mother of a younger school-age child may say, "She has always had difficulty with paper-and-pencil tasks." The father of a 4-year-old child may note, "He only speaks a few words, and even those aren't clear."

In evaluating school problems, it is essential to obtain a detailed educational history. Supplementary materials from the school should be obtained and reviewed. They often will contain not only results of academic and intellectual testing but valuable observations of behavior as well.

The school history should begin with the child's entry into school and proceed to the present. When did the child start school? Did he attend nursery school prior to kindergarten? Did behavior problems interfere with school performance during the early years? How old was he at the end of kindergarten? Did he seem ready for first grade? When were school problems first recognized? What testing or remediation has been carried out? What have been the effects of intervention? Does he seem to be catching up to his classmates, lagging by a fixed amount, or falling farther behind?

A family history of learning problems should be sought. Have other family members (siblings, parents, uncles, aunts) had difficulties in school? The ages and academic status of siblings should be determined and the academic attainments of the parents noted. What was the highest grade level the parents completed in school? Was either parent a slow starter? Were any grades repeated? Does either parent have difficulty now with reading, spelling, handwriting, or arithmetic? Do the parents nowadays read for pleasure, or do they prefer to listen to the radio or watch television? What are the parents' occupations? Did learning problems influence the choice of career?

If, in retrospect, it appears that a parent has had a learning disability, it can be valuable to understand the adult's academic struggles as a child, modes of compensation, and current perception of their child's problem. Not infrequently a parent will say, "I realize now that I had a learning disability. I see the same things in my child and I don't want him to go through what I did."

The parents' academic and career aspirations for their child should also be explored. When the child is just in elementary or junior high school, parents may communicate directly or indirectly their concerns as to his or her making it to a "good" college or to any college at all. Such pressure (which can be severely worsened by comparison with siblings) can set up a "tug-of-war" around learning that has potentially poor results for all parties concerned. On the other hand, parents may have inappropriately low academic or career expectations for their child because of specific reading, writing, or spelling difficulties in elementary school.

Several features of behavior may accompany learning disabilities and should specifically be sought. These include symptoms of attention deficit disorder with or without hyperactivity. This syndrome, described in detail in Chapter 14, generally includes inattentiveness, impulsivity, distractability, and overexcitability. Review of systems should include inquiry about headaches and abdominal pain. They may be psychophysiologic symptoms stemming from the child's frustration, concern, and attempts to compensate by working very hard while anticipating poor results (see Case 11–10).

In evaluating the child with speech delay, current speech and language status as well as earlier development should be noted. What words, phrases, or sentences does the child now say? Specific words or word combinations reported by the parents should be recorded. The child's comprehension and ability to carry out commands (involving one, two, or three steps) should be noted. Hearing, articulation, and quality of voice (hoarse or high-pitched) should be described.

Development of speech and language should begin with the child's responsiveness to sounds. The time of appearance of cooing ("goo-goo, ga-ga") and babbling (more well-defined, rhythmic syllables) should be noted. The age at which the first specific words and word combinations were spoken should also be recorded. Baby books will often help in obtaining the most precise information about such milestones.

Nonverbal modes of communication should also be explored. How does the child make his or her wants known? Does communication involve pointing or taking a parent by the hand? If pointing is involved, is the index finger used as a pointer, or is the entire fist employed? If the child takes a parent by the hand, is the hand manipulated as if it is divorced from the parent's body, or is there some appreciation that a person is attached?

Other relevant inquiry will pertain to the social and home environment. Is English the only language spoken at home? If two languages are spoken, which was introduced first? Does the child have a twin sibling? What is the child's place in the sibship? Does the child merely have to point to have a wish granted?

Development in areas other than speech and language function should also be determined. Is the child globally delayed, or does speech and language impairment far outweigh other deficits? Is the child normally interactive or aloof? Does he play normally with toys or use them in an unusual manner such as spinning or twirling them repetitively? Do bizarre mannerisms such as flicking of the fingers before the eyes occur? Does the child insist on sameness in the environment? Are there any areas of excellence, for example, reciting poetry, naming street signs, or singing? Has the child lost language skills or other milestones?

Past history should include attention to details of pregnancy, delivery, and the neonatal period. Congenital rubella infection, hyperbilirubinemia (with secondary kernicterus), use of ototoxic antibiotics (such as the aminoglycosides kanamycin or gentamicin for suspected or proven neonatal sepsis or meningitis), and prematurity may be associated with sensorineural hearing impairment severe enough to cause speech and language deficit. Any of these can cause hearing impairment that affects primarily high frequencies. Such children may be brought for evaluation because of comprehension difficulties, articulatory problems, and behavior disorders (Matkin, 1968).

Additional history in the speech-delayed child should include significant infectious diseases such as mumps, meningitis (bacterial or viral), or any illness (such as measles) with prolonged high fever. Family history of hearing deficit should also be determined. Familial syndromes involving deafness include those of Waardenburg, Usher, Alport, Pendred, and Jervell-Lange-Nielsen (Fraser, 1964).

In the child with reading disability or loss of language function, head trauma should be inquired about (Shaffer *et al.,* 1980). Severity can be gauged by associated loss of consciousness, skull fracture, posttraumatic seizure, or intracranial hemorrhage.

Examination. The *general description* should describe the most striking aspects of the child's appearance and behavior. Most learning-disabled children will be normal in appearance but may show hyperkinetic behavior and distractability as part of a coexisting attention deficit disorder. The child with speech delay as part of an autistic syndrome will characteristically demonstrate aloof, ritualistic, or otherwise bizarre behavior (see Chapter 5).

The *general physical examination* of the child with a learning disability will usually be essentially normal. In assessing the child with delayed speech, one should note the presence of a white forelock, heterochromia iridis (eyes of different color), and lateral displacement of the medial canthi —features of Waardenburg syndrome. Tympanic membranes should be inspected for signs of chronic middle ear disease. Ear malformations may be associated with hearing impairment (and renal disease) in Alport syndrome. Cataract of the lens can occur secondary to rubella infection *in utero.* Palatal clefts may be obvious or inapparent (as with submucous clefts). They can be associated with chronic middle ear disease because of impaired eustachian tube function. A bifid uvula (shaped like an inverted Y) suggests an underlying submucous cleft of the palate. The head circumference should be measured and plotted. If it is excessively small, prenatal infection (with or without mental retardation) should be suspected.

Neurologic examination of the child with an apparent learning disability or a language problem should focus upon primary perceptual functions (vision and hearing), seek lateralizing findings, and exclude signs of increased intracranial pressure. Testing of visual acuity can be accomplished with a Rosenbaum Vision Screening Card or a Snellen Eye Chart. Visual fields should be tested by confrontation. Careful funduscopic examination should be carried out to detect blurring of optic disk margins and elevation of the optic papillae, both signs of raised intracranial pressure. The maculae and retinal background also should be inspected for signs of macular or other retinal degeneration (for example, with subacute sclerosing panencephalitis or any syndrome with retinitis pigmentosa).

Hearing can be examined by whispering into each ear separately, by rubbing the fingers next to the child's ears, and by measuring the distance at which a watch tick can no longer be heard. Unless hearing deficit has been identified, the Weber and Rinné tuning fork tests need not be done.

The lower cranial nerves play major roles in speech production. Hoarseness, tremulousness, high pitch (squeakiness), or "nasal" quality should be noted. Tremulousness can be brought out by having the child sustain the vowel "ee." Rhythmicity of spontaneous speech should be noted. Repetition of phrases such as "hopping hippopotamus" may elicit dysfluency. The presence of drooling should be noted. Palatal function can be assessed by having the child say "ah." Attention should be given to palatal elevation and symmetry as well as to the gag reflex (absent, diminished, normal, or exaggerated) on both sides of the palate. Swallowing can be assessed by having the child drink from a cup. Regurgitation through the nose, which may occur with inadequate posterior pharyngeal closure, should be noted. Tongue movements can be assessed by having the child stick out his tongue, push it against the inside of his cheeks, and lick his lips to remove a crumb or drop of water. If the child can lick off a real but not an imaginary crumb lying on his lip, an oral apraxia (which may accompany expressive language disorder) is suggested.

"Nasal" speech may, in fact, be hypernasal or hyponasal. Hypernasal speech occurs secondary to incomplete closure of the posterior pharynx. Such palatal insufficiency can occur with cleft palate (including submucous cleft), congenital shortness of the palate, or neuromuscular disorder (such as myasthenia gravis or botulism) in which posterior pharyngeal muscles are paralyzed. Hyponasal speech commonly results from nasal obstruction on an infectious, allergic, or congenital basis.

Testing of language function should include examination of the following: spontaneous speech, naming, repetition, comprehension, and written language. The spontaneous speech of the child should be observed, written down, and perhaps tape-recorded. Maturity of speech and length of utterances should be noted. For example, "wada" and "dare" may be spoken rather than "water" and "there," "free" instead of "three." Speech may be employed not for communication but in an obsessive, self-stimulating fashion. Echolalia should be noted. Naming of both objects and subparts (for example, shoe and lace, watch and band, pencil and eraser) should be carried out. A naming problem often will become evident only when the child tries to name a component part.

Repetition of phrases ("If he comes, I will go," "No if's, and's, or but's," "Methodist, Episcopal") should be requested. Comprehension can be assessed by asking the child to carry out commands of increasing complexity given both in spoken and in written forms where appropriate. In the school-age child, a sample of written language should be obtained. The child can be asked, for example, to write a sentence about the weather or a paragraph on how he spent his summer vacation.

Examination of the motor system should include assessment of both gross and fine motor skills. Hand preference in throwing and writing should be noted (see Case 17–1). Foot preference can be determined by asking the child to kick a ball (or his socks rolled into a ball). Tone and strength should be assessed. The occurrence of drift or flickering distal movements when arms are held outstretched and eyes are closed should be noted. Testing of gait should include walking in regular fashion, on the toes, on the heels, upon outer portions of the feet, and in tandem. More detailed testing of motor functions should be carried out when muscular disorder (such as Duchenne muscular dystrophy or myotonic dystrophy, either of which may be associated with learning problems) is suspected (see Chapter 13). The limbs and nails should be examined for growth asymmetry.

In the learning-disabled child, a number of so-called soft neurologic signs may be found. Examples include dropping or spreading of the outstretched arms when the head is rotated, choreiform movements of the fingers when the arms are held in front of the body, difficulty in hopping on one foot, mirror movements (synkinesias) of the upper extremities, and abnormalities of finger tapping (Denckla, 1973; Peters *et al.,* 1975).

Other neurologic signs that may be found in the learning-disabled child include dysgraphesthesia (inability to recognize letters or numbers drawn upon the child's palm with the examiner's finger), finger agnosia (difficulty in naming the fingers of one's own hand or the examiner's hands), and right-left confusion (Kinsbourne, 1968; Benton, 1968; Benson and Geschwind, 1970).

The *mental status examination* of a child with a learning disability should include assessment of intelligence, attention, and mood. Estimation of intelligence can be made through general conversation in which the examiner notes the child's vocabulary, information, and understanding, and by more formal inquiry about his or her knowledge of definitions, similarities, differences, and verbal absurdities. Additional assessment of intelligence can be carried out by having the child draw a picture of a person, which is scored by use of Goodenough-Harris standards (Schuberth and Zitelli, 1978).

Clearly, this semiformal approach to evaluation of intelligence is less valid when the child has a language disorder. On the other hand, many children with dyslexia or other learning disability do very well in strictly verbal interchanges, demonstrating normal or superior overall intelligence.

Reading performance can be assessed through use of the Gray Oral Reading passages. Levels of achievement in word recognition, spelling, and arith-

CASE 17–1: MIRROR-WRITING AND READING PROBLEMS IN A 7-YEAR-OLD GIRL

C.F. was referred for evaluation because of difficulty learning to read and mirror writing, which included reversal of letters such as *p* and *q*, *b* and *d*. Past history was of a full-term baby weighing 6 pounds, 9 ounces, delivered vaginally without complications after breech presentation. Early development was normal. She sat at 5 months, walked at 13 months, and spoke her first words at 1 year. She consistently preferred to use her left hand since before a year of age. No other family members were left-handed, although one grandparent was ambidextrous. At 18 months, she had a generalized seizure occurring with fever that lasted for 2 minutes.

On examination, she was an attentive, healthy-appearing girl of normal intelligence who was not excessively fidgety for her age. In printing the alphabet she wrote *p* instead of *b* but corrected the error without being prompted. She read the words *boy* and *dog* correctly but had difficulty with *the*. General physical examination was normal. On neurologic examination, visual acuity, optic fundi, visual fields, hearing, and articulation were normal. Deep tendon reflexes were increased on the left side. A left Babinski sign was present. She was better coordinated in using her left hand than her right. She could hop only on her left foot and could wink only her left eye.

Comment. Although it would not be strictly accurate to say that this child in first grade had a learning disability, she clearly did have a learning problem. Her reading ability was at a kindergarten level and she tended to reverse letters, at times to the point of mirror-writing entire words. Individualized educational planning and remediation were considered essential in getting her "off on the right foot" in school so that she did not suffer later emotional consequences of learning failure. Her overall intelligence, motivation, and compensatory skills (already demonstrated) suggested a favorable educational outcome.

In contrast to children with learning problems who have "soft" neurologic signs, this child actually had "hard" neurologic findings: left-sided hyperreflexia, a left Babinski response, poorer coordination on the right side, and "pathologic" left-handedness. The first two signs suggest injury to or dysfunction of the right cerebral hemisphere, whereas the latter two findings indicate cerebral abnormality on the left. Yet her normal intelligence and head circumference hardly support the presence of significant bilateral brain damage. Perhaps dynamic studies of brain such as computer-assisted mapping of cerebral electrical activity or positron emission tomography might help to clarify this confusing picture.

metic can be obtained through the use of the Wide Range Achievement Test (WRAT). As a measure of organization and neatness, the child should be requested to write (or print) his name, the entire alphabet, and the numbers 1

TABLE 17–2. **Investigations to Be Considered in the Child with Learning Problems**

Psychologic testing (including psychometric,
    perceptual-motor, school achievement,
    and projective tests)
Formal speech and language assessment
EEG (in awake and sleep states)
Thyroid function tests
Skull X-rays
Cranial CT scan
Adrenal function tests
Lumbar puncture
Brain electrical activity mapping (BEAM)
Positron emission tomography (PET)

---

through 50 or 100. Hand position (inverted or not inverted) and tilt of the page should be noted (Critchley, 1968; Benson, 1970; Levy and Reid, 1976).

Signs of attention deficit disorder should be sought. They include fidgetiness, easy distractability, brief attention span, impulsivity, overexcitability, and dysphoria. The one-to-one evaluative setting in a highly structured environment may, however, render classroom or home misbehaviors inapparent (see Chapter 14).

Mood disturbance (depression or anxiety) should be noted. It frequently occurs in learning-disabled children, generally secondary to their chronically stressed, failure-ridden academic experiences. It may also occur due to other causes but have an impact on learning.

Investigation (see Table 17–2). Formal psychometric testing is often indicated in assessment of the learning-disabled child to determine the level of overall intelligence and to define areas of strength and weakness. The Wechsler Intelligence Scale for Children (WISC-R) is the standard instrument used for these purposes. Formal speech and language assessment will also be valuable in many instances. It may include the Illinois Test of Psycholinguistic Abilities (ITPA), a diagnostic tool that examines several aspects of language in the school-age child such as auditory memory, auditory discrimination, and visual sequencing (Kirk and Kirk, 1978). Perceptual-motor skills can be assessed through the Bender-Gestalt and Frostig tests as well as the WISC-R (Frostig, 1972; Gofman and Allmond, 1971). Projective testing may be valuable in elucidating emotional aspects of the learning problem.

Electroencephalography and radiography are not routinely indicated in the child with a specific learning disability. Electroencephalography does, however, appear promising as a research and diagnostic tool utilizing computer-assisted brain electrical activity mapping (BEAM) (Duffy *et al.*, 1980). The CT scan has been used for investigation of children with learning disabilities (Hier *et al.*, 1978); and positron emission tomography (PET) may enhance the understanding of learning disabilities through assessing metabolic activity of different brain regions.

When subacute sclerosing panencephalitis or adrenoleukodystrophy is suspected, examination of cerebrospinal fluid and tests of adrenal function, respectively, should be carried out (see Chapter 8).

Neurologic consultation is not generally required in the evaluation of most learning-disabled children, even if they have "soft" neurologic signs, a discrepancy between verbal and performance portions of the WISC-R, or signs of "organicity" on figure drawings. Focal findings, signs or symptoms of increased intracranial pressure, suspected seizures, and evidence of progressive disorder of the nervous system are among the indications for neurologic consultation. When the appropriateness of referral is unclear, the matter can usually be resolved by a telephone call.

For the child with speech delay formal audiologic testing is essential (see Table 17–3). Since definite answers as to adequacy of hearing may not be gained from a single testing session, two or more sessions may be required. Still more specialized testing may be undertaken in evaluating the hearing-impaired child. Investigations might include auditory evoked responses, impedance audiometry, electrocochleography, or tests of dichotic listening.

Electroencephalography in the awake and sleep states is generally indicated in the assessment of the child with speech delay, particularly if seizures have been observed, loss of speech and language function has occurred, or the clinical picture suggests a syndrome of behavioral regression (see Chapter 8).

With speech delay, formal developmental assessment is indicated. The developmental profile of the child should be established with careful attention to the presence of global retardation or specific developmental deficit. Formal speech and language testing should also be carried out.

Further evaluation of speech delay will be determined by the suspected etiology. If mental retardation is suggested, chromosomal analysis, thyroid function tests, assay of blood and urine for amino acids, and blood lead level should be considered (see Chapter 18). Investigation of the child with autism is discussed in Chapter 5.

Plain skull x-rays and computerized tomographic scanning of the head are indicated when the child suffers from an acquired language deficit (such

TABLE 17–3. **Investigations to Be Considered in the Child with a Disorder of Speech and Language**

Audiometry
Tympanometry
Psychologic testing
Formal speech and language assessment
EEG (in waking and sleep states)
Blood lead level, free erythrocyte protoporphyrin (FEP)
Cranial CT scan
Auditory evoked responses
Electrocochleography
Dichotic listening
Blood and urine for amino acid analysis
Chromosomal analysis

TABLE 17–4. **Differential Diagnosis of Learning Disability or Speech Disorder**

Learning failure due to systemic illness, sleep disturbance,
    drug use or abuse, low motivation, or affective disorder
    (depression, anxiety, neurotic underachievement)
Jagged profile of strengths and weaknesses
Soft neurologic signs without learning disability
"Organicity" as indicated on psychologic testing
Mental retardation
Normal disparity between receptive and expressive language
Age-appropriate dysfluency
Loss of language skills with behavioral regression

as following head trauma or other intracranial injury), when increased intracranial pressure is suggested, or when malformation of brain is suspected.

Differential Diagnosis. Several conditions should be kept in mind when assessing the child with a learning disability or speech disorder (see Table 17–4).

Learning disability should not be confused with *learning failure*. A great many causes for failure to progress satisfactorily in school exist, and learning disability is but one of these. Others are intercurrent *medical illness* (including thyroid disease), *sleep disturbance, drug use* (*or abuse*), *low motivation,* and *affective disorder* such as anxiety, depression, or neurotic underachievement ("fear of success").

Several pitfalls in the diagnosis of learning disability should be recognized. The fact that a child does well in one area (manifesting a "talent spike") does not mean that abilities overall are necessarily up to that same high level (Peters *et al.,* 1975). Accordingly, the child should not be assumed to have a learning disability in the *less-than-outstanding areas of achievement.* Conversely, an area of relatively poor achievement (a "downward spike") does not imply low motivation, laziness, or emotional conflict (see Case 17–2).

Another pitfall in approaching the child with a suspected learning disability is to base the diagnosis on *"soft" neurologic signs*. These signs are by no means pathognomonic of a learning disability or even necessarily features of the syndrome.

A further pitfall is diagnosing learning disability or "brain damage" solely on the basis of *"organicity"* felt to be shown on psychologic testing. The diagnosis of learning disability is established by demonstration of a significant gap between intelligence and performance in school subjects. No findings on the standardized tests currently in use correlate consistently with demonstrable abnormalities of brain.

The child with a learning disability or speech delay may, in fact, be *mentally retarded.* Formal developmental and psychologic testing will serve to establish the presence of a more global disturbance.

In a child with suspected speech delay, a *disparity between receptive and expressive language* abilities characteristically occurs between ages 1 and 3 years and should be recognized as normal. Indeed, a normal 18-month-old

CASE 17–2: LEARNING DISABILITY AND ATTENTION DEFICIT DISORDER IN A 9-YEAR-OLD BOY OF SUPERIOR INTELLIGENCE

S.Q. was referred for neurologic evaluation because of underachievement in school. He was noted to have reading problems in first grade, when psychologic testing demonstrated above-average intelligence. In third grade he could read at only a low third-grade level. Mathematics was at grade level or beyond. School evaluation suggested that underachievement was on an emotional basis. Psychosocial history, however, was entirely negative for behavioral or emotional problems. Past history was noncontributory. The boy's father, a truck driver, had difficulties in reading and spelling as a child, which had continued into adulthood.

On examination, the boy was an engaging, energetic child whose superior intelligence was demonstrated by his vocabulary and ability to pursue in depth a topic of conversation. He was fidgety and distractable. Accurate repetition of five digits forward required three trials. Reading a third-grade-level story was a struggle. Elemental neurologic examination for this right-handed, right-footed youngster was normal.

Comment.   Confusion arose in this case because the school had overlooked the possibility of learning disability. This boy's intelligence suggested that he might be reading at least at a fifth- or sixth-grade level while he was barely reading at a third-grade level. Because of his fidgetiness and inattention, he was considered to have emotional problems as the basis for his underachievement. The child's parents disagreed with this assessment and were upset by it. Neurologic evaluation helped to bring parents and school back together. It was clarified for both parties that the child appeared to be a boy of superior intelligence who had a learning disability (probably on a familial basis) associated with an attention deficit disorder. Emotional factors seemed to play a minor secondary role.

Use of psychotropic medication was not recommended in this case. It was suggested that the school carry out further testing in the areas of reading, speech, and language and provide the child with individual or small-group reading assistance. The parents were encouraged to continue their excellent manner of support, which emphasized their child's successes and thus diminished his frustrations from academic difficulties.

child may speak only a few single words and no word combinations but will be able to carry out two-step commands. *Age-appropriate dysfluency* ("the mind working faster than the tongue") should not be interpreted as stuttering.

Loss of language skills should be distinguished from speech delay. It can occur as part of a syndrome of *behavioral regression* or autism (see Chapters 5 and 8).

Etiology.   This section on etiology will focus upon learning disabilities and speech delay, respectively. Most learning disabilities are developmental

TABLE 17–5. **Most Frequent Causes of Speech Delay**

Mental retardation
Deafness
Cerebral palsy
Developmental disorder (including autism)
Environmental deprivation
Verbal auditory agnosia
Psychologic disorder
Seizures

in nature and often have a familial component. Identifiable disease of brain is found infrequently.

Speech delay is likeliest to be associated with, and explained by, *mental retardation* (see Tables 17–5 and 17–6). One must be cautious about establishing the diagnosis of mental retardation based on speech delay, however, particularly because behavioral problems associated with language problems

TABLE 17–6. **Causes of Speech Delay**

Medical	Hearing deficit due to
	    recurrent middle ear infection/effusion
	    viral (mumps) meningitis
	    bacterial meningitis

Neurologic	Anatomic abnormality of brain (as with dyslexia) Cerebral palsy Kernicterus Cerebral injury (trauma or tumor) leading to aphasia Congenital infection (as with rubella) Seizures Verbal auditory agnosia Autism
Toxic	Hearing deficit due to aminoglycoside therapy (gentamicin, kanamycin) Plumbism
Psychologic	Anxiety, depression Elective mutism
Social-Environmental	Twins/triplets Youngest child in sibship Multilingual environment Cultural differences
Genetic-Constitutional	Familial deficits Slower CNS maturation in males
Developmental	Normal behavior for younger age

often render developmental testing inconclusive. It should additionally be kept in mind that a specific language disability may coexist with mental retardation. This combination of problems compounds the retarded child's difficulties, especially when the associated language deficit is unrecognized.

Mild to moderate speech delay is next likeliest to be due to deafness, cerebral palsy, developmental disorders (including autism), environmental deprivation, verbal auditory agnosia, and elective mutism (Rutter, 1977). Though elective mutism is not strictly a cause of speech delay, it is included here since it involves failure to produce adequate speech in certain circumstances.

Medical Causes.   Several medical illnesses have been implicated in causing hearing deficit significant enough to interfere with speech and language development. Chronic, recurrent infections and/or effusions of the middle ear can lead to severe hearing deficit. Sensorineural deafness can also be caused by aseptic meningitis (particularly from mumps) or by bacterial meningitis (as from *H. influenzae, S. pneumoniae,* or *N. meningitidis*).

Neurologic Causes.   The work of Galaburda and Kemper (1979) in analyzing the brain of a young man with developmental dyslexia suggests that *structural abnormalities* of brain may underlie the learning disability of some children (see CORRELATION: ANATOMIC ASPECTS).

Cerebral palsy is a syndrome of nonprogressive motor deficit stemming from demonstrable or presumed injury to brain due to prenatal or perinatal causes. It should be emphasized that although children with cerebral palsy may have severe motor problems (including difficulties in expressive speech) such children cannot be assumed to be mentally retarded. It is of note that children who survive late low Apgar scores (0–3 at 10–20 minutes) without cerebral palsy do not appear to have an increased risk of learning disabilities (Nelson and Ellenberg, 1979).

Kernicterus, a poisoning of the basal ganglia and other portions of the central nervous system with bilirubin, can cause sensorineural deafness and a choreoathetoid form of cerebral palsy.

Cerebral injury due to a variety of causes (including trauma or tumor) may produce aphasia, a loss of previously acquired language function. Children are more likely than adults to develop language disturbance following head injury, but their recovery of language function is usually better. A history of left-handedness in the family or in the child is also generally associated with a better prognosis (see Case 21–4).

Maternal *infection during pregnancy* with rubella virus is an important cause of sensorineural deafness (unilateral or bilateral) and has been associated with a wide variety of behavioral disturbances as well, including autism (see Chapter 5; see Case 8–2).

Several syndromes of speech loss (aphasia) or speech delay in childhood are associated with *seizure disorders* (Landau and Kleffner, 1957; Gascon *et al.,* 1973; Shoumaker *et al.,* 1974; Deuel and Lenn, 1977; Koepp and Lagenstein, 1978). Unfortunately, clinical control of seizures in such cases does not necessarily lead to normalization of language processes. When improved seizure control is accompanied by significant normalization of the electroencephalogram, however, improvement in language function is likelier.

Verbal auditory agnosia is a cause of severe language disturbance among a small group of children (Rapin *et al.*, 1977). Affected children, often considered to be deaf, characteristically have undergone some loss of speech milestones. Their ability to decode language through the auditory route is severely impaired. Electroencephalographic abnormalities are common and appear to reflect bilateral cerebral (particularly temporal lobe) dysfunction.

Neurologic causes of *autism* are discussed in Chapter 5.

Toxic Causes. Sensorineural hearing impairment can result from use of aminoglycoside antibiotics. Included in this group are gentamicin and kanamycin, standard agents in the treatment of neonatal sepsis or meningitis.

Speech and language disturbance is one of several areas of development that may be affected by lead poisoning (see Chapter 14).

Psychologic Causes. Learning-disabled children are frequently thought to underachieve because of emotional disturbance. Such children may indeed be depressed or anxious since school is often such an unrewarding experience. But the primary problem remains the learning disability. Hence the child and family should not be pressured into attributing all problems to emotional causes (see Case 17–2). On the other hand, secondary emotional problems are often significant such that psychiatric or psychologic consultation is indicated (see Case 17–3).

A significant proportion (approximately one-fifth) of children with elective mutism will be found to suffer from specific speech and language problems (Rutter, 1977).

Social-Environmental Causes. The importance of secondary schools themselves in children's behavior and development has been documented and analyzed in an English study (Rutter, 1980). It demonstrated several features that fostered pupil success. These included (1) teachers' ample use of positive feedback (such as praise and demonstration of exemplary work), (2) pleasant and comfortable physical conditions (an environment in class, at lunch, and during breaks that is not unduly restrictive), (3) ample opportunity for student participation and responsibility in the running of their school lives, (4) schoolwide emphasis on scholastic achievement and excellence, (5) models of behavior provided by teachers (as demonstrated, for example, by punctuality and manner of discipline), and (6) staff organization (e.g., coordinated academic and disciplinary approaches).

Several social and environmental factors have been found to be associated with delayed speech and language development (Rutter, 1977). Included among these is diminished stimulation (see Case 20–4). Twins and triplets may have a several-month delay in speech and language development when compared with singletons. Often the problem is one of articulation or clarity of speech; the twins may be comprehensible to each other and to their parents but not to others.

Older siblings who speak for the child and anticipate his or her needs may also contribute to speech delay. The younger child does not develop speech, it seems, because he does not have to.

A multilingual environment is not usually associated with significant language delay, although it may occur if a second language is introduced some months after the first. Delay occurs less often when both languages are intro-

CASE 17–3: ANXIETY AND VISUAL-SPATIAL DYSFUNCTION IN A 17-YEAR-OLD ADOLESCENT WITH NEONATAL BRAIN INJURY

I.J. was referred for neurologic assessment at age 13 years because of learning problems associated with chronic anxiety. He had been hospitalized at 1 month of age for severe dehydration complicated by a right-sided seizure. At 10 years, he was described as restless, anxious, and distractable. Involuntary facial movements (grimacing and blinking) were also noted. Psychometric testing showed a verbal score of 95 and a performance score of 80. At 13 years he was again noted to be anxious. He was unable to copy age-appropriate geometric figures. Throwing, hopping, and walking were poorly coordinated. Facial grimacing and choreiform movements of the outstretched arms were evident. Deep tendon reflexes, strength, and sensation were normal.

At 17 years he had a generalized seizure. Further questioning revealed the possibility of two other seizures in the past. One episode had occurred in a shower and was associated with a fall resulting in scalp laceration. Review of systems indicated what the young man termed "tunnel vision." It involved difficulty in seeing things to his right and led to an automobile accident in which he was unable to see a vehicle approaching from that side.

Examination disclosed a right homonymous hemianopia. The remainder of the cranial nerve examination was unremarkable. Deep tendon reflexes were symmetric in the legs, brisker in the right arm than the left. Plantar responses were normal.

Electroencephalogram showed left-sided slow waves punctuated by left temporal spikes. CT scan demonstrated a porencephalic cyst of the left posterior temporal and anterior parietal regions communicating with the left lat-

duced simultaneously. Cultural differences are occasionally associated with elective mutism. It is manifested by shyness and speech refusal when the child is outside of the familiar home environment (Hayden, 1980).

Genetic-Constitutional Causes. Learning disabilities, like superior drawing skills or musical abilities, often run in families (DeFries *et al.*, 1978). In some parents or other family members, learning disability may never have been recognized but can be suspected on the basis of current or past difficulty in reading and in spelling, poor handwriting, or attentional problems (see Case 17–4).

Genetic factors in language disorders were implicated in the study of Folstein and Rutter (1977) involving twenty-one twin pairs of which at least one member was autistic. Concordance for cognitive difficulty (usually involving language disorder) was found in 82 per cent of monozygotic twins compared with 10 per cent in dizygotic twins.

Like hyperactivity, learning disability occurs more frequently in boys than in girls. This difference has been attributed to the slower rate of neurologic maturation in boys than in girls. Rutter (1977) has noted that girls learn language more quickly than boys but not to a degree that would account for

eral ventricle (see Fig. 17–1). He was placed on anticonvulsant therapy and had no seizures over the next 5 years. During that time he attended college and performed satisfactorily.

Comment. This case demonstrates that early severe illness causing injury to brain does not preclude an excellent outcome. The history suggests that focal seizures at the time of neonatal dehydration were associated with vascular thrombosis. The apparent result was infarction of portions of the left hemisphere leading ultimately to formation of a porencephalic cyst.

The link between this young man's early school behavior—characterized by restlessness, distractability, involuntary movements, and subnormal academic performance—and his later-defined neurologic lesion is speculative. Left hemisphere dysfunction, particularly in association areas, would be expected to be associated with reading or other language difficulty. Left temporal lobe involvement would implicate verbal memory in particular. This young man had evidence of no such difficulty. On the other hand, after an early brain injury perhaps some left hemisphere functions were taken over by the right hemisphere, which was then less able to function effectively in its attentional and visual-spatial roles (see Chapters 7 and 14). The link between the hemispheric defects and the child's anxiety remarked upon throughout much of his life is also unclear, though both probably contributed to his attentional problems.

This young man's two accidents (scalp laceration and automobile collision) serve as a reminder of the value of seeking the cause(s) of apparent accidents. In this case they were seizure and hemianopia, respectively. In another case cerebellar tumor underlay an apparently random mishap (see Case 13–4).

the markedly increased frequency of learning disorders among boys. It has been speculated that because boys are generally larger than girls at birth (in head circumference as well as other parameters), they are potentially more subject to birth injuries, which might result in later learning disabilities.

Developmental Causes. The term "developmental" used with learning disabilities and language disorders might suggest that children outgrow them. As indicated earlier, however, "developmental" is used to indicate behavior that would be considered normal at an earlier age. For example, letter reversals, which are normal at 4 to 6 years of age, are considered abnormal at 7 to 9 years. With developmental learning problems, a failure of maturation is suggested. Indeed, it is often true that the child does not outgrow the problem fully, although strategies for compensation often lessen the degree of disability, and awareness of the problem can minimize secondary complications.

TREATMENT AND OUTCOME

Establishing the diagnosis of *learning disability* in a child who is failing in school does not ensure an unproblematic outcome. A learning disability is,

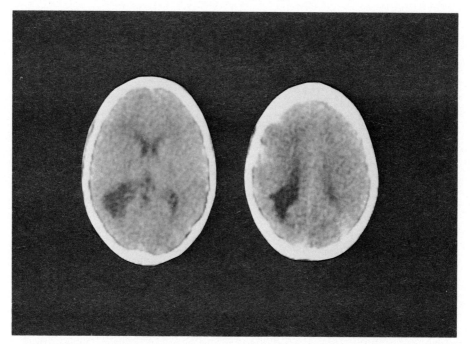

FIGURE 17–1. Porencephalic cyst of left cerebral hemisphere (Case 17–3).

in fact, a handicap with varying degrees of compensation possible. As such, it must be recognized, acknowledged, and dealt with both intellectually and affectively if the best possible adjustment is to be made.

The overall approach to the child with a learning disability should begin with demonstration to child and parents that the problem is a circumscribed disability, not a global impairment. The child is not mentally retarded despite classmates' comments and his own bad feelings about himself when struggling in school. A learning disability can be adjusted to and, in some instances, entirely compensated for through the child's intelligence, persistence, and motivation.

Specific educational remediation is the cornerstone of management (see Table 17–7). The physician will often have a significant role as coordinator, advocate, and support system (Gordon, 1975; Bell *et al.*, 1977; Eisenberg, 1980). Such remediation takes its direction from the psychologic and educational assessment of the child supplemented by medical and sometimes neurologic input. In addition to educational remediation, overall management might include treatment of associated problems such as hyperactivity (found in 25 to 50 per cent of learning-disabled children) and secondary emotional disturbance (depression or anxiety).

The early recognition of learning disability is fraught with some difficulty and potential danger. As defined above, the diagnosis of learning disability is based upon a 2-year gap between anticipated and realized academic performance. A child in kindergarten or first grade thus cannot be said to have a learning disability. Nomenclature notwithstanding, observant teach-

CASE 17–4: POOR MATHEMATICAL PERFORMANCE IN A 16-YEAR-OLD BOY

J.E., a student in eleventh grade, was referred for evaluation because of a long-standing history of poor achievement in mathematics and because of disparity between verbal and performance scores on psychologic testing. On the WISC-R, his full-scale intelligence quotient was 84, with a verbal score of 98 and a performance score of 72. The block design subtest was especially poorly performed.

Past history was of an 8-pound product of an uncomplicated full-term pregnancy. Delivery was unremarkable. Early milestones were on schedule. The child's brother and his father both had difficulty with mathematics.

On examination, the child was a healthy-appearing, articulate adolescent of normal intelligence whose mathematical skills were at a sixth-grade level. The general physical examination was normal. Neurologic examination disclosed an extensor left plantar response and mild coordinative difficulties, left greater than right. Finger-naming and right-left orientation were normal.

Comment. With a marked gap between his year of school (eleventh grade) and his level of mathematical ability (sixth grade), this adolescent certainly qualified as having a specific learning disability in mathematics (dyscalculia), probably on a constitutional-familial basis. His problem did not appear to be part of a Gerstmann syndrome (which implies left hemisphere dysfunction) as finger agnosia, right-left disorientation, and dysgraphia were not found. In fact, the mild left-sided findings suggested right hemisphere dysfunction, which might account for problems in block design, as this hemisphere appears to be specialized in visual-spatial skills.

The task that confronted this young man was to achieve adequacy in mathematical skills (with a pocket calculator certain to be of use) while building upon his obvious verbal and interactional strengths. One had the sense that he would do well.

ers are on the alert for problems such as unusual hyperactivity or marked difficulty with paper and pencil tasks that might suggest such children to be at higher risk for developing learning problems within the next few years. The perceptive teacher will provide individualized remediation within the regular classroom without singling out the child unnecessarily (Lansdown, 1978).

When formal intervention with the learning-disabled child is pursued, the goal should be not only optimizing the child's academic performance but also maintaining a positive self-image and enthusiasm toward learning.

The treatment and outcome of the child with *speech delay* will depend upon the severity of the disorder and associated or contributing factors such as mental retardation, hearing deficit, seizure, behavior disorder, or environmental deprivation (see Table 17–8) (Garvey and Gordon, 1973). Within the category of mental retardation, speech is usually absent when the intelli-

TABLE 17–7. **Treatment of Learning Disabilities**

Medical	Treatment of associated attention deficit disorder
Psychologic	Treatment of associated affective disorder: depression, anxiety Supportive therapy
Social-Environmental	Quiet work area
Educational	Small classes Individualized remediation Multimodal techniques
Mechanical	Typewriters, tape recorders, calculators, dictating machines
Physical	Remediation of associated large and fine motor disabilities

gence quotient is 20 or below. Between 20 and 70, speech is almost always delayed, although it develops to varying degrees.

In considering long-term outcome in the child with language disturbance, one must bear in mind the importance of language in communication. When language does not develop, isolation and secondary behavioral disturbance of severe degree may result (Cantwell *et al.*, 1980). Autism provides an example of severe disturbances in both language and behavior. Though it cannot be said that the interactional difficulties in autism stem entirely from

TABLE 17–8. **Treatment of Speech and Language Disorders**

Medical	Treatment of middle ear infection and/or effusion
Neurologic	Treatment of seizures
Surgical	Tympanostomy tubes Reconstructive palatal surgery
Psychologic	Parental support Treatment of behavioral disturbance
Educational	Individualized remediation
Communication	Manual techniques: finger spelling, gestural language, sign language Speech therapy
Mechanical	Hearing aid

the language deficit alone, it surely plays an important role in contributing to the autistic symptomatology.

Medical Management. Infections of the middle ear, particularly when recurrent, can affect hearing significantly. Such hearing impairment, especially that occurring early in life, may be severe enough to produce language dysfunction. In children with sensorineural hearing deficit, the child may also have a coexisting conductive hearing loss that is specifically remediable. Pneumatic otoscopy or impedance audiometry may indicate the presence of fluid or increased negative pressure within the middle ear, which can diminish mobility of the eardrum and thus hearing.

Antibiotic therapy plus, at times, the use of decongestant medication is the standard pharmacologic approach to ear infections and middle ear effusions. Surgical measures such as placement of tympanostomy tubes may prove necessary in children who have not responded to medical management.

Since inattention and hyperactivity frequently occur in children with learning disabilities, dextroamphetamine (Dexedrine), methylphenidate (Ritalin), or pemoline (Cylert) may be employed in addition to nonpharmacologic modes of therapy (see Chapter 14). Improvement may occur not just in activity level and attentional functions but in other school-related tasks as well, such as handwriting.

In children with disorders of movement involving spasticity or dystonia, such medications as diazepam (Valium) and trihexyphenidyl (Artane), respectively, may improve motor function involved in speech and in handwriting.

Neurologic Management. In the treatment of seizure-related speech delay anticonvulsant therapy is justified, although it may not improve speech and language function. Follow-up electroencephalography, periodic anticonvulsant blood level determinations, and repeat speech and language assessment are components of the ongoing management of this problem.

When aphasia results from brain injury in childhood, recovery of language function is related to the age at which trauma has occurred. Woods and Teuber (1978), in their study of sixty-five children with unilateral hemispheric brain lesions occurring after speech acquisition, found that all of those children who became aphasic before 8 years of age regained language function within weeks to 2 years of the brain injury.

Surgical Management. The treatment of hearing impairment will sometimes involve surgery. Tympanostomy tubes were mentioned earlier. With palatal cleft or other cause of posterior pharyngeal incompetence, reconstructive palatal surgery may be undertaken to restore palatal function. In that way voice quality can be improved and the likelihood of middle ear infection lessened through improved function of the eustachian tubes so that ready reflux of saliva, mucus, and debris from the pharynx into the middle ear can no longer occur.

Psychotherapy. The management of the child with a learning disability or any disorder of speech and language will necessarily involve psychologic measures. As mentioned earlier, formal psychologic or psychiatric assessment will often be an integral part of the evaluation process.

Support is always indicated. It need not be carried out formally by a psychologist or a psychiatrist. Rather, it may take the form of the pediatrician explaining the specific nature of the child's learning disability, the differences between learning disability and mental retardation, and overall goals for developing and using strategies for compensation.

Therapy may also involve active counseling. Parents should be encouraged to support their child's pursuit of success-oriented activities, namely those that have already brought a sense of achievement and reward to the child. Many parents intuitively will have already provided such support. The professional's acknowledgment of the parents' positive actions can serve to offset some of the guilt and doubts they may have accrued over the years. If areas of success and accomplishment have not been identified, they should be sought so that the child's self-esteem can be fortified.

Once educational remediation is in progress, the child should be protected from too much therapy. Balance must be maintained between time spent in remedial classes and that in mainstream activities, including nonacademic pursuits such as sports and the arts. Although it is often helpful for the learning-disabled child to be allowed to complete unfinished assignments at home, an excessive amount of homework should be avoided.

The frustration and fatigue associated with learning disabilities may lead to anxiety, depression, and somatization. Symptoms may take the form of headaches (muscle contraction headaches, migraines, or both), abdominal pain, or listlessness. Depression may be manifested by dysphoria, weight gain, and daydreaming, which may raise the specter of seizures. In fact, daydreaming probably subserves a protective function by providing a mental break from frustrating and fatiguing academic tasks.

Mutual support groups may be of help to learning-disabled teenagers and their families.

Social-Environmental Management.   A quiet study place with minimal visual and auditory distractions will benefit the child with a learning problem. Specifically, radios and television sets should not be in the immediate environment; colorful toys and stimulating wallpaper should be removed or replaced. Adequate sleep arrangements in quiet and comfortable surroundings also may contribute to improved school performance by enhancing daytime attentiveness.

Measures undertaken by the school to foster educational achievement in its pupils along the lines suggested by Rutter (1980) (*vide supra*) should be of significant benefit.

Educational Management.   Many of the measures employed for hyperactive children can be used productively with learning-disabled children. For example, small classes, providing the child with more individualized attention, can be of great help.

Multimodal techniques are often useful. They allow the child quite concretely to get in touch with his or her areas of cognitive difficulty and stimulate the development of adaptive strategies. For example, an 8-year-old child who continues to write letters in reverse or upside-down (for example, M's for W's) can get a better feel for the relationship between the two letters by manipulating sandpaper blocks in the shapes of the letters. The child can thus gain tactile and three-dimensional visual input to supplement his previous two-dimensional perspective.

Assessment of speech and language functions may identify specific areas of difficulty such as auditory discrimination, auditory memory, or visual sequencing that will benefit from specific remediation.

It is often necessary that the learning-disabled child leave regular classes to participate in remedial sessions. Care must be exercised that social stigmata and lack of participation in other, more favored activities do not outweigh benefits gained from special help. The parents and child should be consulted periodically to assess the overall benefits or deficiencies of the educational plan.

For the severely hearing-impaired child, education is an important part of the normalizing process designed to keep the deaf child from becoming isolated and out of the mainstream of society. Use of sign language is discussed below.

Educational treatment of the autistic child is presented in Chapter 5.

Communication Therapy.   Children with severe hearing impairment, verbal auditory agnosia, and developmental language disturbances will often benefit from manual communication: finger spelling, gestures, and sign language (Rapin *et al.,* 1977; Ferry and Cooper, 1978). Such symbolic communication has not always been recommended in the past because of concerns that it limited development of spoken language. It has, however, proved beneficial in providing for increased communication and diminishing the isolation that may result from severe language disturbance. Thus many professionals dealing with language-impaired children now stress the appropriateness of total communication, which implies the use of all available means (oral, visual, or manual) to communicate.

For children with verbal auditory agnosia, communication therapy will involve not only sign language but other visual modalities as well, including written language (Rapin *et al.,* 1977).

Some 5 per cent of school children have been estimated to manifest significant deficits of articulation such as problems in fluency (for example, stuttering) (Cave, 1977). Speech therapy is generally of benefit in such cases. Since comprehension (receptive language function) is often impaired in children with expressive language problems, therapy of the speech-impaired child should not be restricted necessarily to expressive language functions (Bishop, 1979). For children with a severe expressive speech handicap, a communication board may be invaluable (see Fig. 17–2).

Physical Therapy.   Spasticity may be associated with learning disorders or abnormalities of speech and language and may benefit from physical therapy. Athetosis and dystonia are less likely to be benefited, although some improvement may be seen.

When fine motor activities such as tying shoelaces present problems (and embarrassment) to the child, remediation, such as that provided by an occupational therapist, can be directed toward improving these skills of daily living.

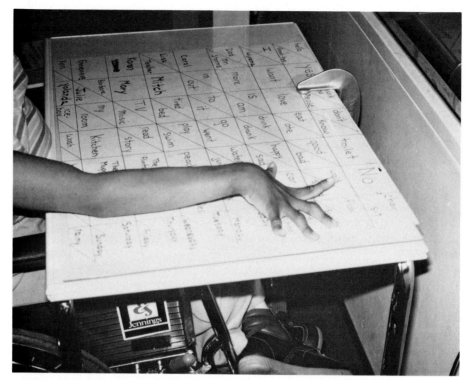

FIGURE 17–2. A child with severe choreoathetoid cerebral palsy "saying" "No" with the use of a communication board.

Neither stimulation of brainstem functions in an effort to enhance integration of cortical activities nor "patterning" techniques have been proved effective in the treatment of learning disabilities (Silver, 1975).

Mechanical Therapy.   Mechanical devices may be useful in attempting to compensate for deficits among learning-disabled and hearing-impaired children. Tape recorders, dictating machines, calculators, and typewriters are often valuable for the learning-disabled child. Amplification devices frequently will benefit the child with hearing impairment.

CORRELATION

Anatomic Aspects.   The superior temporal gyrus of the temporal lobe contains the primary auditory cortex. It receives input from brainstem structures mediating sound perception. Lying just behind the auditory cortex of the temporal lobe is the planum temporale, an auditory association area. Geschwind and Levitsky (1968) demonstrated at autopsy among the brains of 100 adults that the left planum temporale was larger than the right in a significant proportion of cases (see Fig. 17–3). This anatomic difference, evident even to the naked eye, presumably reflects left hemisphere dominance for language functions in most persons.

In 1973 Witelson and Pallie demonstrated such left–right asymmetries of

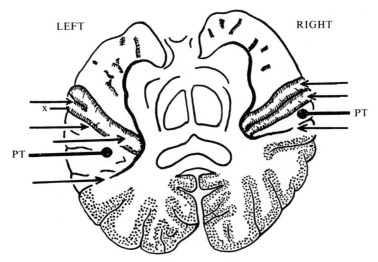

LEFT · RIGHT

FIGURE 17–3. Horizontal section through cerebral hemispheres showing asymmetric (left larger than right) planum temporale (PT). (From Geschwind, N., and Levitsky, W. Human brain: left-right asymmetries in temporal speech region. *Science,* **161:** 186–87, 1968. Copyright 1968 by the American Association for the Advancement of Science.)

the planum temporale in a study of fourteen neonatal brain specimens. They suggested that this neonatal asymmetry, which occurs before the development of speech or of hand preference, underlies the left hemisphere specialization for language seen in most adults.

Computerized tomography has provided evidence for a possible anatomic basis for certain learning disabilities, including developmental dyslexia. Normally, the left parieto-occipital portion of the brain, as represented by CT scan, will be wider than the right. A reversed pattern of this asymmetry occurs in 9 per cent of normal right-handers and 27 per cent of normal left-handers (LeMay, 1977).

Hier and colleagues (1978) examined by CT scan twenty-four persons between ages 14 and 47 years with developmental dyslexia. In only eight was the normal asymmetry found (left parieto-occipital region wider than the right). In six the right and left parieto-occipital regions were of equal size, and in ten the right was greater than the left—a reversal of the usual pattern of asymmetry (see Fig. 17–4). Among this last group, lower verbal intelligence quotient scores were found than among the fourteen other dyslexic persons. It is of further interest that four of the ten persons with reversed hemispheric asymmetry were speech-delayed, as contrasted with only one of the other fourteen dyslexic patients. Evidence that reversal of normal brain asymmetry occurs with infantile autism has been conflicting (see Chapter 5).

Galaburda and Kemper (1979) in their detailed case study of a young man with dyslexia suggested an anatomic basis for this learning disability and

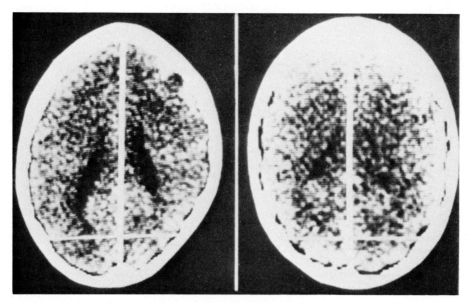

FIGURE 17–4. Computerized tomographic (CT) scans demonstrating normal and reversed cerebral asymmetry. The normal scan (left) shows a wider left than right parieto-occipital region. (Courtesy of P. B. Rosenberger, Boston.)

perhaps others. Their patient was a 20-year-old with well-documented developmental dyslexia and a seizure disorder who died as a result of an accident that did not produce direct trauma to the brain. The most striking abnormality found at postmortem examination of the brain was a small area of malformation, polymicrogyria, in the part of the temporal lobe corresponding to Wernicke's speech area (see Fig. 17–5). In addition, several minute foci of cortical dysplasia were scattered throughout the parietal, temporal, and occipital lobes on the left side only.

The cause or causes for the malformations in this case are unknown. Similar anatomic disturbances have been suggested to result from prenatal injury to brain or from maldevelopment on a familial basis. Whether these malformations could account for the young man's dyslexia must await further studies of learning-disabled persons.

Biochemical Aspects. There are no biochemical aspects unique to learning disabilities or speech delay. Biochemical factors of importance in learning are discussed in the sections on CORRELATION in Chapters 14 ("Hyperactivity and Attentional Disorders") and 16 ("Memory Disturbances").

Physiologic Aspects. The cerebral cortex includes several areas that have been identified as primary perceptual organizers. These include the visual cortex of the occipital lobes, the somesthetic cortex of the parietal lobes, and the auditory cortex of the temporal lobes. Intervening cortical areas function associatively.

Disconnection of one cortical area from another thus will usually permit

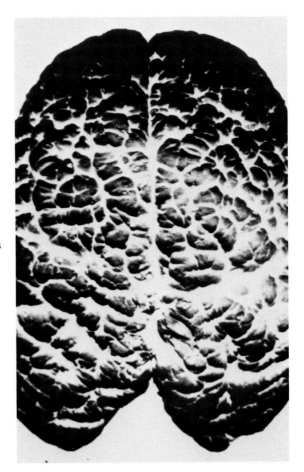

FIGURE 17–5. Brain specimen with extensive areas of polymicrogyria.

maintenance of primary perceptual functions, but with loss of associative functions. For example, injury to the left hemisphere in the region of the angular gyrus (where occipital, parietal, and temporal lobes come together) may be associated with loss of ability to read and write although vision, speech, and motor functions are unaffected.

Several fiber bundles play a crucial role in the interhemispheric transfer of information. They are importantly involved in speech and language functions. The major such fiber bundle is the corpus callosum. As an example of its function, if the posterior-most portion of the corpus callosum is injured, visual information from the left hemifield (which ultimately arrives at the right occipital cortex) cannot be brought over to the left hemisphere, the usual site for language processing. As a result the person so affected can see words in the left hemifield but is not able to read them. Other callosal syndromes may be manifested by an inability to name an object placed in the left hand when the eyes are closed and by failure of the left hand to carry out commands (Geschwind and Kaplan, 1962).

SUMMARY

Learning disabilities and speech delay are common and important problems in childhood. Learning disability is said to occur when a normally intelligent child's performance in a specific school subject (reading or arithmetic, for example) is two grade levels or more below that expected for age. A learning disability can also occur in the child whose intelligence is below or above average should the same gap between school performance and intelligence obtain. Major causes for learning disability are developmental and familial. Brain damage only rarely can be demonstrated in learning-disabled children.

The commonest causes for significant speech delay are mental retardation, deafness, cerebral palsy, developmental disorders of speech and language, environmental deprivation, emotional disturbance, and seizures.

Assessment of the child with a learning problem involves obtaining a careful school history in addition to standard medical data. Evaluation of speech delay should include detailed developmental information with particular focus on whether development is globally impaired or speech and language functions alone are delayed. Causes for deafness should be sought. Behavioral abnormalities seen in syndromes of autism should be inquired about. Formal psychologic testing, speech and language evaluation, and (in the child with speech delay) audiologic assessment are generally indicated.

Treatment of the learning-disabled child is directed toward recognition of the problem, helping the child to compensate for it, and assisting in the adjustment to that which cannot be ameliorated. The speech-delayed child should be evaluated as soon as possible so that treatment can begin promptly. In that way, social isolation and behavioral disturbances can be prevented or minimized.

CITED REFERENCES

Bell, A. E.; Abrahamson, D. S.; and McRae, K. N. Reading retardation: a 12-year prospective study. *J. Pediatr.*, **91**: 363–70, 1977.

Benson, D. F. Graphic orientation disorders of left handed children. *J. Learning Disabilities*, **3**: 6–11, 1970.

Benson, D. F., and Geschwind, N. Developmental Gerstmann syndrome. *Neurology*, **20**: 293–98, 1970.

Benton, A. L. Right-left discrimination. *Pediatr. Clin. North Am.*, **15**: 747–58, 1968.

Bishop, D. V. M. Comprehension in developmental language disorders. *Dev. Med. Child Neurol.*, **21**: 225–38, 1979.

Cantwell, D. P.; Baker, L.; and Mattison, R. E. Psychiatric disorders in children with speech and language retardation. *Arch. Gen. Psychiatry*, **37**: 423–26, 1980.

Cave, D. Assessment and treatment of stuttering in children. *Dev. Med. Child Neurol.*, **19**: 410–12, 1977.

Critchley, M. Dysgraphia and other anomalies of written speech. *Pediatr. Clin. North Am.*, **15**: 639–50, 1968.

DeFries, J. C.; Singer, S. M.; Foch, T. T.; and Lewitter, F. I. Familial nature of reading disability. *Br. J. Psychiatry*, **132**: 361–67, 1978.

Denckla, M. B. Development of speed in repetitive and successive finger-movements in normal children. *Dev. Med. Child Neurol.*, **15**: 635–45, 1973.

Deuel, R. K., and Lenn, N. J. Treatment of acquired epileptic aphasia. *J. Pediatr.*, **90**: 959–61, 1977.

Duffy, F. H.; Denckla, M. B.; Bartels, P. H.; Sandini, G.; and Kiessling, L. S. Dyslexia: automated diagnosis by computerized classification of brain electrical activity. *Ann. Neurol.*, **7**: 421–28, 1980.

Eisenberg, L. Failures in learning and failures in teaching. *Pediatrics*, **65**: 361–62, 1980.

Ferry, P. C., and Cooper, J. A. Sign language in communication disorders of childhood. *J. Pediatr.*, **93**: 547–52, 1978.

Folstein, S., and Rutter, M. Infantile autism: a genetic study of 21 twin pairs. *J. Child Psychol. Psychiatry*, **18**: 297–321, 1977.

Fraser, G. R. Profound childhood deafness. *J. Med. Genet.*, **1**: 118–51, 1964.

Frostig, M. Visual perception, integrative functions and academic learning. *J. Learning Disabilities*, **5**: 5–19, 1972.

Galaburda, A. M. and Kemper, T. L. Cytoarchitectonic abnormalities in developmental dyslexia: a case study. *Ann. Neurol.*, **6**: 94–100, 1979.

Garvey, M., and Gordon, N. A follow-up study of children with disorders of speech development. *Br. J. Disord. Commun.*, **8**: 17–28, 1973.

Gascon, G.; Victor, D.; and Lombroso, C. T. Language disorder, convulsive disorder, and electroencephalographic abnormalities. *Arch. Neurol.*, **28**: 156–62, 1973.

Geschwind, N., and Kaplan, E. A human cerebral deconnection syndrome. *Neurology*, **12**: 675–85, 1962.

Geschwind, N., and Levitsky, W. Human brain: left-right asymmetries in temporal speech region. *Science*, **161**: 186–87, 1968.

Gofman, H. P., and Allmond, B. W., Jr. Learning and language disorders in children. Part II. The school-age child. In *Current Problems in Pediatrics*. Year Book Medical Publishers, Inc., Chicago, 1971.

Gordon, N. Learning difficulties: the role of the doctor. *Dev. Med. Child Neurol.*, **17**: 99–102, 1975.

Hayden, T. L. Classification of elective mutism. *J. Am. Acad. Child Psychiatry*, **19**: 118–33, 1980.

Hier, D. B.; LeMay, M.; Rosenberger, P. B.; and Perlo, V. P. Developmental dyslexia. *Arch. Neurol.*, **35**: 90–92, 1978.

Kinsbourne, M. Developmental Gerstmann syndrome. *Pediatr. Clin. North Am.*, **15**: 771–77, 1968.

Kirk, S. A., and Kirk, W. D. Uses and abuses of the ITPA. *J. Speech Hear. Disord.*, **43**: 58–75, 1978.

Koepp, P., and Lagenstein, I. Acquired epileptic aphasia. *J. Pediatr.*, **92**: 164–65, 1978.

Landau, W. M., and Kleffner, F. R. Syndrome of acquired aphasia with convulsive disorder in children. *Neurology*, **7**: 523–30, 1957.

Lansdown, R. The learning-disabled child: early detection and prevention. *Dev. Med. Child Neurol.*, **20**: 496–97, 1978.

LeMay, M. Asymmetries of the skull and handedness: phrenology revisited. *J. Neurol. Sci.*, **32**: 243–53, 1977.

Levy, J., and Reid, M. L. Variations in writing posture and cerebral organization. *Science*, **194**: 337–39, 1976.

Matkin, N. D. The child with a marked high-frequency hearing impairment. *Pediatr. Clin. North Am.*, **15**: 677–90, 1968.

Moskowitz, B. A. The acquisition of language. *Sci. Am.*, **239**: 92–108, November 1978.

Nelson, K. B., and Ellenberg, J. H. Apgar scores and long-term neurological handicap. *Ann. Neurol.*, **6:** 182, 1979.

Peters, J. E.; Romine, J. S.; and Dykman, R. A. A special neurological examination of children with learning disabilities. *Dev. Med. Child Neurol.*, **17:** 63–78, 1975.

Rapin, I., Mattis, S.; Rowan, A. J.; and Golden, G. G. Verbal auditory agnosia in children. *Dev. Med. Child Neurol.*, **19:** 192–207, 1977.

Rutter, M. Speech delay. Pp. 688–716 in *Child Psychiatry: Modern Approaches.* Rutter, M., and Hersov, L., eds. Blackwell Scientific Publications, Oxford, 1977.

Rutter, M. School influences on children's behavior and development: the 1979 Kenneth Blackfan lecture, Children's Hospital Medical Center, Boston. *Pediatrics,* **65:** 208–20, 1980.

Schuberth, K. C., and Zitelli, B. J., eds. Developmental evaluation. Pp. 87–89 in *The Harriet Lane Handbook,* 8th ed. Year Book Medical Publishers, Inc., Chicago, 1978.

Shaffer, D.; Bijur, P.; Chadwick, O. F. D.; and Rutter, M. L. Head injury and later reading disability. *J. Am. Acad. Child Psychiatry,* **19:** 592–610, 1980.

Shoumaker, R. D.; Bennett, D. R.; Bray, P. F.; and Curless, R. G. Clinical and EEG manifestions of an unusual aphasic syndrome in children. *Neurology,* **24:** 10–16, 1974.

Silver, L. B. Acceptable and controversial approaches to treating the child with learning disabilities. *Pediatrics,* **55:** 406–15, 1975.

Swisher, L.; Wooten, N.; and Thompson, E. D. Biological predictors of language development. Pp. 213–25 in *Topics in Child Neurology.* Blaw, M. C.; Rapin, I.; and Kinsbourne, M., eds. Spectrum Publications, Inc., New York, 1977.

Witelson, S. F., and Pallie, W. Left hemisphere specialization for language in the newborn. *Brain,* **96:** 641–46, 1973.

Woods, B. T., and Teuber, H.-L. Changing patterns of childhood aphasia. *Ann. Neurol.,* **3:** 273–80, 1978.

ADDITIONAL READINGS

Bax, M.; Hart, H.; and Jenkins, S. Assessment of speech and language development in the young child. *Pediatrics,* **66:** 350–54, 1980.

Critchley, M. *The Dyslexic Child,* 2d ed. William Heinemann Medical Books Ltd., London, 1970.

Herron, J.; Galin, D.; Johnstone, J.; and Ornstein, R. E. Cerebral specialization, writing posture, and motor control of writing in left-handers. *Science,* **205:** 1285–89, 1979.

Kinsbourne, M. School problems. *Pediatrics,* **52:** 697–710, 1973.

Kinsbourne, M. Language lateralization and developmental disorders. Pp. 91–107 in *The Neurological Bases of Language Disorders in Children: Methods and Directions for Research.* Ludlow, C. L., and Doran-Quine, M. E., eds. NINCDS Monograph No. 22, Bethesda, Md., 1979.

Levine, D. N.; Hier, D. B.; and Calvanio, R. Acquired learning disability for reading after left temporal lobe damage in childhood. *Neurology* (New York), **31:** 257–64, 1981.

Levine, M. D.; Brooks, R.; and Shonkoff, J. P. *A Pediatric Approach to Learning Disorders.* John Wiley and Sons, New York, 1980.

Levine, M. D.; Oberklaid, F.; and Meltzer, L. Developmental output failure: a study of low productivity in school-aged children. *Pediatrics,* **67:** 18–25, 1981.

Ludlow, C. L. Children's language disorders: recent research advances. *Ann. Neurol.,* **7:** 497–507, 1980.

Rutter, M. Syndromes attributed to "minimal brain dysfunction" in childhood. *Am. J. Psychiatry,* **139:** 21–33, 1982.

Wender, P. H., and Wender, E. H. *The Hyperactive Child and the Learning Disabled Child: A Handbook for Parents.* Crown Publishers, Inc., New York, 1978.

Zinkus, P. W., and Gottlieb, M. I. Patterns of perceptual and academic deficits related to early chronic otitis media. *Pediatrics,* **66:** 246–53, 1980.

18 Mental Retardation

Mental retardation is a problem frequently encountered by the pediatrician, neurologist, and psychologist. Increasingly, children with mental retardation have become of concern to psychiatrists, social workers, and other health professionals as well. This widening area of involvement reflects greater recognition of the many aspects of mental retardation that pertain to the child, family, and community. Commonly associated issues include behavioral and emotional problems of the mentally retarded, the stresses such a child places on the family, and the different kinds of remediation to be considered for the child. Since an estimated 1 to 5 per cent of the population is mentally retarded, the problem is clearly a major one—important not only to affected persons, their families, and health professionals, but also to society at large.

This chapter is of necessity focused on a few areas: the definition and diagnosis of mental retardation, treatable aspects, conditions that might be mistaken for mental retardation, and behavior problems of the mentally retarded.

The following questions will be addressed:

How is the diagnosis of mental retardation established?
What aspects of the examination suggest a specific diagnosis?
What investigations are appropriate?
What conditions must be differentiated from mental retardation?
What specific and symptomatic therapies are available?

MENTAL RETARDATION

DEFINITION

Mental retardation has been defined as general intellectual functioning below the range of normal, beginning during the first 16 years of life and associated with impairment of maturation, learning, or social adjustment (Clarke and Clarke, 1974). These three areas of impairment—maturation,

512

learning, and social adjustment—are especially prominent in three successive periods of development: preschool, school-age, and adulthood. *Maturation* refers to the rate of development of self-help skills in infancy and early childhood. *Learning* is the capacity to acquire new information. *Social adjustment* refers to the individual's ability to adapt within the community to activities of adult life, including those at work and within the home. Mental retardation thus impacts upon intellectual, behavioral, personal, and social functions within the context of family, community, and society.

Mental retardation can be categorized on the basis of intelligence scores derived from formal psychometric testing of individuals. Commonly used tests of intelligence include the Stanford-Binet (for children from 2 through 6 years), the Wechsler Intelligence Scale for Children-Revised (WISC-R) (for children 5 to 16 years), and the Wechsler Adult Intelligence Scale (WAIS).

The World Health Organization Expert Committee has classified mental retardation on the basis of intelligence quotient (IQ) as follows (Clarke and Clarke, 1974):

mild	IQ of 50–70
moderate	IQ of 35–50
severe	IQ of 20–35
profound	IQ of 20 or below

Of the retarded persons in the United States, 85 to 90 per cent fall within the mildly retarded (or educable) range (Chess, 1977). Most such persons live at home and are at least partially self-supporting (see Table 18–1) (Taft, 1973).

Developmental delay is used to describe a lag in one or more areas of development. This term can usefully be employed in the initial stages of diagnostic formulation as a wide range of causes for slow development is being considered. The term "mental retardation," if introduced early in the diagnostic process, may have an upsetting ring of finality and hopelessness to it. Mental retardation can (and usually should) be included in preliminary discussions as *one* of the several causes for developmental delay. There are others to be considered, however, such as deafness or seizure disorder.

DIAGNOSIS

Clinical Process. All three components of the clinical process—history, examination, and investigation—can contribute importantly to establishing the diagnosis of mental retardation and paving the way for the most specific and comprehensive therapy. Frequently, despite extensive evaluation, a specific etiologic diagnosis is not determined. Active pursuit of a specific diagnosis is, however, usually justified, although time, expense, and discomfort must be considered. It should also be remembered that periodic reevaluation may be valuable since newer diagnostic techniques (such as computerized tomographic scanning and chromosomal banding techniques) are continually being developed and undergoing refinement.

History. The chief complaint of the parents will usually focus upon de-

TABLE 18–1. **Mental Retardation and Functional Capacity**

Severity	IQ	Educability	Trainability	Independent Living	Routine Self-care	Vocational Capability
Mild	50–75	yes	yes	often	yes	often
Moderate	25–50	no	yes	with some supervision	yes	in sheltered workshop
Severe	less than 25	no	no	no; custodial or residential care required	limited or none	limited or none

velopment in general or one aspect in particular. "He's not doing everything a 2-year-old should," or "He's 3 years old and still doesn't talk." The chief complaint not only provides a jumping-off point for the history but can also offer clues as to why the parents have sought evaluation at that particular time.

The history of the presenting problem usually begins with the parents' recognition that something is wrong with their child. At other times a physician, grandparent, or friend makes that assessment. Development in various areas (gross motor, fine motor, language, and social-adaptive skills) should be traced. The tempo of development should be noted. Has it always lagged? Does the child do better in some areas than in others? Has acquisition of skills plateaued? Have skills once acquired been lost? This last pattern would suggest a disorder of behavioral regression rather than mental retardation, which is characterized by static or slowed development (see Chapter 8). If the child has undergone prior evaluation, the results of such assessment should be obtained and reviewed.

Past history is especially important in identifying factors that might have caused or contributed to mental retardation. Exposure to rubella in the first trimester of pregnancy can lead to a congenital rubella syndrome. Typical symptoms would include mental retardation (with microcephaly), visual impairment (secondary to cataracts), deafness of sensorineural type, and heart disease (typically patent ductus arteriosus). Contact with cats and their feces may expose the pregnant woman to the protozoan organism *Toxoplasma gondii,* the agent of toxoplasmosis (Krogstad *et al.,* 1972). Cytomegalovirus infection, like toxoplasmosis and rubella infection, may be asymptomatic in the pregnant woman but can cause a wide array of abnormalities in the developing child. These include microcephaly, mental retardation, visual impairment, and hearing deficit. With toxoplasmosis in particular, hydrocephalus often results.

Alcohol abuse, with or without accompanying malnutrition, appears to be associated with an embryopathy ultimately manifested as a fetal alcohol syndrome, which can include mental retardation, poor somatic growth, microcephaly, and a variety of somatic defects, particularly underdevelopment of structures of the mid-face (Ouellette *et al.,* 1977).

In some instances a mother may have recognized something different about her pregnancy such as diminished fetal movement. Suspected lack of intrauterine growth may have been investigated by ultrasound study. Information as to labor and delivery should also be obtained. Was labor prolonged? Was fetal monitoring carried out? Externally? Internally? Was delivery performed vaginally or by cesarean section? If vaginally, did prolapse of the umbilical cord or abruption of the placenta occur? If cesarean section was carried out, what were the indications for doing so? Did the baby breathe right away? What were the Apgar scores?

Birth records often provide much valuable information. Gestational age, weight, height, head circumference, and Apgar scores should specifically be noted. Details of the neonatal course should also be sought. Did illness such as pneumonia, sepsis, meningitis, or urinary tract infection occur? Did the baby have an intracranial hemorrhage? If so, was it large or small? Was examination of cerebrospinal fluid carried out? Was a CT scan obtained?

Family history should be explored in detail. Autosomal dominant ("vertical") transmission may be seen with tuberous sclerosis and neurofibromatosis. An autosomal recessive ("horizontal") pattern of inheritance may be evident with phenylketonuria or homocystinuria. Parental consanguinity should be noted, as it enhances the likelihood of autosomal recessive disorders.

Past hospitalizations of the child (for meningitis, head trauma, or status epilepticus, for example) may suggest a basis for his or her mental retardation. Social history should include the child's position in the family, relationships with other family members, favorite activities, and educational or other programs in which the child participates. Review of systems should include questions as to head trauma, headaches, seizures, medications, birthmarks, and behavior problems such as hyperactivity, withdrawal, aggression, self-injury, stereotyped movements, temper tantrums, and fearfulness (Ando and Yoshimura, 1978).

Examination. The *general description* should include obvious and striking features of the child's examination. These might include unusual facial appearance, short stature, obesity, or other abnormal physical features (Smith, 1976).

Facial appearance often provides a clue to specific diagnosis in the mentally retarded child. The three classic chromosomal disorders in which an extra chromosome is present—trisomies 13, 18, and 21—each have a characteristic appearance that includes the following: bilateral cleft lip and palate, "pixyish" look, and "mongoloid" faces, respectively (see Fig. 18–1).

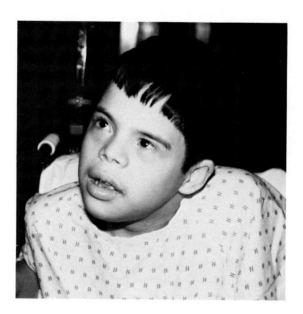

FIGURE 18–1. A 10-year-old boy with Down syndrome and hypothyroidism.

Only with Down syndrome (trisomy 21), however, is survival to adulthood usual.

Congenital hypothyroidism, too, is characterized by a facial appearance that is typical, though the abnormalities are often subtle in early childhood. They include coarsened features, flattened nasal bridge, and prominent tongue. Neonatal screening programs for hypothyroidism have lessened the need for diagnosis to be made on the basis of clinical criteria alone, but such programs are not universal.

The fetal alcohol syndrome is suggested by growth deficiency, microcephaly, facial features that include a hypoplastic upper lip, short palpebral fissures, a small upturned nose, underdeveloped philtrum, and hypoplasia of the midface and jaw combined with other somatic signs such as skeletal, cardiac, and urogenital anomalies.

The Rubenstein-Taybi syndrome has a characteristic facial appearance manifested by antimongoloid slant to the eyes, beaked nose, and elongated nasal septum. The hallmarks of this syndrome are unusually broad thumbs and great toes.

The *general physical examination* should include measurement and plotting of growth parameters on standardized charts. Head size is a most important indicator of brain growth (Nelson and Deutschberger, 1970). Hence, it is essential to measure and plot the head circumference in the evaluation of every child with mental retardation. Although not all persons with microcephaly (defined by head circumference of two or more standard deviations below the mean) are intellectually subnormal, most are (Martin, 1970). If the child is microcephalic, earlier measurements (going back to birth, if possible) will be valuable in determining the time of insult to the central nervous system. A head that is disproportionately small at birth suggests influence of intrauterine or constitutional factors (Gross *et al.,* 1978). If the head circumference is normal at birth (approximately 35 cm for a full-term male and 34 cm for a full-term female) then falls away from the normal curve, a perinatal or postnatal insult (such as asphyxia neonatorum, meningitis, malnutrition, or trauma) should be suspected.

Microcephaly due to diminished brain growth is often associated with craniosynostosis, premature closure of cranial sutures. When multiple sutures are closed prematurely in association with microcephaly, the cause is usually primary failure of brain growth with secondary craniosynostosis. Much less often, multiple sutures close primarily and give rise to secondary impairment of brain growth.

A symmetrically large head, particularly if familial, is usually associated with normal intelligence (Weaver and Christian, 1980). When intelligence is subnormal, hydrocephalus, chronic subdural fluid collection, or storage disorder of brain should be considered.

Examination of the skin may suggest a specific diagnosis. Tuberous sclerosis is characterized by hypopigmented macules that are usually present at birth (see Fig. 4–2). Perception of these macules may be enhanced by use of an ultraviolet lamp. By 2 to 5 years of age, adenoma sebaceum—acneiform lesions of the cheeks, nasal bridge, or chin—may have developed (see Fig.

8–6). Shagreen patches—slightly raised, tawny patches with the dimpled appearance of orange peel—may also be seen over the lower back. Café-au-lait macules occur in some persons with tuberous sclerosis but are more specifically linked with neurofibromatosis (see Fig. 4–1).

Other parts of the general medical examination also may suggest the cause of the child's retardation. Eye examination may disclose cataracts (as seen in congenital rubella, galactosemia, and myotonic muscular dystrophy), dislocation of the lens (characteristic of homocystinuria), or corneal clouding (as seen with the mucopolysaccharidoses).

An infant's cry may itself suggest the diagnosis. A low-pitched, growling cry is typical of the Cornelia de Lange syndrome, while a high-pitched, weak, mewling cry is found with the cri-du-chat ("cat cry") syndrome. The latter is associated with a deletion of the short arm of chromosome 5. Both of these syndromes are characterized by severe retardation; hence, affected children are likely to present for initial assessment before the school-age years.

Skeletal anomalies occur with Apert syndrome (polysyndactyly), homocystinuria (arachnodactyly), Down syndrome (pelvic dysplasia), Laurence-Moon-Biedl syndrome (polydactyly), and the mucopolysaccharidoses (beaked vertebrae).

All parts of the *neurologic examination* may be valuable in determining the cause of the mental retardation, identifying treatable components of a mental retardation syndrome, and excluding conditions that may mimic mental retardation.

Visualization of the optic disks is generally best achieved by dilating the pupils with mydriatic solution. The optic papilla, or nerve head, may be atrophic or swollen. Atrophy may occur with prenatal exposure to toxins or with developmental abnormalities of brain; swelling occurs with raised intracranial pressure (papilledema) or inflammation of the optic nerve (papillitis). Also evident on funduscopy may be macular scarring (chorioretinopathy) occurring with congenital infections such as toxoplasmosis, "salt-and-pepper" pigmentation of the retina seen with congenital rubella syndrome, and pigmentary degeneration of the retina (retinitis pigmentosa) seen with the Laurence-Moon-Biedl syndrome. Extraocular movements may be limited due to external ophthalmoplegia with the Kearns-Sayre syndrome, also associated with short stature and mental retardation.

The facial muscles may be involved bilaterally in mental retardation syndromes to produce a masklike, drooping, expressionless appearance. This pseudo-depressed appearance is characteristic of myotonic muscular dystrophy, associated with mental retardation, as well as other disorders of muscle (such as facioscapulohumeral dystrophy) or neuromuscular junction (myasthenia gravis) that are not associated with mental retardation.

Hearing always should be assessed in the delayed child because of the overlap in symptoms between syndromes of marked hearing impairment and those of mental retardation. Not infrequently, the two coexist, as in congenital syphilis.

Motor examination should note current motor skills and seek abnormalities in tone, strength, bulk, posture, and movement. Although motor function in the infant or younger child does not necessarily mirror intellectual ability or potential, in fact it does frequently reflect such ability. For example, in the child with an atonic form of cerebral palsy, delayed acquisition of motor skills is often only one component of a global delay secondary to widespread brain insult.

Muscle weakness contributes to clumsy walking or inability to run in Duchenne muscular dystrophy. This disorder is characterized also by calves that are enlarged (pseudohypertrophied) because of replacement of muscle tissue with fat. In the older child or adolescent, myotonia, an inability of muscle to relax after percussion or voluntary contraction, may be seen with myotonic muscular dystrophy. Other features of myotonic dystrophy include cataracts, gonadal atrophy (testicular or ovarian), and abnormalities of carbohydrate metabolism (see Chapter 13). Mental retardation frequently accompanies both of these forms of muscular dystrophy (Rosman and Kakulas, 1966). Myotonia also occurs with myotonia congenita (Thomsen disease) and hyperkalemic periodic paralysis, neither of which is associated with mental retardation.

Deep tendon reflexes may be excessively brisk, joining spasticity in reflecting brain damage or dysfunction. A characteristic pattern of involvement is hyperreflexia and spasticity on one side of the body (spastic hemiparesis), often seen with an extensor plantar response (a Babinski sign) on the affected side. Another pattern of abnormal reflexes is hyperreflexia of the lower extremities and a bilateral Babinski sign with lesser spasticity and mildly increased deep tendon reflexes in the arms (spastic diplegia). Spastic hemiparesis usually signifies hemispheric injury. Spastic diplegia suggests injury to deep white matter, as with hydrocephalus or periventricular leukomalacia, the latter found characteristically in prematures (see Chapter 13).

The *mental status examination* of the child suspected of being mentally retarded will include estimation of the child's level of intellectual development. Although formal testing is frequently required, a great deal of information can be gained through office evaluation. Other aspects of the child's mental status such as alertness, attention, memory, orientation, behavior, judgment, and mood should also be assessed. The examiner should recognize that strangeness of the setting may contribute to anxiety, negativism, withdrawal, or other alteration in behavior which may influence the results of intelligence testing. Observed results must therefore be considered along with parents' reports of the child's best level of function. Examining the child in the presence of his parents and carrying out the assessment over two or more sessions often will increase the yield of useful information.

In the older child assessment of intellectual function should include several minutes of conversation to evaluate the child's quality and connectedness of thought, richness of expressive vocabulary, and understanding of words and expressions used by the examiner (receptive vocabulary). In speaking directly with the child, one gains fuller appreciation of him or her as an individual with interests, plans, and feelings. One may get the sense that the matter of mental retardation has been exaggerated or overemphasized to the exclusion of interpersonal or other strengths.

Conversation may make the language-impaired or dysarthric child appear to be unintelligent. The Goodenough-Harris Draw-a-Person Test is a means of assessing overall intelligence that is particularly useful in such cases. It should also be noted that drawing ability in a child with poor graphomotor skills may make him seem dull.

The child's alertness—essentially his or her interest in the environment—is often correlated with intelligence. When a child looks dull, however, the examiner should not assume that the child is mentally retarded but rather should consider what it is that is producing the effect of dullness. For example, the myopathic facial appearance of a child with myotonic muscular dystrophy or Moebius syndrome can convey feelings of sadness or intellectual deficit that are exaggerated or absent.

Attention can be assessed by noting the child's level of distractability, recall of digits, and ability to carry out assigned tasks such as writing the numbers one through twenty. Memory testing should include recall of three or four items after 5 to 10 minutes (short-term memory) as well as past events (long-term memory) (see Chapter 16).

Assessment of orientation should include the child's understanding of why he or she has been brought for examination.

The emotional state of the child is an essential part of the mental status examination. Occasionally a child will be so depressed that a diagnosis of retardation is suggested. More often, a child with mild or moderate retardation will appear additionally delayed because of depression that results from school failure, frustration, teasing, isolation, and lack of opportunities. Aloofness is a manifestation of the emotional disorder that generally coexists with significant mental retardation in childhood autism.

Investigation. Investigation of the mentally retarded child is directed toward identifying treatable causes or components of the mental retardation syndrome and obtaining specific diagnostic data for purposes of genetic counseling (see Table 18–2). No studies are routinely indicated in the evaluation of the mentally retarded child, although a complete blood count and urinalysis can be justified in establishing a complete data base in the child hospitalized for evaluation.

Investigation should be guided by the history and examination. For example, the child with a diagnosis of Down syndrome based upon characteristic appearance and development should generally have chromosome analysis. Serum thyroxine (T_4) level should also be determined because of the increased incidence of hypothyroidism with Down syndrome (see Fig. 18–1). The infant with coarse features suggesting gargoylism (Hurler syndrome) and a cherry red macula should have lysosomal enzyme analysis of blood with specific determination of beta galactosidase—deficient in generalized (GM_1) gangliosidosis—and analysis of urine for mucopolysaccharides.

In children in whom the specific cause for mental retardation has not been established, a number of other investigations should be considered. These include plain skull x-rays, electroencephalogram (with awake and sleep studies), assessment of vision and hearing, blood for amino acid analysis, urine for amino acid and organic acid analysis, serum thyroxine level, blood lead and free erythrocyte protoporphyrin (FEP) levels, serum uric acid, and TORCH titers (that is, measurement of antibodies produced in response

TABLE 18–2. **Investigations to Be Considered in the Child with Mental Retardation**

Thyroid function tests
Psychologic testing
Assessment of hearing and vision
EEG (in awake and sleep states)
Blood lead level, free erythrocyte protoporphyrin (FEP)
Chromosome analysis
TORCH antibody titers in blood
Skull x-rays
Cranial CT scan
Blood and urine for amino acids, urine for organic acids
Urine for mucopolysaccharides
Lysosomal enzyme analyses in blood
Serum uric acid

to prenatal infection with toxoplasma, rubella, cytomegalovirus, *Herpes simplex,* and syphilis). More specialized investigation such as computerized tomographic (CT) scan of the head, lysosomal enzyme determinations, analysis of urine for mucopolysaccharides, and chromosomal analysis will depend upon circumstances in an individual case. An aggressive approach to diagnosis is usually justified in the developmentally delayed child, because early treatment may minimize or prevent some instances of permanent mental retardation (as in phenylketonuria or hypothyroidism) and occasionally can reverse the retardation at least in part (as with seizures accompanying a retardation syndrome).

As indicated above, formal developmental and psychologic testing is frequently valuable, often essential, in the evaluation of the child with developmental delay (Clark, 1974).

Differential Diagnosis.   Several conditions must be differentiated from mental retardation (see Table 18–3). *Normal variation* in the rate of development within a population will result in some children whose development is suspect or delayed with respect to the mean but who prove in the longer run to be normal (Koch *et al.,* 1977). *Cerebral palsy* affecting motor functions alone in the preverbal child may be mistaken for global retardation. In

TABLE 18–3. **Differential Diagnosis of Mental Retardation**

Normal variation in development
Cerebral palsy affecting motor and speech functions
Seizure disorder or excessive anticonvulsant medication
    depressing development
Hearing deficit
Visual impairment
Degenerative disease
Dull facial appearance
Depression
Specific learning disability

later years dysarthria causing slowness in speaking may be misinterpreted as slowness in thinking.

Seizure disorder may be associated with reversible developmental delay. Seizures may have been overlooked if they are subtle (for example, manifested only by brief staring, momentary pausing, or shuddering of the chin). They may be entirely subclinical, evidenced only by spike or spike-and-wave abnormalities on electroencephalogram. In a child treated with *anticonvulsant medication,* overmedication may itself cause developmental delay or even a picture of behavioral regression (see Chapters 8 and 12). Controlling the child's seizures, however, usually does not abolish the developmental delay, for in many children seizures are but one of several manifestations of disordered brain function (e.g., in tuberous sclerosis).

Hearing impairment is an important cause for delayed development that may be mistaken for mental retardation. Such children typically fail to develop language normally, particularly when hearing impairment is severe and present since early life. Since much of our perception of intelligence depends upon language, misdiagnosis of mental retardation in a deaf child can easily result. Associated behavioral problems may make definitive diagnosis even more difficult.

The *visually impaired* child, too, will often manifest developmental lags that cause intelligence to be suspect. For example, sighted children typically elevate themselves in the prone position by 2 months of age by pushing up on their arms, whereas blind children do so at an average of 7 months later. Similarly, the mean age for walking alone across a room is delayed among blind children by some 7 months (19 versus 12 months) (Adelson and Fraiberg, 1977).

Degenerative disease of the nervous system must be differentiated from static mental retardation. History of development and its progression combined with follow-up re-examination will usually clarify this category of developmental disorder.

As noted above, a *dull facial appearance* may be mistaken for intellectual dullness in a child with a myopathic facies associated with muscle disease (myotonic muscular dystrophy, facioscapulohumeral dystrophy), neuromuscular disorder (myasthenia gravis), or central nervous system disorder (Moebius syndrome).

The presence of *depression* with its characteristically associated psychomotor retardation must be considered in the developmentally delayed child as a cause, concomitant, or imitator of delay. Particularly in the younger child, depression may also be manifested in bizarre behavior as with the coprophagia syndrome described by Spitz (1965) (see Chapter 5).

In the school-age child, a *specific learning disability* may raise concerns as to the overall level of the child's intelligence, especially if academic difficulties are compounded by anxiety, depression, or "giving up." Formal psychologic assessment including nonverbal tests will usually clarify this situation (see Chapter 17).

Etiology. Although many causes of mental retardation are recognized, the etiology of mental retardation in many children, perhaps most, remains undetermined (see Table 18–4). Such mental retardation is classified as idio-

TABLE 18–4. **Causes of Mental Retardation**

Medical	Congenital hypothyroidism
Neurologic	Perinatal causes:
	Asphyxia (abruptio placentae, cord prolapse, meconium aspiration)
	Infections (meningitis, encephalitis, TORCH agents, syphilis)
	Trauma (breech delivery)
	Nutritional deprivation
	Postnatal brain injury:
	Trauma
	Drowning
	Heat stroke
	Lightning
Toxic	Lead poisoning
	Fetal alcohol syndrome
	Radiation exposure
Psychologic	Abuse and neglect
Social-Environmental	Deprivation (intentional or unintentional)
Genetic-Constitutional	Autosomal recessive: phenylketonuria, homocystinuria, most mucopolysaccharidoses, galactosemia
	Autosomal dominant: tuberous sclerosis, neurofibromatosis, myotonic muscular dystrophy
	X-linked: Lesch-Nyhan syndrome, Menkes steely hair disease, Hunter syndrome, Lowe syndrome, Duchenne muscular dystrophy

pathic. Many idiopathic disorders of today, however, will find their way into tomorrow's textbooks as specific disorders. Some will prove to be amenable to prevention and treatment as clincal and laboratory research continues to seek causes and cures for disorders of development.

Medical Causes. *Hypothyroidism* is an important preventable cause of mental retardation, affecting one child in every 7,000 live births. Congenital hypothyroidism is usually due to absence (agenesis) or displacement (ectopia) of thyroid gland tissue. It becomes clinically evident insidiously. Infants are generally of normal to somewhat increased birth weight. Coarsening of facial features, prominence of the tongue, low-pitched cry, umbilical hernia, and large anterior fontanelle may suggest the diagnosis in the neonatal period. Less specific features include feeding difficulties, constipation, jaundice, abdominal distention, respiratory difficulties, hypothermia, and mottling of the skin (cutis marmorata) (Rosman, 1976).

Neurologic Causes. Perinatal asphyxia, infections, trauma, and nutritional causes of mental retardation have been recognized. *Infections* affecting the *fetus* include the TORCH group of agents: toxoplasma, rubella, cytomegalovirus, *Herpes simplex,* and the spirochetes of syphilis (Chess *et al., 1978*) (see Case 18–1). Meningitis in the *neonatal period* or meningoencephalitis in *later childhood* (with measles or chickenpox, for example) can result in mental retardation.

Perinatal events such as *abruptio placentae, umbilical cord prolapse, meconium aspiration* with asphyxia, and *difficult breech delivery* each can cause sufficient brain damage to produce mental retardation. Cerebral palsy, a nonprogressive motor deficit of prenatal or perinatal origin, may also be associated (see Chapter 13).

Head trauma associated with vehicular accidents, falls, and inflicted injury is another important neurologic cause of mental retardation (Rosman

CASE 18–1: MENTAL RETARDATION, MICROCEPHALY, AND UNILATERAL BLINDNESS IN AN 11-YEAR-OLD GIRL WITH CONGENITAL INFECTION

B.Q. was brought for evaluation because her mother felt that "age is catching up to her." The child had recently been brought to the United States to rejoin her family, and her mother was concerned about her daughter's continued developmental delay. She had been born at home following an uncomplicated, full-term pregnancy without known infections, rashes, fevers, trauma, drug use, or exposure to cats. Birth weight was unknown. She was recalled to have walked at 8 months, spoken in word combinations between 3 and 4 years, and been toilet-trained by 5 years. She had repeated nearly all elementary school grades prior to leaving her native country. Vision in the right eye was long recognized as poor, but no evaluation had been carried out. Family history was unremarkable.

On examination, the child was a slender, friendly, cooperative, and fidgety girl. She was able to name the days of the week and recognized several letters of the alphabet but could not add 4 + 1. Her figure drawings scored at the 7-year level. On general examination, she was microcephalic. Her head circumference was 50 cm (50th percentile for a 5-year-old girl). On neurologic examination, visual acuity in the right eye was 20/400, in the left eye 20/30. Funduscopic inspection disclosed chorioretinopathy of the right macula, a white patch surrounded by black pigment (see Fig. 18–2).

Investigation included electrolytes, urine culture and analysis, tuberculin skin test, hand films for bone age, urine for amino acid analysis, and chromosome analysis—all normal. Skull x-rays showed microcephaly without intracranial calcification. Viral titers in blood were consistent with past infection with rubella, cytomegalovirus, *Herpes simplex,* and toxoplasma. Formal psychologic testing gave a full-scale intelligence quotient of 46.

Comment. This child appeared to have suffered from an intrauterine infection, probably cytomegalic inclusion disease or toxoplasmosis. Rubella

and Herskowitz, 1982). Brain injury and mental retardation can also result from *drowning, heat stroke,* or *lightning* strike.

Early severe *malnutrition* appears to affect intellectual performance as well as behavior (see Chapter 20).

Toxic Causes. *Lead* poisoning is of major concern in this category, Widespread screening programs appear to have led to a decline in acute encephalopathy (associated almost invariably with permanent mental retardation, sometimes death) because of early detection, prompt treatment with chelating agents, and removal of the child from a leaded environment.

Accumulating evidence indicates that excessive *alcohol* intake during pregnancy can be associated with mental retardation and a variety of physi-

infection could be excluded because of the lack of associated manifestations such as heart disease, cataracts, deafness, and "salt-and-pepper" retinopathy.

The essential features of this case—mental retardation, microcephaly, and chorioretinopathy—are consistent with either cytomegalovirus or toxoplasma infection. Serum antibody levels did not resolve the diagnostic question but did document previous exposure to these organisms, among others. Plain skull x-rays may show characteristic patterns of intracranial calcification—often periventricular with cytomegalovirus infection and more widely scattered with toxoplasmosis—but neither was seen in this case. CT scan, unavailable at the time of assessment, is far more sensitive in detecting intracranial calcification and might have been of diagnostic benefit here (see Fig. 18–3). Toxoplasmosis is often associated with hydrocephalus. It has been linked with ependymal inflammation and elevated levels of cerebrospinal fluid protein. Microcephaly may otherwise result from brain destruction due to infection by toxoplasma organisms as with cytomegalovirus and rubella.

The source of this child's infection was obscure, as it generally is with cytomegalovirus infection and toxoplasmosis. The occurrence of the unicellular protozoan *Toxoplasma gondii* within Toxocara, a gastrointestinal parasite of cats, provides a ready mechanism for infection of man. Persons handling cat feces, within which toxoplasma may exist, are at risk. Improperly cooked meat can also harbor toxoplasma organisms. Toxoplasma and cytomegalovirus, usually asymptomatic when they infect pregnant women, pass through the placenta to the fetus.

Toxoplasmosis often affects both eyes and can significantly affect vision because of the organism's propensity to invade the macular area. Cytomegalovirus infection has been reported to cause chorioretinopathy similar to that seen with toxoplasmosis. Aicardi syndrome, an X-linked dominant disorder involving vertebral anomalies, agenesis of the corpus callosum, chorioretinal lesions, and mental retardation, should be distinguished from both of these infectious causes of chorioretinopathy (Willis and Rosman, 1980).

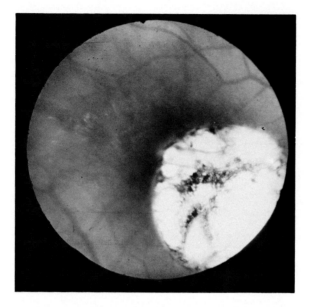

FIGURE 18–2. Destructive chorioretinopathy with congenital toxoplasmosis.

cal anomalies. The role of malnutrition, cigarette smoking, and use of other drugs such as marijuana remains to be clarified.

Radiation exposure before the twentieth week of gestation among pregnant women who survived the nuclear attack in Japan was associated with an increased incidence of mental retardation and microcephaly (Miller and Blot, 1972).

Psychologic Causes. There are probably no exclusively psychologic

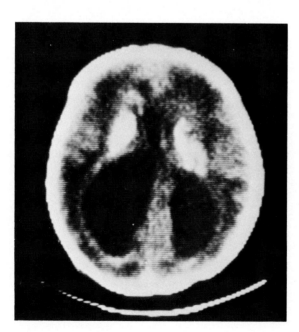

FIGURE 18–3. Computerized tomographic (CT) scan showing intracranial calcifications in congenital toxoplasmosis.

causes for mental retardation. Psychologic contributors to mental retardation are noted below under SOCIAL-ENVIRONMENTAL CAUSES.

Social-Environmental Causes. Psychosocial deprivation may produce developmental delay that is reversible or permanent (see Case 20–4). As documented by Spitz (1965) and others, the result of psychosocial deprivation, even if unintentional, may be not only permanent deficit but in some instances death.

Genetic-Constitutional Causes. Many disorders associated with mental retardation have been identified as familial. Specific biochemical defects have been identified in many but nonetheless a minority of these disorders. Examples in which specific enzymatic deficiencies have been identified are phenylketonuria, homocystinuria, galactosemia, the mucopolysaccharidoses, and X-linked hyperuricemia (Lesch-Nyhan syndrome) (Menkes, 1980) (see Case 18–2).

Genetic-metabolic disorders are most often of autosomal recessive inheritance. This mode of inheritance is seen with phenylketonuria, maple syrup urine disease, galactosemia, all of the mucopolysaccharidoses except for Hunter disease (which is X-linked recessive), and homocystinuria. Autosomal dominant disorders include myotonic muscular dystrophy, tuberous sclerosis, and neurofibromatosis. The Sturge-Weber syndrome occurs on a sporadic basis. Several other disorders are X-linked: Duchenne muscular dystrophy, Menkes (steely hair) disease, and the oculo-cerebral-renal syndrome of Lowe.

Other disorders have been linked with recognizable chromosomal alterations such as the classic trisomies (21, 18, and 13), the cri-du-chat ("cat cry") syndrome (deletion of the short arm of chromosome 5), Klinefelter syndrome (XXY karyotype), Turner syndrome (X0), fragile X syndromes (Gerald, 1981), and various syndromes involving ring chromosome formation (see Case 18–3).

Developmental Causes. There are no truly developmental causes of mental retardation although, as noted above, the broad range of normal development includes some children who, particularly at earlier ages, will be (borderline) delayed in one or more areas.

TREATMENT AND OUTCOME

In many respects the issues confronting a family with a mentally retarded child are those facing the family with a child affected by any other chronic illness (see Chapter 21). These include acute and chronic grief reactions to having a defective child, marital problems related to differences in approaching the retarded child, and associated financial stresses.

Not only are some mental retardation syndromes specifically treatable, but early treatment sometimes will prevent the development of mental retardation (see Table 18–5). Hypothyroidism and phenylketonuria are examples of such disorders. In other disorders the problem may not be so specifically treatable, but certain features may be amenable to therapy. Thus, in the child with a congenital rubella syndrome, hearing impairment might be treated with a hearing aid; cataract by surgical removal and use of corrective lenses; patent ductus arteriosus by surgical ligation. The child with hydro-

CASE 18–2: MENTAL RETARDATION, SEIZURES, AND HYPERACTIVITY IN AN 18-YEAR-OLD GIRL WITH PHENYLKETONURIA

C.S. was born at 7 months gestation following a third trimester hemorrhage that was associated with placenta praevia. Birth weight was 3 pounds, 13 ounces. Perinatal depression did not occur. Development has always been delayed. She fed herself a cookie by 1 year. At 14 months she sat when placed. By 18 months she moved about by rolling and had a pincer grasp. She crawled at $2\frac{1}{2}$ years, walked at 3 years, and said "papa" specifically at $3\frac{1}{2}$ years.

Diagnosis of phenylketonuria (PKU) was made at $2\frac{1}{2}$ years. She was placed on a low phenylalanine diet, which was maintained until age $8\frac{1}{2}$ years. Generalized seizures began at 5 years of age. Electroencephalogram demonstrated diffuse spike, polyspike, and slow-wave activity. Seizures were controlled with phenytoin. Hyperactivity responded to methylphenidate, but parents discontinued it because of persistent sleep disturbance.

At 18 years she was able to sweep a floor upon request, throw a ball into a basket, eat independently with a spoon, brush her hair, and wipe her mouth. She was toilet-trained during the day but usually wet the bed at night unless awakened. Recent behavior had been marked by increased agitation and hyperactivity. Behavior modification had not been of lasting benefit in treating hyperactivity and self-abusive behavior, though some improvement was noted with haloperidol.

On examination, she was a large, fair-haired child without dysplastic features who interacted minimally with others. Left to herself, she rocked back and forth, turned in circles, and occasionally bit her hand. Vocalization was limited to unintelligible sounds. She did not follow one-step commands consistently. She placed simple figures into a formboard by trial and error. She stacked several blocks and scribbled with a pencil.

Comment. This child illustrates a condition that, fortunately, is seen relatively rarely (about 1 in 14,000 births). Institution of mandatory screening programs for phenylketonuria and other metabolic disorders has identified many such children and spared them profound retardation and behavioral disturbances through the use of a low phenylalanine or other special diet begun early in life (see CORRELATION: BIOCHEMICAL ASPECTS).

Since phenylalanine is a precursor of tyrosine, which itself is a precursor of norepinephrine and epinephrine, it is reasonable to speculate that the hyperactivity occurring in persons with PKU stems from catecholamine deficiency, as has been purported to occur in some children with hyperactivity and attentional disorders (see Chapter 14). Indeed, she did respond to methylphenidate, although treatment was not maintained.

cephalus due to congenital toxoplasmosis or bacterial meningitis, for example, might undergo ventriculoperitoneal shunting. Seizures occurring in mentally retarded persons are generally treated in conventional fashion (see Chapter 12). Case 18–4 illustrates the specific treatment of a problem (severe hearing impairment) associated with another mental retardation syndrome (myotonic muscular dystrophy).

Building upon the retarded person's positive features and relative strengths was emphasized by Langdon Down in 1866 in his original description of the syndrome that bears his name (Wilkins and Brody, 1971):

> They [persons with the "mongolian type of idiocy"] are humorous, and a lively sense of the ridiculous often colours their mimicry. This faculty of imitation may be cultivated to a very great extent, and a practical direction given to the results obtained. They are usually able to speak; the speech is thick and indistinct, but may be improved very greatly by a well-directed scheme of tongue gymnastics. The coordinating faculty is abnormal, but not so defective that it cannot be greatly strengthened. By systematic training, considerable manipulative power may be obtained.

Most mentally retarded persons are in the mildly retarded category and will be able to care for themselves and to contribute to society, though often in a less than fully independent manner (see Table 18–1) (Taft, 1973). The outlook for the mentally retarded child in later life may be brighter than parents may anticipate during early periods of gloom. For even with Down syndrome (which is usually associated with moderate mental retardation) the child is likely to walk and talk. Such an outcome may not fit the stereotype of the mentally retarded person held by many parents and professionals and is useful to consider in the early, difficult phases of decision-making when a child is recognized as being defective (Solnit and Stark, 1961; Golden and Davis, 1974).

Medical Management.   The cornerstone of treatment of hypothyroidism is thyroid replacement. The prognosis of athyrotic cretinism depends largely upon the time that replacement therapy is begun (Klein *et al.,* 1972; Rosman, 1976). If treatment is begun within the first 6 months of life, about half the children will ultimately show normal mental development (see Figs. 18–6 and 18–7). If begun within the first 3 months, most will achieve mental normalcy.

Dietary management is an important part of treatment in several neurologic disorders of genetic-metabolic origin. Phenylketonuria (PKU) is the most widely known. The child recognized as having PKU early in life (generally through a neonatal screening program) is placed on a low phenylalanine diet. With regular follow-up and ongoing communication between family, physician, and nutritionist, mental subnormalcy can be avoided altogether in many instances. When the diagnosis of PKU has been made later in childhood, dietary therapy may help associated behavioral problems (such as hyperactivity), but the mental retardation, now well established, persists.

Dietary management of PKU is not without dangers, however. Too low a level of phenylalanine in the diet can result in hypoglycemia, seizures, osteo-

CASE 18–3: MENTAL RETARDATION WITH RING CHROMOSOME 22 MALFORMATION IN A 3-YEAR-OLD BOY

I.F. was evaluated because of developmental delay. He weighed 5 pounds, 4 ounces at birth following a full-term pregnancy, the first for a 35-year-old woman. The pregnancy had been complicated by spontaneous rupture of membranes 1 month prior to delivery. Antibiotics were given prophylactically. Birth occurred after 23 hours of labor without cardiorespiratory depression. The placenta showed amnionitis. Despite irritability and poor feeding in the immediate neonatal period, the child was discharged at 5 days of age.

Development was generally delayed, though less so in gross motor skills than in language and other areas. He walked at 15 months. First words were spoken at 18 months but were lost 6 months later. Following a language enrichment program begun at 2 years, he spoke nearly 20 single words and a few word combinations by 3 years of age. He engaged in some repetitive behaviors, but twirling, spinning, or other bizarre behaviors, were not seen. He demonstrated no "islands of excellence." Past history and family history were unremarkable.

On examination, the child was a small, cute, young-appearing boy who showed little anxiety with strangers and interacted minimally with parents or others. He vocalized little; but when his father left the room, he said, "Dad go work." He showed no bizarre mannerisms. Palate was high-arched. Head circumference was at the second percentile, height and weight at the 10th to 25th percentiles. Head circumferences of both parents and a normal sibling were around the 50th percentile. Funduscopic examination was unremarkable. Elemental neurologic examination was normal, including deep tendon reflexes and plantar responses. He showed no consistent hand preference. Developmental testing showed gross motor skills at a 2-year level, fine motor skills at 1 year, and personal-social and language skills at a 1½-year level.

Investigation included blood lead level, serum thyroxine level, and anal-

porosis, and mental retardation itself. Although dietary restriction can be relaxed in adolescence and adulthood, a pregnant woman with PKU must resume a low-phenylalanine diet to minimize the risk of damage to the fetal brain, for a high-phenylalanine environment *in utero* is associated with microcephaly and mental retardation in offspring.

Other disorders of amino acid metabolism are treated according to similar dietary principles. Maple syrup urine disease, a disorder of branched-chain amino acid metabolism, is effectively treated by a diet low in valine, leucine, and isoleucine. Homocystinuria is treated by a low-methionine diet, usually in combination with pyridoxine (vitamin B_6,) folic acid, and/or vitamin B_{12}.

When a hyperkinetic syndrome (attention deficit disorder) occurs with mental retardation, a trial of dextroamphetamine (Dexedrine) or methyl-

ysis of blood and urine for amino acids. All were normal. Electroencephalogram showed no evidence for seizures. Skull x-rays and CT scan were normal. Audiology assessment showed no hearing deficit. Chromosome analysis disclosed a ring 22 chromosome (presumed to result from a deletion with rejoining of "sticky" ends) (see Fig. 18–4).

At follow-up examination one year later development continued to lag significantly, particularly in speech and language, although continued progress was evident.

Comment. In this case several causes for the child's developmental delay seemed reasonable to consider. Complications of pregnancy and delivery could have amply accounted for this child's problems. Membranes ruptured a month prior to delivery and provided a fine opportunity for microorganisms to gain access to the amniotic fluid, an excellent culture medium. Labor itself was prolonged, which might have compromised blood supply to the fetal brain.

The child's relatively small head and developmental delay were consistent with congenital infection by cytomegalovirus, rubella virus, or toxoplasma organisms. The examination and investigation did not, however, support any of these possibilities. Funduscopic examination disclosed no cataract or chorioretinitis, skull x-rays were without intracranial calcification, and viral studies were negative.

Particularly with speech and language delay and interactional difficulties, infantile autism was a consideration. The degree of aloofness was not great, however, nor did the child manifest bizarre behavior or show "islands" of normal or superior performance.

Chromosomal analysis was pursued because of several factors: mother's age, the child's dysplastic features (though mild), and the lack of defined etiology for the child's delayed development. A ring 22 chromosome syndrome was not anticipated; but such surprises are occurring with increased frequency as techniques of chromosome analysis have become further developed and more widely utilized.

phenidate (Ritalin) may be justified (see Chapter 14). Hyperactive mentally retarded children may, however, respond better to a phenothiazine such as thioridazine (Mellaril) or chlorpromazine (Thorazine) (see Chapter 5).

Intercurrent medical problems such as obesity, asthma, or diabetes mellitus should be treated as indicated.

Neurologic Management. Infectious diseases associated with mental retardation (such as measles, rubella, and toxoplasmosis) usually cause nonprogressive effects rather than ongoing disease. Measles and rubella, both viral infections, have not been amenable to specific antiviral treatment. Congenital toxoplasmosis, a protozoan infection, can be treated with sulfadiazine and pyrimethamine. This is in contrast to diseases due to infectious agents associated with behavioral regression such as subacute sclerosing

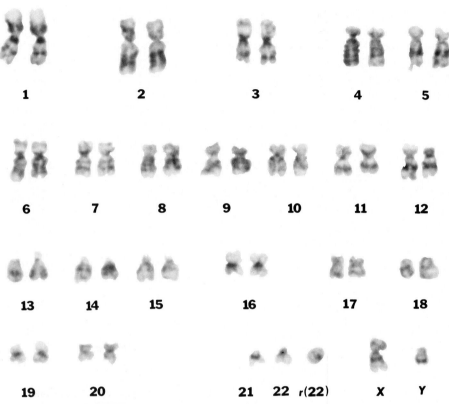

FIGURE 18–4. Chromosome analysis showing ring 22 chromosome [r (22)] (Case 18–3).

panencephalitis (a late complication of measles) and progressive rubella panencephalitis (a delayed complication of earlier rubella infection) (see Chapter 8).

Management of seizures is presented in Chapter 12.

Surgical Management. Neurosurgical treatment of hydrocephalus is presented in Chapter 11.

In Down syndrome several conditions that may require surgical treatment commonly occur. These include congenital heart disease, duodenal atresia, and cataract—treatment of which often involves difficult ethical issues.

A feeding gastrostomy can greatly facilitate adequate nutrition of some mentally retarded children.

Psychotherapy. Individual as well as family therapy should not be overlooked in the management of mentally retarded persons. It should be reemphasized that most retarded persons fall into the mildly retarded category. Thus, many of them attain the intellectual and academic abilities of grade-school children and can express well (if not verbally, then affectively or otherwise behaviorally) some of their fears and frustrations.

Psychotherapy will often take the form of supportive counseling provided by the primary physician, who is in a uniquely favorable position to support

TABLE 18–5. **Selected Aspects of Treatment of Mental Retardation**

Medical	Thyroid hormone replacement for hypothyroidism
	Dietary therapy for phenylketonuria, maple syrup urine disease
	Vitamin B_6, B_{12}, or folic acid plus dietary therapy for homocystinuria
	Pharmacotherapy (among other measures) for associated hyperactivity
	Treatment of intercurrent medical problems
Neurologic	Anticonvulsant medication for associated seizures
Surgical	Shunt for hydrocephalus
	Feeding gastrostomy
Psychologic	Family support
	Counseling regarding behavior problems
	Individual therapy for retarded person
	Group therapy
	Behavior modification
Social-Environmental	Group homes in community
	Respite care
	Day-hospital programs
	Chronic institutionalization
Educational	Special education
Physical	Remedial (to maintain and improve skills)
	Fitness
	Socialization, emotional outlet

the mentally retarded individual and his family (Davis, 1973; Freeman, 1978). Such ongoing therapy may be supplemented by consultation with a psychiatrist or psychologist attuned to problems of mentally retarded persons (Chess, 1962; Menolascino, 1968; Freeman, 1973). Group therapy may be especially valuable among retarded adolescents in whom concerns about sex, marriage, and jobs are frequent (Kaldeck, 1958; Oliver *et al.*, 1965; Slivkin and Bernstein, 1970).

In more severely retarded persons behavior modification may be valuable in shaping behaviors that are of increased adaptive value (Gardner, 1970; Simmons *et al.*, 1974; Kiernan, 1974). An example of such behavioral shaping was seen with a profoundly retarded boy whose caretakers were becoming increasingly alienated from him because of his lack of interaction, accentuated by his diminishing degree of eye contact. Through a system of food rewards, the child was trained to look first in the general direction of the therapist's face, then at the face in particular, then at the midface, next the eyes, and finally at the eyes for several seconds. Eye contact was thereby

CASE 18–4: MENTAL RETARDATION AND HEARING DEFICIT IN A 10-YEAR-OLD GIRL WITH MYOTONIC MUSCULAR DYSTROPHY

S.R. was the 7 pound, 4 ounce product of a term gestation, born to a 28-year-old woman, gravida 6, para 3, abortus 2. Apgar scores were 7 at 1 minute, 9 at 5 minutes. Head circumference at birth was 34.5 cm. As a neonate, the child was tachypneic, fed poorly, was markedly hypotonic, and had an unusual facial appearance. After gaining weight with difficulty, she was discharged to home at 3 weeks of age. She was hospitalized at 2 months because of failure to thrive. She suffered nearly continuous middle ear infections during her first 2 years, which led to severe bilateral hearing impairment. Language and motor milestones were delayed. Family history was negative for muscle disease. A paternal uncle was said to be mentally retarded. Evaluation during the first 2 years of life included a thyroxine level of 9.5 mcg/dl (normal), electromyography (showing "dive bomber" potentials typical of myotonia), and muscle biopsy consistent with myotonic dystrophy. At 10 years of age, she attended an ungraded classroom in a school for the deaf.

On examination, she was an alert, active girl with a transverse smile and a twinkle in her eye but an otherwise sad-looking, masklike facial appearance (see Fig. 18–5). Wearing a hearing aid, she responded to a loud voice. Resting pulse rate was 130/minute. Tympanic membranes were thickened and scarred. She spoke in three to four-word combinations with a hypernasal voice. She counted to ten, recognized many letters, and named three colors. Overall, she functioned at a 4- to 5-year level. Percussion and grasp myotonia

reestablished, and the relationship between child and institutional staff was enhanced.

Social-Environmental Management. Group homes within the community have been established for mildly retarded adolescents and young adults. Thus these persons have been taken out of institutions or, if they had not been institutionalized, given the opportunity to leave their families of origin in a developmentally appropriate fashion, a normalizing experience.

Respite care is an important aspect of social-environmental management. Such care gives the family of a retarded child an opportunity to place the child with skilled professionals for brief periods of time (a few days or weeks) while parents or other caretakers become "revitalized," devoting some time exclusively to themselves. When a parent is ill or convalescing, some form of respite care generally becomes necessary.

Day-hospital programs may offer a workable and cost-effective substitute for long-term institutionalization. Physical therapy, nutritional counseling, social service support, and medical monitoring are carried out, generally on weekdays, along with special education individualized to the needs of the child.

was absent. Deep tendon reflexes were quiet and symmetric throughout. A Gowers sign was not present.

Comment. This child got off to a particularly slow and enigmatic start. Indeed, her prognosis appeared to be so bad within the first year of life that institutionalization was discussed with the family, who refused to consider the possibility at that time. Despite the child's serious difficulties as a neonate and infant, a strong parent-child bond was formed. She has been greatly assisted by committed parents who have followed through with the complicated medical, neurologic, and educational management that she needs.

As is obvious from this case, myotonic muscular dystrophy does not involve muscles in the same way as does Duchenne muscular dystrophy. The latter most prominently affects proximal musculature, and children with Duchenne muscular dystrophy are usually wheelchair-bound by adolescence. Myotonic dystrophy, by contrast, involves distal as well as proximal muscles, the latter less severely than with Duchenne muscular dystrophy. In this case involvement of pharyngeal muscles was the most important manifestation of her muscle disease. It interfered with eating during infancy. Within her first 2 years it contributed to severe middle ear disease, as she was unable to close her eustachian tube adequately. As a result, saliva, mucus, food, and bacteria were permitted to flow from the nasopharynx to her middle ear.

Myotonia, the inability of muscle to relax, was not seen clinically in this case. With electromyography, however, a characteristic myotonic "dive bomber" pattern was heard, resulting from amplification of potentials generated on needle insertion.

Institutionalization may be, in some circumstances, the best choice among those available to the family. Discussing institutionalization should never be carried out in a heavy-handed or premature manner. Rather it should be offered as an option to be explored at a time the family feels is best. Since many pediatric nursing homes or other chronic care facilities have a waiting list of months to years, the family should be so informed and encouraged to take such preliminary steps (such as visiting the institution or putting their name on its waiting list) as seem appropriate.

Educational Management. Many persons with mild mental retardation will be able to learn to read at a third- to fifth-grade level (Cohen, 1973). This academic potential, among others, should be recognized so that the skills of the retarded person can be maximized and his role within family and society enhanced. With comprehensive educational planning mandated in many parts of the United States, not only educational but also occupational, social, and emotional needs of mentally retarded persons are being addressed increasingly.

The education of the mentally retarded child, like that of any other, will be based upon the child's profile of strengths and weaknesses as determined

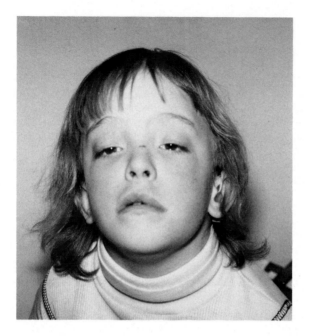

FIGURE 18–5. Bilateral ptosis with paucity of facial expression in a girl with myotonic muscular dystrophy (Case 18–4).

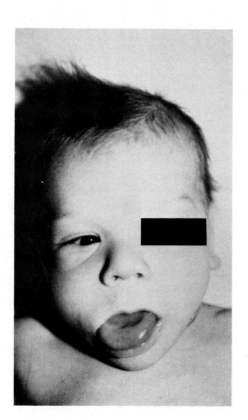

FIGURE 18–6. A 5-month-old with untreated congenital hypothyroidism.

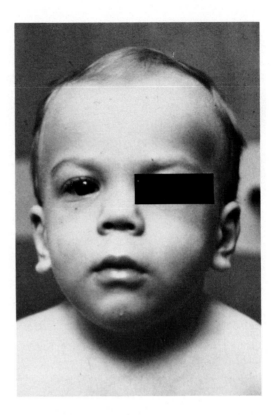

FIGURE 18–7. A 1-year-old boy (the same child as in Fig. 18–6) treated with thyroid hormone replacement.

by testing. It should never be assumed that the mentally retarded child is equally impaired in all areas (Chess and Hassibi, 1970). Language skills particularly often are depressed. And, it should be recalled, if reading performance falls 2 or more years behind the level predicted by the child's intelligence, the child with mental retardation should be considered to have a learning disability as well (see Chapter 17).

Physical Therapy. Because motor function is often compromised in mentally retarded persons, physical therapy often is employed to maintain range of motion, improve general fitness as well as specific skills, build social capabilities, and provide a physical outlet for emotions.

Sensorimotor patterning therapy does not appear to be more effective than enlightened supportive and symptomatic treatment (Sparrow and Zigler, 1978; Fremont *et al.,* 1978)

CORRELATION

Anatomic Aspects. Although many (if not most) mentally retarded persons have normal-appearing brains, central nervous system malformations are recognized in many mental retardation syndromes. The brain in Down syndrome, for example, is slightly smaller than normal and has a globular rather than elongated shape. There is underdevelopment of cerebellum, brainstem, frontal lobes (described as "short"), and superior temporal gyri, which are tucked into the Sylvian fissures (Lemire *et al.,* 1975).

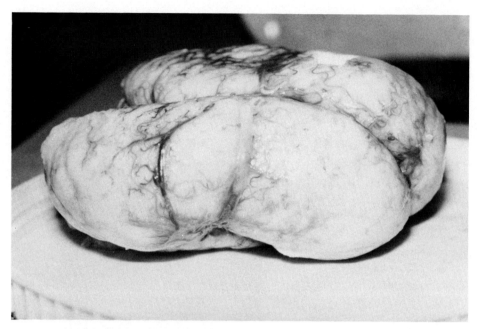

FIGURE 18–8. Lissencephaly (smooth brain) from a severely retarded child with a seizure disorder.

The trisomy 13 syndrome is typically associated with a much more striking brain malformation than either Down syndrome or trisomy 18. The most severe form is holoprosencephaly in which the olfactory tracts and bulbs are absent and the frontal lobes are fused, containing a single ventricle in lieu of paired lateral ventricles.

Trisomy 18 is characterized by a variety of brain defects. These include distorted gyral patterns, agenesis of the corpus callosum, encephalocele, and hypoplasia of cerebellum and brainstem.

Other malformations that have been associated with mental retardation of varying degrees are lissencephaly, ulegyria (sclerotic microgyria), polymicrogyria, congenital porencephalic cyst, schizencephaly, and hydranencephaly (Yakovlev, 1959) (see Figs. 17–5, 18–8, and 18–9).

Biochemical Aspects. Phenylketonuria provides a prototype of genetic-metabolic diseases that produce mental retardation. The underlying biochemical defect is deficiency of the enzyme phenylalanine hydroxylase. Phenylalanine, thus, cannot be hydroxylated to form tyrosine (see Fig. 18–10). Hence, it accumulates in large amounts in blood where it is converted (by transamination) to phenylpyruvic acid. This substance, a phenylketone, is excreted into the urine, giving the disorder its original name (phenylpyruvic oligophrenia) and its current name, phenylketonuria (PKU). Phenylpyruvic acid is the substance responsible for production of a green color when ferric chloride is added to the urine of a person with PKU.

The cause for mental retardation, seizures, and hyperactivity seen in children with PKU has not been clearly identified. It is thought that phenylala-

FIGURE 18–9. Plain computerized tomographic (CT) scan in an infant with hydranencephaly. Arrow indicates remaining brain tissue.

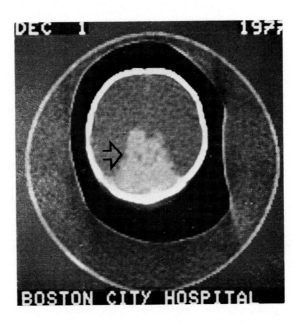

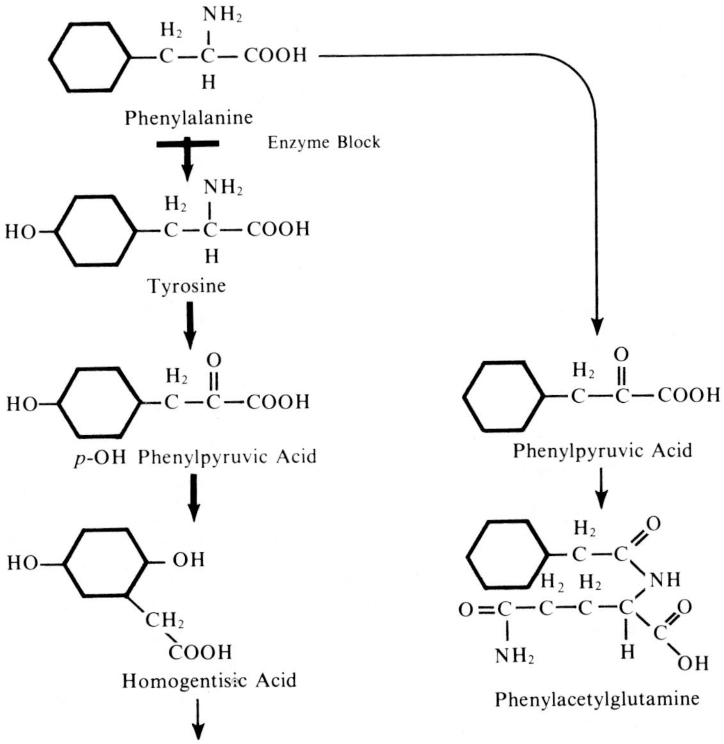

FIGURE 18–10. Metabolic pathways involving phenylalanine, proceeding normally to tyrosine or—with enzyme block (lack of phenylalanine hydroxylase)—proceeding to phenylpyruvic acid and other phenylketones.

nine in excess, phenylpyruvic acid, and their metabolites exert a toxic effect on the developing central nervous system. In addition, the child is deprived of tyrosine, a semiessential amino acid important in the synthesis of melanin, norepinephrine, thyroxine, and many proteins.

In the classic form of homocystinuria, the hepatic enzyme cystathionine synthase is deficient. Consequently, homocysteine cannot readily combine with serine, another amino acid, to form cystathionine. Homocysteine builds up in the blood and is rapidly oxidized to homocystine, which spills into the urine. A beet-red color of urine tested with cyanide-nitroprusside reagent indicates homocystinuria. Quantitative amino acid analysis of urine and blood will define more specifically the locus of the enzyme block, which will influence the specific (vitamin) therapy employed (Nyhan, 1980).

Physiologic Aspects. Errors in the distribution of genetic material (deoxyribonucleic acid, DNA, organized into chromosomes) underlie Down syndrome and other chromosomal disorders. Two mechanisms are employed to distribute genetic material to "daughter" nuclei: mitosis and meiosis (Herskowitz, 1979). Mitosis involves the orderly separation of replicated chromosomes to produce two daughter nuclei identical to the parent nucleus in number of chromosomes (46, or 23 pairs).

Whereas mitosis occurs in all human tissues, meiosis occurs only with the formation of gametes. Unlike mitosis, meiosis reduces the number of chromosomes per cell (through separation of chromosome pairs) so that each daughter nucleus contains an unpaired complement of chromosomes (see Fig. 18–11). Union of egg and sperm, the process of fertilization, thus restores the paired condition.

The meiotic distribution system breaks down in producing trisomy 21 (the most frequent form of Down syndrome at any age), in which the pair of number 21 chromosomes fails to separate during gamete formation. This failure is termed nondisjunction. One gamete thus has no number 21 chromosome; the other has two. When the former gamete is fertilized, the resulting zygote, exhibiting monosomy, is unable to develop into an organism with prolonged survival. When the latter gamete (usually, though not invariably, the ovum) is fertilized by a normal gamete, the fertilized egg (zygote) has three number 21 chromosomes, hence, the term "trisomy."

This error in distribution occurs with increased frequency with advancing maternal age. The risk of a 50-year-old woman bearing a child with Down syndrome is about 2 per cent, as contrasted with the risk of about 0.2 per cent in the general population. The precise pathophysiology of nondisjunction has not been fully clarified. Aging of oocytes and exposure to toxins have been suggested, since oocytes are produced only before birth, whereas spermatozoa are made continually throughout a male's reproductive life. On the other hand, the male gamete has been implicated in carrying the extra 21 chromosome in nearly one-quarter of cases of Down syndrome (Holmes, 1978). Consequently, mothers should not be assumed to bear the sole responsibility for producing a child with Down syndrome. It is best shared.

Nondisjunction also occurs in trisomy 18, trisomy 13, Klinefelter syndrome (XXY), Turner syndrome (X0), and the XYY syndrome.

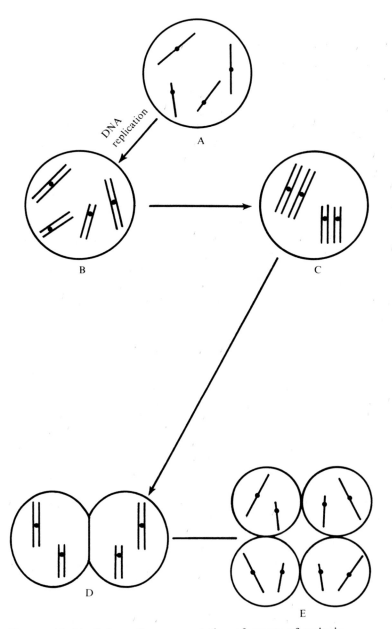

FIGURE 18–11. Schematic representation of events of meiosis, demonstrating formation of four gametes with half the original number of chromosomes following a single DNA replication. (From Herskowitz, I. H. *The Elements of Genetics*. Macmillan Publishing Co., Inc., New York, 1979.)

SUMMARY

Mental retardation is a common problem, affecting some 1 to 5 per cent of the population to varying degrees. Before the diagnosis of mental retardation has been established and while specific etiologies are being sought, the problem is often best considered as one of developmental delay of unknown cause. Evaluation should include determining areas of delay and of more normal performance, if such do exist. The tempo of development should be noted, since a falloff in development can result from seizures, drugs, intercurrent illness, and emotional stress or may herald the presence of a degenerative neurologic disorder.

The approach to the child with delayed development is directed toward differentiating the child's condition from those which mimic mental retardation, identifying treatable parts of the mental retardation syndrome (such as deafness, seizures, emotional disturbance, hyperactivity, or visual deficit), and, whenever possible, treating the cause of the retardation itself.

A comprehensive approach to treatment that includes attention to medical, psychologic, social, and educational needs will maximize the mentally retarded person's degree of happiness, self-sufficiency, and contributions to society.

CITED REFERENCES

Adelson, E., and Fraiberg, S. Gross motor development. Pp. 198–220 in *Insights from the Blind: Comparative Studies of Blind and Sighted Infants.* Fraiberg, S., and Fraiberg, L., eds. Basic Books, Inc., New York, 1977.

Ando, H., and Yoshimura, I. Prevalence of maladaptive behavior in retarded children as a function of IQ and age. *J. Abnorm. Child Psychol.,* **6:** 345–49, 1978.

Chess, S. Psychiatric treatment of the mentally retarded child with behavior problems. *Am. J. Orthopsychiatry,* **32:** 863–69, 1962.

Chess, S. Evolution of behavior disorder in a group of mentally retarded children. *J. Am. Acad. Child Psychiatry,* **16:** 4–20, 1977.

Chess, S.; Fernandez, P.; and Korn, S. Behavioral consequences of congenital rubella. *J. Pediatr.,* **93:** 699–703, 1978.

Chess, S., and Hassibi, M. Behavior deviations in mentally retarded children. *J. Am. Acad. Child Psychiatry,* **9:** 282–97, 1970.

Clark, D. F. Psychological assessment in mental subnormality: general considerations, intelligence and perceptual-motor tests. Pp. 387–438 in *Mental Deficiency: The Changing Outlook,* 3d ed. Clarke, A. M., and Clarke, A. D. B., eds. The Free Press, New York, 1974.

Clarke, A. M., and Clarke, A. D. B. Criteria and classification of subnormality. Pp. 13–30 in *Mental Deficiency: The Changing Outlook,* 3d ed. Clarke, A. M., and Clarke, A. D. B., eds. The Free Press, New York, 1974.

Cohen, H. J. Treatment of mental retardation. *Pediatr. Annals,* **2:** 64–80, 1973.

Davis, J. G. A pediatrician's approach to counseling families of mentally retarded children. *Pediatr. Annals,* **2:** 59–63, 1973.

Freeman, B. J. Appraising children for mental retardation: the usefulness and limitations of IQ testing. *Clin. Pediatr.* (Philadelphia), **17:** 169–73, 1978.

Freeman, R. D. Psychological management of the retarded child and the family. *Pediatr. Annals,* **2:** 53–58, 1973.

Fremont, A. C.; Halpern, D.; Merrill, R. E.; and Taft, L. T. Patterning treatment for retarded children. *Pediatrics*, **62:** 274, 1978.

Gardner, W. I. Use of behavior therapy with the mentally retarded. Pp. 250–75 in *Psychiatric Approaches to Mental Retardation*. Menolascino, F. J., ed. Basic Books, Inc., New York, 1970.

Gerald, P. S. X-linked mental retardation and the fragile-X syndrome. *Pediatrics*, **68**, 594–95, 1981.

Golden, D. A., and Davis, J. G. Counseling parents after the birth of an infant with Down's syndrome. *Children Today*, pp. 7–11, March–April 1974.

Gross, S. J.; Kosmetatos, N.; Grimes, C. T.; and Williams, M. L. Newborn head size and neurologic status. *Am. J. Dis. Child.*, **132:** 753–56, 1978.

Herskowitz, I. H. Genetic recombination in eukaryotes: I. mitosis, meiosis, and segregation. Pp. 137–71 in *The Elements of Genetics*. Macmillan Publishing Co., Inc., New York, 1979.

Holmes, L. B. Genetic counseling for the older pregnant woman: new data and questions. *N. Engl. J. Med.*, **298:** 1419–21, 1978.

Kaldeck, R. Group psychotherapy with mentally defective adolescents and adults. *Int. J. Group Psychotherapy*, **8:** 185–92, 1958.

Kiernan, C. C. Behaviour modification. Pp. 729–803 in *Mental Deficiency: The Changing Outlook*, 3d ed. Clarke, A. M., and Clarke, A. D. B., eds. The Free Press, New York, 1974.

Klein, A. H.; Meltzer, S.; and Kenny, F. M. Improved prognosis in congenital hypothyroidism treated before age three months. *J. Pediatr.*, **81:** 912–15, 1972.

Koch, R.; Strickland, G.; and Graliker, B. A 17-year longitudinal study of 117 children with mental retardation, starting in infancy. *Clin. Pediatr.* (Philadelphia), **16:** 1015–20, 1977.

Krogstad, D. J.; Juranek, D. D.; and Walls, K. W. Toxoplasmosis: with comments on risk of infection from cats. *Ann. Intern. Med.*, **77:** 773–78, 1972.

Lemire, R. J.; Loeser, J. D.; Leech, R. W.; and Alvord, C. A., Jr. *Normal and Abnormal Development of the Human Nervous System*. Harper and Row, Publishers, Hagerstown, Md., 1975.

Martin, H. P. Microcephaly and mental retardation. *Am. J. Dis. Child.*, **119:** 128–31, 1970.

Menkes, J. H. Metabolic diseases of the nervous system. Pp. 1–109 in *Textbook of Child Neurology*, 2d. ed. Lea and Febiger, Philadelphia, 1980.

Menolascino, F. J. Emotional disturbances in mentally retarded children. *Arch. Gen. Psychiatry*, **19:** 456–64, 1968.

Miller, R. W., and Blot, W. J. Small head size after in-utero exposure to atomic radiation. *Lancet*, **2:** 784–87, 1972.

Nelson, K. B., and Deutschberger, J. Head size at one year as a predictor of four-year IQ. *Dev. Med. Child Neurol.*, **12:** 487–95, 1970.

Nyhan, W. L. Understanding inherited metabolic disease. *Clin. Symp.*, **32:** 1–36, 1980.

Oliver, B. E.; Simon, G. B., and Clark, B. Symposium on psychotherapy with the mentally subnormal: I. group discussions with adolescent female patients in a mental subnormality hospital. *J. Ment. Subn.*, **11:** 53–57, 1965.

Ouellette, E. M.; Rosett, H. L.; Rosman, N. P.; and Weiner, L. A. Adverse effects on offspring of maternal alcohol abuse during pregnancy. *N. Engl. J. Med.*, **297:** 528–30, 1977.

Rosman, N. P. Neurological and muscular aspects of thyroid dysfunction in childhood. *Pediatr. Clin. North Am.*, **23:** 575–94, 1976.

Rosman, N. P., and Herskowitz, J. Trauma to the central nervous system. In *The Practice of Pediatric Neurology,* 2d ed. Swaiman, K. F., and Wright, F. S., eds. C. V. Mosby Co., Saint Louis, 1982.

Rosman, N. P., and Kakulas, B. A. Mental deficiency associated with muscular dystrophy: a clinicopathological study. *Brain* **89:** 769–88, 1966.

Simmons, J. Q., III; Tymchuk, A. J.; and Valente, M. Treatment and care of the mentally retarded. *Psychiatric Annals,* **4:** 38–69, 1974.

Slivkin, S. E., and Bernstein, N. R. Group approaches to treating retarded adolescents. Pp. 435–54 in *Psychiatric Approaches to Mental Retardation.* Menolascino, F. J., ed. Basic Books, Inc., New York, 1970.

Smith, D. W. *Recognizable Patterns of Human Malformation,* 2d ed. W. B. Saunders Co., Philadelphia, 1976.

Solnit, A. J., and Stark, M. H. Mourning and the birth of a defective child. *Psychoanal. Study Child,* **16:** 523–37, 1961.

Sparrow, S., and Zigler, E. Evaluation of a patterning treatment for retarded children. *Pediatrics,* **62:** 137–50, 1978.

Spitz, R. A. *The First Year of Life: A Psychoanalytic Study of Normal and Deviant Development of Object Relations.* International Universities Press, Inc., New York, 1965.

Taft, L. T. Mental retardation: an overview. *Pediatr. Ann.,* **2:** 10–24, 1973.

Weaver, D. D., and Christian, J. C. Familial variation of head size and adjustment for parental head circumference. *J. Pediatr.,* **96:** 990–94, 1980.

Wilkins, R. H., and Brody, I. A. Down's syndrome. *Arch. Neurol.,* **25:** 88–90, 1971.

Willis, J., and Rosman, N. P. The Aicardi syndrome versus congenital infection: diagnostic considerations. *J. Pediatr.,* **96:** 235–39, 1980.

Yakovlev, P. I. Anatomy of the human brain and the problem of mental retardation. Pp. 1–43 in *Mental Retardation.* Bowman, P. W., and Mautner, H. V., eds. Grune and Stratton, New York, 1959.

ADDITIONAL READINGS

Donaldson, J. Y., and Menolascino, F. J. Past, current, and future roles of child psychiatry in mental retardation. *J. Am. Acad. Child Psychiatry,* **16:** 38–52, 1977.

Frankenburg, W. K.; Fandal, A. W.; Sciarillo, W.; and Burgess, D. The newly abbreviated and revised Denver Developmental Screening Test. *J. Pediatr.,* **99:** 995–99, 1981.

Friedman, P. R. *The Rights of Mentally Retarded Persons: The Basic ACLU Guide for the Mentally Retarded Persons' Rights.* Avon Books, New York, 1976.

Hecht, F.; Glover, T. W.; and Kaiser-Hecht, B. Fragile sites on chromosomes. *Pediatrics,* **69:** 121–23, 1982.

Madow, L. (Chairman, Committee on Mental Retardation). *Mild Mental Retardation: A Growing Challenge to the Physician.* Group for the Advancement of Psychiatry, New York, Vol. VI, Report No. 66, 1967.

Riccardi, V. M. Von Recklinghausen neurofibromatosis. *N. Engl. J. Med.,* **305:** 1617–26, 1981.

Roberts, N., and Roberts, B. *David.* John Knox Press, Richmond, Virginia, 1968. A written and pictorial account of a boy with Down syndrome made by his parents.

Szymanski, L. S. Psychiatric diagnostic evaluation of mentally retarded individuals. *J. Am. Acad. Child Psychiatry,* **16:** 67–87, 1977.

Warkany, J.; Lemire, R. J.; and Cohen, M. M., Jr., *Mental Retardation and Congenital Malformations of the Central Nervous System.* Year Book Medical Publishers, Chicago, 1981.

19 Drug Abuse

Drug use is a fact of everyday life. Drinking coffee for its alerting and stimulating effects is a typical example of the use of a drug (in this instance, caffeine), whether it is recognized as such or not. Alcohol is another drug used widely for its effects upon the brain. When used judiciously, such drugs can assist or even enhance the everyday life of an individual. The line between drug use and drug abuse can be a fine one, however. When the drug exerts a harmful effect on the person, when energies are diverted inappropriately so that continued use of the drug can be assured, or when cessation or diminution of use produces physical symptoms or signs, most would agree that the term drug abuse is applicable.

This chapter will address several general and specific aspects of the abuse of drugs. Definitions of drug abuse, addiction, dependence, and tolerance will be presented. Pertinent features of the history will be outlined and medical, neurologic, and mental status portions of the examination described. Investigations such as blood and urine tests, electroencephalography, and computerized tomography will be outlined and management considered. The section on CORRELATION will include discussion of naturally occurring opioid substances found within the central nervous system and their relevance to the subject of drug abuse.

A number of questions will be addressed:

How are drug abuse, addiction, dependence, tolerance, and withdrawal defined?
What features of the medical, neurologic, and mental status examinations should be stressed in evaluating the person suspected of drug abuse?
What investigations, if any, are indicated?
What treatments are available for drug abuse? What outcome can be anticipated?
What are the anatomic, biochemical, and physiologic substrata for drug abuse and dependence?

545

DRUG ABUSE

Definition

A *psychoactive drug* is a substance taken into the body for its known or presumed effect upon the central nervous system. Some of these drugs, such as caffeine and alcohol, are essentially "nonmedical," whereas others (including opiates and barbiturates) are more conventionally grouped within the medical category.

Drug abuse, as indicated above, is defined by deleterious effects of the substance upon the user's body or mind, alteration of usual behavior such that ongoing effort is made to assure a continuous supply of the drug, and the occurrence of an abstinence syndrome when drug use is discontinued or curtailed.

The term *drug addiction* has now been largely supplanted by the more encompassing term *drug dependence,* closely related to the above definition of drug abuse. Drug dependence is a psychic state—sometimes also a physical state—which results from the interaction between a person and a drug to cause behavior that includes a compulsion to take the drug on a continuous or periodic basis in order to experience its psychic effects or to avoid the discomfort of abstinence (World Health Organization, 1969).

The distinction between effects of drugs upon behavior and behaviors that center upon obtaining and maintaining drug supply must always be kept in mind in any consideration of drug use or abuse. For example, the effects of morphine in producing euphoria and sedation (symptoms of drug *use*) are to be contrasted with the drug-oriented behaviors devoted to ensuring a supply of the drug (manifestations of drug *abuse*).

The effects of drugs (including alcohol) upon behavior are subsumed under the category of *organic mental syndrome* (*DSM*-III, 1980). The behavioral syndrome associated with drug use is termed most broadly a *substance use disorder*. This latter category is defined by social consequences of use (such as failure to meet important obligations, erratic and impulsive behavior, and inappropriate expression of aggressive feelings) and a pathologic pattern of use (as distinguished from so-called recreational use of a substance). Typical pathologic patterns of use are as follows: remaining intoxicated or under the influence of a drug throughout the day; daily use of the substance for a month; or having several episodes of complications of drug use—overdosage, delusional syndrome, or loss of consciousness.

Drug addiction generally refers to physical and/or psychologic addiction. These two can overlap, but they do not necessarily coexist. *Physical addiction* is characterized by tolerance and physical dependence. *Tolerance* refers to the biologic process in which increasing doses of drug are required for the desired drug effect to be maintained. Alternatively, the drug effect diminishes as the dosage is held constant. *Habituation* is essentially synonymous with tolerance as it applies to drug effects. *Physical dependence* refers to the state of necessity for continued drug administration in order to prevent a withdrawal or abstinence syndrome (Jaffe, 1980). A relatively safe interval between opiate injections in man at which tolerance and dependence do not occur appears to be 2 to 3 days (Snyder, 1979).

TABLE 19–1. **Key Terms Pertaining to Drug Abuse**

Psychoactive drug
Drug abuse
Organic mental syndrome
Substance use disorder
Drug addiction or dependence
   Physical addiction (tolerance or habitua-
     tion and physical dependence)
   Psychologic addiction
Drug effects
  Idiosyncratic
  Dose-related
  Overdose
  Withdrawal

Psychologic addiction refers to a behavioral pattern of compulsive drug use characterized by overwhelming involvement with the use of the drug, the securing of a supply, and the high tendency to relapse after withdrawal (World Health Organization, 1969).

Overall, *drug effects* can be categorized as follows: idiosyncratic, dose-related, overdosage, and withdrawal. An *idiosyncratic* effect is exemplified by acute dystonic reaction, e.g., torticollis occurring with trifluoperazine (Stelazine), a phenothiazine that can produce an extrapyramidal syndrome at low dosage. *Dose-related* side effects are typified by gaze-evoked nystagmus (which is asymptomatic) and somnolence occurring with standard anticonvulsant agents such as phenobarbital within the usual therapeutic range. *Overdosage* is illustrated by ataxic gait with phenytoin (Dilantin) toxicity or severe respiratory depression with opiate excess. *Withdrawal* may be manifested by tremulousness, hallucinosis, and seizures as part of an alcohol abstinence syndrome. When approaching a person suspected of using drugs, one should keep these categories in mind and also be aware that several drugs may be taken at the same time, for example, amphetamines (''uppers'') and barbiturates (''downers'') (see Table 19–1).

DIAGNOSIS

Clinical Process. *History.* The chief complaint of the person evaluated for possible drug abuse may be related to a direct drug effect such as hallucinosis (''Ants are crawling under my skin'') or to a more behavioral and situational reason (''The court sent me here''). History should be obtained not only from the patient but from the referring party (parent, teacher, or legal authority) as well, because negativism or unreliability may limit the value of information obtained directly.

In interviewing the patient, the examiner is—in addition to obtaining information—conducting a mental status examination and developing a relationship with the person being interviewed. Therefore, overly direct questioning such as, ''How much acid did you take?'' or ''What did you shoot up with this time?'' may provoke stony silence or an angry response that yields little information and further alienates the child or adolescent. A gentler approach to questioning should be taken, for example, "Have you taken any LSD recently?" or "Have you ever tried speed?"

A nonjudgmental attitude is particularly important when interviewing the child (usually a teenager) implicated in drug abuse. Once confidence in the interviewer has been gained (which may take several sessions), then, in the context of a trusting relationship, additional information may be divulged as to the extent of drug use. Also, associated effects such as delusions or other psychic disturbances may be discussed more comfortably.

When the child manifests acute effects indicative of drug use, more direct questioning is generally indicated. This information can be supported by examination, by analysis of urine and blood for drugs, by learning of previous drug use from friends and family, by reviewing past medical records, and by knowing the "epidemiology of the street." One must not only be aware of current drugs in use but also of agents with which drugs may have been "cut," or diluted. These include such noxious substances as phencyclidine (PCP) and strychnine. At times lack of dilution leads to increased danger, as when morphine and heroin are "uncut" and the threat of overdosage is thereby increased.

The history of the presenting problem should begin with the onset of drug use. It should be determined whether such use has been on an experimental or recreational basis, what has been the influence of peer pressure on drug-taking behavior, and whether emotional disturbance such as depression or anxiety has been associated. The pattern of drug use also should be determined, for example, whether alcohol is taken on a daily basis or during weekend binges only.

Examination. Because the history is often incomplete or unreliable, the examination of the person suspected of using psychoactive drugs is especially important in confirming such use and in identifying the specific agent(s) used (see Case 19–1).

The *general description* should note the most striking aspects of the examination. Is the child or adolescent lethargic or "spaced out?" Is activity level increased? Is he hallucinating? Is he relaxed and unconcerned?

The *general physical examination* should include assessment of vital signs, altered in many syndromes involving drug use. The pulse rate is often increased with marijuana, atropine, or amphetamine (Vachon *et al.,* 1973). Blood pressure may be increased with amphetamines and phencyclidine (Liden *et al.,* 1975). Respirations may be depressed by barbiturates or opiates. Temperature elevation can be seen with atropine poisoning. Subnormal temperature can occur with phenothiazines or secondary to exposure, should the person have fallen asleep or lain comatose in cool surroundings.

The head, eyes, ears, nose, and throat should be examined for evidence of head trauma: scalp swelling or laceration, periorbital ecchymosis, hemotympanum, or broken teeth, among other signs. The conjunctivae are typically reddened with marijuana use and may be icteric secondary to serum hepatitis. The nasal septum may be eroded with chronic cocaine use. The pharynx may be very dry in association with drug withdrawal.

Examination of the skin may show needle tracks in the antecubital fossa

CASE 19–1: PHENCYCLIDINE ("ANGEL DUST") USE IN A 14-YEAR-OLD BOY

R.L. was brought to the emergency room by friends who recognized him to be "dazed" and acting strangely after ingesting 15 small yellow tablets known to them as "THC." On examination an hour later, he was lethargic and took no interest in his surroundings. He opened his eyes and mouth upon request and muttered "Yes" to questions, but was unwilling or unable to give his name. He did not appear to be hallucinating.

Blood pressure was 100/60, pulse rate 80 per minute, and temperature normal. Cheeks were red, nasal mucosa injected, tongue dry, and lacrimation increased. On neurologic examination, eye movements were strikingly abnormal. Bursts of irregular, shuddery, jerk nystagmus were seen upon vertical and horizontal gaze. Pupils were 5.5 mm and reacted briskly to light. The optic fundi were normal. Tone was increased in a paratonic manner (see Chapter 13). He stood with a broad base and toppled when his legs were brought together. Deep tendon reflexes and plantar responses were normal.

He was treated supportively and showed rapid improvement in mental status. Nystagmus was still evident on the fourth hospital day. Inpatient management included psychiatric consultation, after which arrangement was made for follow-up at a community mental health center.

Comment. Diagnosis in this case was facilitated (as well as hindered) by information provided by the boy's friends. They referred to the drug mistakenly at first as "THC" (tetrahydrocannabinol, the active principle of marijuana), though they later identified it correctly as "angel dust" (phencyclidine). They also brought in one of the pills so that it could be identified.

This adolescent had been brought to the hospital with another boy who had ingested the same drug. Both boys manifested the same clinical picture: altered mental state, ataxia, hypertonia, autonomic changes, and strikingly abnormal eye movements. Gaze-evoked nystagmus is widely recognized with alcohol or barbiturate intake. Those drugs, however, are not associated with the extremely rapid, shuddery nystagmus that was seen in these teenagers. For that reason, such nystagmus may prove useful in identifying phencyclidine toxicity since this drug can produce a variable and confusing mixture of excitation and depression, rendering prompt, accurate clinical diagnosis difficult.

or on the back of the hand as a result of intravenous drug use. Subcutaneous or intramuscular abscesses often follow injection into soft tissues. The skin may be widely excoriated from intense scratching in response to tactile hallucinations occurring with cocaine abuse. The skin may be jaundiced from hepatitis, which may be associated with hepatic tenderness.

On *neurologic examination,* abnormal level of consciousness, seizures, or focal neurologic signs should be noted. Coma is discussed in this section, other alterations in consciousness under MENTAL STATUS EXAMINATION.

TABLE 19–2. **Ophthalmologic Examination with Drug Abuse**

Pupils	Dilated with cocaine, LSD, atropinic agents, amphetamines, acute anxiety
	Pinpoint (1–2 mm) with narcotics such as heroin, morphine, meperidine (Demerol), methadone
Extraocular Movements	Nystagmus (jerky, gaze-evoked): phenytoin (Dilantin), barbiturates, phencyclidine (PCP)
	Oculocephalic reflex, caloric vestibular responses: may be depressed or abolished with barbiturates or other sedatives

Drug overdosage must always be considered in the comatose child, particularly in the adolescent. Other major considerations are postictal state, head trauma, and meningitis or other severe infection. Since reliable history is often lacking, careful examination and judicious use of laboratory tests are essential in establishing the diagnosis.

Examination of the eyes is a key part of the assessment of the comatose child (see Table 19–2). Pupils are characteristically "pinpoint" (1–2 mm) and reactive to light with opiates such as heroin, morphine, meperidine (Demerol), and methadone. In such circumstances, magnification may be required to detect pupillary responses. Dilated pupils that are poorly reactive to light occur typically with atropinic agents and cocaine. These drugs interfere with the normal balance between cholinergic and adrenergic influences that determine pupillary size. Dilated pupils may also be seen with hallucinogenic drugs such as lysergic acid diethylamide (LSD) or amphetamines.

Testing of extraocular movements also provides important information in the comatose patient. Integrity of a significant portion of the brainstem is implied by normal responses to the oculocephalic maneuver or to caloric testing. The oculocephalic maneuver consists of turning the head rapidly from one side to the other or up and down. It should be done only if one can be certain that the neck has not been injured. A normal response is conjugate deviation of the eyes opposite to the direction of head turning (see Fig. 19–1).

Cold caloric testing involves irrigation of an ear canal with ice water with the head elevated to 30 degrees above the horizontal. Patency of the canal and integrity of the tympanic membrane must be determined prior to instillation of cold water. In the comatose person with intact brainstem pathways for conjugate lateral gaze, both eyes will deviate to the side of cold irrigation and remain there for 1 or more minutes. Eye movements induced by head turning or caloric stimulation can be diminished or abolished by drugs such as barbiturates.

Nystagmus often occurs in the awake patient as a side effect of a drug. Symmetric, gaze-evoked nystagmus is commonly seen with phenytoin or phenobarbital when used as an anticonvulsant. Barbiturates will also produce this effect. Phencyclidine (PCP), or "angel dust," has been associ-

COLD CALORIC
IRRIGATION

DOLL'S HEAD REFLEX

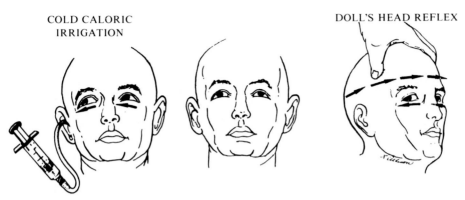

FIGURE 19–1. Normal vestibular responses in the comatose person. Sustained deviation of the eyes toward the side of cold irrigation; conjugate eye deviation opposite to direction of head-turning. (From Glaser, J. S. *Neuro-ophthalmology.* Harper and Row, Publishers, Hagerstown, Md., 1978.)

ated with a peculiar, shuddery gaze-evoked nystagmus that occurs in bursts (Herskowitz and Oppenheimer, 1977) (see Case 19–1).

It should be emphasized that drug-induced nystagmus is generally gaze-evoked, bilateral, and symmetric. One should be reluctant to make this diagnosis when the nystagmus occurs in the primary position of gaze (with eyes centered and gaze directed straight ahead at a distance), when the rapid phase of nystagmus is always to the same side regardless of the direction of gaze, when vertical nystagmus occurs without horizontal nystagmus, or when the amplitude of nystagmus is clearly greater in one eye than the other. Conditions in which these kinds of nystagmus occur include visual loss early in life, multiple sclerosis, pontine tumor, and spasmus nutans, respectively.

Seizures, usually generalized, typically occur following abrupt withdrawal from sedative drugs that have been abused, such as barbiturates or alcohol. Seizures may also result from head trauma associated with focal brain injury (contusion) or with metabolic derangement such as might be associated with dehydration (occurring as part of an alcohol withdrawal syndrome, for example).

Peripheral nerve damage may occur during coma in which compressive injury takes place. The radial nerve, coursing behind the humerus, is particularly vulnerable to this kind of injury, which is manifested by wrist drop. Muscle tissue also may suffer crush injury with resultant liberation of muscle enzymes and myoglobin. The latter can produce severe kidney damage and lead to acute renal failure.

Abnormalities in movement or posture should suggest ingestion of major tranquilizers (see Case 19–2).

The *mental status examination* may show a wide variety of alterations with drug abuse. Of these, hallucinations are among the most striking. LSD, mescaline, and psilocybin typically cause visual hallucinations (Hyde *et al.*, 1978). LSD and mescaline can also produce synesthesia, the sensation of "hearing" colors, "seeing" sounds, or both (Jaffe, 1980). Tactile (or haptic)

CASE 19–2: DRUG-RELATED DYSTONIA IN A 17-YEAR-OLD MALE

V.R. came to the emergency room complaining, "I can't seem to straighten out." For several hours he had had discomfort in his shoulders, neck, and back. In addition, he experienced what he called a "drawing sensation" of his tongue and face that was unassociated with dysphagia, dysphonia, or diplopia. He denied drug use or the possibility that he might have been given any drugs. He had no history of similar problems in the past. He acknowledged recent situational stresses but denied suicidal thoughts or actions.

On examination, he appeared markedly uncomfortable, diaphoretic, and tachycardic. His head was turned rigidly to one side, but he could voluntarily bring it to the opposite side with considerable effort. Involuntary grimacing, chewing movements, and teeth grinding were seen. Elemental neurologic examination was remarkable only for inability to retract fully the corners of the mouth or to contract the platysma voluntarily. On mental status testing, he was alert and oriented without evidence of thought disorder.

Although drug ingestion had been denied, drug-related dystonia was considered the likeliest diagnosis. Urine was obtained for drug analysis, and he was given intramuscular diphenhydramine (Benadryl), 25 mg, which relieved his symptoms within 15 minutes.

Additional history was forthcoming. Earlier that day, he had ingested three pills he believed to be "downers," provided him by an acquaintance. The nature of the drug reaction was explained, and outpatient psychiatric involvement was arranged.

Comment. The strange appearance of this adolescent's motor dysfunction might have caused it to be mistaken as hysterical or even catatonic in nature. Indeed, disorders of the basal ganglia—e.g., Wilson disease, dystonia musculorum deformans, and Sydenham chorea—can easily be mistaken as hyseria (see Chapter 13).

In this case, the diagnosis was suggested by the examination. The young man had denied drug use (or had forgotten it), and review of his medical record did not disclose antipsychotic drug therapy or other psychiatric treatment. Nor did the laboratory provide immediate assistance. The most likely offending agents were trifluoperazine (Stelazine) and haloperidol (Haldol), antipsychotic drugs with relatively high potential for producing extrapyramidal reactions. Prochlorperazine (Compazine), a phenothiazine antiemetic, can also cause severe extrapyramidal reactions. Symptoms, including opisthotonus, can be so severe as to mimic tetanus (see Chapter 5).

hallucination frequently occurs with cocaine intoxication (Siegel, 1978). Such hallucinations may involve the sensation of ants crawling underneath or on top of the skin, formication, from the Latin *formica*, meaning ant. Olfactory and gustatory hallucinations also may be seen with cocaine intoxication.

Mental status changes with intravenous heroin use follow a characteristic progression (Dole, 1980). Beginning some 10 seconds after injection of the drug, the user feels a "rush." It consists of euphoria, visceral sensations like orgasm, facial flushing, and a deepening of the voice. This effect lasts for a few minutes only and is followed by 2 to 4 hours of calm, contented detachment during which the user is responsive to questioning. Thereafter, restlessness and craving for another injection ensue.

Paranoia as part of a full-blown paranoid psychosis can occur with amphetamine abuse (Snyder, 1973). In addition to auditory hallucinations with amphetamine psychosis, visual, tactile, and olfactory hallucinations are frequently seen. These hallucinations are often accompanied by stereotyped and compulsive behaviors such as pacing, grimacing, and taking things apart and putting them back together. Aggressive behavior may also occur, as can be seen with alcohol and with diazepam (Valium) (see Chapter 15).

Laughing and giddiness can result from inhalation of nitrous oxide ("laughing gas"). This gas is readily available at supermarkets in certain aerosols, which provide a "grocery store high" (Block, 1978).

Panic, an acute state of severe disorganizing anxiety, may occur in some persons with use of hallucinogenic drugs (a "bad trip"). This response does not appear to be the direct effect of the drug but rather seems to result largely from lack of knowledge of the drug's hallucinogenic and autonomic properties. As a consequence, the person misinterprets what is happening and experiences a sense of confusion, fear of losing control, then panic (Weil, 1970).

Depersonalization is a common acute effect of marijuana use. It has been reported to occur also for a prolonged period, lasting for up to several months, when marijuana use was combined with psychosocial stress (Szymanski, 1981).

Investigation (see Table 19–3). Alcohol, amphetamines, barbiturates, cocaine, and opiates can be detected by analysis of serum and urine in many laboratories. Other substances such as phencyclidine, LSD, and marijuana are not routinely assayable at this time. When intake of specific drugs (such as alcohol, a barbiturate, or another anticonvulsant) is suspected, measurement of serum levels (rather than simply screening blood or urine for the presence of the drug) should be obtained when available.

The importance of supervised voiding of urine for analysis is emphasized because the patient may substitute a bottle of someone else's urine. Urine

TABLE 19–3. **Investigations to Be Considered in Evaluation of Drug Abuse**

Analysis of serum and urine for drugs (qualitative
   and/or quantitative analysis)
Renal and hepatic function tests
Lead level
Anticonvulsant blood levels
Naloxone (Narcan) administered parenterally under
   medical supervision

testing is generally qualitative. It does not reveal the magnitude of the dosage taken, nor does it indicate whether the individual is drug-dependent or a sporadic user (DeAngelis, 1973).

The diagnosis of drug dependence can be facilitated by the use of subcutaneous injection of naloxone (Narcan), an opiate antagonist, which may precipitate symptoms of withdrawal (dilated pupils, yawning, "goose flesh," abdominal cramps, and irritability) in the opioid-dependent person. The abstinence syndrome thus produced can be so severe, however, that naloxone should be given in this manner only under close medical supervision if at all.

Liver function tests should be obtained in persons suspected of taking drugs by injection because of frequently associated hepatitis. Glue-sniffing and nutmeg intoxication can also be associated with hepatic damage (Litt and Cohen, 1969; Faguet and Rowland, 1978). Renal function tests should be obtained following muscle crush injury, because myoglobinuria can lead to kidney failure. In cases involving inhalation of leaded gasoline, blood lead level should be measured (Boeckx *et al.*, 1977).

Differential Diagnosis.   Several conditions should be differentiated from drug abuse (see Table 19–4). *Mania*, occurring as part of unipolar or bipolar affective disturbance, may be mistaken for acute cocaine, phencyclidine, or amphetamine intoxication because of symptoms of excitement, elation, grandiosity, and loquacity (Slavney *et al.*, 1977; Jaffe, 1980). Pupillary dilation, tachycardia, elevated blood pressure, and inflammatory changes of the nasal mucosa seen with cocaine use should assist in distinguishing cocaine intoxication from mania. Phencyclidine poisoning is often associated with a clinical picture that includes depression as well as excitation. Abnormal eye movements may provide a clue to diagnosis (see Case 19–1). Amphetamine toxicity may be manifested as acute paranoid schizophrenia (see below).

Acute *paranoid psychosis* without identifiable cause may mimic precisely the paranoid psychosis caused by amphetamines (Snyder, 1973). A careful drug history and examination for signs of adrenergic drug effects should aid in differentiating these two conditions.

Infection of the central nervous system (meningoencephalitis or meningitis) should be considered in the evaluation of persons whose behavior suggests drug abuse. Herpes simplex *encephalitis*, with its predilection for limbic portions of the brain, can be associated with behavioral and emotional disturbances consistent with organic mental syndromes secondary to drug

TABLE 19–4. **Differential Diagnosis of Drug Abuse**

Mania
Paranoid psychosis
Meningitis or encephalitis
Temporal lobe epilepsy (ictal or postictal)
Anticonvulsant medication overdosage
Migraine (aura; confusional state; basilar artery syndrome)
Metabolic-endocrine disorder
Sporadic drug use
Cultural differences in perception of drug use

use. Acute *meningitis,* too, may suggest drug abuse when it presents with a fulminant picture of lethargy or coma.

Seizures of temporal lobe origin may be associated with bizarre behavior such that drug abuse is suspected (see Chapters 5 and 12, Cases 5–5 and 12–11). Postictal lethargy and confusion can also readily be mistaken for drug effects. Attempts to assist a person who has just had a seizure or otherwise to intervene may provoke aggressive behavior that additionally suggests the influence of drugs (see Chapter 15).

Overdosage of anticonvulsant medication can occur inadvertently due to a variety of errors (see Chapter 12) or secondary to intentional overdosage (see Case 6–5). Measurement of anticonvulsant levels in blood will usually clarify the matter.

The visual auras of *migraine* may resemble the visual hallucinations of cocaine intoxication (Siegel, 1978). Also, confusional migraine, associated with altered mental state and at times agitation, may suggest drug abuse (see Chapter 11).

Metabolic or endocrine disorders such as hypo- or hyperthyroidism (which may be manifested as "myxedema madness' or "thyroid storm," respectively), hypoglycemia, or diabetic ketoacidosis may also be associated with behavioral syndromes mistakenly thought to be drug-induced.

Sporadic drug use should be distinguished from drug abuse and dependence. Criteria for abuse and dependence are presented in the section on DEFINITION.

Cultural differences will influence whether or not use of a particular substance is considered to be abuse. Alcohol provides a well-known example. Few persons in most cultures would term the use of alcohol in moderation as drug abuse. On the other hand, even occasional use of marijuana is considered by some to be a form of drug abuse.

Etiology. The etiology of drug abuse is complex and incompletely understood (see Table 19–5). Clearly, a psychologic need (anxiety, depression, peer pressure) must be felt and must override personal and societal proscriptions. In addition the drug must be available and obtainable. Individual susceptibility to drug use varies and in some instances appears to be influenced by familial factors (Mendelson and Mello, 1979).

Medical Causes. Though use of pain medication under medical supervision can be associated with tolerance, such pharmacologic drug use is not generally accompanied by mental effects such as euphoria that appear to be important in syndromes of drug abuse.

Neurologic Causes. Used as an anticonvulsant, phenobarbital is not addictive. Tolerance does not develop; that is, the desired effect of altering seizure threshold does not require continuing increases in medication. Nor does a marked withdrawal syndrome occur with discontinuance of phenobarbital used as an anticonvulsant. It should nonetheless be withdrawn gradually (over several weeks to months) because of the possibility of severe nightmares or seizure recurrence as the dosage is reduced (see Chapter 9). It should be noted that phenobarbital dosages among persons who abuse that drug usually far exceed dosages taken for anticonvulsant purposes.

The supervised medical use in childhood of the psychoactive drugs dex-

TABLE 19–5. **Causes of Drug Abuse**

Psychologic	Depression
	Anger
	Boredom
	Anxiety
	Curiosity
	Sensation-seeking
Social-Environmental	Family disorganization
	Peer group pressure
	Chronic stress
Genetic-Constitutional	(?) Individual and familial susceptibility
Developmental	Adolescence

troamphetamine (Dexedrine) and methylphenidate (Ritalin) does not appear to lead to increased frequency of drug abuse in later life (Beck *et al.*, 1975).

Psychologic Causes. No specific personality disorder has been identified as a substrate for drug abuse. It is, however, widely recognized that depression, anger, and boredom may provide the affective backdrop for drug experimentation on a one-time, occasional, or more extensive basis. Other psychologic factors that have been cited as contributing to drug use include curiosity, sensation-seeking, a desire to experience altered states of consciousness, anxiety, and a wish for a general reduction in drive (Forrest and Tarala, 1973; Blumberg, 1977; Pope, 1979).

Social-Environmental Causes. Social and environmental factors appear to play major roles in drug abuse (Jaffe, 1980). Family disorganization has been cited as a contributing factor. Peer group pressures to experiment with drugs can be especially intense during adolescence. A chronically stressful military setting can contribute significantly to drug use. Postwar stresses appeared to contribute to a massive epidemic of methamphetamine abuse in Japan (Brill and Hirose, 1969). Drug use among persons in lower socioeconomic groups often has been felt to be influenced by their perception of having little possibility for upward socioeconomic mobility.

Genetic-Constitutional Causes. Males outnumber females in most reported series of drug abusers. The reasons are unclear.

The occurrence of alcoholism in a biologic parent seems to be the most reliable predictor of later alcoholism among offspring (Mendelson and Mello, 1979). Studies of adoptive persons have attempted to clarify whether such influences are mainly environmental or more strictly biologic. The data are not yet conclusive.

Developmental Causes. Adolescence is a stage of development frequently associated with drug use and, at times, abuse (see PSYCHOLOGIC CAUSES and SOCIAL-ENVIRONMENTAL CAUSES earlier). Difficulty in tolerating increased sexual and aggressive drives and feelings of depression may prompt the adolescent, striving for identity and independence, to use drugs (Blumberg, 1977) (see Cases 19–3 and 19–4).

CASE 19–3: ALCOHOL ABUSE AND HYPERVENTILATION ATTACKS IN A 19-YEAR-OLD WOMAN WITH AN APPARENT SEIZURE

R.L. was referred for neurologic evaluation because of a "seizure." While in her usual state of health, she became upset during a party and began to breathe rapidly and deeply. She next recalled awakening on the floor with a spoon in her mouth. She was told that her whole body had shaken for 5 minutes. She had not been incontinent of urine or feces, nor had she bitten her tongue. Previous episodes of hyperventilation had not been associated with loss of consciousness.

Past history included head trauma sustained in a bicycle accident 4 years previously, during which she was dazed but not "knocked out." Family history was negative for seizures. Review of systems was negative for unexplained muscle soreness in the morning, enuresis, or tongue-biting.

Social history was significant. After graduation from high school, she worked at a business while continuing to live with her parents. Issues of independence and her relationship with her mother were sources of considerable stress. She had gained 20 pounds over several months and had begun to drink alcohol to the point of inebriation to control her rage and calm her fear of losing control. She denied sleep disturbance, suicidal thoughts, or self-destructive actions.

On examination, she was a composed young woman eager to discuss her psychosocial difficulties. She did not appear depressed or anxious. General physical and neurologic examinations were normal. Her electroencephalogram showed no abnormalities.

Comment.   Whether or not this young woman did indeed have a seizure was not clearly determined. Her episode of hyperventilation might have led to syncope, although 5 minutes of generalized shaking would be unusual for a simple faint. Hyperventilation itself can produce a peculiar tightening sensation across the face and body (in addition to carpopedal spasm). Trembling and anxiety may be associated as well, but unconsciousness does not usually result. Another possibility was hysterical seizure (see Chapter 7). To clarify as precisely as possible what actually occurred that evening, it would have been valuable to speak directly with persons who witnessed the episode.

The normal EEG did not rule out seizure; for seizure discharges deep within the brain (inaccessible to recording by conventional scalp electrodes) can trigger a focal or generalized convulsion. In fact, she might have bruised her temporal lobe(s) in the bicycle accident several years previously, thereby setting up a seizure focus (see Chapter 12).

Management in this case did not involve pharmacotherapy. Clues as to the occurrence of nighttime seizures were discussed, and seizure precautions were reviewed. The major thrust of management was directed toward having the young woman begin psychologic or psychiatric counseling promptly because of the explosive psychosocial situation that had led to her abuse of alcohol.

CASE 19–4: MEMORY LAPSES, AGGRESSIVE BEHAVIOR, AND POLYDRUG ABUSE IN A 16-YEAR-OLD ADOLESCENT

O.G. was referred for neurologic evaluation because of memory lapses. He recalled that beginning 8 years earlier he frequently had gotten into fights but he did not remember details of them. At 12 years he began using drugs (including marijuana, methamphetamine, cocaine, and LSD). As many as ten memory lapses would occur daily, each lasting several minutes to 2 hours; these were not associated with fighting. Most recently he had had frequent episodes of déjà vu and had experienced premonitory dreams that allegedly came true. Attacking behavior (after uncertain provocation) followed episodes of intense anger during which his hands felt cool, he heard his heart pounding, and he felt like exploding. He did not recall these bouts of violence. Past history of birth and development was unremarkable. The boy's father had a history of violent outbursts unassociated with alcohol intake.

On examination, the boy was an articulate adolescent of normal intelligence who did not appear to be under the influence of any drugs. Affect was bland. General physical examination was normal. Neurologic examination, including visualization of optic disks and assessment of visual fields, was notable only for exaggerated deep tendon reflexes and equivocal plantar responses.

Comment. This young man's history was indeed troubling. His recurrent memory lapses, déjà vu, and rage attacks suggested temporal lobe dysfunction. The episodes were not clearly ictal in nature, however, and he lacked other symptoms suggesting temporal lobe epilepsy such as staring spells, semipurposeful behavior, or disturbances in perception. On the other hand, the episodes were ones in which his mental state was clearly altered and he was amnestic for the episodes themselves, both characteristic features of psychomotor (or temporal lobe) seizures. The episodic memory lapses and behavioral outbursts were unlike the alterations seen in confusional or basilar artery migraine (see Chapter 11).

Although it seemed most likely that the symptoms were related to drug intake, it was not certain. Thus, a wide diagnostic net was recommended: measurement of thyroid hormone, calcium, phosphorus, and sugar levels in serum; CT scan with and without contrast; and EEG in the awake and sleep states with nasopharyngeal recordings. Since the presence of a seizure disorder could not be excluded, it was suggested that regardless of the EEG results consideration be given to a trial of phenytoin or carbamazepine if adequate monitoring of such therapy and its effects could be assured.

TREATMENT AND OUTCOME

The treatment of drug dependence has been divided into five categories: (1) maintenance of drug dependence, (2) treatment of acute intoxication and other drug emergencies, (3) withdrawal of drug of dependence, (4) treatment of the early abstinence phase, and (5) long-term treatment and rehabilitation (see Table 19–6) (Blumberg, 1977).

TABLE 19–6. **Selected Aspects of Treatment of Drug Abuse**

Acute Intoxication	Ensuring adequate airway and ventilation
	Treatment of shock
	Recognition and treatment of raised intracranial pressure
	Naloxone (Narcan) for opiates
	Physostigmine for atropine
	Chlorpromazine (Thorazine) or haloperidol (Haldol) for amphetamine psychosis
	Phentolamine (Regitine) for amphetamine-related hypertension
	Haloperidol (Haldol) or diazepam (Valium) for agitation with phencyclidine (PCP)
	Anticonvulsant medication as indicated
	Treatment of intercurrent medical and surgical problems (as with head trauma)
Abstinence or Withdrawal Syndrome	Treatment of coexisting problems such as pneumonia, hepatitis, dehydration, head trauma
	Substitution for drug of dependence
	Methadone for opiate
	Pentobarbital for other barbiturate
	Chlordiazepoxide (Librium) or other drug (plus thiamine) for alcohol
	Clonidine (Catapres)
Long-term	Maintenance (methadone)
	Support group (Alcoholics Anonymous)
	Disulfiram (Antabuse)

The outcome of persons who have used drugs will depend upon the specific drugs used, the circumstances under which they have been used, and the pattern of use. Available data indicate that only 30 to 45 per cent of persons withdrawn from opiate dependency abstain entirely from further use (Stimson *et al.,* 1978). Those who do "outgrow" their dependence do so about 9 years after onset of drug use (*DSM*-III, 1980). A disproportionate number of persons addicted to opiates in the United States die before the age of 40.

A history of dependence on opiates does not necessarily predict a poor outcome. Follow-up studies of American servicemen who had been drug dependent in Vietnam showed that few continued or resumed their drug dependent behavior upon returning to the United States (Snyder, 1979). Furthermore, a majority of persons maintained on methadone in lieu of heroin became productively employed in the series reported by Dole (1980). Criminal activity that had been part of the drug abuse syndrome diminished concurrently.

McLellan and colleagues (1979), in a 6-year-study of fifty-one adults who abused drugs, found evidence that the choice of drug was associated with later development of specific psychiatric illness. A significant number of stimulant users became psychotic, and depressant users became depressed. The role of preexisting personality structure in such outcomes is unclear (Pope, 1979).

In approaching the person with known or suspected drug abuse, it is important to remember that several drugs may be used concurrently or in succession and that problems such as hepatitis, malnutrition, and head trauma may complicate the clinical situation.

Medical Management.   The person presenting in coma should first receive basic supportive care. An airway must be established, ventilation assured, and shock recognized and treated immediately. Acutely raised intracranial pressure (secondary to intracranial hemorrhage due to trauma, for example) may likewise demand urgent diagnostic and therapeutic measures (see Chapter 20).

Specific pharmacotherapy may include agents directed toward symptoms of overdosage, those used to reverse symptoms of withdrawal, and those employed to prevent further drug use.

Naloxone hydrochloride (Narcan) is a key drug in the treatment of opioid overdosage. Given intravenously or intramuscularly, usually in a dosage of 0.4 mg (1 ml), it promptly reverses the respiratory depression induced by opiate drugs. This dose is repeated as needed, up to three times, at 2- to 3-minute intervals (Abramowicz, 1980). Physostigmine, a cholinesterase inhibitor, is a specific antidote for atropine intoxication.

Standard antipsychotic agents such as chlorpromazine (Thorazine) or haloperidol (Haldol) are utilized for treatment of amphetamine psychosis, and antihypertensive agents such as phentolamine (Regitine), an alpha adrenergic blocking agent, can be used to control associated blood pressure elevation (Angrist, 1978). Haloperidol or diazepam (Valium) appears to be preferable to a phenothiazine in treating agitation associated with acute phencyclidine (PCP) poisoning, because phenothiazines may cause severe postural hypotension and increased muscle ridgidity (Abramowicz, 1980).

Treatment of abstinence syndromes is essentially symptomatic and supportive. The major features of an opioid withdrawal syndrome run their course within 7 to 10 days. By contrast, abstinence syndromes with phenobarbital, diazepam (Valium), or glutethimide (Doriden) are longer, lasting up to several weeks (Abramowicz, 1980). Lacrimation, rhinorrea, yawning, and sweating usually appear 8 to 10 hours after the last dose of opioid. They are followed by restlessness, irritability, tremor, and dilated pupils. These symptoms are maximal at 2 to 3 days. Nausea, vomiting, and diarrhea are also commonly seen during the first few days of withdrawal. Another characteristic autonomic manifestation of opiate withdrawal is the appearance of "goose flesh." Since the skin thus affected resembles that of a plucked turkey, the expression "cold turkey" has been used to describe abrupt opiate withdrawal (Jaffe, 1980). Purposive behavior, manifested as compulsive drug-seeking, peaks at $1\frac{1}{2}$ to 3 days following the last dose, after which it subsides gradually.

After the acute withdrawal period, more subtle behavioral and emotional symptoms arise, constituting a "protracted abstinence syndrome" that can last for several weeks. Features include poor tolerance of stress, low threshold for discomfort, and diminished self-esteem. The risk of returning to drug abuse appears to be increased during this time.

As a general strategy in treating withdrawal, adequate amounts of whatever drugs are necessary are given to suppress major withdrawal symptoms, and the dose is gradually reduced (Dole, 1980; Jaffe, 1980). Coexisting medical problems such as hepatitis or pneumonia are also treated.

In practice, methadone is often substituted for whatever narcotic the patient had been using: heroin, morphine, or meperidine (Demerol). Methadone, given orally, is then reduced in dosage by about 20 per cent per day to achieve withdrawal. This withdrawal process is associated generally with symptoms no worse than that of a moderately severe "flu" syndrome and is rarely fatal (Connell, 1974; Jaffe, 1980). Some persons are maintained on relatively low doses of methadone for several months. Following maintenance at this level, methadone is gradually withdrawn on an ambulatory basis.

The euphoric effects of intravenous narcotics such as heroin and morphine are blocked by methadone, which, as noted above, can be used as a maintenance drug in lieu of other narcotics (Jaffe, 1980). Like other narcotics, methadone can be associated with an abstinence syndrome when dosage is lowered too rapidly or abruptly cut off. Unlike other narcotics, it is effective when taken by mouth.

Because methadone can itself cause dependence, methadone maintenance is considered by some to be of little value. In many persons, however, methadone maintenance removes the need for compulsive drug-seeking and diminishes associated antisocial activities such as theft and prostitution, previously required in order to maintain the drug habit (Verebey *et al.*, 1978; Dole, 1980).

Clonidine (Catapres), a centrally acting antihypertensive drug that is nonnarcotic, has shown considerable promise in diminishing symptoms of opiate withdrawal (Gold *et al.*, 1980; Riordan and Kleber, 1980; Blaschke and Melmon, 1980).

Withdrawal from drugs is a multifaceted process that usually is best carried out in a hospital (Blumberg, 1977). Withdrawal syndromes characteristically occur following dependence on opiates, alcohol, barbiturates, benzodiazepines, other sedative-hypnotic drugs, and amphetamines. As a general rule withdrawal symptoms are manifested as "rebound" effects when contrasted with the physiologic effects of the drug. For example, amphetamine withdrawal is characterized by hyperphagia, depression, and lack of energy, whereas use of amphetamines suppresses appetite, elevates mood, and reduces fatigue. Barbiturates, which prevent seizures, are associated in the withdrawal phase with a lowering of seizure threshold, resulting in an increased tendency to develop convulsions.

The management of barbiturate withdrawal involves gradual reduction of dosage over a somewhat longer period than is generally required for opiates or alcohol—that is, up to 3 weeks. Oral pentobarbital can be substituted for the barbiturate of dependence during the withdrawal phase (Jaffe, 1980).

The treatment of alcohol withdrawal generally involves substitution of chlordiazepoxide (Librium), a barbiturate, paraldehyde, or diazepam (Valium) for alcohol followed by gradual reduction in drug dosage (Jaffe, 1980). Acute management should include careful attention to vital signs and fluid and electrolyte status. With delirium tremens, an acute alcohol withdrawal syndrome, life-threatening hyperthermia and dehydration may occur.

Management of the chronic alcoholic must also include attention to the nutritional status of the patient. Deficiency of thiamine is of particular concern, since it can be manifested acutely by confusion, ataxia, and ophthalmoplegia, which are reversible by treatment with thiamine (usually given by injection). The memory deficit of Wernicke-Korsakoff syndrome (retrograde amnesia and severe impairment in short-term memory, anterograde amnesia) is, by contrast, largely irreversible (see Chapter 16).

Prevention of a return to alcohol abuse can be facilitated by use of disulfiram (Antabuse), a drug that produces an altered response to alcohol. Disulfiram interferes with the intermediary metabolism of alcohol in such a way that acetaldehyde, a toxic by-product, is produced. As a result, within 5 to 10 minutes after alcohol ingestion, acetaldehyde causes an intense throbbing headache followed by nausea, vomiting, diaphoresis, blurred vision, hypotension, and confusion.

Neurologic Management.   Alcohol withdrawal seizures usually take place within the first 12 to 24 hours of alcohol withdrawal. They may occur unexpectedly, as when a person has been hospitalized for elective surgery and information as to alcohol use has not been disclosed. Alcohol withdrawal seizures are typically brief and generalized, and usually do not require acute treatment with anticonvulsant medication.

The management of seizures is discussed in Chapter 12. When alcohol abuse is suspected in a person who is actively convulsing, attention should be given to the possibility of complicating hypoglycemia, head trauma, or meningitis. Chronic anticonvulsant therapy should be based upon the particular aspects of an individual case. Past history of head trauma, focal neurologic signs, and electroencephalographic results will enter into such considerations (see Chapter 12).

Barbiturate withdrawal seizures may be difficult to treat. They do not respond to intravenous phenytoin (Dilantin), a drug used regularly in treating status epilepticus, but are usually controlled by intravenous barbiturates. Phenobarbital or pentobarbital are the drugs of first choice.

Psychotherapy.   It is important to provide the young drug abuser with straightforward, factual information and not to approach him in a punitive or rejecting manner. For example, the teenager using barbiturates might be informed that while tolerance develops to the sedative effects of the drug, respiratory depression and death continue to be major dangers to which tolerance does not develop. Alternatives to drug-induced sensory and affective experiences can be offered as well in a supportive setting (Cohen, 1977).

In situations of panic, such as may be associated with use of LSD or other hallucinogens, psychotherapeutic management should take the form of continuous reassurance. The person suffering from acute, disorganizing anxiety should be told that the symptoms are drug-related and will pass within a few hours and that he is not losing his mind (Weil, 1970). Persons under the influence of hallucinogenic agents must be watched carefully to prevent damage to themselves as a result of delusions of being able, for example, to fly or to walk on water. A phenothiazine may be employed as a therapeutic adjunct but is not often necessary.

Mutual support groups (e.g., involving adolescents who abuse alcohol) can be valuable in furthering understanding of the reasons for drug abuse and in preventing a return to such behavior.

Social-Environmental Management. A quiet, unstimulating environment (not an emergency room teeming with people) is the most favorable setting for treatment of a person suffering the effects of an hallucinogen. Calm reassurance can best be carried out in such circumstances.

Hospitalization is itself a form of social-environmental therapy: a highly structured environment where drug use is controlled, and which is devoid of the social contacts and other influences that had contributed to drug abuse.

Self-help groups and halfway houses are other social-environmental modes of therapy (Alonzi and Faigel, 1972). Of the former, Alcoholics Anonymous has been particularly successful.

CORRELATION

Anatomic Aspects. The limbic system has been implicated as playing a major role in the effects of psychoactive drugs. Specifically, opiate receptors in high density have been demonstrated in the amygdala, thalamus, and hypothalamus. Other opiate receptors have been found intimately associated with spinothalamic pathways that mediate pain sensation. Thus, opiate receptors appear to be involved not only in the primary sensory aspect of pain (spinothalamic) but also in its emotional (limbic) component (Snyder, 1977; Fields, 1981). This link between analgesic and affective properties of opioids is underscored by the euphoric effects of opiates when taken exogenously.

Other areas of spinal cord and regions of brainstem also appear to have opiate receptors. These anatomic findings allow for correlation between opiate analgesia, depression of the cough reflex, and effects upon gastrointestinal function.

Biochemical Aspects. Proteins are complicated molecules composed of chains of amino acids. They may be very long, as with enzymes, or shorter, as with polypeptides (or simply peptides). Peptides have been found to play key roles throughout the body. For example, antidiuretic hormone, consisting of only nine amino acids, is one such peptide.

Snyder (1977) and others have identified specific opiate receptors in vertebrates at the sites mentioned above. The presence of these receptors suggested that morphine-like substances might be present naturally in brain, perhaps functioning as neurotransmitters at these sites. Hughes and colleagues (1975) isolated two morphine-like peptides from pig brain. Each was composed of five amino acids and differed only in a terminal amino acid (leucine or methionine). These substances, endogenous opioids, were named enkephalins. These enkephalins and related compounds have since been found in many other organisms, including man. Fluorescent antibody studies have demonstrated that the distribution of enkephalins closely parallels that of opiate receptors: the substantia gelatinosa of the spinal cord, the amygdala of the limbic system, and central portions of the thalamus (Snyder, 1977).

Beta-endorphin, another endogenous opioid, is more potent than either enkephalin. It is a polypeptide consisting of 31 amino acids, the first five of which are identical to methionine enkephalin. Beta-endorphin itself is identical to amino acids 61 through 91 of beta-lipotropin, a pituitary hormone that may act as precursor to several of the endogenous opioids (Murad and Haynes, 1980; Cooper and Martin, 1980).

Physiologic Aspects.   Snyder (1977, 1979) has suggested how enkephalin-containing neurons may play a role in opiate addiction. Normally, enkephalins (endogenous opioids) act upon opiate receptors to carry out functions that are not currently well understood (Willer *et al.*, 1981). When an exogenous opioid such as heroin is taken into the body, opiate receptors become saturated. Through a presumed neuronal feedback loop, the release and/or production of endogenous opioids is then curtailed. If the exogenous opiate is then discontinued or the dosage diminished, the opiate receptors are now saturated with neither heroin nor enkephalin. Thus, withdrawal symptoms develop.

A hypothesis for development of tolerance suggested by animal studies is that exogenous opiates increase the activity of enkephalin-degrading enzymes ("enkephalinases") (Snyder, 1979). As a result, less opiate is available through endogenous sources and more must be supplied from outside the organism.

The influence of endogenous opioids in behavior has been demonstrated in experimental studies. When animals are given beta-endorphin, they manifest "wet dog shaking" behavior, which is similar to behavior occurring with opiate withdrawal in dependent animals. Also seen are hypothermia, akinesia, and muscular rigidity (like catatonia), lasting for hours. These effects upon movement and temperature have suggested a link between endorphins and antipsychotic agents such as phenothiazines and butyrophenones (Cooper *et al.*, 1978). A possible connection between endogenous opioids and schizophrenia has been discussed by Jacquet and Marks (1976), Comfort (1979), Verebey and colleagues (1978), and Judd and colleagues (1981).

SUMMARY

Drug abuse, a complex subject, includes both the behavior of the drug-user and the effects of the drug itself. Because information obtained by history is often unreliable, examination and investigation are especially important in assessing the person with suspected drug use or abuse.

Drug abuse must be differentiated from mania, schizophrenia, encephalitis, seizure disorder, migraine, and endocrine-metabolic disease. Causes for drug abuse include self-treatment of anxiety, depression, and boredom; sensation-seeking; peer pressure; and difficult or intolerable social circumstances. Treatment is directed toward the adverse effects of a drug as well as behavior associated with its use. Management of withdrawal is symptomatic and supportive. Long-term management may include group therapy, residence in a halfway house, and, with narcotic abuse, methadone mainte-nance.

An explosion of knowledge about brain peptides, including those that function as endogenous opioids, has increased understanding of drug actions and mechanisms of dependence. Possible links between endogenous opioids and antipsychotic agents have suggested exciting avenues for future investi-gation of major psychiatric disorders.

CITED REFERENCES

Abramowicz, M. Diagnosis and management of reactions to drug abuse. *Med. Lett. Drugs Ther.*, **22:** 73–76, 1980.

Alonzi, J., and Faigel, H. C. A structured, therapeutic approach to drug abuse. *Pediatrics*, **50:** 754–59, 1972.

Angrist, B. M. Toxic manifestations of amphetamine. *Psychiatric Annals*, **8:** 443–46, 1978.

Beck, L.; Langford, W. S.; MacKay, M.; and Sum, G. Childhood chemotherapy and later drug abuse and growth curve: a follow-up study of 30 adolescents. *Am. J. Psychiatry*, **132:** 436–38, 1975.

Blaschke, T. F., and Melmon, K. L. Antihypertensive agents and the drug therapy of hypertension. Pp. 793–818 in *The Pharmacological Basis of Therapeutics*, 6th ed. Gilman, A. G.; Goodman, L. S., and Gilman, A., eds. Macmillan Publishing Co., Inc., New York, 1980.

Block, S. H. The grocery store high. *Am. J. Psychiatry*, **135:** 126–27, 1978.

Blumberg, H. Drug taking. Pp. 628–45 in *Child Psychiatry: Modern Approaches*. Rutter, M., and Hersov, L., eds. Blackwell Scientific Publications, Oxford, 1977.

Boeckx, R. L.; Postl, B.; and Coodin, F. J. Gasoline sniffing and tetraethyl lead poisoning in children. *Pediatrics*, **60:** 140–45, 1977.

Brill, H., and Hirose, T. The rise and fall of a methamphetamine epidemic: Japan 1945–55. *Semin. Psychiatry*, **1:** 179–92, 1969.

Cohen, S. Alternatives to adolescent drug abuse. *JAMA*, **238:** 1561–62, 1977.

Comfort, A. Morphine as antipsychotic drug. *Lancet*, **1:** 95, 1977.

Connell, P. H. Addiction in adolescence: some comments about its diagnosis, treatment, and vulnerable groups. *Community Health*, **6:** 29–31, 1974.

Cooper, J. R.; Bloom, F. E.; and Roth, R. H. *The Biochemical Basis of Neuropharmacology*, 3d ed. Oxford University Press, New York, 1978, pp. 264–71.

Cooper, P. E., and Martin, J. B. Neuroendocrinology and brain peptides. *Ann. Neurol.*, **8:** 551–57, 1980.

DeAngelis, G. G. Testing for drugs: II. techniques and issues. *Int. J. Addict.*, **8:** 997–1014, 1973.

Diagnostic and Statistical Manual of Mental Disorders, 3d ed. Organic mental disorders and substance use disorders. American Psychiatric Association, Washington, D.C., 1980, pp. 101–79.

Dole, V. P. Addictive behavior. *Sci. Am.*, **243:** 138–54, 1980.

Faguet, R. A., and Rowland, K. F. "Spice cabinet" intoxication. *Am. J. Psychiatry*, **135:** 860–61, 1978.

Fields, H. L. Pain II: new approaches to management. *Ann. Neurol.*, **9:** 101–6, 1981.

Forrest, J. A. H., and Tarala, R. A. Abuse of drugs "for kicks": a review of 252 admissions. *Br. Med. J.*, **4:** 136–39, 1973.

Gold, M. S.; Pottash, A. C.; Sweeney, D. R.; and Kleber, H. D. Opiate withdrawal using clonidine: a safe, effective, and rapid non-opiate treatment. *JAMA*, **243:** 343–46, 1980.

Herskowitz, J., and Oppenheimer, E. Y. More about poisoning by phencyclidine ("PCP," "angel dust"). *N. Eng. J. Med.*, **297:** 1405, 1977.

Hughes, J.; Smith, T. W.; Kosterlitz, H. W.; Fothergill, L. A.; Morgan, B. A.; and Morris, H. R. Identification of two related pentapeptides from the brain with potent opiate agonist activity. *Nature*, **258:** 577–79, 1975.

Hyde, C.; Glancy, G.; Omerod, P.; Hall, D.; and Taylor, G. S. Abuse of indigenous psilocybin mushrooms: a new fashion and some psychiatric complications. *Br. J. Psychiatry*, **132:** 602–4, 1978.

Jacquet, Y. F., and Marks, N. The C-fragment of beta-lipotropin: an endogenous neuroleptic or antipsychotogen. *Science*, **194:** 632–35, 1976.

Jaffe, J. H. Drug addiction and drug abuse. Pp. 535–84 in *The Pharmacological Basis of Therapeutics*, 6th ed. Gilman, A. G.; Goodman, L. S.; and Gilman, A., eds. Macmillan Publishing Co., Inc., New York, 1980.

Judd, L. L.; Janowsky, D. S.; Segal, D. S.; Parker, D. C.; and Huey, L. Y. Behavioral effects of methadone in schizophrenic patients. *Am. J. Psychiatry*, **138:** 243–45, 1981.

Liden, C. B.; Lovejoy, F. H., Jr.; and Costello, C. E. Phencyclidine: nine cases of poisoning. *JAMA*, **234:** 513–16, 1975.

Litt, I. F., and Cohen, M. I. "Danger . . . vapor harmful": spot-remover sniffing. *N. Engl. J. Med.*, **281:** 543–44, 1969.

McLellan, A. T.; Woody, G. E.; and O'Brien, C. P. Development of psychiatric illness in drug abusers: possible role of drug preference. *N. Engl. J. Med.*, **301:** 1310–14, 1979.

Mendelson, J. H., and Mello, N. K. Biologic concomitants of alcoholism. *N. Engl. J. Med.*, **301:** 912–21, 1979.

Murad, F., and Haynes, R. C., Jr. Adenohypophyseal hormones and related substances. Pp. 1388–89 in *The Pharmacological Basis of Therapeutics*, 6th ed. Gilman, A. G.; Goodman, L. S.; and Gilman, A., eds. Macmillan Publishing Co., Inc., New York, 1980.

Pope, H. G. Drug abuse and psychopathology. *N. Engl. J. Med.*, **301:** 1341–43, 1979.

Riordan, C. E., and Kleber, H. D. Rapid opiate detoxification with clonidine and naloxone. *Lancet*, **1:** 1079–80, 1980.

Siegel, R. K. Cocaine hallucinations. *Am. J. Psychiatry*, **135:** 309–14, 1978.

Slavney, P. R.; Rich, G. B.; Pearlson, G. D.; and McHugh, P. R. Phencyclidine abuse and symptomatic mania. *Biol. Psychiatry*, **12:** 697–700, 1977.

Snyder, S. H. Amphetamine psychosis: a "model" schizophrenia mediated by catecholamines. *Am. J. Psychiatry*, **130:** 61–67, 1973.

Snyder, S. H. Opiate receptors and internal opiates. *Sci. Am.*, **236:** 44–56, March 1977.

Snyder, S. H. Receptors, neurotransmitters and drug responses. *N. Engl. J. Med.*, **300:** 465–72, 1979.

Stimson, G. B.; Oppenheimer, E.; and Thorley, A. Seven-year follow-up of heroin addicts: drug use and outcome. *Br. Med. J.*, **1:** 1190–92, 1978.

Szymanski, H. V. Prolonged depersonalization after marijuana use. *Am. J. Psychiatry*, **138:** 231–33, 1981.

Vachon, L.; FitzGerald, M. X.; Solliday, N. H.; Gould, I. A.; and Gaensler, E. A. Single-dose effect of marihuana smoke. *N. Engl. J. Med.*, **288:** 985–89, 1973.

Verebey, K.; Volavka, J.; and Clouet, D. Endorphins in psychiatry: an overview and a hypothesis. *Arch. Gen. Psychiatry*, **35:** 877–88, 1978.

Weil, A. T. Adverse reactions to marihuana: classification and suggested treatment. *N. Engl. J. Med.*, **282:** 997–1000, 1970.

Willer, J. C.; Dehen, H.; and Cambier, J. Stress-induced analgesia in humans: endogenous opioids and naloxone-reversible depression of pain reflexes. *Science,* **212:** 689–91, 1981.

World Health Organization. *Sixteenth Report of the WHO Expert Committee on Drug Dependence.* Technical report series no. 407, Geneva, 1969.

ADDITIONAL READINGS

Altura, B. T., and Altura, B. M. Phencyclidine, lysergic acid diethylamide, and mescaline: cerebral artery spasms and hallucinogenic activity. *Science,* **212:** 1051–52, 1981.

Chou, S. N. Acupuncture, *Mayo Clin. Proc.*, **55:** 775–76, 1980.

Hofmann, A. The discovery of LSD and subsequent investigations on naturally occurring hallucinogens. In *Discoveries in Biological Psychiatry.* Ayd, F. J., Jr., and Blackwell, B., eds. J. B. Lippincott Company, Philadelphia, 1970.

Jaffe, J. H., and Martin, W. R. Opioid analgesics and antagonists. Pp. 494–534 in *The Pharmacological Basis of Therapeutics,* 6th ed. Gilman, A. G.; Goodman, L. S.; and Gilman, A., eds. Macmillan Publishing Co., Inc., New York, 1980.

Snyder, S. H. *Biological Aspects of Mental Disorder.* Oxford University Press, New York, 1980.

Wikler, A. *Opioid Dependence: Mechanisms and Treatment.* Plenum Press, New York, 1980.

Wynder, E. L., and Hoffmann, D. Tobacco and health: a societal challenge. *N. Engl. J. Med.,* **300:** 894–903, 1979.

20 Child Abuse and Neglect

All professionals who work with children—physicians, nurses, teachers, and day care workers—should have been sensitized by now to the prevalence of child abuse and neglect and their importance in childhood morbidity and mortality. They account for some 80,000 injuries and 800 deaths annually in the United States and approximately one-half those figures in England and Wales (Schmitt and Kempe, 1975; Collingwood and Alberman, 1979).

Child abuse involves inflicted injury. An example is the "battered child" who has suffered head trauma and broken bones. Child neglect is often evidenced as failure to thrive. Medical, neurologic, social, and psychologic factors each may play contributing roles in producing these two disorders, which not infrequently coexist. This chapter looks broadly at child abuse and neglect with particular attention to their neurologic aspects, particularly the effects of head injury and nutritional deprivation upon the brain.

Several questions will be addressed:

What physical and neurologic signs should be sought in evaluation of the child suspected of being abused or neglected?
What conditions mimic child abuse or neglect and must be differentiated from it?
What investigations are necessary or useful?
What kinds of head injury can be seen in an abused child?
What is the effect of nutritional deprivation upon the brain?
How are the neurologic complications of child abuse or neglect treated?
What is the long-term outcome for the child whose brain has been damaged by abuse or neglect?

CHILD ABUSE AND NEGLECT

DEFINITION

Child abuse is defined by nonaccidental inflicted physical injury, whereas *neglect* is defined by failure to provide adequately for physical and psychologic growth of the child. As described by Kempe and colleagues (1962) in

568

their germinal paper on "The Battered Child Syndrome," child abuse should be suspected in any child (particularly when 3 years of age or younger) with bone fracture(s), subdural hematoma, unexplained soft tissue swelling, skin bruising, or sudden death. It should also be considered whenever the apparent injuries do not match the accounts of parents or other caretakers. Neglect refers not only to material neglect but to emotional neglect as well (Helfer, 1975). Material neglect applies to lack of basic necessities such as adequate food, clothing, shelter, medical care, education, and supervision. Emotional neglect refers to lack of understanding of, or empathy toward, the child's needs so that interactions with the child reflect the adult's needs to an exaggerated degree.

DIAGNOSIS

The diagnosis of child abuse or neglect can be established by evidence seen at a single examination or upon observations made over time. Information provided by the index child and family is, of course, important; but its validity is often uncertain. Hence, the diagnosis frequently must be based upon physical findings and results of investigation. In many instances information obtained by the physician, who has had initial contact with the abused or neglected child and his family, will be turned over to a multidisciplinary child protection team that is hospital- or community-based.

Clinical Process. *History.* The chief complaint of the child may express particulars of abuse or neglect: "My mother beats me." "We never have enough to eat." "They dropped us off at a friend's house and never picked us up." On the other hand, the child may cover up or refuse to acknowledge a parent's wrongdoings through a desire to protect mother or father or because of prior threats intended to maintain secrecy.

The child should be interviewed separately from the parents or other caretakers in an unhurried fashion so that difficult and troubling material can be brought to the surface and dealt with. A trusting relationship often will need to be established before the child is able to discuss sensitive material; the same is true for the parents as well.

The parents' perception of their child's problems should be recorded. What are the problems? When did they begin? What measures (diagnostic or therapeutic) have been undertaken to deal with the situation? How successful have they been? The particulars of caretaking arrangements (included as part of the child's daily schedule) should be determined.

Discipline of the child should be asked about. Do both parents discipline the child or only one? What forms of discipline are employed? In what circumstances have disciplinary measures been used? Have they been effective? How were the parents themselves disciplined as children? Is the child hyperactive, provocative, or destructive?

Past history should note events that may have interfered with mother-child bonding. Early attachment may have been impaired by separation of child from mother because of prolonged hospitalization of the newborn due to prematurity or illness (Klein and Stern, 1971; Collingwood and Alberman, (1979). The severity of the baby's illness (especially as perceived by the parents) should be determined, since bonding may have been weakened by anticipatory grieving. Parental concerns as to persisting defectiveness should be explored. Postpartum depression may have interfered with bonding as well.

Evaluation of the child who is failing to thrive should include attention to both somatic growth and development. A careful nutritional history is essential. Such accounts are often unreliable, however. In such circumstances opportunity to observe eating behavior and weight gain in the child hospitalized for evaluation is especially valuable. Major illnesses and separations beyond the neonatal period should also be noted.

Examination. The *general description* should mention the most striking features of the child's examination. Is he unusually small for age? Is he withdrawn? Is he hyperactive? In what condition are the child's clothing and hygiene? Are bruises about the face and limbs readily apparent?

The *general physical examination* should include careful attention to growth. Height, weight, and head circumference should be measured and plotted on standard growth curves. Previous growth measurements, including those from birth, if available, are especially useful. These data may suggest a syndrome of postnatal neglect or growth retardation of prenatal origin. Nutritional deprivation typically affects weight more than length or head size, although all three can be affected with long-term malnutrition (Brown, 1966). Small head measurements since birth suggest that failure to thrive is, at least in part, on a cerebral basis.

Skin markings and injuries must be sought in the child suspected of being abused or neglected (Gillespie, 1965; Sussman, 1968; Kempe, 1975). The entire skin must be examined and lesions carefully recorded (e.g., through drawings upon preprinted anatomic maps, such as those used in children with burns or through photographs).

Inflicted injury may be manifested by several kinds of skin injuries: linear marks in parallel due to a switch or a fork; teeth marks; ligature marks around the limbs, neck, or penis; scald marks of the buttocks and perineum secondary to immersion in hot water; small, rounded lesions due to cigarette burns; or multiple ecchymoses ("black and blue marks") occurring widely (see Figs. 20–1 and 20–2).

The distribution of the skin lesions and the child's age may provide clues as to whether or not the injuries are inflicted. A toddler who is just learning to walk or a clumsy older child often will have multiple ecchymoses. These, however, are generally found on the lower extremities only. In children with widespread ecchymoses, hematologic abnormalities such as thrombocytopenia should be considered in addition to inflicted injury. Multiple petechiae (pinpoint hemorrhages) would support the possibility of hematologic disorder (see Case 20–1).

With syndromes of neglect, different skin manifestations are found. The diaper area may show an ammoniacal rash (erythematous or excoriated) due to infrequent diaper changes. Chronic nutritional deprivation may be evidenced by loss of subcutaneous fat (in marasmus), pitting edema (in kwashiorkor), areas of depigmentation (in vitamin A deficiency), and cracking of the corners of the mouth (cheilosis, in riboflavin deficiency). With kwashiorkor, the hair is brittle, sparse, and easily pulled out in tufts.

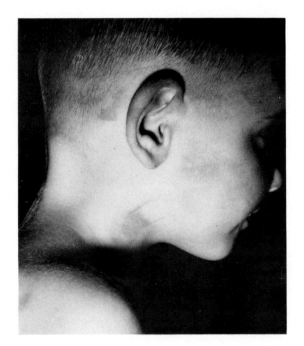

FIGURE 20–1. Multiple abrasions of shoulder, neck, and face in an abused child.

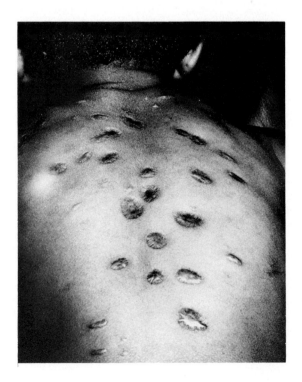

FIGURE 20–2. Multiple cigarette burns of back in a case of child abuse.

CASE 20–1: APPARENT CHILD ABUSE IN A 2-YEAR-OLD GIRL WITH HEMATOLOGIC DISORDER

M.F. was brought to the hospital because of fever and rash. For 2 days she had suffered from a "cold" with cough, rhinitis, and fever. She had received no medication. Past history was unremarkable.

On examination, the child was an alert, shy 2-year-old with a large "black eye," sucking a pacifier warily (see Fig. 20–3). Ecchymoses were scattered widely over her body, and an apparent bite mark was evident on the leg. Temperature was 101.8 degrees F. The optic fundi were normal. The pharynx was injected without exudate. The abdomen was soft and nontender. Further examination of the skin disclosed multiple pinpoint hemorrhages (petechiae) of the extremities and trunk.

Investigations included a complete blood count (including a white blood cell count and differential), which was normal except for diminished platelets on smear of peripheral blood. Platelet count was markedly depressed (15,000 per cubic mm). Bone marrow was consistent with idiopathic thrombocytopenic purpura, apparently secondary to a viral illness. Psychosocial evaluation revealed no evidence of abuse or neglect. Recovery from the viral process was uneventful. Because thrombocytopenia persisted, corticosteroid therapy was begun. It was interrupted several weeks later for approximately 10 days because the girl developed chickenpox. Platelet count dropped below 50,000 during this period but rose again to normal levels when steroids were reinstituted. Within several months, prednisone was discontinued and the platelet count remained normal.

Comment. Upon inspection from across the room, this child with a prominent periorbital ecchymosis and widespread black-and-blue marks appeared battered. Examination of the entire skin, however, disclosed petechiae that suggested hematologic disorder rather than inflicted injury. Laboratory studies showed a low platelet count. The bone marrow examination ruled out leukemia. The apparent bite mark was unaccounted for. Though no fully satisfactory explanation was forthcoming, the child was not considered to be at high risk for abuse or neglect based upon inpatient psychosocial evaluation. Pediatric follow-up confirmed this impression.

Examination of the abdomen may disclose evidence for trauma (in child abuse) or hepatomegaly (in protein-calorie malnutrition). Abdominal distention would be consistent with hemorrhage due to a ruptured viscus in the former or with ascites in the latter.

One form of inflicted injury involves parents creating medical or surgical illness in their child (Kohl *et al.,* 1978; Taylor and Newberger, 1979). For example, foreign bodies have been inserted into the child's urethra in an effort to mimic kidney stones, and feces have been injected into a child in order to produce an infectious illness.

The *neurologic examination* may show a wide variety of findings (Baron

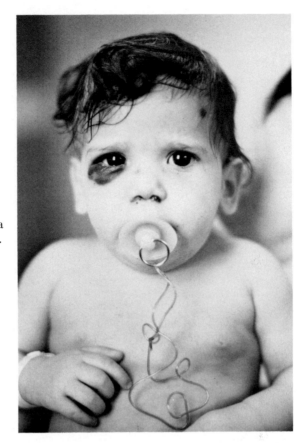

FIGURE 20–3. "Black eye" and multiple ecchymoses in a child with platelet deficiency.

et al., 1970; Silber and Bell, 1971). Head injury is the most important component of child abuse, since such injury may cause permanent brain damage or death.

Housed within the skull, the brain is protected from head trauma to a considerable degree. The skull and overlying scalp are often involved in head injuries and provide objective evidence that trauma has occurred. Head injuries can cause scalp swelling due to local *bruising* (*contusion*) or *laceration*. A large, boggy area of scalp swelling may be due to *subgaleal hemorrhage* (see Fig. 20–4) (see CORRELATION: ANATOMIC ASPECTS). The amount of blood within the subgaleal space may be considerable and can be associated with anemia or even shock. Subgaleal hemorrhage can result from a child's being grabbed by braids or pigtails, which provide convenient "handles" for an angry parent (Hamlin, 1968).

Cephalohematoma (subperiosteal hemorrhage) is another cause of traumatic scalp swelling in the child. It occurs most frequently in the parietal area and is associated with an area of locally diminished transillumination. Calcification around its base may produce the false impression of an underlying depressed skull fracture, which is only rarely associated. Linear skull fracture, however, occurs in 5 to 25 percent of cases.

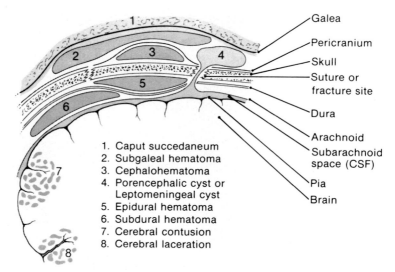

1. Caput succedaneum
2. Subgaleal hematoma
3. Cephalohematoma
4. Porencephalic cyst or
   Leptomeningeal cyst
5. Epidural hematoma
6. Subdural hematoma
7. Cerebral contusion
8. Cerebral laceration

FIGURE 20–4. Schematic representation of tissue layers from scalp to brain that may be affected by head trauma. (From Rosman, N. P.; Herskowitz, J.; Carter, A. P.; and O'Connor, J. F. Acute head trauma in infancy and childhood: clinical and radiologic aspects. *Pediatr. Clin. North Am.*, **26:** 707–36, 1979.)

TABLE 20–1. **Clinical Features of Acute Subdural Hematoma in Infants and Children***

Supratentorial

Frequency	Greater (5–10x) than acute epidural hematoma
Skull fracture	<25%
Bleeding	Venous
Age	<2 years; peak age 4–6 months
Laterality	Mostly bilateral
Seizures	75%
(Pre)retinal hemorrhages	75%
Intracranial hypertension†	Present
Mortality	<25%
Morbidity	High

Infratentorial

Frequency	Less than supratentorial
Skull fracture	Frequent
Bleeding	Venous
Clinical signs	Varied

* Adapted from Rosman, N. P.; Herskowitz, J.; Carter, A. P.; and O'Connor, J. F. Acute head trauma in infancy and childhood: clinical and radiologic aspects. *Pediatr. Clin. North Am.*, **26:** 707–36, 1979.
† For signs of acutely increased intracranial pressure, see Table 11–12.

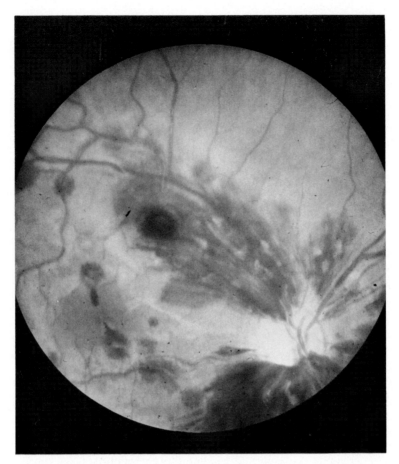

FIGURE 20–5. Fundus photograph showing retinal and preretinal hemorrhages. (From Rosman, N. P.; Herskowitz, J.; Carter, A. P.; and O'Connor, J. F. Acute head trauma in infancy and childhood: clinical and radiologic aspects. *Pediatr. Clin. North Am.*, **26:** 707–36, 1979.)

Subdural hematoma is a most serious consequence of head trauma in the abused child (see Table 20–1) (see CORRELATION: ANATOMIC ASPECTS). The child with acute subdural hemorrhage characteristically presents with signs of acutely raised intracranial pressure (see Chapter 11). Mental status is usually altered and may be manifested by extreme irritability, obtundation, or frank coma. Blood pressure may be elevated, with pulse rate diminished and respirations slowed and/or irregular. Persistent vomiting may occur. A sixth cranial nerve palsy can be seen. Seizures and retinal hemorrhages are found in at least 75 per cent of cases (see Fig. 20–5) (Mushin, 1971; Tomasi and Rosman, 1975; Rosman *et al.*, 1979).

Subdural hemorrhage can occur without direct trauma to the head. For example, the infant who has been forcibly shaken or hit upon the back may sustain a whiplash injury associated with this complication (Ommaya *et al.,* 1968; Guthkelch, 1971; Caffey, 1974). Since the neck muscles of infants are weak, shaking an infant by the trunk causes the head to be thrown violently backward and forward. These whiplike movements can shear bridging cortical veins that connect vessels upon the brain's surface to the superior sagittal sinus. Blood thus accumulates in the subdural space. Such an injury may be inflicted as disciplinary excess, by inappropriate resuscitative efforts (for example, in an effort to aid a choking child), or through overvigorous burping (Caffey, 1972) (see Case 20–2).

Acute epidural hemorrhage is another life-threatening complication of head trauma. It tends to occur in somewhat older children (above 2 years of age) than acute subdural hemorrhage, which usually occurs in young infants. Signs of acutely raised intracranial pressure and, at times, localizing findings such as hemiparesis are characteristic. A rapidly evolving clinical picture typically results from tearing of the middle meningeal artery associated with fracture of the overlying temporal bone. Skull fracture is found in approximately three-quarters of children with epidural hematomas (in contrast with less than one-quarter of those with subdural hematomas).

Subdural hemorrhage that does not cause a fatal outcome or lead to prompt surgical attention undergoes breakdown and resorption over several days to weeks. The result may be a chronic subdural fluid collection. *Chronic subdural hematoma* is characterized by failure to thrive, pallor, irritability, and fever (Rosman *et al.,* 1979). The skull is typically large for age and tends to be box-shaped when viewed from above. The anterior fontanelle is often enlarged and may be full. Funduscopic examination may disclose blurring of optic disk margins (papilledema) associated with elevated intracranial pressure. Pallor of the skin, nail beds, and conjunctivae is due to associated anemia secondary to blood loss and poor nutrition. Fever is often present without identifiable infectious cause.

Characteristic neurologic findings in infants with chronic subdural hemorrhage include irritability, jitteriness, hypertonia, and hyperreflexia. Increased muscle tone may be evident in the infant who comes to a stand rather than to a sit when pulled forward by arms or shoulders. Lateralizing signs such as asymmetric limb movements, muscle tone, or deep tendon reflexes reflect contusion of brain that commonly underlies the subdural fluid collection.

Acute subdural and epidural hematomas are neurologic emergencies. Though generally not an emergency, chronic subdural hematoma merits prompt and definitive treatment (which may include protective custody). Diagnosis and treatment of these conditions are discussed below.

Fractures of the skull in childhood most often occur in the absence of complicating intracranial hemorrhage. They may take several forms: linear, depressed, compound, comminuted, basal, diastatic, and "growing." Linear fractures are commonest, making up about 75 per cent of childhood skull fractures. Such fractures may be suggested by overlying scalp swelling. They can be diagnosed definitively only by radiography (see Fig. 20–6) (see INVESTIGATION below). There are no clinical features typically associated with linear skull fracture unless the fracture has involved the temporal bone, lacerating the middle meningeal artery to produce an acute epidural hema-

CASE 20–2: ACUTE SUBDURAL HEMATOMA IN A
4-MONTH-OLD BOY

D.L. was the full-term product of a pregnancy complicated by gestational diabetes mellitus in a 19-year-old married woman. Delivery was by cesarean section because of cephalopelvic disproportion. The child was noted in the nursery to have congenitally dislocated hips. He was treated at first with triple diapers, then with a lower limb brace. At 4 months of age, the child's parents brought him to the hospital because of focal and generalized seizures. His anterior fontanelle bulged, and bilateral subdural taps yielded fresh blood. Skull x-rays were negative, but radiographs of the wrists and clavicles disclosed fractures. Upon discharge from the hospital several weeks later, he was placed with a foster family. He did well for 3 months, when he was hospitalized for fever and irritability found to be due to pneumococcal meningitis with subdural empyema. He responded well to parenteral antibiotic treatment in high dosage and was again discharged to foster care. At 2 years, he was returned to his parents' home while maintained in the legal custody of the state. Social service involvement continued. Several months later, when a chest x-ray was obtained to evaluate a respiratory infection, a new rib fracture was detected incidentally. At 26 months, development was delayed to a 15-month level. The child was again placed in foster care, and an adoptive home was sought.

Comment. This unfortunate child illustrates complications of acute subdural hemorrhage that can make it a severe form of head injury. Subdural hemorrhage, commonly seen among battered infants, is estimated to account for several hundred deaths annually in the United States.

Seizures—focal and generalized, acute and recurrent—result from cerebral contusion underlying the acute subdural hemorrhage. Indeed, acute subdural hemorrhage should be suspected in any infant with seizures, especially if accompanied by signs of raised intracranial pressure (bulging fontanelle, retinal hemorrhages, papilledema). Developmental retardation and/or spasticity may result from damage to one or both cerebral hemispheres. Infection of the subdural space is rare in childhood. In this case it appeared to result from a respiratory pathogen that had spread by the bloodstream to infect the subdural and subarachnoid spaces.

The cause for the initial injury in this child was not established with certainty. As noted above, the infant was being treated with a brace for congenital hip dislocations. Perhaps one or both parents, attempting to comply with the orthopedic management, had lost control while trying to put the fussing child into this device. Though careful medical and social service monitoring of the family was not fully successful, it did limit further injury, for the child received prompt treatment for a medical illness at which time an additional unsuspected fracture was detected. At times it may be possible to return the child to his or her natural parents despite a well-defined inflicted injury. In this case, despite intensive social service input, it became necessary to remove the child permanently from his home.

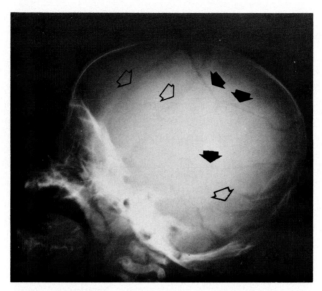

FIGURE 20–6. Plain skull x-ray showing multiple linear fractures (closed arrows). Open arrows indicate cranial sutures. (From Rosman, N. P.; Herskowitz, J.; Carter, A. P.; and O'Connor, J. F. Acute head trauma in infancy and childhood: clinical and radiologic aspects. *Pediatr. Clin. North Am.*, **26:** 707–36, 1979.)

toma (described above), or starts to "grow" because of a protruding cyst (described below).

Because of the extreme vulnerability of infants, a linear (or other) skull fracture in a child below 1 year of age should be considered evidence of abuse or neglect until proved otherwise. Radiologic examination of the skull should be supplemented in such cases by a skeletal survey.

Depressed skull fracture involves disruption and displacement of a portion of the cranium. It is of particular concern because underlying brain may have been bruised or lacerated. Such focal brain injury may be manifested clinically by lateralizing neurologic signs, including focal seizures.

Compound fracture involves laceration of scalp down to bony fracture. It is a medical and surgical emergency because of the danger of complicating infection to the central nervous system. When there has been delay in the child's being brought to medical attention, meningitis may already be in progress; hence, the clinician may need to "work backward" to identify unsuspected or unreported head trauma. Comminuted fracture is defined by the presence of multiple bony fragments.

Basal skull fracture refers to a fracture involving one or more bones making up the base of the skull: frontal, ethmoid, sphenoid, temporal, and occipital. Although other kinds of fractures are diagnosed most readily and definitively by radiography, basal skull fractures are usually not seen on skull x-ray because of the complicated normal radiologic features of the base of the skull. The diagnosis is therefore usually established through characteristic clinical features. These include hemorrhage into the nose, nasopharynx, or middle ear (the last producing a hemotympanum when bleeding occurs behind an intact tympanic membrane) and hemorrhage overlying the mastoid bone (Battle sign) or about the eyes ("raccoon eyes" sign). Cranial nerves, particularly the first (olfactory), eighth (vestibuloauditory), and seventh (facial), may be injured in basal skull fractures. They may be complicated further by a cerebrospinal fluid (CSF) leak through the nose (CSF rhinorrhea) or ear (CSF otorrhea). CSF rhinorrhea occurs secondary to fracture of the cribriform plate of the ethmoid bone, CSF otorrhea from fracture of the petrous portion of the temporal bone. The former is more common than the latter and is likelier to persist. Basal skull fracture may also be complicated by meningitis (most often due to *S. pneumoniae* or *H. influenzae*) because of ready access of bacterial pathogens to the subarachnoid space.

Diastatic fractures are traumatic separations of cranial bones at one or more suture sites. They most commonly affect the lambdoid suture and usually occur within the first 4 years of life.

"Growing fractures" result from development of CSF-containing cysts at the site of linear or diastatic skull fracture, which prevent fusion of fracture margins. These cysts are usually porencephalic in type, communicating with the lateral ventricles. Less often they are leptomeningeal (Kingsley *et al.*, 1978). Growing fractures usually occur in children under 3 years of age, most often affect the parietal bone, and typically develop within 2 to 6 months of head injury. Diagnosis is suggested by palpable skull defect and cyst formation (with focally increased transillumination) in a child with a previous linear or diastatic skull fracture. The head may have grown excessively large. In circumstances of abuse or neglect, the child may not have been brought for medical attention at the time of initial trauma. Hence, the diagnosis of linear or diastatic skull fracture must be made retrospectively.

Other forms of injury associated with abuse or neglect do not involve head injury directly but result in damage to the central nervous system nonetheless. Such injury may be associated with strangulation, burns, and trauma to the spine. Subdural hemorrhage and cervical spine injury can occur secondary to shaking.

Strangulation can be manifested by acute as well as by later neurologic symptoms and signs. Acutely, the child may be agitated, drowsy, or comatose. These effects are primarily due to blockage of blood supply to the brain. Spinal cord injury (associated with fracture or dislocation of the cervical spine) can further complicate the child's physical state (Herskowitz and Rosman, 1982).

Late deterioration may follow apparent recovery from strangulation and fit the picture of behavioral regression (see Chapter 8). Dooling and Richardson (1976) described an 11-year-old boy who was "blue, shivering, and delirious" on the day of strangulation but was considered to behave normally the next day. Within 1 week, his behavior changed markedly, as mutism, emotional lability, and flailing of the arms were seen. These symptoms were felt at first to be an emotional reaction to his assault. Within several days, however, drooling, somnolence, and involuntary jerking movements of the body began. Over the next several weeks, extrapyramidal motor signs

CASE 20–3: STRANGULATION IN A 7-YEAR-OLD BOY

C.B. was brought to the hospital emergency room comatose, having been found hanging by a sheet around his neck from a curtain rod for an undetermined period of time. As the story was reconstructed, the child had been playing "Spider Man" wearing a self-made cape, attempted to jump from a dresser onto a bed, and inadvertently became caught by the cape. His younger brother found him and called for help. Police found the child obtunded and limp, but breathing spontaneously. Previous history was negative for depression or suicide attempt.

On examination in the emergency room, the child was stuporous. He responded to painful stimulation upon the sternum by flexing his arms across the chest, but did not respond to voice. Pulse rate, blood pressure, and respirations were normal. No sign of head trauma was seen. The skin of the neck was reddened. Dislocation of the cervical spine was not evident by inspection or gentle palpation. On neurologic examination, pupils measured 5 mm and reacted briskly to light. Optic disks were normal and the retinal background showed no hemorrhages. Eye movements were disconjugate and roving, although excursions were full. Flexor tone of the arms was increased. Deep tendon reflexes were 2+ at the biceps, 3+ at the knees, and 4+ (clonic) at the ankles. Plantar responses were bilaterally extensor. Cervical spine x-rays showed no fracture or dislocation. Arterial blood gas determinations showed normal pH and bicarbonate. Blood glucose was normal.

The child was managed supportively. Treatment included fluid restriction and intravenous steroids because of asphyxic insult to brain and anticipated cerebral edema. The day after injury the child recognized his mother. Such lucidity alternated with periods of somnolence. Tone and deep tendon reflexes continued to be increased in all extremities. Plantar responses remained abnormal. By the third hospital day, the child was continuously alert and complained of being hungry and thirsty. Deep tendon relfexes in the

progressed. Swallowing difficulties, fever, and bronchopneumonia ensued, leading to death 14 weeks after strangulation (see Case 20–3).

Burn injury is one of the commonest forms of child abuse, and neurologic problems are recognized in 10 to 20 per cent of affected children (Antoon *et al.,* 1972). Seizures (generalized or focal), obtundation, or hallucinosis are typical presenting manifestations of burn encephalopathy. Electrolyte abnormalities (especially hyponatremia) caused or accentuated by treatment with topical silver nitrate, hypoxia associated with smoke inhalation, shock, and central nervous system infection such as meningitis or encephalitis are the major causes of such encephalopathy.

Treatment with a hexachlorophene-containing solution such as "pHiso-Hex" may also produce an encephalopathy that complicates management of the burn patient. It can be manifested by irritability, seizures, and other focal neurologic findings caused by absorption through injured skin of toxic amounts of hexachlorophene (Larson, 1968; Herskowitz and Rosman,

lower extremities were exaggerated as before. Only the left plantar response remained extensor.

A week after the injury, CT scan was normal. Electroencephalogram showed slowing of background activity. By a week later, mental status had returned to normal. The only neurologic abnormalities were hyperreflexia of the left ankle and a left Babinski sign. Psychiatric evaluation failed to disclose evidence of serious psychologic problems, including depression. Social service assessment revealed generally satisfactory caretaking arrangements.

One month later, neurologic status was unchanged.

Comment. The major concerns here were twofold: acute and delayed effects. Acute effects of strangulation in this case as in others appeared to result not from injury to the cervical spinal cord but from impediment to blood flow to brain caused by vascular compression. Compromise of this child's cerebral blood flow was evidenced acutely by his state of obtundation, hyperreflexia, and abnormal plantar responses.

Once he recovered from the acute insult, attention was directed toward possible development of a delayed syndrome of cognitive, motor, and behavioral deterioration that can follow asphyxic injury of various kinds. Such late neurologic deterioration typically has its onset within several weeks of an acute asphyxic insult. Fortunately, this child appeared to have been spared this complication.

Strangulation is included in this chapter on child abuse and neglect because such an injury (as a homicidal or suicidal action) may be inflicted or may result from inadequate supervision. It is conceivable that the initial insult would not be reported by the child and might be suspected only by later neurologic deterioration (see Chapter 8). The CT scan may be of diagnostic help in such cases by showing characteristic lucent areas within the globus pallidus bilaterally that reflect asphyxic injury to brain.

1979). Encephalopathic symptoms of irritability, excitement, and delirium may, of course, also be caused by burn-related pain, separation from family members, and fear of injury to relatives involved in the fire.

The spine, like other portions of the skeletal system, may show injury as part of a child abuse syndrome (Swischuk, 1969; McGrory and Fenichel, 1977; Dickson and Leatherman, 1978). Unsuspected fracture or dislocation may be detected upon radiologic survey of the skeleton. Spine injury may otherwise have been suggested by signs of overlying skin damage (ecchymosis, swelling, tenderness) or by neurologic abnormality (gait disturbance, reflex asymmetry).

The *mental status examination* of the abused or neglected child may show several abnormalities. Abused children tend to interact too readily with strangers (Wolkind, 1974). Further, such children appear to have an impaired ability to enjoy play, manifesting little pleasure or exuberance (Martin and Beezley, 1977). An abused child may be excessively fearful. Hyperki-

TABLE 20–2. **Investigations to Be Considered in Abused or Neglected Children**

CBC
Skeletal survey (skull, long bones, chest, spine)
Cranial CT scan
Bleeding/clotting studies
Blood lead, free erythrocyte protoporphyrin (FEP)
  levels
Serum for total protein, albumin, globulin, calcium,
  phosphorus, vitamins A and D, electrolytes
Urinalysis
Urine, blood for toxic screen
Tuberculin skin test
Stool for ova and parasites
EEG (in awake and sleep states)
Lumbar puncture

netic behavior or other features of attention deficit disorder should be noted since they may have contributed to the circumstances of inflicted injury.

Chronically neglected children tend to be overly compliant. For example, a 2-year-old child may tolerate passively an ear examination that, under normal circumstances, would provoke active resistance. In addition, the chronically neglected child who is hospitalized usually will not manifest the typical behavioral changes of protest, despair, and detachment characteristic of most children when separated from parents.

Developmental delay may be caused by understimulation, depression, or interference with brain growth due to nutritional inadequacy. With severe protein-calorie malnutrition, characteristic changes in mental state are irritability, apathy, lack of interest in the environment, and lack of exploratory behavior.

Investigation.   Investigation of the child with suspected abuse or neglect will depend upon the age of the child and the nature of the apparent or suspected injury (see Table 20–2).

The infant should have a complete skeletal survey: skull, long bones, chest, and spine. Multiple fractures, particularly those found in different stages of healing, are characteristic of child abuse (see Fig. 20–7) (Kempe *et al.*, 1962). Metaphyseal angle fragments are characteristically seen in abused children. They appear to result from torsional and accelerative influences upon long bones rather than direct trauma (Caffey, 1972).

If bruises are prominent (especially when they affect the upper as well as the lower body), bleeding and clotting studies should be carried out. These would include platelet count, bleeding time, prothrombin time, and partial thromboplastin time. A complete blood count, blood lead level (for the child 1 through 6 years of age), and urinalysis are indicated routinely.

When subdural or epidural hematoma is being considered, computerized tomography (CT scan) of the head will usually be diagnostic (see Figs. 20–8 and 20–9). With acutely raised intracranial pressure, however, the

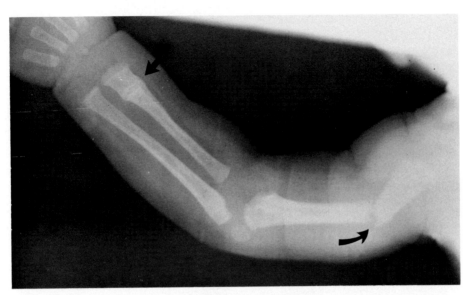

FIGURE 20–7. X-ray of arm in a battered child showing recent (curved arrow) and old (straight arrow) fractures. (Courtesy of W. Cranley, Wakefield, Mass.)

clinical situation may be so precarious that immediate treatment must be undertaken if death is to be averted.

In the older child a full skeletal survey is not always indicated. It may, however, be valuable in detecting healing fractures that are not suggested by history or examination. When administration of drugs to the child is suspected, blood and urine should be analyzed for toxic substances (Dine, 1965).

Lumbar puncture should be performed in the child with basal skull fracture or burn when complicating meningitis is suspected. Serum electrolytes should be measured early in the treatment of children who have suffered burns and periodically thereafter. Electroencephalography (EEG) in awake and sleep states should be carried out in evaluating the child with post-traumatic seizures.

In cases of malnutrition a complete blood count should be obtained and serum levels of total protein, albumin, globulin, calcium, phosphorus, vitamin A, and vitamin D measured (Chase *et al.*, 1980). Blood lead and free erythrocyte protoporphyrin (FEP) levels should be obtained. Tuberculin skin testing should be carried out and stool examined for ova and parasites. Evaluation of developmental delay and mental retardation is discussed in Chapter 18.

Differential Diagnosis. Several conditions must be differentiated from syndromes of abuse and neglect (see Table 20–3). *Hematologic disorders* such as idiopathic thrombocytopenic purpura can easily be mistaken for inflicted injury, since the child may be covered with ecchymoses, and parents may be unaware of how these marks were acquired. Petechiae or anemia may suggest the hematologic nature of the problem (see Case 20–1).

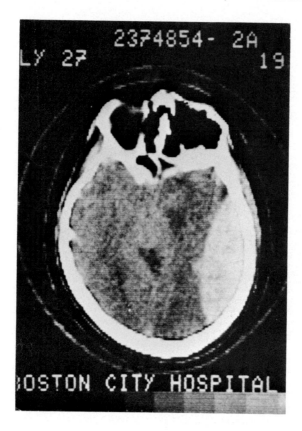

Figure 20–8. Plain computerized tomographic (CT) scan showing lens-shaped epidural hematoma. (From Rosman, N. P.; Herskowitz, J.; Carter, A. P.; and O'Connor, J. F. Acute head trauma in infancy and childhood: clinical and radiologic aspects. *Pediatr. Clin. North Am.,* **26**: 707–36, 1979.)

Hypersensitivity vasculitis is another medical cause for purpuric lesions, which characteristically are palpable (Waskerwitz *et al.,* 1981).

Clumsy children may also have multiple bruises. Their skin lesions typically affect the extremities, legs more than arms. Significant head trauma is uncommon. Developmental clumsiness, of course, occurs in children learning to walk—their "black and blue marks" providing medallions for their efforts.

Bone diseases such as osteogenesis imperfecta or osteopetrosis are associated with brittle bones. Affected children readily may sustain multiple fractures.

Failure to thrive has many medical causes other than chronic neglect. These include such relatively insidious diseases as chronic urinary tract infection, cardiac disease, and cystic fibrosis as well as more obvious causes such as ulcerative colitis, chronic asthma, and neoplastic disease. Idiopathic hypopituitarism with short stature may closely mimic a syndrome of emotional deprivation (Patton and Gardner, 1962; Powell *et al.,* 1967).

Scurvy may also be mistaken for child abuse or neglect because of associated malnutrition, bruising, and bones that are abnormal by x-ray (Berant and Jacobs, 1966).

Etiology. Schmitt and Kempe (1975) have emphasized the multiplicity of factors that come together to cause child abuse (see Table 20–4). It requires

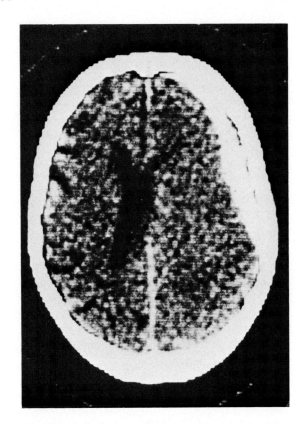

FIGURE 20–9. Plain computerized tomographic (CT) scan demonstrating curvilinear subdural hematoma and shift of midline structures to opposite side. (From Rosman, N. P.; Herskowitz, J.; Carter, A. P.; and O'Connor, J. F. Acute head trauma in infancy and childhood: clinical and radiologic aspects. *Pediatr. Clin. North Am.*, **26:** 707–36, 1979.)

the "right" child at the "right" place at the "right" time with the "right" parents (or other caretakers). The child may be unusually irritable due to illness. The father may have just been laid off from work, is feeling angry and depressed about that, and finds himself exposed to the child much more than usual. The parents themselves may have been abused as children.

Medical Causes. An ill child's behavior frequently is altered for the worse during an illness and often for a while afterward, particularly when returning home after hospitalization. The child may be irritable despite efforts to console or distract him. He may cling more than usual. Previously

TABLE 20–3. **Differential Diagnosis of Abuse and Neglect**

Hematologic disorder associated with multiple ecchymoses (idiopathic thrombocytopenic purpura)
Vasculitis (causing purpura)
Bone disease associated with brittle bones and multiple fractures (osteogenesis imperfecta, osteopetrosis)
"Organic" failure to thrive (chronic urinary tract infection, heart disease, cystic fibrosis, ulcerative colitis, asthma, neoplastic disease, hypopituitarism)
Scurvy
Clumsiness (developmental or constitutional)

TABLE 20–4. **Causes of Child Abuse and Neglect**

Medical	Medical illness rendering child irritable
Neurologic	Impaired child, unable to "give" to parent(s)
Toxic	Drug abuse rendering parent abusive or unavailable Prenatal influences of alcohol and other drugs
Psychologic	Role reversal
Social-Environmental	Unemployment, drug abuse Parent abused or neglected as child Prolonged separation from mother at birth, causing impaired parent-child bonding
Developmental	Parent unable to adjust to new developmental stage as child grows up

gained skills such as toilet-training may be lost. When medicine (e.g., for an ear infection) needs to be given several times daily and a battle is involved with each dose, parents may feel guilty or angry if the child refuses to take the medicine or spits it out.

Even as "simple" a task as fever control may generate anxiety. A parent may find it extremely difficult and frustrating to take the temperature rectally of a howling, squirming infant at 3:00 A.M. If tepid bathing is required because of a very high temperature, frustration may become intensified further.

Neurologic Causes. The neurologically impaired child is often less able than the normal child to "give" to the mother who may then feel unrewarded. As a result, bonding may suffer. Social smiling, which usually begins at 2 to 4 weeks of age, and cooing, which begins slightly later, are among the first reinforcers of maternal behavior. They are characteristically delayed in retarded children. Poor feeding, jitteriness, and increased muscle tone, which may be other signs of neurologic disorder, may also impair bonding. Specific neurologic defects such as blindness or deafness may be mistaken for global cognitive dysfunction. Hence they must be identified as early as possible so the infant's development can be fostered and appropriate adjustments in the attachment process made.

Toxic Causes. The abuse of alcohol or other drugs often plays a role in child abuse and neglect. For example, alcohol intoxication can lessen impulse control and increase the likelihood of inflicted injury. Chronic drug abuse may also render a parent unavailable to nurture or supervise the child, either because of direct drug effects or because of time consumed in maintaining a supply of the drug. Alcohol and other drugs may also exert adverse prenatal influences (see Chapter 18) (see Case 20–4).

Psychologic Causes. Role reversal between parent and child is often seen in families with an abused child (Steele, 1975; Green, 1978). A child, however, is poorly equipped to meet all the emotional needs of a deprived

CASE 20–4: MARASMUS AND MENTAL RETARDATION DUE TO CHRONIC NEGLECT IN A 6-YEAR-OLD BOY

C.V. was brought to the hospital because of extreme malnutrition and developmental retardation. It was learned that he had been placed in a dimly lighted room for several years prior to hospitalization. The child had been discovered upon a home visit by school authorities because he had not been registered for school. History was limited and of doubtful reliability. At the time of the child's hospitalization his mother also was hospitalized, with severe alcoholic cirrhosis. Father alleged that the child "ate a normal diet." He had received no immunizations.

On examination the boy was dirty, cachectic, and apathetic. He smelled of urine and feces. His abdomen was protuberant. Subcutaneous tissues and muscles were profoundly wasted. All growth parameters were far below the second percentile for age. Weight was 22 pounds, 12 ounces (fiftieth percentile for a 1-year-old male), height 34⅔ inches (fiftieth percentile for 2 years, 3 months), and head circumference 40 cm (fiftieth percentile for a 3-month-old). Neurologic examination showed marked psychomotor retardation without focal findings or evidence for increased intracranial pressure. The child did not walk. Spontaneous speech was minimal.

Investigation included a normal serum total protein of 6.8 gm/dl, hematocrit of 29 per cent, generalized osteoporosis on skull x-ray, and bone age of 3 years. During his 6-week hospitalization, he gained 6 pounds. Apathy diminished dramatically. He learned to walk and was able to speak in sentences by the time of discharge to a foster family.

At 9 years, weight was 48 pounds, 12 ounces (fiftieth percentile for 7 years), height 45¾ inches (fiftieth percentile for 6 years), and head circumference 49.5 cm (fiftieth percentile for 2½ years). Overall function was between the 4- and 6-year levels, poorest in language skills and best in fine motor abilities. Tested 2 years later, he showed further improvement with a full-scale intelligence quotient of 66.

Comment. This child, who suffered greatly from prolonged nutritional and emotional deprivation, benefited greatly from medical, social, and educational intervention. One wonders why this child was "selected" for such extreme neglect. His head circumference at 6 years and the mother's medical illness may provide clues. Although all growth parameters were depressed, the head was disproportionately small, suggesting early—probably prenatal—insult to the central nervous system. Maternal malnutrition combined with potentially teratogenic effects of alcohol may have played important prenatal roles here, accentuated by postnatal effects of physical and emotional unavailability due to continuing maternal alcoholism.

The apathy that was so marked early in this child's hospital course demonstrated how malnutrition can foster psychosocial deprivation. Such children lack interest in their environment. They are further limited in seeking out stimulation by weakness and fatigue. Hence they provide little attraction to the attention of a mother who may be struggling to meet the needs of other children who are more obviously viable, more truly "alive" than the malnourished one.

parent. Hence an isolated, needy mother is particularly vulnerable to being frustrated when her child provides insufficiently for her.

Social-Environmental Causes. As has repeatedly been demonstrated, child abuse and neglect cut across socioeconomic and educational boundaries to affect all groups (Kempe *et al.*, 1962). Unemployment, drug abuse, and a parental history of abuse in childhood all predispose to child abuse and neglect (Chase and Martin, 1970; Clancy and McBride, 1975; Schmitt and Kempe, 1975; Chase *et al.*, 1980) (see Case 20–5).

Illegitimacy, low birth weight (2,000 grams or less), and immediate separation from mother at birth for at least 14 days are among other factors contributing to disturbed mother-child interaction and impaired bonding.

The profound effect of (unintentional) institutional neglect was documented by Spitz (1945) in his studies of "hospitalism." The outcome was especially poor among infants raised in the "foundling home," a meticulously clean setting where the children received essentially all their care from a limited number of women. Though these caretakers were described as "unusually motherly, baby-loving women," the infants nevertheless lacked human contact for most of the day. Development of infants in the foundling home group lagged behind that of children in all the other groups by 1 year, and the rate of illness and mortality among the foundling home children during the first 2 to 3 years of life was markedly increased.

CASE 20–5: DRUG INTOXICATION AND HEAD TRAUMA IN A 2-YEAR-OLD BOY

I.S., the 2-year-old son of an unemployed 25-year-old man, a chronic alcoholic, so distressed his father by crying that his father fed him several diazepam (Valium) tablets. The boy became drowsy, stumbled, and fell, striking his head and lacerating his scalp. He was brought to an emergency room where he was examined and his wound sutured. His father acknowledged giving the boy diazepam to quiet him. The child was hospitalized for observation, protection, and psychosocial assessment. Recovery was uneventful, with the parents actively involved during the child's hospital stay. He was discharged home, but only after visiting nurse arrangements were made, referral of the father to an alcoholic rehabilitation center carried out, a clinical nursery program arranged for the child, and state protective services notified.

Comment. This case illustrates the importance of asking, "Why did it occur?" in evaluating a child who has sustained head trauma. This child was well beyond the toddler stage, so that competency in walking had long been established. In another case (13–4), a fall from a porch apparently was associated with incoordination due to a cerebellar tumor. Papilledema and ataxia of gait provided the major clues to diagnosis in that instance. In this case ataxia and drowsiness suggested drug ingestion, acknowledged by the father and confirmed by analysis of the urine.

In chronically malnourished children, fatigue, apathy, and immobility lead to restricted and monotonous behaviors. As a result a parent receives little stimulation in, and reward for, interacting with such a child. Hence understimulation of the child is accentuated and social deprivation worsened (Latham, 1974; Pollitt and Thomson, 1977).

Developmental Causes. As children develop, their behavior changes. A parent who was able to deal with the challenges of one developmental stage may be overwhelmed, temporarily or for a longer period, when the child enters a new phase of development.

For the first year of life, for example, a parent may have been quite successful in meeting the needs of an essentially helpless, totally dependent infant. By 1 or 2 years of age, however, the child has become much more independent. He is able to crawl or to walk away from a parent, demands to feed himself, and is starting to develop an unerring eye for the dangerous or provocative. A parent may respond to these changes in behavior by "child-proofing" the home and setting firm, consistent limits. Alternatively—in order to control the child—a parent may resort to physical punishment, particularly if that was the manner in which the parent was raised. In other circumstances, the child with newly acquired motor skills may be allowed to roam relatively unsupervised: exploring open windows, chewing on moldings that contain lead paint, walking downstairs, or wandering into busy streets.

Misunderstandings of normal child development may also contribute to abuse and neglect (Steele, 1975; Taylor and Newberger, 1979). A parent may feel that the crying child is angry at him or her or that a child can and should be toilet-trained by 6 months of age. The result can be frustration, coercive measures, and frank abuse.

TREATMENT AND OUTCOME

Ultimately, the goal of the professional who works with abused or neglected children is that they be provided the opportunity for an optimal quality of life. Treatment must necessarily begin by ensuring the child's survival. Then a comprehensive approach to assessment and treatment can be pursued, respecting the rights of the family while intervening on behalf of the relatively defenseless child (Markham, 1980; Solnit, 1980).

Emergency medical, neurologic, or surgical care may be required for life-threatening head injuries or abdominal trauma. Even without such obviously grave injuries, child abuse or severe neglect should be considered a social emergency and hospitalization or other form of protective custody effected.

The long-term consequences of malnutrition upon the human brain are not clear, although it generally appears to have a deleterious effect (Latham, 1974). The work of Stoch and Smythe (1963, 1967) showed that severe malnutrition in infancy was associated with diminished physical growth and intellectual development over an 11-year period of follow-up. Hertzig and colleagues (1972) also found that boys who had been severely malnourished during the first 2 years of life showed diminished intelligence when compared with siblings or peers.

Studies of the Dutch famine of 1944–45 investigated the effects of nutritional deprivation during pregnancy upon intelligence at age 19 years (Stein *et al.*, 1972). No significant differences in mental performance were found between offspring in the famine and nonfamine groups, although the mean birth weight was significantly lower in the former.

Lloyd-Still and colleagues (1974) studied the effects of severe malnutrition in infancy upon later development and intelligence. Their study involved 41 persons with cystic fibrosis whose weight was below the third percentile during at least 4 of the first 6 months of life. When evaluated before 5 years of age, affected children performed significantly less well than sibling controls. Tested after 5 years, however, no differences in intelligence were found.

Although the precise effects of undernutrition on the brain are unclear, an approach emphasizing prevention or early intervention appears to minimize behavioral consequences, including intellectual subnormalcy (Chase and Martin, 1970; Winick *et al.*, 1975; Evans *et al.*, 1980).

Winick and colleages (1975) studied the relationship of nutritional status in Korean adoptees less than 3 years of age upon intelligence during later childhood. The malnourished group (below the third percentile for height and weight according to Korean norms) had a mean intelligence quotient of 102. Though normal, this figure was significantly lower than the mean intelligence quotient (112) of adoptees who were well nourished at the time of admission to the adoption service.

Evans and colleagues (1980) demonstrated a beneficial effect upon intelligence of early nutritional intervention in children at risk for malnutrition. Their study involved children from families in which one child had suffered from kwashiorkor. These children were given supplementary feedings for the first 2 years of life. They scored significantly higher 6 to 7 years later in tests of intelligence than did control groups of siblings (with or without a history of kwashiorkor) within their own family.

Medical Management (see Table 20–5). Undernutrition, incomplete or absent routine health care, and inadequate medical treatment are medical problems commonly seen in neglected and abused children (see Case 20–6).

Undernutrition usually involves both protein and caloric deprivation. In their severest forms such deficiency states take the form of kwashiorkor and marasmus, respectively. The latter only rarely occurs in pure form; hence marasmus is often used synonymously with protein-calorie malnutrition. Vitamin deficiencies may also occur. Rickets can result from vitamin D deficiency, night blindness and corneal damage from vitamin A deficiency, changes in skin and other epithelia from lack of riboflavin and thiamine. Scurvy results from vitamin C deficiency.

The malnourished child should be fed three balanced meals daily. Small, nutritious snacks can be given between meals and before bedtime. Care must be taken that signs and symptoms of overly rapid nutritional rehabilitation such as diarrhea do not develop. Standard multivitamin preparations should be given routinely and specific vitamin deficiencies treated in pharmacologic doses. Rickets, for example, is treated with vitamin D. Care must be taken to avoid vitamin D excess. Overdosage is manifested by symptoms

TABLE 20–5. **Selected Aspects of Treatment of Abuse and Neglect**

Nutrition	Calories
	Protein
	Vitamins
Routine health care	Immunizations
	TB skin testing
	Lead, FEP levels
	Dental care
	Vision and hearing screening
Acute problems	Infection
	Head trauma
	Seizures
	Burns
Protection	Acute hospitalization
	Placement in foster family
	Return to natural home with supervision
	Mandatory reporting to governmental agency
Education	Remedial, as necessary
Social-environmental	Homemaking services
	Babysitting
	Visiting nurse arrangements
	Respite care

of hypercalcemia (weakness, fatigue, and diarrhea). Measurement of serum calcium and phosphorus levels should be carried out periodically when vitamin D is used in high dosage. Overdosage of vitamin A is associated with signs and symptoms of increased intracranial pressure (see Chapter 11).

High-protein feeding of previously starved children may be associated with splitting of cranial sutures that may be unaccompanied by other manifestations of intracranial hypertension (Capitanio and Kirkpatrick, 1969; De Levie and Nogrady, 1970). The increased protein intake apparently leads to excessively rapid brain growth, with which enlargement of the skull does not keep pace.

Immunization against diphtheria, pertussis, tetanus, polio, and measles is of high priority in the abused or neglected child. He or she is likely to be unimmunized or behind schedule and, if malnourished, at increased risk of contracting a severe case of any of these preventable illnesses. Interruption of immunizations does not require that the full series be restarted. They can be continued where left off, regardless of the time elapsed. Schedules for primary immunization of children not immunized in early infancy are summarized in Table 20–6.

The fully immunized child who has had a clean wound cared for promptly need not have a tetanus booster if one has been received within 10 years of the injury. On the other hand, a "dirty" penetrating wound that has been

CASE 20–6: ABUSE AND NEGLECT IN A 9-MONTH-OLD BOY

I.V. was brought to the emergency room because of leg burns allegedly sustained accidentally while he was being bathed. He was the 5 pound, 8 ounce product of a gestation of unknown duration born to a woman without prenatal care. Head circumference at birth was 31.75 cm (below the third percentile). In recent months, he was said to have lost weight despite being offered wholesome food in adequate amounts. Immunizations were incomplete.

On examination, the infant appeared marasmic, frightened, and irritable. Lack of subcutaneous fat made him look like a "wizened old man." Weight was 9 pounds. Temperature was 102 degrees. Second degree burns were present over both legs. There were flexion contractures at the hips and knees. Investigations included a serum total protein of 5.7 gm/dl with albumin of 2.6 gm/dl. Blood culture grew beta hemolytic streptococcus. Stool culture grew Shigella. X-ray revealed a healing femoral fracture.

Therapy was necessarily multifaceted. Septicemia was treated with parenteral penicillin, burns with topical mafenide acetate (Sulfamylon), and contractures with daily physical therapy. After a slow start the child gained 3 pounds during a 5-week hospital stay. Development advanced to a 6- to 8-month level. The child was placed in the custody of the state but allowed to return home after biweekly visits by a visiting nurse, regular social service appointments, and ongoing pediatric care had been arranged.

Comment. This case illustrates the multiplicity of problems with which an abused or neglected child may present, even as an infant. In this case problems included burns, septicemia (probably secondary to superinfection of the burns), healing fracture, malnutrition, and incomplete immunizations. With this child one sensed that as new problems emerged the parents became increasingly reluctant to bring the child for medical attention, perhaps because of fear that they would be prosecuted.

neglected for longer than 24 hours should be treated by passive immunization with human tetanus immune globulin in addition to active immunization with tetanus toxoid (Committee on Infectious Diseases, 1977).

Other aspects of routine preventive health care in the medical management of abused or neglected children should include regular dental care, tuberculin skin testing, measurement of blood lead and FEP levels, and testing of vision and hearing.

Specific medical problems that have received inconsistent medical attention (or none at all) should be pursued. These might include chronic middle ear disease, asthma, impetigo, urinary tract infection, or venereal disease such as syphilis or gonorrhea.

Neurologic Management. The treatment of head injury will be directed toward affected portions of the scalp, skull, brain, or its coverings. Localized swelling of the scalp is usually due to bruising (contusion). Specific therapy is generally not required unless laceration has occurred. In these cir-

TABLE 20–6. **Recommended Schedule for Active Immunization of Normal Infants and Children**[*]

2 mo	DTP[1]	TOPV[2]
4 mo	DTP	TOPV
6 mo	DTP	[3]
1 yr		Tuberculin Test[4]
15 mo	Measles,[5] Rubella[5]	Mumps[5]
1½ yr	DTP	TOPV
4–6 yr	DTP	TOPV
14–16 yr	Td[6]—repeat every 10 years	

[*] Committee on Infectious Diseases, from *Report of the Committee on Infectious Diseases,* 18th ed. Copyright American Academy of Pediatrics, Evanston, Ill., 1977.
[1] DTP = diphtheria and tetanus toxoids combined with pertussis vaccine.
[2] TOPV = trivalent oral poliovirus vaccine.
[3] A third dose of TOPV is optional but may be given in areas of high endemicity of poliomyelitis.
[4] Frequency of repeated tuberculin tests depends on risk of exposure of the child and on the prevalence of tuberculosis in the population group. The initial test should be done at the time of, or preceding, the measles immunization.
[5] May be given at 15 months as measles-rubella or measles-mumps-rubella combined vaccines.
[6] Td: combined tetanus and diphtheria toxoids (adult type) for those more than 6 years of age, in contrast to diphtheria and tetanus (DT) toxoids, which contain a larger amount of diphtheria antigen.

cumstances thorough cleansing is necessary, suturing may be required, and tetanus prophylaxis must be assured. Subgaleal hematoma or cephalohematoma does not require specific therapy other than measures to achieve hemostasis (such as localized pressure). Aspiration of either kind of hematoma is contraindicated because of the risk of introducing infection. When blood loss to the subgaleal space causes anemia or shock, specific treatment, such as iron or blood transfusion, should be pursued.

In general, any child who has suffered significant head trauma (associated, for example, with loss of consciousness, skull fracture, posttraumatic seizure, or focal neurologic findings) should be admitted to hospital and observed for 24 to 48 hours for recurrent seizures, signs of increased intracranial pressure, and other complications of head injury (Rosman *et al.,* 1979). When circumstances of the head trauma are unclear, hospitalization should be prolonged pending further evaluation.

Uncomplicated linear skull fracture does not require specific treatment. Surgical elevation of a depressed skull fracture will depend upon particulars of the individual case. Treatment of compound skull fracture involves meticulous debridement of the wound and administration of parenteral antibiotics. Basal skull fracture with complicating bacterial meningitis is treated with large doses of intravenous antibiotics, usually ampicillin. The use of prophylactic antibiotics in children with basal skull fracture has been recommended, although its efficacy has not been clearly established (Einhorn and Mizrahi, 1978). A persistent CSF leak with basal skull fracture will require neurosurgical repair. "Growing" fracture is treated by removal of the porencephalic or leptomeningeal cyst, dural closure, and cranioplasty.

Focal or generalized seizures resulting from direct injury to brain itself (contusion or laceration) should be treated with anticonvulsant medication (see Chapter 12).

Treatment of acute subdural or epidural hemorrhage is an emergency. Acutely raised intracranial pressure poses an immediate threat to life due to progressive or impending herniation of brain through the tentorial notch or foramen magnum. Treatment of acute intracranial hypertension is based upon those factors which normally determine intracranial pressure: the intracranial vascular system, cerebrospinal fluid system, skull, and brain tissue itself. Hyperventilation acts promptly to cause vasoconstriction that limits intracranial blood supply. Osmotically active agents such as mannitol shrink the brain to lower intracranial pressure. Ventricular drainage of cerebrospinal fluid can be lifesaving in treating acute hydrocephalus. Occasionally decompressive surgery is performed to provide extra space for an increase in intracranial mass (inaccessible hematoma, swollen brain) and thus avert compression of vital brainstem structures.

Definitive therapy of acute intracranial hemorrhage in the older child involves craniotomy and surgical removal of the blood clot (Milhorat, 1978). In the infant with a subdural hematoma it may be possible to remove significant quantities of subdural blood by tapping the subdural space at the lateral margins of the anterior fontanelle. In the older child without open fontanelles and in the infant with suspected subdural hemorrhage in whom standard subdural taps have not been effective, craniotomy and clot removal may be required.

Treatment of strangulation is essentially supportive (see Case 20–3).

Surgical Management.   Prompt neurosurgical removal of an acute epidural hematoma generally allows for an excellent outcome. Neurologic morbidity is usually greater with acute subdural hematoma than with acute epidural hematoma because of cerebral contusions that typically are associated with the former. Motor deficits, recurrent seizures, and developmental delay not infrequently result.

Orthopedic surgery may be necessary in treating long bone fractures. Closed fractures usually require casting or stable splinting following reduction. Open fractures generally necessitate debridement, antibiotic treatment, and, at times, internal stabilization.

In cases of abdominal or thoracic trauma, emergency surgical consultation is indicated and operation may be required (for example, removal of a ruptured spleen) (Touloukian, 1968).

Treatment of burns will generally include correction of associated fluid and electrolyte disturbance, topical antibiotic therapy, reverse precautions to prevent superinfection of wounds, and treatment of complications such as meningitis and/or seizures.

Psychotherapy.   Older children should generally be engaged in individual therapy because of complicated feelings associated with parents who have abused or neglected them (Martin and Beezley, 1977; Green, 1978). Even though removed from an unsafe environment, the child may nevertheless worry about father or mother out of habit (reversal of parent-child roles), because of concern that he has been responsible for getting his parents into legal difficulty, or because of fears that he has disclosed family secrets (which threats previously had been kept hidden).

Parents, too, will often benefit from supportive and insightful therapy with a psychiatrist or psychologist experienced in dealing with issues of abuse and neglect. Individual or group-based therapy may include discussion of ways in which the parents themselves were disciplined as children, behaviors that render them as parents out of control, and strategies for changing their behavior so that they do not reinjure their children. Parents Anonymous is a mutual support group that may benefit (potentially) abusing parents.

Social-Environmental Management. Social-environmental management is an important part of the treatment of child abuse and neglect. Ensuring that an ill child can obtain prompt and regular medical care without undue financial hardship to the family may be crucial in preventing further injury. Homemaking, babysitting, and visiting nurse services can provide some relief for a mother who is chronically stressed and on the verge of being overwhelmed. Such "time off" may be used, for example, for shopping, social activities, or formal psychotherapy.

If the safety of the child at home cannot be assured, placement with relatives or foster parents (otherwise, hospitalization) is generally required. In the United States and in many, if not most, other countries of the world it is required by law that children suspected of being abused or neglected be reported to governmental authorities by professional persons such as physicians, nurses, teachers, social workers, and day care workers. Custody (physical and/or legal) may be granted to the state and an evaluation of the family mandated following such notification.

It is important to remember that involvement of the court does not necessarily place the involved physician or other professional in an adversarial role with regard to the child's parents. The legal process often enables children to remain with their parents by providing for needed structure and services. As a father involved in a child abuse case said wistfully prior to a court appearance, "I wish somebody had done this (gone to court) when I was growing up." Shunted from one relative to another as a child, he had himself apparently been neglected, if not abused.

Educational Management. Remedial education is a necessary component in the treatment of abused and neglected children. In some school systems the child may receive psychotherapy during the day, either at school or at a nearby office.

CORRELATION

Anatomic Aspects. Head trauma in childhood can very usefully be approached by considering the anatomic structures involved. Figure 20–4 depicts a portion of the brain and surrounding structures. The scalp lies outermost and is bounded on its inner surface by the galea aponeurotica, a tendinous sheath that connects the frontalis muscle anteriorly with the occipitalis muscle posteriorly. Underlying the galea is the subgaleal compartment, a potential space containing loosely arrayed connective tissue. Hemorrhage within this space thus is associated with widespread boggy swelling of the scalp.

Next lies the skull, the outermost portion of which is the periosteum. Because the periosteum is an integral part of the bone and since the skull in young children is an unfused set of bones, a subperiosteal hemorrhage (cephalohematoma) is localized—limited by the cranial sutures that demarcate the bones that make up the calvarium.

The dura lies just below the inner table of the skull. In the infant it is more closely adherent to the cranium than in the older child or adolescent. As a result, epidural hemorrhage—lying between skull and dura—is encountered less often in infancy than in later years. The middle meningeal artery, a branch of the external carotid artery crossing the petrous portion of the temporal bone, is the usual source of bleeding in acute epidural hemorrhage. Laceration of a large venous sinus may also cause epidural hemorrhage, in which circumstance clinical manifestations may be less fulminant than those associated with arterial bleeding.

The sources of bleeding in acute subdural hemorrhage, by contrast, are small-caliber veins within the leptomeninges that traverse the subdural space to drain into dural sinuses. These bridging veins within the subdural space may be torn as a result of differential shearing forces from whiplash or other accelerative injury.

Biochemical Aspects.   Human beings eat to provide energy for growth and activity. Thus the chronically malnourished child will manifest characteristic abnormalities of both. Carbohydrates and fats are the primary sources of energy (measured in calories), while proteins provide the building blocks for enzymes and other proteins.

Daily caloric requirements vary with growth and activity, increasing from infancy through adolescence. About 500 calories are required daily in the neonate, while some 2,500 calories per day are needed by the teenager. The daily caloric requirement per kilogram of body weight declines, however, with increasing age: 100 to 120 calories per kilogram per day required for growth in the infant, 40 to 60 calories per kilogram per day in the school-age child, and 30 to 50 in the adolescent.

Amino acids, subunits for structural proteins, are also used as building blocks for enzymes that catalyze bodily activities. About 20 amino acids are needed for these purposes. The body is able to make one-half of these amino acids from other compounds. The other half, those amino acids which cannot be synthesized, are termed "essential." Essential amino acids in man are valine, leucine, isoleucine, lysine, threonine, tryptophan, phenylalanine, and methionine. Tyrosine and cystine are semiessential, since they can be synthesized but only through the essential amino acids phenylalanine and methionine.

Amino acids also serve as precursors for hormones and neurotransmitter substances. Tryptophan is metabolized to serotonin; phenylalanine and tyrosine to thyroxine, norepinephrine, and epinephrine (Fernstrom, 1977). The influence of diet upon levels of neurotransmitter substances in brain has been demonstrated by experimental studies in rats in whom a tryptophan-poor diet caused a marked reduction in brain serotonin. This reduction was prevented by dietary supplementation with tryptophan (Fernstrom and Wurtman, 1974; Fernstrom and Lytle, 1976).

Physiologic Aspects. Malnutrition affects not only growth but also behavior, including attention. Studies of normal and malnourished children have utilized analysis of changes in cardiac rate to assess reaction and habituation to novel stimuli (Latham, 1974; Pollitt and Thompson, 1977). Novel auditory stimuli among normally nourished children characteristically produce a deceleration in heart rate (part of the orienting response) that indicates habituation to the sound stimulus. Investigation of 20 malnourished children subjected to sounds of 400 and 750 Hz at 90 decibels (equal in intensity to a radio that is uncomfortably loud) found that they failed to show an orienting response to such auditory stimuli. Tested again after treatment of malnutrition, these infants had improved but still showed abnormalities in attention. Such attentional problems have been suggested to contribute to poor performance on psychologic testing among previously-malnourished children.

SUMMARY

The diagnosis of child abuse or neglect is often suggested by inadequate explanation for the problem or problems for which the child was brought to medical attention. Examination can establish the diagnosis through recognition of characteristic skin markings, signs of head injury, or failure to thrive. Investigation can play an important role in establishing or confirming the diagnosis. Particularly helpful are x-rays that detect unsuspected earlier fractures. Differential diagnosis includes hematologic disorders that render the child easily bruisable, bone disease associated with brittle bones, developmental or constitutional clumsiness affecting gait, and systemic disease causing failure to thrive.

Causes of child abuse or neglect are rooted in disturbed interpersonal relationships that often stem from parents' own early experiences. Treatment generally involves the working together of medical, psychiatric, neurologic, surgical, nutritional, social service, and legal specialists. The goal is to provide the child an optimal environment for physical and psychologic growth with ongoing professional involvement, evaluation, and therapy as needed.

CITED REFERENCES

Antoon, A. Y.; Volpe, J. J.; and Crawford, J. D. Burn encephalopathy in children. *Pediatrics,* **50:** 609–16, 1972.

Baron, M. A., Bejar, R. L.; and Sheaff, P. J. Neurologic manifestations of the battered child syndrome. *Pediatrics,* **45:** 1003–7, 1970.

Berant, M., and Jacobs, J. A "pseudo" battered child. *Clin. Pediatr.* (Philadelphia) **5:** 230–37, 1966.

Brown, R. E. Organ weight in malnutrition with special reference to brain weight. *Dev. Med. Child Neurol.,* **8:** 512–22, 1966.

Caffey, J. Some traumatic lesions in growing bones other than fractures and dislocations: clinical and radiological features. *Br. J. Radiology.* **30:** 225–38, 1957.

Caffey, J. On the theory and practice of shaking infants. *Am. J. Dis. Child.*, **124:** 161–69, 1972.

Caffey, J. The whiplash shaken infant syndrome: manual shaking by the extremities with whiplash-induced intracranial and intraocular bleedings, linked with residual permanent brain damage and mental retardation. *Pediatrics,* **54:** 396–403, 1974.

Capitanio, M. A., and Kirkpatrick, J. A. Widening of the cranial sutures: a roentgen observation during periods of accelerated growth in patients treated for deprivation dwarfism. *Radiology,* **92:** 53–59, 1969.

Chase, H. P., and Martin, H. P. Undernutrition and child development. *N. Engl. J. Med.,* **282:** 933–39, 1970.

Chase, H. P.; Kumar, V.; Caldwell, R. T.; and O'Brien, D. Kwashiorkor in the United States. *Pediatrics,* **66:** 972–76, 1980.

Clancy, H., and McBride, G. The isolation syndrome in childhood. *Dev. Med. Child Neurol.,* **17:** 198–219, 1975.

Collingwood, J., and Alberman, E. Separation at birth and the mother-child relationship. *Dev. Med. Child Neurol.,* **21:** 608–18, 1979.

Committee on Infectious Diseases. *Report of the Committee on Infectious Diseases,* 18th ed. American Academy of Pediatrics, Evanston, Ill., 1977.

De Levie, M., and Nogrady, M. B. Rapid brain growth upon restoration of adequate nutrition causing false radiologic evidence of increased intracranial pressure. *J. Pediatr.,* **76:** 523–28, 1970.

Dickson, R. A., and Leatherman, K. D. Spinal injuries in child abuse: case report. *J. Trauma,* **18:** 811–12, 1978.

Dine, M. S. Tranquilizer poisoning: an example of child abuse. *Pediatrics,* **36:** 782–85, 1965.

Dooling, E. C., and Richardson, E. P., Jr. Delayed encephalopathy after strangling. *Arch. Neurol.,* **33:** 196–99, 1976.

Einhorn, A., and Mizrahi, E. M. Basilar skull fractures in children. The incidence of CNS infection and the use of antibiotics. *Am. J. Dis. Child.,* **132:** 1121–24, 1978.

Evans, D.; Bowie, M. D.; Hansen, J. D. L.; Moodie, A. D.; and van der Spuy, H. I. J. Intellectual development and nutrition. *J. Pediatr.,* **97:** 358–63, 1980.

Fernstrom, J. D. Effects of the diet on brain neurotransmitters. *Metabolism,* **26:** 207–23, 1977.

Fernstrom, J. D., and Lytle, L. D. Corn malnutrition, brain serotonin and behavior. *Nutr. Rev.,* **34:** 257–62, 1976.

Fernstrom, J. D. and Wurtman, R. J. Nutrition and the brain. *Sci. Am.,* **231:** 84–91, February 1974.

Gillespie, R. W. The battered child syndrome: thermal and caustic manifestations. *J. Trauma,* **5:** 523–34, 1965.

Green, A. H. Psychopathology of abused children. *J. Am. Acad. Child Psychiatry,* **17:** 92–103, 1978.

Guthkelch, A. N. Infantile subdural haematoma and its relationship to whiplash injuries. *Br. Med. J.,* **2:** 430–31, 1971.

Hamlin, H. Subgaleal hematoma caused by hair-pull. *JAMA,* **204:** 129, 1968.

Helfer, R. E. *The Diagnostic Process and Treatment Programs.* U.S. Department of Health, Education and Welfare. DHEW Publication No. (OHD) 75-69, 1975.

Herskowitz, J., and Rosman, N. P. Acute hexachlorophene poisoning by mouth in a neonate. *J. Pediatr.,* **94:** 495–96, 1979.

Herskowitz, J., and Rosman, N. P. Other trauma to the central nervous system. In *The Practice of Pediatric Neurology,* 2d ed. Swaiman, K. F., and Wright, F. S., eds. C. V. Mosby Co., Saint Louis, 1982.

Hertzig, M. E.; Birch, H. G.; Richardson, S. A.; and Tizard, J. Intellectual levels of school children severely malnourished during the first two years of life. *Pediatrics*, **49**: 814–24, 1972.

Kempe, C. H.; Silverman, F. N.; Steele, B. F.; Droegemueller, W.; and Silver, H. K. The battered-child syndrome. *JAMA*, **181**: 105–12, 1962.

Kempe, C. H. Uncommon manifestations of the battered child syndrome. *Am. J. Dis. Child.*, **129**: 1265, 1975.

Kingsley, D.; Till, K.; and Hoare, R. Growing fractures of the skull. *J. Neurol. Neurosurg. Psychiatry*, **41**: 312–18, 1978.

Klein, M., and Stern, L. Low birth weight and the battered child syndrome. *Am. J. Dis. Child.*, **122**: 15–18, 1971.

Kohl, S.; Pickering, L. K.; and Dupree, E. Child abuse presenting as immunodeficiency disease. *J. Pediatr.*, **93**: 466–68, 1978.

Larson, D. L. Studies show hexachlorophene causes burn syndrome. *Hospitals*, **42**: 63–64, 1968.

Latham, M. C. Protein-calorie malnutrition in children and its relation to psychological development and behavior. *Physiol. Rev.*, **54**: 541–65, 1974.

Lloyd-Still, J. D.; Hurwitz, I., Wolff, P. H.; and Shwachman, H. Intellectual development after severe malnutrition in infancy. *Pediatrics*, **54**: 306–12, 1974.

Markham, B. Child abuse intervention: conflicts in current practice and legal theory. *Pediatrics*, **65**: 180–85, 1980.

Martin, H. P., and Beezley, P. Behavioral observations of abused children. *Dev. Med. Child Neurol.*, **19**: 373–87, 1977.

McGrory, B. E., and Fenichel, G. M. Hangman's fracture subsequent to shaking in an infant. *Ann. Neurol.*, **2**: 82, 1977.

Milhorat, T. H. *Pediatric Neurosurgery*. F. A. Davis Co., Philadelphia, 1978.

Mushin, A. S. Ocular damage in the battered-baby syndrome. *Br. Med. J.*, **3**: 402–5, 1971.

Ommaya, A. K.; Faas, F.; and Yarnell, P. Whiplash injury and brain damage. *JAMA*, **204**: 285–89, 1968.

Patton, R. G., and Gardner, L. I. Influence of family environment on growth: the syndrome of "maternal deprivation." *Pediatrics*, **30**: 957–62, 1962.

Pollitt, E. P., and Thomson, C. Protein-calorie malnutrition and behavior: a view from psychology. Pp. 261–306 in *Nutrition and the Brain*, Vol. 2. Wurtman, R. J., and Wurtman, J. J., eds. Raven Press, New York, 1977.

Powell, G. F.; Brasel, J. A.; Raiti, S.; and Blizzard R. M. Emotional deprivation and growth retardation simulating idiopathic hypopituitarism: II. endocrinologic evaluation of the syndrome. *N. Engl. J. Med.*, **276**: 1279–83, 1967.

Powell, G. F.; Brasel, J. A.; and Blizzard, R. M. Emotional deprivation and growth retardation simulating idiopathic hypopituitarism: I. clinical evaluation of the syndrome. *N. Engl. J. Med.*, **276**: 1271–78, 1967.

Rosman, N. P.; Herskowitz, J.; Carter, A. P.; and O'Connor, J. F. Acute head trauma in infancy and childhood: clinical and radiologic aspects. *Pediatr. Clin. North Am.*, **26**: 707–36, 1979.

Schmitt, B. D., and Kempe, C. H. The battered child syndrome. Pp. 603–8 in *Handbook of Clinical Neurology*, Vol. 23. Vinken, P. J., and Bruyn, G. W., eds. North-Holland Publishing Co., Amsterdam, 1975.

Silber, D. L., and Bell, W. E. The neurologist and the physically abused child. *Neurology*, **21**: 991–99, 1971.

Solnit, A. J. Child abuse: least harmful, most protective intervention. *Pediatrics*, **65**: 170–71, 1980.

Spitz, R. A. Hospitalism: an inquiry into the genesis of psychiatric conditions in early childhood. *Psychoanal. Study Child*, **1**: 53–74, 1945.

Steele, B. F. *Working with Abusive Parents from a Psychiatric Point of View*. DHEW publication No. (OHD) 75-70, 1975.

Stein, Z.; Susser, M.; Saenger, G.; and Marolla, F. Nutrition and mental performance. *Science,* **178:** 708–13, 1972.

Stoch, M. B., and Smythe, P. M. Does undernutrition during infancy inhibit brain growth and subsequent intellectual development? *Arch. Dis. Child.,* **38:** 546–52, 1963.

Stoch, M. B., and Smythe, P. M. The effect of undernutrition during infancy on subsequent brain growth and intellectual development. *S. Afr. Med. J.,* **41:** 1027–35, 1967.

Sussman, S. J. Skin manifestations of the battered-child syndrome. *J. Pediatr.,* **72:** 99–101, 1968.

Swischuk, L. E. Spine and spinal cord trauma in the battered child syndrome. *Radiology,* **92:** 733–38, 1969.

Taylor, L., and Newberger, E. H. Child abuse in the International Year of the Child. *N. Engl. J. Med.,* **301:** 1205–12, 1979.

Tomasi, L. G., and Rosman, N. P. Purtscher retinopathy in the battered child syndrome. *Am. J. Dis. Child.,* **129:** 1335–37, 1975.

Touloukian, R. J. Abdominal visceral injuries in battered children. *Pediatrics,* **42:** 642–50, 1968.

Waskerwitz, S.; Christoffel, K. K.; and Hauger, S. Hypersensitivity vasculitis presenting as suspected child abuse: case report and literature review. *Pediatrics,* **67:** 283–84, 1981.

Winick, M.; Meyer, K. K.; and Harris, R. C. Malnutrition and environmental enrichment by early adoption. *Science,* **190:** 1173–75, 1975.

Wolkind, S. N. The components of "affectionless psychopathy" in institutionalized children. *J. Child Psychol. Psychiatry,* **15:** 215–20, 1974.

ADDITIONAL READINGS

Asnes, R. S., and Wisotsky, D. H. Cupping lesions simulating child abuse. *J. Pediatr.,* **99:** 267–68, 1981.

Bauman, W. A., and Yalow, R. S. Child abuse: parenteral insulin administration. *J. Pediatr.,* **99:** 588–91, 1981.

Bowlby, J. B. *Attachment and Loss,* Vols. I–III. Basic Books, Inc., New York, 1969, 1973, and 1980.

Feldman, K. W., and Simms, R. J. Strangulation in childhood: epidemiology and clinical course. *Pediatrics,* **65:** 1079–85, 1980.

Kempe, C. H., and Helfer, R. E., eds. *Helping the Battered Child and His Family*. J. B. Lippincott Company, Philadelphia, 1972.

O'Doherty, N. *The Battered Child: Recognition in Primary Care*. Macmillan Publishing Co., Inc., New York, 1982.

Rimsza, M. E., and Niggemann, E. H. Medical evaluation of sexually abused children: a review of 311 cases. *Pediatrics,* **69:** 8–14, 1982.

Schmitt, B. D., ed. *The Child Protection Team Handbook. A Multidisciplinary Approach to Managing Child Abuse and Neglect*. Garland STPM Press, New York, 1978.

Suskind, R. M., ed. *Textbook of Pediatric Nutrition*. Raven Press, New York, 1980.

21 Chronic Illness and the Dying Child

Chronic illness (or, to use a more broadly applicable term, a chronic handi-capping condition) will have, in almost every instance, major effects upon the child and his or her family. Diabetes mellitus, asthma, and cystic fibrosis are examples of chronic medical illness. A wide spectrum of neurologic disorders that are chronically handicapping includes epilepsy, cerebral palsy, multiple sclerosis, posttraumatic brain injury, muscular dystrophy, meningomyelocele, learning disability, attention deficit disorder, and mental retardation. Some of these (e.g., cerebral palsy) reflect static effects upon the nervous system. Others tend to remit and relapse (e.g., multiple sclero-sis), while still others pursue a relentlessly downhill course (e.g., muscular dystrophy). Within the latter two groups are diseases to which issues of death and dying are added to those of chronic illness.

This chapter will consider certain aspects of chronic illness in childhood with primary focus upon disorders affecting the nervous system and with particular attention to the following questions:

What issues confront the child with a chronic neurologic illness and his or her family?
What behavioral and emotional problems are associated?
What medical, neurologic, or psychologic factors can cause or contribute to such problems?
What is the role of the psychologist, physician, and other health profes-sional in managing the child with a chronic illness? The child who is dying?
What setting (home, hospice, or hospital) is most appropriate for a dying child?

CHRONIC ILLNESS AND THE DYING CHILD

Definition

Chronic illness can be defined as disorder or disability of a physical or psychologic nature that persistently reduces a child's level of function to below that appropriate for his or her chronologic age. Duchenne muscular

601

dystrophy, for example, is associated with a progressive motor deficit beginning in early childhood that usually renders the child wheelchair-bound by adolescence. Pulmonary and cardiac complications of the disease usually will appear and progress over the next one to two decades along with continuing decline in muscle strength. Thus, the child is removed increasingly from activities of his peers.

With muscular dystrophy, as with other chronic disorders, the child's illness will also have major effects upon the entire family. These, in turn, will secondarily affect the handicapped child, further complicating the effects of the illness itself.

DIAGNOSIS

Diagnosis is usually not an issue in the child with a chronic illness. Presumably it has been established already and a treatment plan initiated. On the other hand, when a specific diagnosis has not been determined (for example, in a child with mental retardation of unknown cause), periodic reassessment, or at least diagnostic reconsideration, may be worthwhile, for recent diagnostic techniques (such as increasingly sophisticated chromosome analysis and newer biochemical analyses of blood and urine) may shed further light on the nature of the disorder. In general, important issues (and problems) will frequently surface when a 6-month or yearly follow-up visit is not restricted to the specific medical or neurologic problem alone, within limits imposed by a 15- to 20-minute time slot. In other words, sufficient time should be scheduled so that one can learn about what is happening in the person's life, not just with his disease.

Clinical Process. *History.* The complaints of a child with a chronic illness or those of his parents will often reflect behavioral aspects of the condition. "My parents won't let me out of their sight because they're afraid I'll have a seizure." "He refuses to take his medication because he says there's nothing wrong with him." "We think he's becoming too dependent on us because we find it so hard not to baby him." "We're worried about who will take care of him when we're gone."

Consideration should be given to intercurrent illnesses and their effect upon the child. School progress should be noted. Disturbances in mood, acting-out, and other behavioral difficulties should be sought. Relationships with family members and peers should be determined. With motor-handicapping conditions, transportation problems need to be addressed.

It is valuable to review periodically the perceptions of the child and parents as to the nature of the illness. Such inquiry should include thoughts as to what has caused it and what is (or is not) being done about it. Oftentimes a family will ask about causes or cures based upon their readings in the lay press or conversations they have had with others. Such discussion will often permit the family to question aspects of management in a manner that should be nonthreatening to family and health professional alike. It may also serve to strengthen the relationship between family and physician or other therapist.

If a child is deteriorating, it is useful to interview the parents apart from the child to learn of their perception as to the imminence of death and whether the child has asked (directly or indirectly) about dying. Parents should be encouraged to direct the physician as to what the child should be told about his or her illness, when it should be told, and how that information should be conveyed. The knowledge and experience of the professional can guide the family in such difficult matters, but final decisions should rest with the family.

Examination. The *general description* should note the overall feeling the child conveys, both physically and emotionally. Is he robust or emaciated? Cheerful, euphoric, apathetic, or depressed?

The *general physical examination* should include attention to intercurrent problems such as pneumonia or urinary tract infection that are specifically treatable complications of underlying conditions such as muscular dystrophy or multiple sclerosis.

The *neurologic examination* should focus upon pertinent portions of the examination. For example, gait, coordination, vision, and bladder function should receive careful attention in the child with multiple sclerosis.

The *mental status examination* should note in particular the child's outward emotional state. The subjective emotional state should be noted as well. Partially directed conversation should permit the child to express current interests, preoccupations, and fears. Stemming from this conversation, further discussion can be directed toward the child's illness, his perception of its causes and cures, and issues of dying and death.

One should seek to determine the degree to which the illness influences the life of the child and family. Does family life center upon the child's illness? Or does life go on, with adaptation to the disability? The spectrum of influence is broad. It ranges from total preoccupation with the defective part of the child to a family focused upon the normal aspects of the child (Herskowitz and Marks, 1977).

Investigation. Investigations, if any, will depend upon the particular illness and changes taking place. For example, follow-up investigation of the child with a seizure disorder will commonly involve electroencephalogram, anticonvulsant blood level(s), complete blood count, and liver function tests. In a person with multiple sclerosis and bladder dysfunction, urine should be obtained for culture and analysis. When a child is affected by muscular dystrophy, electrocardiogram and chest x-ray may be indicated. The child who is being tested for leukemia and who has undergone a change in mental status or has developed severe headaches should have a computerized tomographic (CT) scan of the head and may require cerebrospinal fluid examination (see ETIOLOGY).

When the diagnosis of developmental delay or behavioral regression is being reconsidered or the evaluation extended, lysosomal enzyme determinations, chromosomal fragility studies, or electron microscopic analysis of skin fibroblasts are examples of investigations that might be pursued.

When emotional problems in the child or family have been identified or are suspected, formal psychiatric or psychologic diagnostic consultation should generally be sought. At the very least the case should be discussed with a mental health professional experienced in the problems of children with chronic illness.

When a dying child is suspected of being brain-dead, several investigations (electroencephalogram, radioisotope brain scan, evoked potential studies, and arteriography) may be undertaken to confirm the clinical diagnosis. The essential clinical criteria are no cortical function (evidenced by absence of volitional movements and of response to painful stimulation), no brainstem function (manifested by absence of pupillary reactions, corneal reflexes, and responses to caloric stimulation), and no spontaneous respirations (Beecher *et al.*, 1968; Black, 1978; Powner and Fromm, 1979). In order that such criteria be interpreted as reflecting brain death, drug overdose (e.g., with glutethimide [Doriden] or barbiturates) and hypothermia must be excluded.

Etiology.   Several causes of chronic illness were mentioned earlier. This section will focus upon behavioral and emotional problems that can be associated with chronic illness. These may stem directly from the disease itself, its treatment, or as a reaction to the associated disability (see Table 21–1).

Medical Causes.   Systemic illness in any child, but especially one already affected by a chronic illness, can be associated with fatigue, lassitude, and loss of interest in usual activities—symptoms that suggest a depressive syndrome that may in fact coexist. Pain due to the illness itself or its treatment may have a particularly adverse effect. With multiple sclerosis or myelomeningocele, urinary tract infection should be suspected first when an intercurrent illness is being considered. With Duchenne muscular dystrophy, respiratory disease is a particular risk.

Neurologic Causes.   The central nervous system can be affected by the disease process itself, by complications of the disease, or by the therapies utilized (see Case 21–1).

With leukemia the meninges may be infiltrated by malignant cells to pro-

TABLE 21–1. **Causes of Affective and Behavioral Problems Associated with Chronic Illness**

Medical	Fatigue, lassitude, and pain associated with illness or its treatment
Neurologic	Involvement of central nervous system by disease, complications of disease, or its treatment
Toxic	Anticonvulsant overdosage Analgesic overdosage Side effects of chemotherapeutic agents in treatment of malignancy
Psychologic	Depression (from loss of function) Anxiety (concerning diagnostic procedures, operation, impending death)
Social-Environmental	Physical, social, and financial stresses Social isolation
Developmental	Failure to progress along developmental lines of peers

duce mental status changes and headache. Meninges or brain can be infected by bacteria or opportunistic organisms such as fungi because of immunologic suppression due to leukemia or its treatment. Widespread brain disease of viral etiology—progressive multifocal leukoencephalopathy (PML)—may also occur with leukemia as well as with other childhood malignancies. Because of blastic crises or low platelet levels (which often result from the disease itself or from bone marrow suppression caused by chemotherapy), intracranial hemorrhage (subarachnoid, cerebral, subdural, or epidural) should be suspected in the child with leukemia who undergoes a change in mental state or manifests a worsening of another elemental neurologic function such as gait (see Fig. 21–2) (see Table 21–2).

A week to 2 weeks of somnolence following radiation to the head is commonly seen following prophylactic treatment of neoplastic disease (Freeman *et al.*, 1973). This effect should not be confused with a more long-lasting subacute leukoencephalopathy, a white matter degeneration that can be clinically manifested by dementia and confusion following treatment with cranial irradiation with or without intrathecal methotrexate (McIntosh and Aspnes, 1973; Price and Jamieson, 1975; Gangji *et al.*, 1980).

Toxic Causes. Anticonvulsant overdosage must always be considered in the child being treated for seizures who manifests a change in mental state (or, more concretely, school performance). Many of the possible causes of overdosage (including physician, pharmacist, parent, or patient error) are discussed in Chapter 12.

Analgesic drugs (such as morphine) and chemotherapeutic agents (such as methotrexate) may also alter the child's mental state.

Psychologic Causes. Depression and anxiety are important manifestations of behavioral change in children with chronic illness. The child may be depressed, for example, because of loss of previous physical, linguistic, or memory capabilities (e.g., following head injury). With intermittent or progressive disease such as multiple sclerosis or muscular dystrophy, the child may be anxious about anticipated diagnostic procedures, surgery, and issues pertaining to death. The child may become fearful, withdrawn, and isolated if these concerns are not addressed. Depression of other family members may cause the child's mood and behavior to deteriorate still further.

Social-Environmental Causes. Many of the chronic handicapping conditions of childhood such as muscular dystrophy, spina bifida, cerebral palsy, and mental retardation cause physical and social limitations that may further stress both the child and the rest of the family. Financial pressures are commonly an additional stress.

Developmental Causes. The developmental problems of children with chronic illness should be approached by considering the child's developmental status in comparison with chronologic age. It is well recognized that the development of walking is an important step in acquiring a sense of autonomy. Most children with Duchenne muscular dystrophy, confined to a wheelchair by adolescence, will have their feelings of self-sufficiency severely compromised unless adaptations such as motorized wheelchairs are effected.

In some circumstances parents and child come to focus upon the disabil-

CASE 21–1: MULTIPLE SCLEROSIS IN AN 18-YEAR-OLD FEMALE

B.C. developed weakness of the right leg and difficulty with balance at age 14 years. Investigation at that time included a normal myelogram and a cerebrospinal fluid examination, which showed 30 lymphocytes per ml and had a protein content of 47 mg/dl. She was treated with dexamethasone for several weeks and returned essentially to her previous level of functioning within a few months. Six months after her first symptoms, weakness in the right leg recurred and again appeared to respond to dexamethasone therapy.

At 15 years she was hospitalized because of double vision and difficulty walking. Examination showed diminished adduction of the right eye. She was treated with ACTH by injection, and the problem resolved within several weeks. Six months later she complained of diminished vision and pain in the left eye. Evaluation disclosed retrobulbar neuritis. While being treated with prednisone, visual function returned to normal, but she developed urinary frequency and incontinence. She did not always feel the need to void. At 16½ years, the prednisone dosage was raised because of increasing gait difficulty. Motor function deteriorated, however, and she was again hospitalized.

On examination, she was a weak young woman with obvious signs of Cushing syndrome: flushed skin, mooned facial appearance, purple striae, truncal obesity, and buffalo hump. She was alert and oriented but showed surprisingly little concern about her worsened status. She was unable to recall any of three items after 10 minutes. Visual acuity was normal. Optic disks were pale bilaterally. The right pupil reacted briskly to light but "escaped." A swinging flashlight sign was evident as light was brought from the left eye to the right. Proximal muscle weakness was so severe that she was unable to rise from a seated to a standing position. Deep tendon reflexes were exaggerated throughout, more so on the right than the left. Both plantar responses were extensor. Proprioception and perception of vibration were diminished in both legs. Gait was widely based and could be accomplished only with assistance.

Investigation included cerebrospinal fluid examination, which showed 2 lymphocytes per ml and a protein content of 110 mg/dl (3 per cent of which was IgG). CT scan showed cerebral atrophy (see Fig. 21–1). Prednisone was tapered, and gradual improvement in muscle strength was seen. By the time of discharge from hospital 3 weeks after admission, she could walk with use of a walker. Two weeks later she could ambulate aided only by a cane, and a

ity to an unhelpful and unhealthful degree. Further, on occasion, the disability may be used by the child for manipulative purposes (see Case 21–2).

In other circumstances parents have been able to provide the handicapped child with means for developing independence in other than an ambulatory manner. Thus, the child can learn to exert influence over his en-

month later she walked without any device or assistance. Urinary incontinence continued. Suppressive antibiotic therapy was begun and a program of self-catheterization instituted.

Comment. This teenager manifested a characteristic clinical picture of multiple sclerosis. As is typical with "disseminated sclerosis," the lesions of multiple sclerosis affect multiple sites within the central nervous system (brain, spinal cord, or both) at different times (see Fig. 13–8). Since areas of demyelination tend to become remyelinated, the result is a clinical picture of relapse and remission.

As is unfortunately true in about one-third of cases, the course of the illness may be characterized by progressive loss of function. Such has occurred in this case; for following nearly every relapse, a return to previous levels of function was not achieved.

This young woman suffered several deficits typical of multiple sclerosis: ataxia of gait, visual loss, and urinary dysfunction. Ataxia generally results not only from demyelination within the cerebellum but within the cerebrum, brainstem, and spinal cord as well, affecting pyramidal, proprioceptive, and spinocerebellar fibers. Visual loss is common in multiple sclerosis because of the many myelinated fibers that make up the visual system. In this case, she experienced retrobulbar neuritis (demyelination of the optic nerve), manifested by a painful eye with diminished vision. Because the inflammatory process occurred behind the eye, funduscopic examination disclosed a normal disk, without blurred margins. Her abnormal pupillary reaction to light on the right was a residuum of past optic nerve involvement on that side. Urinary incontinence appeared to be primarily on an afferent basis, as she had lost the sensation of bladder fullness necessary to control urination.

This case was severely complicated by effects of prednisone, which earlier had seemed to help but had made her profoundly weak and had altered her physical appearance.

Longer-range issues in this case involved clarifying what this young woman was to do with her life, her neurologic illness permitting. After graduation from high school, she contented herself with staying at home and watching television. Her urinary problem increased her reluctance to leave home even briefly. A family-based approach to counseling was attempted in addition to individual supportive therapy. It was further suggested that she contact her local chapter of the Multiple Sclerosis Society.

vironment in a positive, nonmanipulative fashion and thereby develop a better sense of self.

Adolescence is a time of considerable peer group pressure. Having a chronic, handicapping deformity (such as limp due to polio or infantile hemiplegia) or needing to take chronic medication (as with epilepsy) will set the child apart from his or her crowd in a way that can be upsetting (Wol-

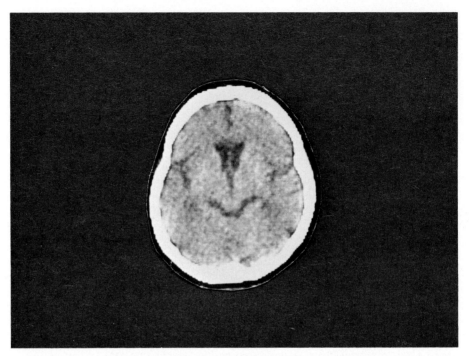

FIGURE 21–1. Plain computerized tomographic (CT) scan of the head showing enlargement of lateral ventricles and mild cortical atrophy (Case 21–1).

fish and McLean, 1974). The adolescent with a seizure disorder, for example, may therefore decide to discontinue anticonvulsant medication (resulting in a return of seizures) or, as a manifestation of more serious emotional disturbance, ingest anticonvulsant pills in overdosage (see Case 21–3).

Overall, adolescents appear to handle chronic illness surprisingly well, perhaps due in part to their adaptive use of denial (Kellerman *et al.*, 1980; Zeltzer *et al.*, 1980).

TREATMENT AND OUTCOME

The overall goal of treatment is to maintain at the highest level those functions that have been acquired and to restore to the highest level possible those functions that have declined (see Table 21–3). A further goal is to keep the child in the developmental mainstream of his peers insofar as is achievable (see Case 21–4).

The specifics of management will be determined by the particulars of the chronic handicapping condition. For example, the therapy of cerebral palsy differs markedly from that of acute lymphoblastic leukemia. Of note, however, the latter disorder has become, in many instances, a chronic illness, often with long-term survival and even "cures" (rather than an acute life-taking illness). Indeed, leukemia or other malignant disease of childhood can be viewed increasingly as something that one lives with rather than dies from. With improved survival, problems of depression, anxiety, and low

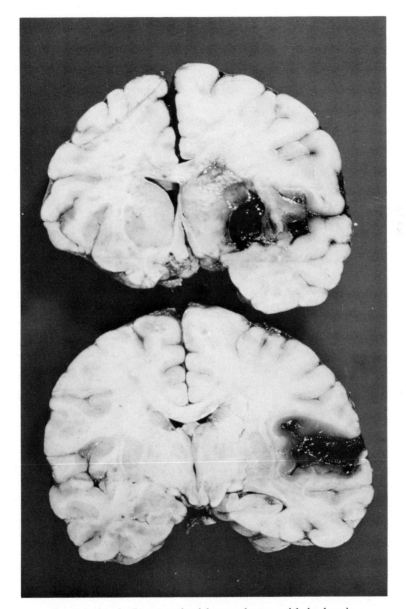

FIGURE 21–2. Intracerebral hemorrhages with leukemia.

self-esteem have been identified among survivors of cancer in childhood (Koocher *et al.*, 1980; D'Angio, 1980).

In approaching the child with a chronic illness, it is important that the child's strengths be identified and built upon. Otherwise the child's illness or defectiveness can become the focal point of his or her existence and a disturbed sense of self can result (Herskowitz and Marks, 1977).

Medical Management. Medical management will involve the treatment of intercurrent illness such as urinary tract infection (e.g., with multiple sclero-

TABLE 21–2. **Central Nervous System
Complications of Leukemia**

Leukemic infiltration of meninges
Infection of brain (abscess) and/or meninges due
    to bacteria and opportunistic organisms (such as
    fungi)
Progressive multifocal leukoencephalopathy (PML)
Intracranial hemorrhage (subarachnoid, intra-
    cerebral, subdural, epidural) associated with
    blastic crisis or bleeding diathesis (platelet
    deficiency)
Leukoencephalopathy (radiation-related; ? effects
    of methotrexate or other medications)

sis), pneumonia (e.g., with Duchenne muscular dystrophy in its later stages), and pain (e.g., with malignant disease of bone). Effective analgesia may include the use of narcotic agents. Drug dependency does not appear to be a problem in such circumstances of medical supervision (Hackett, 1976; Krant, 1978; Potter, 1980). Sedation with chloral hydrate, flurazepam (Dalmane), or diazepam (Valium) may assist the child in getting to sleep and can

CASE 21–2: MENINGOMYELOCELE IN A 17-YEAR-OLD MALE

L.W. was born with a meningomyelocele at the third to fourth lumbar level. It was removed on day two of life. A ventriculoperitoneal shunt was placed at 8 months because of excessively rapid head growth. Development included speaking in sentences at 2 years and walking at 3 years, aided by braces and crutches. He had never been continent of urine or feces. Urinary drainage was accomplished through an ileostomy, necessitated by frequent bouts of pyelonephritis and diminishing renal function. Bowel management consisted of suppositories, mineral oil, enemas, and use of diapers. Past medical history was notable for multiple orthopedic operations including derotational osteotomy and adductor tenotomy. Family history was negative for meningomyelocele or other form of spina bifida.

On examination, the young man was an immature, articulate, large-headed adolescent sitting in a wheelchair. He explained that his neurologic problem resulted from too much pressure upon his spine and brain. As a consequence a hole in his back blew out at the time of birth. Once this defect was repaired, pressure built up once again and a shunt was required to bring it down to normal. He indicated long-standing difficulties in expressing anger for fear of "blowing his top" and "going crazy." He was passive, somewhat angry about his disabilities, and had no definite plans for the future other than finishing school. He recognized many of the medical, surgical, and fi-

ease the anxiety and physical discomfort associated with necessary procedures such as lumbar puncture or bone marrow aspiration. Antidepressant
medication may be employed in conjunction with psychotherapy.

Ensuring adequate nutrition is another important aspect of medical
management.

Neurologic Management. Care must be taken not to overmedicate the patient with a seizure disorder. The benefits of therapy (seizure control) must
always be titrated against the side effects (sedation, for example). In many
instances therapy can be discontinued after several years if the child has
been seizure-free and the electroencephalogram is normal or nearly so (see
Chapter 12).

Diazepam (Valium) may be helpful in treating spasticity.

Surgical Management. Surgical treatment may be of benefit to persons
with chronic handicapping conditions. The gait of persons with spastic
cerebral palsy may be improved through lengthening of the heel cords.
Spinal fusion has been used to advantage in some persons with muscular
dystrophy to prevent further scoliosis and additional cardiorespiratory compromise. Feeding gastrostomy can facilitate adequate nutrition in children
with severe posttraumatic encephalopathy. Thus the hours previously
spent laboriously feeding the child become available to be used more productively.

nancial implications of his condition and derived some satisfaction from the
influence it had given him over others.

Comment. This young man's physical defects were integrally interwo-
ven with his personality and behavior. Indeed, there had been such focus in
his life upon what was wrong with him that he appeared to identify himself
more as a defect than as a person. The reason for this identification was unclear. Perhaps it stemmed from a disturbance in early bonding as his parents
reacted to the birth of their defective child. The many operations that followed and the necessities of home management surely must have strained
the family physically, emotionally, and financially. The developing child
may have come to view his defective body as a medium of interaction with
his family and, by extension, with others.

Around the time of his ileostomy, this young man had been aided in preparation for surgery by an ongoing psychotherapeutic relationship with a
child psychiatrist. Sessions lasting 15 minutes to 1 hour were relatively
informal and covered a wide range of topics. His fantasies and fears were
explored, his many confusions about sexuality addressed, and his thoughts
about the future discussed.

One hopes that with increased understanding of a family's reactions to the
birth of a defective child, further refinements in the care of children with severe spina bifida, and enhanced opportunities for handicapped persons, parents will be able to relate increasingly to the more normal aspects of a multi-
ply handicapped child.

CASE 21–3: POSTTRAUMATIC SEIZURES AND BEHAVIORAL DISTURBANCE IN A 14-YEAR-OLD BOY

S.L., at $2\frac{1}{2}$ years of age, fell out of a moving car and was struck by another vehicle. When he regained consciousness 3 weeks later, he had a right hemiparesis. Seizures began 6 months after the head trauma. They consisted of a blank expression, eye blinking, and clicking of the mouth followed by a period of confusion. They were controlled by a combination of anticonvulsant medicines. Disruptive behavior in school led to neurologic reassessment at age 14 years.

On examination, the boy was a pleasant, cooperative, muscular adolescent with an evident right hemiparesis. Head circumference was normal. The right hand and nails were smaller than the left. He was able to recall six digits forward and read at a fourth grade level. No hemianopia was demonstrable on testing of visual fields. Optokinetic nystagmus was absent when the tape was moved to his left. The right heel cord was tight, and he limped upon that leg. All modalities of sensation were diminished over the right half of his body. Deep tendon reflexes were exaggerated in the right arm and in both legs.

Comment. Several problems appeared to come together to precipitate this boy's disruptive behavior. He had entered pubescence recently with a growth spurt and development of secondary sexual characteristics. Schoolmates had been teasing him by calling him "cripple." Mother described her son as "spoiled" and indicated that much parental guilt remained from the time of the early childhood accident.

Management in this case was directed toward emphasizing this youngster's strengths (which were significant) while not ignoring his weaknesses, about which he clearly was sensitive. Intellectual limitation, although not severe, and social immaturity had made sexual issues especially confusing and troubling. As a result it was suggested that they be explained to him in simple and concrete terms that he could understand.

In some children anticonvulsant medication may produce behavioral alterations such as irritability or lethargy that can lead to disruptive behavior. These effects, which may be dose-related or idiosyncratic, did not appear to play a role in this case.

Psychotherapy. Psychotherapy involving child and family is generally valuable in the treatment of chronic diseases of childhood. Treatment will often take the form of supportive therapy. It should be remembered that this mode of treatment is by no means trivial or effortless. Further, it is often much more appreciated by patient and family than the most intensive diagnostic and therapeutic measures. Supportive therapy can involve clarification of goals, discussion of past successes and failures, and encouragement during periods of stress. Parents may benefit from support in allowing greater independence of their affected child. Mothers may respond to urging to develop interests

TABLE 21–3. **Selected Aspects of Treatment of the Child with a Chronic Illness**

Medical	Treatment of intercurrent illness (such as urinary tract infection, pneumonia) Maintenance of adequate nutrition Analgesia Sedation as needed for sleep
Neurologic	Anticonvulsant therapy Pharmacologic agents for spasticity
Psychologic	Individual therapy for depression (plus pharmacotherapy as indicated) Family therapy including support Counseling as to issues of death and dying
Surgical	Heel cord lengthening Spinal fusion Gastrostomy
Social-Environmental	Home, hospice, or hospital
Educational	Individualized assistance at school Tutoring at home
Physical	Maintenance of motor function (prevent contracture, improve mobility) Aid in respiratory functioning
Mechanical	Wheelchairs and other devices to enhance motor capacity and independence

outside the family, and fathers may need to be encouraged to involve themselves further with their chronically ill child (Boyle *et al.,* 1976).

Explanation of the illness to the child should be developmentally appropriate. Children's concepts of illness appear to undergo a progression of change analogous to that recognized with other aspects of cognitive development (Bibace and Walsh, 1980). In follow-up visits, it will be valuable to learn what the child and parents have understood about previous explanations, since omissions and distortions frequently occur (Steinhauer *et al.,* 1974).

With regard to the dying child and his or her family, much has been written within the last decade about the importance of the physician's or other professional's being available to discuss critical issues that form a constant part of their daily lives. The physician should seek to break through the isolation that typifies patients approaching death and should strive to have the parents and child discuss, rather than retreat from, issues that should be faced (Hackett, 1976) (see Case 21–5).

The therapist should be aware that anticipatory grieving by parents may weaken their bonds of attachment to the child (Lindemann, 1944). This de-

CASE 21–4: ACUTE HEMIPLEGIA AND APHASIA IN A 14-YEAR-OLD BOY

F.E. collapsed suddenly while running to first base during a baseball game. He was unable to move his right limbs and his speech was slurred. He had previously been well and had not experienced any recent trauma. Past history was entirely unremarkable. He was right-handed. On examination at the hospital, he was stuporous and had an obvious right hemiparesis. Blood pressure, pulse, and the remainder of the cardiovascular examination were normal. On neurologic examination, he responded to verbal stimuli but was mute. The right arm was weaker than the right leg. The face was also mildly affected on that side. Sensory examination was normal.

Initial laboratory data included a normal platelet count, electrocardiogram, and clotting studies. Sedimentation rate was 7 mm/hour, and serum antinuclear antibody was normal. Analysis of blood and urine for amino acids (including homocystine) was normal. Cerebrospinal fluid examination and echocardiogram were normal. CT scan obtained within hours of collapse was normal, but a scan repeated 2 days later showed a wedge-shaped portion of brain with decreased density in the area of distribution of the left middle cerebral artery (see Fig. 21–3). Cerebral arteriogram showed occlusion of the left middle cerebral artery at its point of origin from the internal carotid artery.

During initial hospitalization, marked improvement occurred. He rapidly regained the ability to walk. Speech became telegraphic. He was able to speak in short phrases but was obviously frustrated because of difficulty in expressing himself. Praxis was impaired. For example, he was much better able to blow out a real match than to blow out an imagined one.

He returned to school 5 months later. Spontaneous speech was still sparse and he rarely used more than two words at a time. Motor function had continued to improve, particularly proximal functions of the right arm. Precise hand movements remained markedly impaired. Ten months after the stroke he used longer word combinations. He could walk without a cane and dribble a basketball with his right hand but could not use that hand for writing. A picture of himself playing basketball was drawn in left profile, omitting entirely the right (hemiplegic) part of his body (see Fig. 21–4).

At age 16 years, two years after the initial incident, further improvement in motor and language functions was apparent. As before, motor deficit was more marked in the arm than in the leg. Proximal movements of the right

tachment can intensify the child's feelings of isolation; if survival extends beyond what is anticipated, behavioral disturbance may result (Green and Solnit, 1964).

Therapy may be individual or family-based. Treatment of associated depression may involve the use of antidepressant medication. In approaching

upper extremity were much better performed than distal movements. Speech was improved although still dysfluent. When asked if he had a good winter, he replied, "Oh, not really." He qualified this remark by saying, "No. . . . A bad winter, because, the snow, the snow, oh, the snow is, there is no snow."

He has continued in a regular classroom with individual tutoring that includes speech and language therapy. He also participates in regular physical therapy. At night he wears a splint for the right arm and a bivalved cast for the right leg. His parents have noted continued frustration and occasional angry outbursts linked with his language difficulty and loss of motor skills.

Comment. This young man illustrates the origin of the word "stroke," as his paralysis and language disturbance arose suddenly without warning. Extensive evaluation detailed above disclosed no identifiable cause for occlusion of the left middle cerebral artery.

This case demonstrates also that recovery from hemispheric brain injury in childhood and adolescence does not necessarily cease after 6 months or a year. In this case it has continued beyond 2 years. The prognosis for this boy in terms of language skills was enhanced by his age. The younger the child is at the time of damage to the dominant hemisphere (usually the left), the better is the amount of recovery of useful language. At 16 years this boy continued to manifest significant language impairment, but he fared much better than would have been expected had he been 30 or 40 years old at the time of the stroke.

This young man's language disturbance was an anterior (or Broca's) aphasia, typically associated with a right hemiparesis with impaired praxis. Speech is characteristically nonfluent and comprehension relatively well preserved. As is usual with cortical injuries, fine hand movements suffered significantly more than crude, more proximal movements.

This case provides an example of multispecialty participation in the treatment of a child with a chronic handicapping condition. Neurologic management has involved determining—insofar as possible—the causes of the young man's disability, following his progress, and coordinating various aspects of his overall treatment. Physical therapy and speech and language therapy were directed toward specific areas of difficulty. Psychotherapy has been advised as the boy and his parents continue their adjustment to his ongoing disabilities while he attempts to negotiate adolescence in as normal a manner as possible.

the dying child, one should be aware that the child's perception of death (like that of illness) changes with age. The child may, for example, perceive illness and death as punishment (White *et al.,* 1978; Share, 1980).

It is also useful to keep in mind the successive stages of attitude toward dying and death as described by Kübler-Ross (1969): denial and isolation,

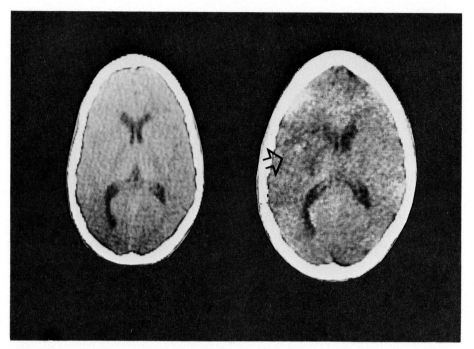

FIGURE 21–3. Plain computerized tomographic (CT) scans of the head obtained on the day of the stroke (left) and eight days later (Case 21–4). Open arrow indicates area of tissue loss.

anger, bargaining, depression, and acceptance. One should not always expect, however, to see this prototypical progression during childhood (or in later life for that matter).

Kübler-Ross (1969) has stressed the importance of supporting the dying person in maintaining hope. Such an approach should not be construed as false optimism, for much remains unknown and unpredictable. As exemplified by the treatment of neoplastic diseases in childhood, more effective therapies are continuously being sought and are emerging (Honn *et al.*, 1981). Furthermore, denial often has adaptive value in the dying person, enabling him to keep on living without being engulfed in gloom.

In addition to assisting the child, the professional also should devote attention to the parents. They must be able to deal with their own feelings of anxiety, depression, and guilt in order to be of greatest help to their child, who characteristically is grappling with many of these same emotions.

Fischhoff and O'Brien (1976), Adams (1978), and others have emphasized the value of parental involvement in self-help groups consisting of families with a chronically ill or dying child. These include Muscular Dystrophy Associations, Epilepsy Societies, Mental Retardation Associations, and groups for parents who have recently lost a child to illness.

Social-Environmental Management. Many persons with severe chronic illnesses such as muscular dystrophy can be maintained well at home. Wheelchairs to aid in mobility and special devices to ensure safety in the

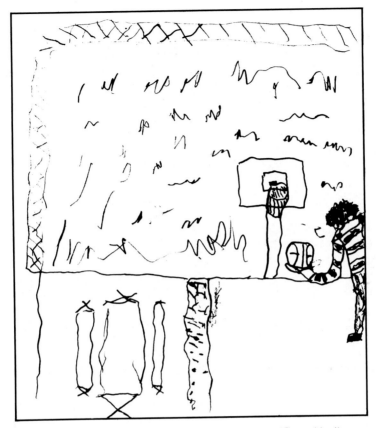

FIGURE 21–4. Drawing by 14-year-old boy (Case 11–4)
omitting right (hemiplegic) portion of his body.

bathroom will often help in adaptation. Professional nursing assistance in
the home also may be beneficial. Hospitalization may nonetheless be necessary at times for medical reevaluation or treatment of intercurrent medical
problems.

The best environment for the dying child—home, hospice, or hospital—is an issue that often must be addressed (Keyser, 1977; Ruymann
et al., 1977; Lauer and Camitta, 1980; Potter, 1980). Krant (1978), citing
the "rescue mode" of hospital medicine, has described how the hospice system has much to offer the person with a fatal illness. Used for years in England, hospices are intermediate facilities whose primary focus is upon pal-
liative therapy. Much can be said as well for home management, since taking
one's meals, sleeping, and bathing at home are generally more comfortable
within familiar surroundings than in an institutional setting (Keyser, 1977).

Decisions as to home, hospice, or hospital treatment should be made only
after careful consideration of issues such as prognosis, comfort, cost, and the
need (if any) for a setting whose orientation is more active diagnostically and
therapeutically.

Educational Management. Schooling should continue in as normal a

CASE 21–5: SPINAL CORD TUMOR IN A 14-YEAR-OLD BOY

L.R. was referred for neurologic evaluation at 12 years of age because of progressive weakness of the right arm. He had complained 2 years previously of intermittent pain in the neck and right forearm, which subsided after a year. Decrease in size of muscles of the right chest was noted, and he began having difficulty controlling a pencil with his right hand. Aching of the right shoulder and numbness of the right arm followed. Gait became increasingly unsteady. Occasionally morning headaches were associated with nausea but not with vomiting. He had no bowel or bladder problems. Previous medical history was unremarkable.

On examination, the boy was an alert, cooperative adolescent with obvious wasting of the right pectoral muscles. Right arm weakness was readily demonstrable, and strength in the right leg was decreased as well. Tone and deep tendon reflexes were diminished in the right arm. Deep tendon reflexes in the legs were exaggerated. Plantar responses were normal. Temperature sensation was decreased over the ulnar aspect of the right arm. Finger-to-nose movements on the right were dysmetric, out of proportion to weakness.

Investigation included normal x-rays of skull and spine. Myelography showed an intramedullary mass of the spinal cord extending from the first cervical vertebra to the first thoracic vertebra. Upon exploratory surgery, tissue for biopsy was obtained, which proved to be a grade III astrocytoma. He was treated with antineoplastic chemotherapy and radiation delivered to the posterior fossa, cervical cord, and upper thoracic cord.

Over the next several months weakness, diminished tone, and hyperreflexia progressed to affect the left arm; spasticity increased in the legs. There was no deterioration in intellect. Physical therapy was employed to maintain function as much as possible. A priest played a major role in providing support to the child and his parents. Eighteen months after initial diagnosis, he developed respiratory failure and died.

Comment. The management of this child's fatal illness was necessarily multifaceted. Medically, he received antibiotic therapy for pneumonia while efforts were made to maintain adequate nutrition. Surgical treatment was limited to diagnostic measures since the tumor was within the substance of the spinal cord; hence, definitive resection was impossible. Mechanical therapy took the form of a wheelchair, employed because of diminishing capacity for self-ambulation. The important role of the family priest in this case was noted above.

manner as possible as part of the overall goal of normalizing the life experience of the child with a chronic illness. Obviously, the profoundly weakened child should not be carried off to school. In many instances, home or hospital-based tutoring will be the most appropriate form of educational involvement. The commitment to appropriate educational assistance for handicapped children in the United States is defined by Public Law 94-142 (Palfrey *et al.*, 1978).

Physical Therapy. The goal of physical therapy is first to maintain function. With the cerebral-palsied child, for example, active and passive range-of-motion exercises are often valuable and may help to avoid or delay surgery. With a disorder such as multiple sclerosis, it is particularly important that exercises be carried out so that irreversible muscle contracture may not develop before the episode has remitted.

Physical therapy will often have a valuable role to play in the treatment or prevention of pneumonia (for example, with Duchenne muscular dystrophy or motor neuron disease).

In some circumstances physical therapy can facilitate acquisition of new motor functions, especially those associated with mechanical devices (see below).

Mechanical Therapy. Braces, crutches, and wheelchairs (propelled by hand or by motor) are forms of mechanical therapy that may be helpful in individual cases.

CORRELATION

Anatomic, biochemical, and physiologic aspects of chronic handicapping conditions such as seizure disorders and mental retardation are discussed within the sections on CORRELATION in earlier chapters.

SUMMARY

Chronic illness in childhood has important effects upon the child's behavior and emotions. Some effects may result directly from the disease itself, others from its treatment, still others from limitation and isolation related to associated disability.

In approaching the child with a chronic handicapping condition, the illness itself must be attended to—but not to the exclusion of the person who is suffering from the disorder. The meaning of the illness to the child, its causes and its cures, should be explored in sessions that allow ample time for pursuit of such subjects. Issues of dying and death, whether or not imminent or even applicable to the clinical circumstances, may then surface so that they can be dealt with. An understanding of the parents' perceptions of the illness and their expectations will help the professional to appreciate the child's view and will assist in establishing a treatment plan. Formal psychiatric or psychologic consultation can be valuable in elucidating further important areas of concern for the child and family that may have been given lesser priority because of pressing medical needs.

Management will often be multifaceted, involving several disciplines and modes of therapy. Treatment of intercurrent problems such as urinary tract infection may assist in restoring the child's energy. Adequate nutrition should be assured to maintain strength and minimize fatigue. Pain medication should be used in full dosage when needed. Seizure medication should be monitored so that it does not diminish alertness or worsen coordination through overdosage. Psychotherapy (individual, family, or group) may be indicated at any phase of the illness from the time of initial diagnosis to the end of life. Overall, the goal of the professional is to maximize the child's quality of life, to reduce suffering, and—when necessary—to help ensure that death is met without undue pain, fear, or isolation.

CITED REFERENCES

Adams, M. A. Helping the parents of children with malignancy. *J. Pediatrics,* **93:** 734–38, 1978.

Beecher, H. K., *et al.* A definition of irreversible coma: report of the Ad Hoc Committee of the Harvard Medical School to examine the definition of brain death. *JAMA,* **205:** 337–40, 1968.

Bibace, R., and Walsh, M. E. Development of children's concepts of illness. *Pediatrics,* **66:** 912–17, 1980.

Black, P. McL. Brain death. *N. Engl. J. Med.,* **299:** 338–44, 393–401, 1978.

Boyle, I. R.; di Sant'Agnese, P. A.; Sack, S.; Millican, F.; and Kulczycki, L. L. Emotional adjustment of adolescents and young adults with cystic fibrosis. *J. Pediatr.,* **88:** 318–26, 1976.

D'Angio, G. J. Late sequelae after cure of childhood cancer. *Hosp. Pract.,* pp. 109–11, 114, 115, 119, 120, 121, November, 1980.

Fischhoff, J., and O'Brien, N. After the child dies. *J. Pediatr.,* **88:** 140–46, 1976.

Freeman, J. E.; Johnston, P. G. B.; and Voke, J. M. Somnolence after prophylactic cranial irradiation in children with acute lympoblastic leukaemia. *Br. Med. J.,* **4:** 523–25, 1973.

Gangji, D.; Reaman, G. H.; Cohen, S. R.; Bleyer, W. A.; and Poplack, D. G. Leukoencephalopathy and elevated levels of myelin basic protein in the cerebrospinal fluid of patients with acute lymphoblastic leukemia. *N. Engl. J. Med.,* **303:** 19–21, 1980.

Green, M., and Solnit, A. J. Reactions to the threatened loss of a child—a vulnerable child syndrome: pediatric management of the dying child, part III. *Pediatrics,* **34:** 58–66, 1964.

Hackett, T. P. Psychological assistance for the dying patient and his family. *Annu. Rev. Med.,* **27:** 371–78, 1976.

Herskowitz, J., and Marks, A. N. The spina bifida patient as a person. *Dev. Med. Child Neurol.,* **19:** 413–17, 1977.

Honn, K. V.; Cicone, B.; and Skoff, A. Prostacyclin: a potent antimetastatic agent. *Science,* **212:** 1270–72, 1981.

Kellerman, J.; Zeltzer, L.; Ellenberg, L.; Dash, J.; and Rigler, D. Psychological effects of illness in adolescence: I. anxiety, self-esteem, and perception of control. *J. Pediatr.,* **97:** 126–31, 1980.

Keyser, M. At home with death: a natural child-death. *J. Pediatr.,* **90:** 486–87, 1977.

Koocher, G. P.; O'Malley, J. E.; Gogan, J. L.; and Foster, D. J. Psychological adjustment among pediatric cancer survivors. *J. Child Psychol. Psychiatry,* **21:** 163–73, 1980.

Krant, M. J. The hospice movement. *N. Engl. J. Med.,* **299:** 546–49, 1978.

Kübler-Ross, E. *On Death and Dying.* The Macmillan Company, New York, 1969.

Lauer, M. E., and Camitta, B. M. Home care for dying children: a nursing model. *J. Pediatr.,* **97:** 1032–35, 1980.

Lindemann, E. Symptomatology and management of acute grief. *Am. J. Psychiatry.,* **101:** 141–48, 1944.

McIntosh, S., and Aspnes, G. T. Encephalopathy following CNS prophylaxis in childhood lymphoblastic leukemia. *Pediatrics,* **52:** 612–15, 1973.

Palfrey, J. S.; Mervis, R. C.; and Butler, J. A. New directions in the evaluation and education of handicapped children. *N. Engl. J. Med.*, **298:** 819–24, 1978.

Potter, J. F. A challenge for the hospice movement. *N. Engl. J. Med.*, **302:** 53–55, 1980.

Powner, D. J., and Fromm, G. H. The electroencephalogram in the determination of brain death. *N. Engl. J. Med.*, **300:** 502, 1979.

Price, R. A., and Jamieson, P. A. The central nervous system in childhood leukemia: II. subacute leukoencephalopathy. *Cancer,* **35:** 306–18, 1975.

Ruymann, F. B.; Mease, A. D.; and Mosijczuk, A. D. At home with death: antidote for anxiety. *J. Pediatr.,* **91:** 354–55, 1977.

Share, L. Family communication in the crisis of a child's fatal illness: a literature review and analysis. Pp. 30–44 in *Caring Relationships: The Dying and the Bereaved.* Kalish, R. A., ed. Baywood Publishing Co., Inc., Farmingdale, N.Y., 1980.

Steinhauer, P. D.; Mushin, D. N.; and Rae-Grant, Q. Psychological aspects of chronic illness. *Pediatr. Clin. North Am.,* **21:** 825–40, 1974.

White, E.; Elsom, B.; and Prawat, R. Children's conceptions of death. *Child Dev.,* **49:** 307–10, 1978.

Wolfish, M. G., and McLean, J. A. Chronic illness in adolescents. *Pediatr. Clin. North Am.,* **21:** 1043–49, 1974.

Zeltzer, L.; Kellerman, J.; Ellenberg, L.; Dash, J.; and Rigler, D. Psychologic effects of illness in adolescence: II. impact of illness in adolescents—crucial issues and coping styles. *J. Pediatr.,* **97:** 132–38, 1980.

ADDITIONAL READINGS

Bluebond-Langner, M. *The Private Worlds of Dying Children.* Princeton University Press, Princeton, N.J., 1978.

Cooper, I. S. *Living with Chronic Neurologic Disease: A Handbook for Patient and Family.* W. W. Norton and Company, Inc., New York, 1976.

Eissler, R. S.; Freud, A.; Kris, M.; and Solnit, A. J., eds. *Physical Illness and Handicap in Childhood.* Yale University Press, New Haven, Conn., 1977.

Featherstone, H. *A Difference in the Family: Life with a Disabled Child.* Basic Books, Inc., New York, 1980.

Fiore, N. Fighting cancer: one patient's perspective. *N. Engl. J. Med.,* **300:** 284–89, 1979.

Fulton, R.; Markusen, E.; and Owen G., eds. *Death and Dying: Challenge and Change.* Addison-Wesley Publishing Co., Reading, Ma., 1979.

Garfield, C. A. *Psychological Care of the Dying Patient.* McGraw-Hill Book Co., New York, 1978.

Kemp, E., Jr. Aiding the disabled: no pity, please. *New York Times,* September 3, 1981, p. A 19.

Kübler-Ross, E. *Living with Death and Dying.* Macmillan Publishing Co., Inc., New York, 1981.

Kushner, H. S. *When Bad Things Happen To Good People.* Schocken Books, New York, 1981.

Part Three

Conclusion

22 Prevention, Early Intervention, and New Directions

To this point this book has focused on the common ground between pediatrics, neurology, and psychiatry: the structure and function of the nervous system, developmental aspects of behavior, the clinical process, and major clinical problems of concern to those dealing with children. Prevention and early intervention, important issues in maximizing the health of children, and new directions in investigation and treatment are discussed in this concluding chapter.

PREVENTION

Pediatrics is intrinsically a prevention-oriented specialty. A great many preventive measures instituted in this century have impacted forcefully upon behavioral and affective problems of childhood and adolescence. Such effects have been seen, for example, in the area of mental retardation (as with hypothyroidism and phenylketonuria) and other chronic handicapping conditions (such as poliomyelitis). Table 22–1 lists disorders typifying different stages of development that are potentially preventable.

The earliest time for prevention is *before conception*. Many disorders affecting the nervous system are of known inheritance. With Tay-Sachs disease, for example, the pattern of inheritance is autosomal recessive. Since carriers can be detected through a blood test, the chance of having an affected child can be determined. Two carriers (heterozygotes) would have a risk of one in four. If this risk is too great for the prospective parents, they may choose to avoid pregnancy. Prevention could be pursued otherwise during the intrauterine period of development. Amniocentesis can be performed during the first trimester of pregnancy, fetal cells analyzed for hexosaminidase A activity, and elective abortion carried out if the fetus is affected.

Immunization against rubella has been demonstrated to be effective in preventing the congenital rubella syndrome with its wide variety of physical, neurologic, and psychiatric manifestations. Before pregnancy, a woman

TABLE 22–1. **Preventable Disorders**

Stage of Development	Disorder	Treatment Options
Before Conception	Tay-Sachs disease	Genetic counseling, contraception
	Congenital rubella syndrome	Maternal immunization (or prenatal abortion)
Prenatal	Kernicterus (bilirubin encephalopathy)	RhoGAM, intrauterine transfusion, exchange transfusion
	Down syndrome, X-linked disorders (such as Duchenne muscular dystrophy)	Elective abortion after amniocentesis and karyotyping
	Dysraphic states	Elective abortion after ultrasound examination and amniocentesis
	Methylmalonic acidemia	Megadoses of vitamin B_{12} to mother during pregnancy
	Hydrocephalus	Through ultrasound diagnosis; in utero treatment possible
	Birth asphyxia causing cerebral palsy Brain damage from birth asphyxia	Placenta previa detected by ultrasound; fetal monitoring to detect stress patterns indicating need for cesarean section
Birth	Brain damage from birth trauma	Use of fetal monitoring, ultrasound, elective cesarean section in obstetrical management
Postnatal	Phenylketonuria, maple syrup urine disease, congenital hypothyroidism	Neonatal screening of blood with early therapy (diet; thyroid hormone)
	Fabry disease	Enzyme replacement through kidney transplantation
Infancy	Child abuse/neglect	Diminish neonatal separation; enhance contact; home visiting especially beginning prenatally; child abuse hotlines

TABLE 22–1. (Cont.)

Stage of Development	Disorder	Treatment Options
Early Childhood	Accidents, poisoning	"Accident-proofing" home
	Head trauma	Use of appropriate car seats
	Child abuse/neglect	As above Early intervention
	Lead encephalopathy	Lead screening, treatment, removal from leaded environment
School Age	School failure	Recognition and treatment of attentional problems, learning disabilities
	Head trauma	Use of seat/shoulder belts; pedestrian education and safety; swimming instruction; "drown-proofing"
Adolescence	Head trauma	Driver education, use of automobile restraint devices
	Suicide	Early recognition and treatment of depression
	Drug abuse	Education, referral, treatment

should have a measurable level of antibodies to rubella, whether due to naturally acquired infection or immunization. If she does not have demonstrable rubella titers before pregnancy, the appearance of antibody levels at any time during the first few months of that gestation may provide the basis for elective abortion because of the high risk of significant fetal damage (such as microcephaly, deafness, cataract, and heart disease).

During the *prenatal period,* many opportunities for prevention exist. With Rh or ABO blood group incompatibility between mother and child, for example, bilirubin at excessively high levels may poison the nervous system to produce sensorineural deafness, choreoathetoid cerebral palsy, or both. Prevention of bilirubin encephalopathy can occur in several ways. Administration of RhoGAM (an anti-Rh gamma globulin) to an Rh-negative mother soon after delivery of an Rh-positive baby can prevent the build-up of mother's own anti-Rh antibodies so that future pregnancies will not be jeopardized by Rh incompatibility. If Rh sensitization has occurred previously, then other measures such as intrauterine transfusion or exchange transfusion early in the neonatal period can be pursued.

With known chromosomal disorders such as Down syndrome or with X-linked disorders such as adrenoleukodystrophy or Duchenne muscular dystrophy, chromosomal analysis (karyotype) of fetal cells obtained at amniocentesis can provide information of preventive importance (Golbus et al., 1979; Powledge and Fletcher, 1979). Down syndrome due to trisomy 21 or translocation may be found in women in whom amniocentesis was carried out because of relatively advanced age or a previously affected child.

With X-linked disorders, mothers are carriers, male offspring have a 50 per cent chance of being affected, and female offspring have a 50 per cent chance of being carriers.

Amniocentesis can also provide fluid for measurement of alpha fetoprotein (abnormally elevated with dysraphic states such as anencephaly and meningomyelocele) as well as lysosomal enzyme activity in fetal cells. Blood from placental vessels may also be obtained for analysis by use of a small fiberoptic endoscope.

Successful treatment of a metabolic defect has been carried out in utero. Large doses of vitamin B_{12} were given by injection to the mother of a fetus affected with methylmalonic acidemia, a rare disease that characteristically is associated with failure to thrive, developmental retardation, and often death (Ampola et al., 1975). Treatment resulted in sufficient amounts of the vitamin crossing the placenta to compensate for the inborn error of metabolism. Postnatal treatment (limited to dietary protein restriction) in such cases has been associated with normal developmental outcome.

Other prenatal studies may help prevent problems that otherwise might be associated with brain injury incurred during delivery. Ultrasound evaluation may show the placenta to be overlying the entrance to the birth canal (placenta previa). Were labor and vaginal delivery to proceed without intervention, the blood supply to the fetus would be interrupted as the placenta was compressed or dislodged during labor. This potentially damaging outcome can be avoided through delivery by cesarean section.

Ultrasound has also been used to diagnose anencephaly, meningomyelocele, and hydrocephalus in utero. The antenatal treatment of hydrocephalus has recently been described (Birnholz and Frigoletto, 1981).

Use of fetal monitoring during labor to record the pattern of fetal heart rate in relation to intrauterine pressure can detect signs of fetal distress. With severe or sustained distress due to umbilical cord compression or placental insufficiency, delivery by cesarean section can, in some circumstances, prevent brain damage. The outcomes of birth trauma may include cerebral palsy, mental retardation, and epilepsy.

Much can be done preventively in the immediate postnatal period. Neonatal screening of blood obtained by heel prick has been effective in identifying children with phenylketonuria and other disorders of amino acid metabolism such as homocystinuria and maple syrup urine disease (Menkes, 1980). Urine is also generally screened for amino acids several weeks after birth. Once the diagnosis of amino acid disorder is established, an affected child is placed on a diet designed to prevent the adverse effects of the enzyme deficiency. The potential for normal development is thereby maximized.

Neonatal screening of blood for congenital hypothyroidism (cretinism) has allowed for early diagnosis and treatment with thyroid hormone. Testing of just over 1 million newborns in North America detected 277 infants with hypothyroidism (Fisher *et al.*, 1979). If treatment is begun within the first 3 months of life, mental subnormality due to thyroid hormone deficiency will be minimized and often prevented (Rosman, 1976).

Enzyme replacement therapy is another model of treatment for metabolic disorders. It has been accomplished in later life with Fabry disease through transplantation of a kidney from a nonaffected person. In these circumstances the "new" kidney is able to produce the previously deficient enzyme.

The *period of infancy* is another time during which prevention can be practiced. The effects upon later behavior of increased early contact between mother and child (within the first few hours of life) have become widely recognized (Klaus and Kennell, 1976; Lozoff *et al.*, 1977). Rooming-in has also been recommended to foster maternal-infant bonding (O'Connor *et al.*, 1980). For the ill neonate, visits by parents to the intensive care nursery where they can receive ample explanation and psychologic support have been advised.

The increased frequency of later child abuse in children who were born prematurely is among the evidence that has linked interference with early bonding and later disorders of mother-child interaction. Prolonged neonatal hospitalization due to any cause, illness of the mother, and even routine hospital newborn policies can interfere with the attachment process (Lozoff *et al.*, 1977).

Child abuse hotlines have been established for purposes of prevention as well as early intervention.

When medical or emotional problems render a mother unable to care adequately for her newborn, alternative caretaking arrangements (including foster care) may be necessary, particularly when previous children of the mother have been abused, neglected, or removed from her custody.

Home visiting appears to have beneficial effects upon child health and development. In a controlled study Larson (1980) demonstrated a reduced accident rate among the children, improved mother-child interaction, and increased paternal involvement—but only when home visiting began prenatally, not just 6 weeks after birth.

In *early childhood,* accidents, poisoning, child abuse, and neglect are major threats to the health and optimal development of children. Head trauma with associated brain injury can be prevented by use of age-appropriate automobile restraint devices, monitoring of children's activities near windows and stairs, pursuing measures to avoid abuse and neglect, and accident-proofing the home. Aspirin, iron tablets, furniture polish, and other toxic substances should be kept inaccessible to children and stored in child-resistant containers. Syrup of ipecac and instructions for its use should be at hand. The telephone number of the local poison center should be immediately available.

Several measures should be pursued to prevent lead poisoning, associated with seizures, mental retardation, or death in its acute encephalopathic form, attention deficit disorder in its chronic asymptomatic form (Needleman *et al.*, 1979). The child between 1 and 4 years of age should undergo periodic screening of blood for lead and free erythrocyte protoporphyrin (FEP). In older homes paint chips from window sills and other reachable areas should be tested for lead. Lead screening programs in the United States have identified many thousands of children with low levels of lead poisoning and have provided for their treatment and removal from the leaded environment prior to development of encephalopathic symptoms.

In the *school-age child* syndromes of attention deficit disorder and learning disability are common. Prevention in the former should be directed toward minimizing the secondary effects of inattention and hyperactivity: poor school performance, impaired peer relationships, and loss of self-esteem (see Chapter 14). With learning disabilities, behavioral and emotional problems frequently overshadow the academic ones. As discussed in Chapter 17, preventive intervention might include defining the problem for child and family (ensuring that it is not viewed as lack of motivation or as global retardation) and constructing an individualized plan of educational remediation.

As in the younger child, brain injury in the child of school age is an important concern. It can result in a variety of ways: automobile, skateboard, or bicycle accidents; athletic injuries; falls from heights; and drowning. Child safety education (including encouragement in the use of seat and shoulder belts and instruction in ''drown-proofing'') and appropriate supervision are measures that can reduce the number of such tragic accidents.

In *adolescence,* head trauma, depressive illness, and abuse of alcohol or other drugs can lead to preventable injuries that have implications for behavior and emotions. Head trauma can result from athletic injuries, fights, vehicular accidents, or failure to use automobile safety devices (seat belts and shoulder harnesses) (Christophersen, 1977). Driver education has sought to impact upon the last two of these causes of preventable injuries. Depression, which can be associated with suicidal or aggressive behavior, may be overlooked because of more prominent behavioral symptoms that mask the underlying affective component (see Chapter 6). Education as to the effects of various drugs and the availability of treatment are important means of preventing drug abuse and its many associated problems (see Chapter 19).

EARLY INTERVENTION

Early intervention can be viewed in many instances as a form of prevention. For example, treatment of lead poisoning in an asymptomatic child can be considered preventive in terms of brain damage that might later have occurred had the problem not been recognized and effectively dealt with earlier. Elevation in blood lead and free erythrocyte protoporphyrin levels through a screening program indicates that hematologic and biochemical systems already are affected. Hence the term ''early intervention'' applies just as well as prevention.

Early intervention in cases of child abuse or neglect has undoubtedly improved (and sometimes actually saved) the lives of many children. To help the child and his or her parents maximally, the diagnosis of abuse or neglect cannot rest solely upon flagrant signs of inflicted injury. Rather, it must be based whenever possible upon more subtle findings that allow for timely intervention that respects the rights of the family while it protects the vulnerable child.

Malnutrition is another problem where early intervention has impacted upon later behavior and development. The work of Winick and colleagues (1975) and Evans and colleagues (1980) has documented the beneficial effects upon intelligence of nutritional intervention within the first 2 or 3 years of life in children who were malnourished or at risk for malnutrition (see Chapter 20).

In many instances (lead poisoning again providing a good example) the value of early intervention has been clearly demonstrated. The pain of a few fingerpricks to permit blood samples to be obtained is a small price to pay for identification of a potentially handicapping, even lethal, toxin in the child's body and environment. In other circumstances early intervention cannot be viewed as being of clear benefit. For example, the difficulties with identifying kindergarten or first-grade students as being "learning-disabled" and singling them out for remediation are discussed in Chapter 17. Indeed, early intervention may have potentially negative effects. For example, children who will outgrow developmentally based difficulties may suffer stigmatization and a negative self-image needlessly as a result of premature or inaccurate diagnosis.

Early intervention with the high-risk infant is an extremely important and controversial subject (Piper and Pless, 1980; Leib et al., 1980; Haggerty, 1980; Denhoff, 1981; Ferry, 1981; Bricker et al., 1981; Browder, 1981). The term "high-risk" refers to influences (maternal, gestational, obstetric, and/or neonatal) that might affect a child's physical and mental attainments adversely during childhood and later years. For example, a small-for-gestational-age infant who experienced hypoglycemia on the first day of life would be at increased risk of manifesting significant developmental disability.

Darlington and colleagues (1980) have concluded that early intervention, stimulation, and head start programs seem to help both child and family. Benefits, at least in part, appear to be through family education and support that enhance parenting skills. Denhoff (1981) has also concluded that early intervention programs emphasizing infant stimulation and parental involvement do make a difference in the child's developmental outcome, most notably in emotional and social behavior.

Many questions remain unanswered as to the benefits of early intervention and stimulation programs: the cost effectiveness of a multidisciplinary team approach as compared with that emphasizing pediatrician support of the family combined with physical, occupational, or speech and language therapy as needed; the impact of home-based versus center-based programs. Controlled prospective studies, though extremely difficult to carry out, must be viewed as most crucial in answering these and other important questions (Haggerty, 1980).

NEW DIRECTIONS

This book has emphasized a comprehensive, often multidisciplinary diagnostic and therapeutic approach to the behavioral and affective problems of childhood and adolescence. This approach has been justified by the several levels (from the molecular to the societal) at which such disorders usually are expressed. A person with a seizure disorder, for example, will receive therapy (anticonvulsant medication) that has effects at the molecular level, while social ramifications may include restrictions in operating a motor vehicle and the choice of occupation.

Further progress in diagnosis and treatment is anticipated as the common ground shared by pediatrics, neurology, and psychiatry is enlarged and explored. New refinements in the nomenclature of behavioral and affective disorders should foster meaningful communication between practitioners and researchers in multiple disciplines, facilitating collaborative studies in which populations of sufficient size can be assessed so that statistically significant conclusions can be drawn.

Structural, biochemical, and physiologic studies of the central nervous system are clarifying to an increasing degree the extraordinarily complex workings of brain, the organ of behavior. Detailed postmortem analysis of the brains of individuals with well-characterized disorders (dyslexia being a recent example) remains a cornerstone of the neurologic method. Investigational tools such as computerized tomography of brain, neurophysiologic studies of evoked potentials, ultrasonography, noninvasive techniques to assess regional cerebral blood flow, neuroendocrine investigations of increasing subtlety, brain electrical activity mapping, positron emission tomography, nuclear magnetic resonance, and new methods in detecting metabolic disorders will continue to increase our understanding of normal and abnormal brain functioning (see Table 22–2) (Greenberg *et al.*, 1981).

These often breathtaking examples of technology supplement but do not replace the ears and eyes of the clinician, who begins with the words and actions of pediatric patients and their parents in addressing their problems, seeking their causes, and formulating treatment plans.

The concluding decades of this century promise to be extraordinarily rich and exciting times of discovery, certain to have profound implications for the behavioral and emotional well-being of our children.

TABLE 22–2. **Newer Diagnostic Techniques**

Computerized tomography (CT)
Evoked potential studies
Ultrasonography
Noninvasive measurement of regional cerebral blood flow
Neuroendocrine investigations
Brain electrical activity mapping (BEAM)
Positron emission tomography (PET)
Nuclear magnetic resonance (NMR)
Lysosomal and other enzyme determinations

CITED REFERENCES

Ampola, M. G.; Mahoney, M. J.; Nakamura, E.; and Tanaka, K. Prenatal therapy of a patient with vitamin-B_{12}-responsive methylmalonic acidemia. *N. Engl. J. Med.,* **293:** 313–17, 1975.

Birnholz, J. C., and Frigoletto, F. D. Antenatal treatment of hydrocephalus. *N. Engl. J. Med.,* **303:** 1021–23, 1981.

Bricker, D.; Carlson, L.; and Schwarz, R. A discussion of early intervention for infants with Down syndrome. *Pediatrics,* **67:** 45–46, 1981.

Browder, J. A. The pediatrician's orientation to infant stimulation programs. *Pediatrics,* **67:** 42–44, 1981.

Christophersen, E. R. Children's behavior during automobile rides: do car seats make a difference? *Pediatrics,* **60:** 69–74, 1977.

Darlington, R. B.; Royce, J. M.; Snipper, A. S.; Murray, H. W.; and Lazar, I. Preschool programs and later school competence of children from low-income families. *Science,* **208:** 202–4, 1980.

Denhoff, E. Current status of infant stimulation or enrichment programs for children with developmental disabilities. *Pediatrics,* **67:** 32–37, 1981.

Evans, D.; Bowie, M. D.; Hansen, J. D. L.; Moodie, A. D.; and van der Spuy, H. I. J. Intellectual development and nutrition. *J. Pediatr.* **97:** 358–63, 1980.

Ferry, P. C. On growing new neurons: are early intervention programs effective. *Pediatrics,* **67:** 38–41, 1981.

Fisher, D. A.; Dussault, J. H.; Foley, T. P., Jr.; Klein, A. H.; LaFranchi, S.; Larsen, P. R.; Mitchell, M. L.; Murphey, W. H.; and Walfish, P. G. Screening for congenital hypothyroidism: results of screening one million North American infants. *J. Pediatr.* **94:** 700–705, 1979.

Golbus, M. S.; Loughman, W. D.; Epstein, C. J.; Halbasch, G.; Stephens, J. D.; and Hall, B. D. Prenatal genetic diagnosis in 3,000 amniocenteses. *N. Engl. J. Med.,* **300:** 157–63, 1979.

Greenberg, J. H.; Reivich, M.; Alavi, A.; Hand, P.; Rosenquist, A.; Rintelmann, W.; Stein, A.; Tusa, R.; Dann, R.; Christman, D.; Fowler, J.; MacGregor, B.; and Wolf, A. Metabolic mapping of functional activity in human subjects with the [^{18}F]fluorodeoxyglucose technique. *Science,* **212:** 678–80, 1981.

Haggerty, R. J. Damn the simplicities. *Pediatrics,* **66:** 323–24, 1980.

Klaus, M. H., and Kennell, J. H., eds. *Maternal-Infant Bonding.* C. V. Mosby Co., Saint Louis, 1976.

Larson, C. P. Efficacy of prenatal and postpartum home visits on child health and development. *Pediatrics,* **66:** 191–97, 1980.

Leib, S. A.; Benfield, D. G.; and Guidubaldi, J. Effects of early intervention and stimulation on the preterm infant. *Pediatrics,* **66:** 83–90, 1980.

Lozoff, B.; Brittenham, G. M.; Trause, M. A.; Kennell, J. H.; and Klaus, M. H. The mother-newborn relationship: limits of adaptability. *J. Pediatr.,* **91:** 1–12, 1977.

Menkes, J. H. Metabolic diseases of the nervous system. Pp. 1–109 in *Textbook of Child Neurology,* 2nd ed. Menkes, J. H., ed. Lea and Febiger, Philadelphia, 1980.

Needleman, H. L.; Gunnoe, C.; Leviton, A.; Reed, R.; Peresie, H.; Maher, C.; and Barrett, P. Deficits in psychologic and classroom performance of children with elevated dentine lead levels. *N. Engl. J. Med.,* **300:** 689–95, 1979.

O'Connor, S.; Vietze, P. M.; Sherrod, K. B.; Sandler, H. M.; and Altemeier, W. A., III. Reduced incidence of parenting inadequacy following rooming-in. *Pediatrics,* **66:** 176–82, 1980.

Piper, M. C., and Pless, I. B. Early intervention for infants with Down syndrome: a controlled trial. *Pediatrics,* **65:** 463–68, 1980.

Powledge, T. M., and Fletcher, J. Guidelines for the ethical, social and legal issues in prenatal diagnosis. *N. Engl. J. Med., 300:* 168–72, 1979.

Rosman, N. P. Neurological and muscular aspects of thyroid dysfunction in childhood. *Pediatr. Clin. North Am., 23:* 575–94, 1976.

Winick, M.; Meyer, K. K.; and Harris, R. C. Malnutrition and environmental enrichment by early adoption. *Science, 190:* 1173–75, 1975.

ADDITIONAL READINGS

Anderson, W. F., and Fletcher, J. C. Gene therapy in human beings: when is it ethical to begin? *N. Engl. J. Med., 303:* 1293–27, 1980.

Bronfenbrenner, U. *Is Early Intervention Effective?* Department of Health, Education and Welfare, Office of Child Development, Washington, D.C., Publication No. (OHD) 74-25, 1974.

Eisenberg, L. Psychiatry and society: a sociobiologic synthesis. *N. Engl. J. Med., 296:* 903–10, 1977.

Ellenberg, J. H., and Nelson, K. B. Early recognition of infants at high risk for cerebral palsy: examination at age four months. *Dev. Med. Child Neurol., 23:* 705–16, 1981.

Epstein, F. H. Nuclear magnetic resonance: a new tool in clinical medicine. *N. Engl. J. Med., 304:* 1360–61, 1981.

Eto, Y.; Tahara, T.; Koda, N.; Yamaguchi, S.; Ito, F.; and Okuno, A. Prenatal diagnosis of metachromatic leukodystrophy: a diagnosis by amniotic fluid and its confirmation. *Arch. Neurol., 39:* 29–32, 1982.

Fischer, T. J. The pediatrician and the deaf child: perspectives of a pediatrician-parent. *Pediatrics, 67:* 313–14, 1981.

Fredrickson, D. S. Biomedical research in the 1980s. *N. Engl. J. Med., 304:* 509–17, 1981.

Goldman-Rakic, P. S. Plasticity of the primate telencephalon. Pp. 55–62 in *Neonatal Neurological Assessment and Outcome.* Report of the Seventy-seventh Ross Conference on Pediatric Research. Brann, A. W., and Volpe, J. J., eds. Ross Laboratories, Columbus, Ohio, 1980.

Hecox, K. E.; Cone, B.; and Blaw, M. E. Brainstem auditory evoked response in the diagnosis of pediatric neurologic diseases. *Neurology* (*New York*), *31:* 832–40, 1981.

Mercola, K. E., and Cline, M. J. The potentials of inserting new genetic information. *N. Engl. J. Med., 303:* 1297–1300, 1980.

Olton, D. S., and Noonberg, A. R. *Biofeedback: Clinical Applications in Behavioral Medicine.* Prentice-Hall, Englewood Cliffs, N.J., 1980.

Ramsey, J. The little girl who was saved before she was born. *Family Circle,* pp. 12, 14, 43, January 8, 1980.

Reisinger, K. S.; Williams, A. F.; Wells, J. K.; John, C. E.; Roberts, T. R.; and Podgainy, H. J. Effect of pediatricians' counseling on infant restraint use. *Pediatrics, 67:* 201–6, 1981.

Rosenzweig, M. R., and Bennett, E. L. Experiential influences on brain anatomy and brain chemistry in rodents. Pp. 289–327 in *Studies on the Development of Behavior and The Nervous System:* Early Influences. Gottlieb, G., ed. Academic Press, New York, 1978.

Ter-Pogossian, M. M.; Raichle, M. E.; and Sobel, B. E. Positron-emission tomography. *Sci. Am. 243:* 170–81, October 1980.

Zinkus, P. W., and Gottlieb, M. I. Patterns of perceptual and academic deficits related to early chronic otitis media. *Pediatrics, 66:* 246–53, 1980.

Index

(c) Indicates case, (f) figure, and (t) table.

685